Clinical Laboratory
Blood Banking and Transfusion Medicine
Principles and Practices

Gretchen Schaef Johns, MD

Elizabeth A. Gockel-Blessing, series editor

William Zundel, MS

Lisa Denesiuk, BSc

PEARSON

Boston   Columbus   Indianapolis   New York   San Francisco   Upper Saddle River
Amsterdam   Cape Town   Dubai   London   Madrid   Milan   Munich   Paris   Montreal   Toronto
Delhi   Mexico City   Sao Paulo   Sydney   Hong Kong   Seoul   Singapore   Taipei   Tokyo

Publisher: Julie Levin Alexander
Publisher's Assistant: Regina Bruno
Editor in Chief: Marlene McHugh Pratt
Executive Editor: John Goucher
Editorial Program Manager: Monica Moosang
Editorial Assistant: Ericia Vivani
Director of Marketing: David Gesell
Marketing Manager: Katrin Beacom
Marketing Coordinator: Alicia Wozniak
Marketing Specialist: Michael Sirinides
Project Management Team Lead: Cindy Zonneveld
Project Manager: Patricia Gutierrez
Art Director: Mary Siener

Text Designer: Christine Cantera
Cover Designer: Carly Schnur
Cover/Chapter Opener image: Sebastian Kaulitzki/
    Shutterstock.com
Media Producer: Amy Peltier
Lead Media Project Manager: Lorena Cerisano
Full-Service Project Management:
Composition: Laserwords, Inc
Printer/Binder: LSC Communications
Cover Printer: LSC Communications
Text font:

Notice: The author and the publisher of this book have taken care to make certain that the information given is correct and compatible with the standards generally accepted at the time of publication. Nevertheless, as new information becomes available, changes in treatment and in the use of equipment and procedures become necessary. The reader is advised to carefully consult the instruction and information material included in each piece of equipment or device before administration. Students are warned that the use of any techniques must be authorized by their medical advisor, where appropriate, in accordance with local laws and regulations. The publisher disclaims any liability, loss, injury, or damage incurred as a consequence, directly or indirectly, of the use and application of any of the contents of this book.

Many of the designations by manufacturers and seller to distinguish their products are claimed as trademarks. Where those designations appear in this book, and the publisher was aware of a trademark claim, the designations have been printed in initial caps or all caps.

Library of Congress Cataloging-in-Publication Data
Clinical laboratory blood banking and transfusion medicine: principles and
practices / [edited by] Gretchen Schaef Johns . . . [et al.].—1st ed.
    p. ; cm.
Includes bibliographical references and index.
ISBN-13: 978-0-13-083331-0
ISBN-10: 0-13-083331-2
I. Johns, Gretchen Schaef.
 [DNLM: 1. Blood Group Antigens—classification.   2. Blood
Banks–standards.   3. Blood Grouping and Crossmatching—classification.
4. Blood Transfusion.   5. Safety Management. WH 420]
 RM172
 615.3'9–dc23   2013016008

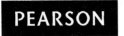

ISBN 10: 0-13-083331-2
ISBN 13: 978-0-13-083331-0

33 2019

In loving memory of Linda Dolan Jasper, who set out to be the primary author of this book, designed the initial structure, and drafted several early chapters. Due to illness and her subsequent untimely death, Linda was unable to complete her part of the project. With this book, her memory lives on and her vision is realized.

To my husband, Dr. Thomas Davant Johns, for his patience and understanding while I labored on this book every weekend and during most of our vacations. Many thanks to Dr. Michael Creer and Dr. Edahn Isaak, for your examples of exceptionally high standards in teaching, integrity, and excellence in medicine and my wonderful residents and students.   —*Gretchen Schaef Johns, MD*

To my entire family for their unending patience, love, and support during this entire project. Special thanks to my husband, Bob, who understood the importance of me completing my portion of this book and made numerous sacrifices to ensure that I did. He kept me focused and on track. He is indeed my "Blessing." Bob, I love you!   —*Elizabeth A. Gockel-Blessing, PhD*

To my wife, Jenise, for her undying love and support and our six extraordinary children: Jason, Andrew, Taylor, Katie, Heidi, and Jacob. Special thanks to Janet Vincent for providing me with roots and wings. To all the students—past, present, and future—who make teaching and learning a daily adventure.   —*Bill Zundel, MS*

For all the remarkable laboratorians out there—be proud of what you accomplish each day and be fearless in grabbing opportunities. This is dedicated to my parents, Ruth and Russ; my sister, Marci; and especially my nephew, Marlowe.   —*Lisa Denesiuk, BSc*

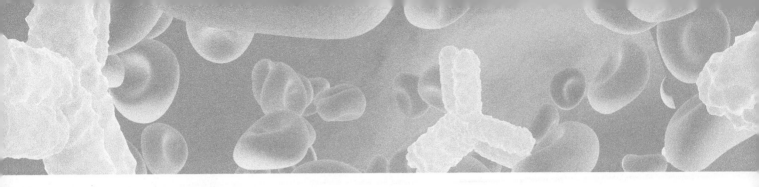

Contents

CHAPTER 9   DONOR SELECTION, PHLEBOTOMY, AND REQUIRED TESTING   153

CHAPTER 10   BLOOD PRODUCTS: PREPARATION, STORAGE, AND SHIPMENT OF BLOOD COMPONENTS   175

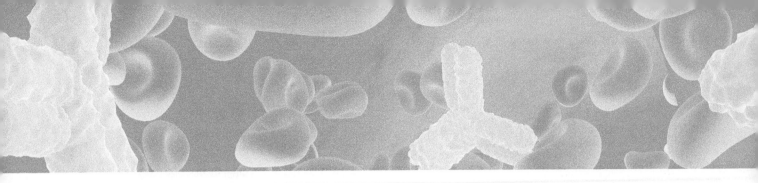

Foreword

Clinical Laboratory Blood Banking and Transfusion Medicine is part of Pearson's Clinical Laboratory Science series of textbooks, which is designed to balance theory and practical applications in a way that is engaging and useful to students. The authors and contributors of *Clinical Laboratory Blood Banking and Transfusion Medicine* present detailed technical information and real-life case studies that help learners envision themselves as members of the health care team, providing the laboratory services specific to transfusion medicine that assist in patient care. The mixture of theoretical and practical information relating to transfusion medicine in this text allows learners to analyze and synthesize information and, ultimately, to answer questions and solve problems and cases. Additional instructional resources are available at www.pearsonhighered.com/healthprofessionsresources.

We hope that this book, as well as the entire series, proves to be a valuable educational resource.

Elizabeth A. Gockel-Blessing (formerly Zeibig), PhD, MLS(ASCP)^{CM}
Clinical Laboratory Science Series Editor
Pearson Health Science
Associate Dean for Graduate Education
Interim Associate Dean for Student and Academic Affairs
CLS Program Director | Associate Professor | Clinical Laboratory Science
Doisy College of Health Sciences
Saint Louis University

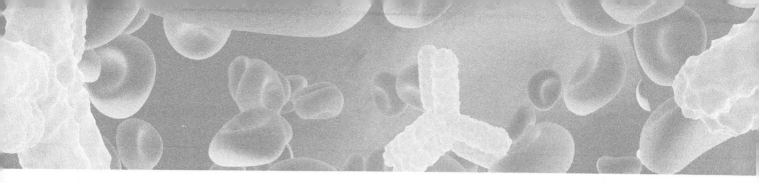

Preface

BACKGROUND AND PURPOSE

The laboratory discipline of transfusion medicine (also known as immunohematology or blood banking) has a rich and fascinating history. In fact, interest in the mystery surrounding the human body and the practice of bloodletting to rid the body of unwanted toxins dates back to the time period between 2500 BCE and 999 CE. It wasn't until the 17th century that the first known animal-to-animal and animal-to-human blood transfusions took place. In spite of the fact there were no recorded medical benefits, a significant number of these individuals apparently survived! Human-to-human blood transfusions were initiated and gained popularity between the 18th and early 20th centuries. Unfortunately, the success rate in these cases was marginal at best. Reasons for the high rate of blood transfusion failures began to unfold in 1901 when Dr. Karl Landsteiner discovered the existence of three different types of human blood: A, B, and C (now known as O). The fourth blood type, AB, was discovered in 1902 by two of Dr. Landsteiner's colleagues: Alfred Von DeCastello and Adriano Sturli. In the years that followed, a number of significant contributions to the field were made that are still valid today. Highlights of representative important events follow. Blood collection, processing, and storage processes were developed. Blood depots, now known as blood banks, were established. The Rh factor, named for the rhesus monkey that was used in the initial testing, along with numerous other red blood cell proteins (known as *antigens*), were discovered. Laboratory tests, procedures, and protocols designed to minimize adverse effects of blood transfusions were developed and refined. Most recently, the advent and implementation of automation in the transfusion medicine laboratory has advanced the discipline into previously uncharted territories.

Transfusion medicine is considered by many to be the area of the clinical laboratory where "life-and-death" decisions occur based on the laboratory results generated. For it is here where blood types are determined and blood is tested prior to transfusion. The goal is to prevent individuals from rejecting transfused blood that in some cases may cause a fatal reaction in a patient (a concept known as *blood incompatibility*). It is important to point out here that laboratory tests are performed *in vitro* and predict what is or will happen *in vivo* and that no test result is 100% foolproof. As long as laboratorians practice proper procedures and techniques and remain alert during the pre-examination (preanalytical), examination (analytical), and post-examination (postanalytical) phases of testing, the chances of laboratory error are greatly reduced. It is thus of paramount importance that laboratorians are educated in the theoretical and pathophysiological considerations associated with transfusion medicine testing. Furthermore, didactic

and psychomotor components on specimen collection, processing and analysis, and result interpretation are critical components of effective laboratorian training. This text was developed to assist in this effort by providing readers with the didactic foundation, background, and tools to successfully function in a typical transfusion medicine laboratory.

ORGANIZATION AND FEATURES OF THE BOOK

The content of this book is organized into 21 chapters, beginning with an in-depth discussion of the origins and interactions between antigens and antibodies. The successive chapters cover the most common blood groups, pretransfusion testing protocols, donor considerations, reactions to transfusions, special populations and testing, safety and regulatory issues, and quality assurance. The book is written at a level adaptable for multiple categories of students and professionals. Instructors and readers are encouraged to utilize the sections and chapters pertinent to their needs.

Each chapter begins with a general content outline, content-specific learning objectives, and a list of key terms (and phrases). Each key term and phrase is **bold** where the term is described. References to a term or phrase prior to its description appear in the text in *italics*. A real-world "running" case study with initial questions for consideration, called ***Case In Point***, is designed to introduce the chapter content. Subsequent installments of the "running" case study, each with pertinent questions for consideration, are strategically placed throughout the rest of the chapter. The introduction for each chapter is titled ***What's Ahead?*** and is comprised of an introductory paragraph followed by a series of questions with the answers covered in the body of the chapter. The chapter content is presented in a logical order under appropriate headings and subheadings. Periodic self-assessment questions, known as ***Checkpoints***, are strategically placed and are designed to provide opportunities for students to evaluate their understanding of the material. Tables, figures, and boxes are incorporated into the chapters as appropriate. The text portion of each chapter concludes with a section termed ***Review of Main Points*** that consists of a bulleted list of the key "take-home" content points of the chapter. A set of review questions, each coded to the corresponding chapter learning objective, allows readers to assess their knowledge over the entire chapter content. A list of references concludes each chapter.

There are four appendices found in the back of this text, three of which consist of answers to chapter-posed questions: (1) Case In Point questions, (2) Checkpoint questions, and (3) Review questions.

The fourth appendix is comprised of an alphabetized glossary of the key terms and phrases identified within the chapters. Two features have been embedded into the glossary to assist readers. First, each glossary entry includes the one or more chapter number(s) in which the entry is designated as a key term. Second, there are numerous terms in the glossary that are synonyms. To help readers learn them, full definitions are provided for each entry with reference to the synonymous entries rather than an entry instructing the reader to look under a synonymous entry for its definition.

Although the terms Blood Bank (Banking) and Transfusion Medicine are often used interchangeably, this book primarily considers them as two different entities. Blood Bank refers to a blood collection and processing center whereas completion of the associated tasks is known as Blood Banking. Transfusion Service is the laboratory area responsible for pre-transfusion testing and blood product distribution (typically located in a hospital setting).

A COMPLETE TEACHING AND LEARNING PACKAGE

The book is complemented by a variety of ancillary materials designed to help instructors be more effective and students more successful.

- The *Instructor's Resource Manual* is a guide designed to equip faculty with necessary teaching resources regardless of the level of instruction. Features include lecture outlines, classroom discussion questions, and suggested learning activities. The *Test Bank* includes over 400 questions to allow instructors to design customized quizzes and exams.

- The *PowerPoint Lectures* contain key discussion points, along with color images, for each chapter. This feature provides dynamic, fully designed, integrated lectures that are ready to use and allows instructors to customize the materials to meet their specific course needs.

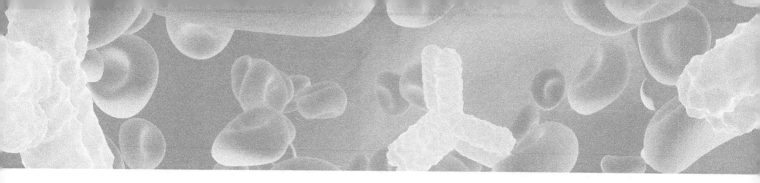

Acknowledgments

This book was truly a team effort. The beauty of multiple editors is that whenever one of us needed assistance, which happened on many occasions, the others were *always* there to help out. Each of us put our heart and soul into this book and it was truly a pleasure working together.

The editors would like to extend their thanks to all of the authors and chapter contributors who worked tirelessly to draft and revise chapters. Special thanks to Susan Conforti for writing and refining the Chapter Objectives, Checkpoints, and Review Questions and to Stephanie Codina for writing the majority of the chapter case study entries and corresponding questions. Most of the wonderful illustrations in this text were done by our coeditor Lisa Denesiuk, who is terrifically talented. Thanks to each of the chapter reviewers who provided the team with invaluable suggestions. Thanks also to Laura Mayer who assisted on numerous logistical and clerical aspects of assembling manuscript for this book—her speed and accuracy are amazing!

We would like to especially thank Mark Cohen for his role in the approvals required to develop this book. Special thanks as well to Cynthia Mondgock who served as our developmental editor by orchestrating all of the various components and individuals associated with this book—we could not have done this without her! The other members of the book development team—Marion Waldman, Melissa Kerian, John Goucher, and everyone behind the scenes at Pearson Education—assisted the team in numerous ways throughout the process. Thanks for providing project guidance and helping to keep us on track.

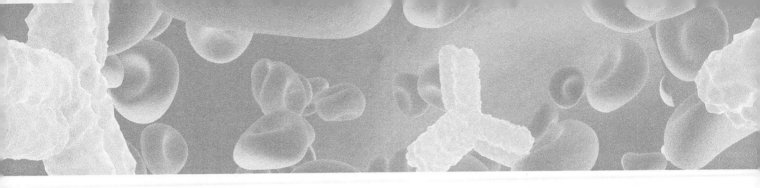

Reviewers

Megan V. Brown, BS, MLS(ASCP)^{CM}
Creighton Medical Center
Omaha, Nebraska

Karen Burgess MSEd, BS MT(ASCP)^{CM}
Valdosta Technical College
Valdosta, Georgia

Mildred K. Fuller, PhD, MT(ASCP), CLS(NCA)
Norfolk State University
Norfolk, Virginia

Michelle Lancaster Gagan, MSHS, BSMT (ASCP), CLS (NCA)
York Technical College
Rock Hill, South Carolina

Karen Gordon, CLS(NCA), MT(ASCP)SLS, PBT(ASCP)
Northern Virginia Community College, Medical Education Campus
Springfield, Virginia

Candace Grayson, MEd, MT(ASCP)
Community College at Baltimore County
Baltimore, Maryland

Mary Madden, BS, MLS(ASCP)^{CM}
BJC Healthcare
St. Louis, Missouri

William C. Payne, MS, MT(ASCP)
Arkansas State University
Jonesboro, Arkansas

Thomas Patterson, MS, BS, MT(ASCP)
Texas State University
San Marcos, Texas

Deirdre D. Parsons, MS, MT(ASCP) SBB
University of Maryland, School of Medicine
Baltimore, Maryland

Christine Pitocco, MS, MT(ASCP), BB
Stony Brook University
Stony Brook, New York

Teri Ross, MS, MT(ASCP) SBB, CLS (NCA)
Loma Linda University
Loma Linda, California

Sandra S. Rothenberger MS, MT(ASCP) SBB
Clarian Health
Indianapolis, Indiana

Diane L. Schmaus, MA, MT(ASCP)
McLennan Community College
Waco, Texas

Sarah Schumacher, BS, MLS(ASCP)^{CM}
BJC Healthcare
St. Louis, Missouri

DEVELOPMENT TEAM
EDITORS

Gretchen Schaef Johns, MD
Medical Director/Assistant Professor of Medicine
Division of Laboratory Medicine and Pathology
Mayo Clinic, Jacksonville Florida

William B. Zundel, MS, MLS (ASCP)^{CM}, SBB
Associate Teaching Professor
Brigham Young University
Provo, Utah

Elizabeth A. Gockel-Blessing (formerly Zeibig), PhD, MLS(ASCP)^{CM}
Interim Associate Dean for Student and Academic Affairs
Program Director | Associate Professor, Clinical Laboratory Science
Doisy College of Health Sciences
Saint Louis University
St. Louis, Missouri

Lisa Denesiuk, MLT, ART, MLS^{CM} (ASCP) SBB^{CM}, BSc (MLS)
Learning Management System and Website Content Specialist
DynaLIFE$_{DX}$
Edmonton, AB, Canada

CONTRIBUTORS

Hannah Acevedo, MS, MT(ASCP)SBB
Manufacturing Processes Specialist
Blood Systems
Phoenix, AZ
Chapter 9

Robert W. Allen, PhD
Chair, Department of Forensic Sciences
Director, Graduate Program in Forensic Sciences
Director, Human Identity Testing Laboratory
Professor of Forensic Sciences
Adjunct Professor of Biochemistry
Director of the Human Identity Testing Laboratory
Chapter 19

Brenda Colleen Barnes, MSEd, MLS(ASCP)^{CM} SBB^{CM}
Director, Medical Laboratory Science Program
Associate Professor
Distance Education Facilitator
Allen College
Waterloo, IA
Chapter 1 and Chapter 3

Stephanie Codina, MA, MT(ASCP)
Gaithersburg, MD
Chapter 8

Susan Conforti EdD, MLS(ASCP) SBB
Assistant Professor
Medical Laboratory Technology
Farmingdale State College
Farmingdale, NY
Chapter 12 and Chapter 13

Patricia Davenport, MT(ASCP) SBB
Donor Notification Manager
Medical Services
Carter BloodCare
Bedford, TX
Chapter 21

Lisa Denesiuk, MLT, ART, MLS^{CM} (ASCP), SBB^{CM}, BSc (MLS)
Learning Management System and Website Content Specialist
DynaLIFE$_{DX}$
Edmonton, AB, Canada
Chapter 4, Chapter 7, and Chapter 20

Brian F. Duffy, MA CHS(ABHI)
Technical Coordinator
HLA Laboratory
Barnes-Jewish Hospital
St. Louis, MO
Chapter 18

Deanna C. Fang, MD
Fellow, Blood Banking/Transfusion Medicine
Department of Laboratory Medicine and Pathology
University of Minnesota
Minneapolis, Minnesota
Chapter 12

Joshua J. Field, MD, MS
Blood Center of Wisconsin
Chapter 17

Mark K. Fung, MD, PhD
Associate Professor of Pathology, University of Vermont College
   of Medicine
Medical Director, Blood Bank, Stem Cell and Tissue Typing Laboratories,
   Fletcher Allen Health Care
Fletcher Allen Health Care
Burlington, VT
Chapter 15

Ralph J. Graff, MD
St. Louis, MO
Chapter 18

Elizabeth A. Hartwell, MD, MT(ASCP) SBB
Medical Director, Gulf Coast Regional Blood Center
Houston, TX
Chapter 14

Beverly Hoover, BA
St. Louis, MO
Chapter 18

Michael R. Lewis, MD, MBA
Associate Professor of Pathology, University of Vermont College of Medicine
Medical Director, Flow Cytometry Laboratory, Fletcher Allen Health Care
Fletcher Allen Health Care
Burlington, VT
Chapter 15

Larisa Kay Maristany, MT(ASCP) SBB
Medical Technologist
Ivinson Memorial Hospital
Laramie, WY
Chapter 11

Mary M. Mayo, PhD, DABCC, MT(ASCP)
Director of Clinical Chemistry, Special Chemistry, POCT
Associate Professor of Pathology
Co-Director-Clinical Pathology, Pathology Residency Training Program
Saint Louis University School of Medicine
St. Louis, MO
Chapter 1

Karen McClure, PhD, MLS(ASCP) SBB
Vice-President, Global Health Partnerships, Clinical and Laboratory
   Standards Institute
Philadelphia, PA
Chapter 5

Karen Nielson
Chapter 20

Elaine J. Scott, MT(ASCP) SBB
St Louis, MO
Chapter 8

Mary F. Signaigo, MT(ASCP)
Clinical Laboratory Educator—Blood Bank
Mercy Hospital Saint Louis
St. Louis, MO
Chapter 2

Margaret A. Spruell, MT(ASCP) SBB
Retired
Gulf Coast Regional Blood Center
Immunohematology Reference Laboratory
Houston, TX
Chapter 6

Andrij E. Sverstiuk, MD
Vanderbilt University Hospital
Nashville, Tennessee
Chapter 16

Janet L. Vincent, MS, SBB(ASCP)
Education Coordinator
Specialist in Blood Bank Program
University of Texas Medical Branch
Galveston, Texas
Chapter 14

Collen Young, BSc (MLS)
Production Manager, Edmonton Centre
Canadian Blood Services
Edmonton, AB, Canada
Chapter 7, Chapter 10, and Chapter 12

Pampee E. Young, MD, PhD
Associate Professor
Medical Director, Transfusion Medicine
Vanderbilt University Medical Center
Nashville, Tennessee
Chapter 16

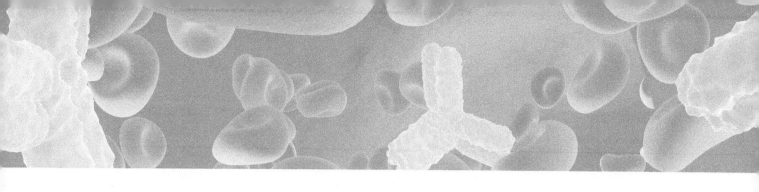

1

The Immune Process
The Origin and Interaction between Antigens and Antibodies

BRENDA COLLEEN BARNES AND MARY M. MAYO

Chapter Objectives

Upon completion of this chapter, the student will be able to:

1. Define the key terms presented in this chapter.
2. Summarize each of the key historical events that contributed to the understanding of the immune system.
3. Construct a timeline that chronologically details the historical events that contributed to the current understanding of antibodies.
4. Compare and contrast the following types of immunity: innate (natural) immunity, adaptive (acquired) immunity, and passive immunity.
5. Identify and describe the purpose of the cells and molecules involved in the immune system.
6. Define, compare, and contrast the key antigen and antibody characteristics that play a role in determining the extent of an immune response.
7. Explain the structural characteristics and function of immunoglobulins.
8. State and differentiate the structure and role of the five classes of immunoglobulins: IgA, IgD, IgE, IgG, and IgM.
9. Explain how the law of mass action affects antigen–antibody interactions.
10. Name the types of noncovalent bonds involved in sensitization.
11. Diagram the process of agglutination.
12. Identify and describe the factors that affect sensitization.
13. Identify and describe the factors that affect lattice formation.
14. Compare and contrast sensitization and lattice formation.
15. State the purpose of the complement system.
16. Summarize the process of hemolysis.
17. State the purpose of each of these complement pathways: (a) classical, (b) alternative, and (c) lectin.
18. Compare and contrast the three complement pathways: (a) classical, (b) alternative, and (c) lectin.
19. Construct a flowchart that diagrams how the complement system is regulated on cell surfaces and in the fluid phase.
20. Describe the role of complement in antigen–antibody interactions.
21. Explain the purpose of the membrane attack complex (MAC).

(continued)

Chapter Objectives *(continued)*

22. Select the effects of storage and anticoagulants on complement activity.
23. Explain the purpose of complement fixation testing.
24. Paraphrase the steps, including the use of and reason for including controls when performing complement fixation testing.
25. Analyze case studies involving the origin of antigens and/or antibodies and:
    a. Identify the process taking place (innate immune response, generation of antibody diversity, or primary/secondary immune responses).
    b. Explain the process taking place.
    c. Choose the next logical step with justification in the process taking place.
26. Analyze case scenarios involving antigen–antibody interactions and:
    a. Identify the process(es) taking place.
    b. Explain the process(es) taking place.
    c. Identify sources of error.
    d. Choose next logical step(s) with justification in the process(es) taking place.

Key Terms

Activation of complement	IgD
Adaptive immunity (acquired immunity)	IgE
	IgG
Affinity	IgM
Agglutination	Immunogen(s)
Alloantibody (alloantibodies)	Immunogenicity
Alternative pathway	Immunoglobulin(s) (Ig)
Amplification loop	Innate immunity
Anamnestic	Intravascular
Antibody (antibodies)	Isotype switching
Antigen(s)	Isotype(s)
Avidity	Lattice formation
C3 convertase	Law of mass action
C5 convertase	Lectin-binding pathway (mannose-binding pathway)
Catabolize	
Cation(s)	Lymphocyte(s)-T, B, and NK
Chemokine(s)	Major histocompatibility complex (MHC)
Classical pathway	
Clonal deletion	Membrane attack complex (MAC)
Clonal selection theory	
Complement	Neutralization
Cytokine(s)	Noncovalent bond(s)
Endothermic	Opsonization
Epitope	Passive immunity
Exothermic	Phagocytosis
Extravascular	Plasma cell(s)
Hapten(s)	Sensitization
Hemolysis	Somatic hypermutation
Humoral immunity	Zeta potential
IgA	Zymogen(s)

CASE IN POINT

This case study will be referred to throughout this chapter.

LC is a 69-year-old woman who was seen in the hospital after she slipped on an overturned rug and fell on her right side. During examination, the physician noted swelling and bruising to her right hip area. She was diagnosed with a femoral head fracture and brought to the operating room for hemiarthroplasy, a surgery in which the head and neck of the femur was removed and a prosthesis was implanted. During surgery, she was transfused with 2 units of red blood cells.

Question for consideration:

1. Name some characteristics that red blood cell antigens may possess that will help to elicit an immune response.

What's Ahead?

The human body is exposed to foreign substances, organisms, and toxins on a daily basis. Most of these invaders never cause clinical disease, and those that do are usually not able to cause disease upon reinfection. The body is equipped with remarkable immune defense mechanisms that dispose of most of these foreign offenders. This chapter examines the origin of and the interactions between **antigens**, substances that are recognized as foreign by the body triggering a response, and proteins that are designed to attack specific foreign invaders known as **antibodies**. A general discussion of antigens and antibodies along with concepts pertinent to blood banking is presented to answer the following questions:

- How is the body able to respond quickly upon first exposure to an invader?
- How is the body able to respond to an almost limitless number and variety of potential invaders?
- How is reinfection prevented or attenuated on a subsequent exposure to an invader?
- What are the cells and molecules that carry out the body's immune defense?
- What antigen characteristics play a role in determining the extent of an immune response?
- What are the functions of antibodies?
- What are the five classes of antibodies?
- What classes of antibodies are important in antigen–antibody interactions?
- What is the nature of antigens and antibodies in blood bank testing?
- What are the key considerations that must be taken into account when dealing with antigen–antibody reactions?
- What is the difference between affinity and avidity?
- What is agglutination and how does it occur?
- What occurs during and what factors affect sensitization?
- What occurs during and what factors affect lattice formation?
- What is the purpose of the complement system?

- What role does complement play in antigen–antibody interactions?
- What complement activation pathways occur and how is each pathway activated?

- What is the purpose of the membrane attack complex (MAC)?
- How is the complement system regulated?
- How does storage and anticoagulants affect complement activity?
- How is complement fixation testing performed?

HISTORICAL BACKGROUND

The immune system serves as the body's sophisticated defense mechanism against infection. The origin of the study of the immune system, known as *immunology*, is usually attributed to British physician Edward Jenner, who in 1798 discovered that exposure to cowpox (the vaccinia virus) could provide protection against the otherwise fatal disease human smallpox virus. Jenner called the process *vaccination*, the term that is still used today to describe the inoculation of healthy individuals with attenuated organisms or recombinant components to confer protection against infection with the virulent natural organism. Although Jenner introduced vaccination, it was not until a century later that Robert Koch proved that infections were caused by microorganisms. Other major developments in immunology occurred around this time, including the development of a rabies vaccine by Louis Pasteur. *Complement*, a concept that is described in more detail later in the chapter, was discovered by Jules Bordet in 1894 and Robert Kaus discovered precipitins in 1897.

In the late 1800s, researchers began to elucidate the mechanism of host immunity. A Russian scientist by the name of Elie Metchnikoff introduced foreign objects into transparent starfish larvae and observed that the offending objects were surrounded by motile cells that attempted to destroy them. He called this phenomenon "**phagocytosis**," which literally means cell eating. The theory of **humoral immunity** (a type of response against foreign particles present that the body initiates through the production and secretion of targeted antibodies) was born out of work done by Emil von Behring and for which he was awarded the first Nobel Prize in Physiology or Medicine in 1901. In 1890, he along with Erich Wernicke, developed the first effective therapeutic serum against diphtheria. Working with Shibasaburo Kitasato, he developed an effective therapeutic serum against tetanus. The scientists immunized animals with attenuated forms of diphtheria and tetanus organisms. They then injected serum from these immune animals into other animals that had been exposed to live organisms. The serum from the immunized animals provided protection from infection. This phenomenon is known today as **passive immunity**, that is, immunity that is not generated by the host's own system but is transferred passively from another. We now know that the protection from infection came from antibodies produced by the immune animals.

Paul Ehrlich postulated that specialized cells carried antibodies and that the molecular structure of antibodies had receptor sites for the antigens that had stimulated their formation, a so-called lock-and-key concept. It was not until 1948 that **plasma cells** were found to be the producers of soluble antibodies, followed in the 1950s and 1960s by the identification of **T lymphocytes** and **B lymphocytes**, (members of a group of white cells whose primary function is to assist the body in fending off unwantered foreign particles) and the subsequent determination that plasma cells were derived from B lymphocytes.[1, 2]

Immunoglobulin, abbreviated as **Ig**, (that is, antibody) structure was elucidated by Gerald Edelman and coworkers in 1969, an accomplishment for which Edelman and Rodney Porter were awarded the Nobel Prize in Physiology or Medicine in 1972.[3]

☑ CHECKPOINT 1-1

Jules Bordet's contribution to the study of immunology was the discovery of:

A. Antibodies
B. Antigens
C. Complement
D. Passive Immunity

COMPONENTS OF THE IMMUNE SYSTEM

As previously indicated, a foreign substance that is capable of triggering an immune response is known as an antigen. Three general properties of antigens are: (1) they are chemically complex; (2) they are foreign or nonself; and (3) they are usually of high molecular weight.

The immune system must be able to distinguish self from nonself and to eliminate nonself components such as infectious organisms. The immune system also eliminates tumor cells and senescent cells, which are old cells at the end of their lifespan.

The natural or innate immune system acts within minutes or hours of exposure to rid the host of potentially infectious organisms. This type of immune response is nonadaptive and does not generate immunological memory. Defense mechanisms involved in the innate immune response typically belong to one of these categories:

- Anatomical (e.g., skin, mucus membranes, and respiratory tract cilia)
- Cellular (e.g., NK cells)
- Humoral (chemicals found in body fluids such as enzymes, fatty acids, and complement)
- Microbiological (host's resident flora)

Adaptive immunity, also known as learned or **acquired immunity**, is the specific response to an antigen and is accomplished by cells of the immune system known as B and T lymphocytes. Adaptive immunity has the property of immunological memory so that when an antigen is reintroduced to the host, the response to the antigen the second and subsequent times is significantly faster.

All of the cells of the immune system, as well as the other cellular elements of blood (erythrocytes, leukocytes, and platelets), arise in the bone marrow from pluripotent hematopoietic stem cells.

These pluripotent hematopoietic stem cells produce two types of stem cells upon division: lymphoid progenitors and myeloid progenitors. The common lymphoid progenitor gives rise to T and B lymphocytes of adaptive immunity as well as **NK lymphocytes** (which are natural killer cells found in the bone marrow and the spleen that are capable of destroying virus infected and select tumor cells) of the type of protection in which the body naturally utilizes its own physiologic capabilities to attack unwanted invaders known as **innate immunity**. Additionally, the common lymphoid progenitor cell gives rise to lymphoid-related dendritic cells, which are important for presenting antigen to T lymphocytes. The common myeloid progenitor gives rise to monocytes, macrophages (the mature tissue form of monocytes), myeloid-related dendritic cells, mast cells, granulocytes, erythrocytes, and megakaryocytes, which produce platelets (Figure 1-1 ■). This chapter is primarily concerned with the properties of B lymphocytes, as these are the cells that produce antibodies. B lymphocytes originate and mature in the bone marrow. T lymphocytes also originate in the bone marrow, but the precursor T lymphocytes migrate to the thymus and mature there. Mature lymphocytes that have not encountered a specific antigen are known as "naïve" lymphocytes.

ANTIGEN CHARACTERISTICS

The term **immunogen** refers to a substance capable of eliciting the formation of an antibody. An antigen is a substance that reacts with an antibody, but may or may not be able to evoke an immune response. Therefore, all immunogens are antigens, but not all antigens are immunogens.

Certain antigen characteristics play a role in determining the extent of an immune response. Foreign particles that are large in size make better immunogens than smaller substances. A weight of 100,000 kD is usually the minimum molecular weight for recognition as an immunogen.[4] **Haptens** are substances that are too small

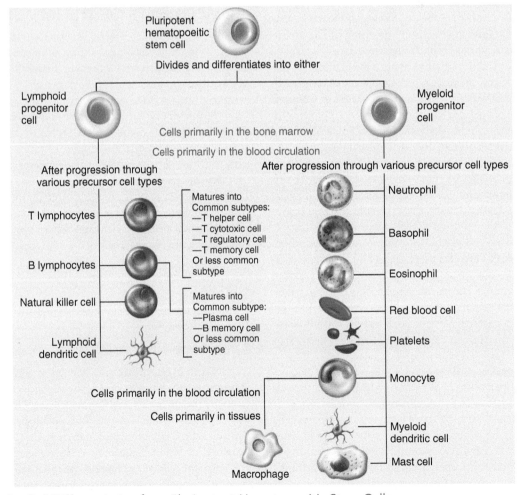

■ **FIGURE 1-1** • Cell Differentiation from Pluripotent Hematopoeitic Stem Cells

to be recognized on their own, but can potentially combine with a carrier molecule to create a new antigenic determinant able to elicit the formation of an antibody.

Chemical composition and molecular complexity also play a role in the ability of an antigen to elicit the formation of an antibody, also known as its **immunogenicity**. Proteins are the best immunogens because they are made up of many amino acids resulting in a complex structure. Carbohydrates can stimulate an immune response, but they are less immunogenic than proteins because sugar molecules are inherently less complex.

The degree of foreignness is also a determining factor in immunogenicity. Generally, the greater the difference between a host and nonhost substance (i.e., the higher the degree of foreignness), the better the immunogenic stimulus it provides. Finally, a substance must be able to be enzymatically digested to create small peptides that can be complexed to **major histocompatibility complex (MHC)**, molecules for presentation to lymphocytes. The MHC consists of a group of genes located on chromosome 6 that play a significant role in blood and tissue compatibility (Chapter 18). Antigens associated with blood bank testing consist of proteins that sit on the surface of blood cells. Although white blood cells (Chapter 18) and platelets (Chapter 16) possess antigens, most antigens of interest in blood bank testing reside on the surface of red blood cell (RBC) membranes. It is important to point out here that if RBCs from one individual are transferred to another individual and the recipient does not see the incoming cells as self, the recipient considers them as foreign and mounts an appropriate immune response. Rather than improving, often the recipient in these cases gets worse instead of better. Specific blood bank testing is available and routinely done to reduce the risk of recipients mounting such a response to transfused cells.

☑ CHECKPOINT 1-3

Immunogenicity is enhanced by which of these characteristics?

A. Chemical simplicity
B. Less than 80,000 kD
C. Increased molecular complexity
D. Low degree of foreignness

ANTIBODY (IMMUNOGLOBULIN) STRUCTURE AND FUNCTION

Immunoglobulins (Ig) are the antigen-recognition molecules of B lymphocytes. Immunoglobulins bound to the membrane of the B cell surface are known as B cell receptors. Secreted immunoglobulins are known as antibodies and are secreted by plasma cells, which are terminally differentiated B lymphocytes. Each plasma cell clone secretes antibody of one particular antigen specificity.

The immunoglobulins are roughly "Y"-shaped molecules comprised of two identical heavy chains (each approximately 50 kDa MW) and two identical light chains (each approximately 25 kDa MW) linked by disulfide bonds (Figure 1-2 ■). There are two regions on each

antibody molecule: (1) the variable region, also known as the antigen binding site, and (2) the constant region, which engages the effector functions. Each heavy chain and each light chain have variable and constant regions. It is important to keep in mind that proteolytic digestion of the molecule by the papaya-derived enzyme known as papain results in two identical Fab fragments (the antigen-binding fragments) and one Fc fragment (the crystallizable or the constant portion of the heavy chain).

There are five different classes or **isotypes** of antibody molecules, which are distinguished by the differences in their constant heavy chains. The heavy chains are designated by Greek letters, with the corresponding intact immunoglobulin (heavy or light chain) designated by the appropriate capital of the English alphabet. The isotypes are alpha (α) in IgA, delta (δ) in IgD, epsilon (ε) in IgE, gamma (γ) in IgG, and mu (μ) in IgM. Each of the particular isotypes has a unique location and function, which is discussed in the following section. There are two types of light chains, lambda (λ) and kappa (κ). Each antibody formed has a particular type of light chain, either kappa or lambda, never one of each. The ratio of kappa-producing plasma cells in humans is approximately twice that of lambda-producing cells.

There are three main functions of antibody molecules: (1) **neutralization**, in which antibodies bind to pathogens or toxins and prevent their entry into cells; (2) **opsonization**, a process in which the antibodies bind to the bacteria coating them, allowing phagocytes to recognize the Fc portion of the antibody molecule and eliminate the bacteria; and (3) **activation of complement**, which enhances the bactericidal actions of phagocytes.

Antibodies associated with blood bank testing reside in the plasma *in vivo* and in the plasma or serum *in vitro*. Most blood bank testing involves antibodies against antigens on the surface of RBCs. With only a few exceptions, individuals make antibodies against red blood cell antigens they lack when they are exposed to cells containing such antigens via pregnancy or transfusion.

☑ CHECKPOINT 1-4

The primary region that distinguishes the five immunoglobulin isotypes are the:

A. Constant heavy chains
B. Constant light chains
C. Variable heavy chains
D. Variable light chains

THE FIVE CLASSES OF IMMUNOGLOBULINS[1, 5]

IgA is the principal isotype in mucosal secretions. IgA-secreting plasma cells are found predominantly in the lamina propria, which lies directly below the basement membrane of many surface epithelial layers. IgA is transported across the epithelium to the external surface and secreted as a dimer, with the two monomers linked by a "J" chain. The principal sites of synthesis of IgA are the gut, respiratory

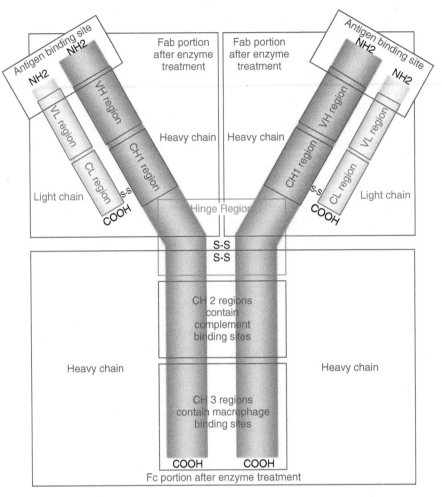

Immune globulin is a protein consisting of 2 heavy chains and 2 light chains joined together by disulfide bonds.

Each heavy chain has a variable region (VC) and a constant region encompassing functional domains named CH1, CH2, and CH3.

Each light chain has a variable (VL) and a constant (VC) region.

The carboxy (-COOH) ends of both the light chain and the heavy chain are highly conserved; the amino acid sequence is very similar for all antibodies of the same class: IgA, IgD, IgE, IgG, or IgM.

Both the heavy and light chains at the amino (-NH₂) end of the proteins are highly variable, which allows for the development of specific antigen binding sites.

Certain enzymes will cleave the immune globulin molecule at several points in the hinge region, resulting in 3 fragments- 1 Fc or fraction crystalizable and 2 Fab or fraction antigen binding.

■ **FIGURE 1-2**   Basic Antibody Schematic

epithelium, lactating breast, and exocrine glands such as salivary and tear glands. IgA does not activate complement.

IgD is found predominantly bound to the surface of naive B lymphocytes along with surface IgM. Although its function is not clear, recent studies suggest that it has been preserved over evolutionary time since the inception of the adaptive immune system.[6]

IgE was officially recognized in 1968 by the World Health Organization as the factor in serum that causes allergies. IgE is unique in its ability to activate mast cells. First exposure to an antigen or allergen causes production of a large amount of IgE specific for that antigen. The IgE molecules attach to the Fc receptors for IgE on mast cells. Upon subsequent exposure with that allergen, the IgE-primed mast

cells release the contents of their granules, including histamine and heparin. This cross-linking and granule release results in a hypersensitivity or allergic reaction.[7]

IgG is the principal isotype in blood and extracellular fluid, and is formed after **isotype switching** (a process in which B cells are able to switch the class of antibody molecules they produce) and the process that allows the immune system to adapt to the antigens that confront it known as **somatic hypermutation**. There are four subclasses of IgG: IgG1–4, which may vary in their hinge region and disulfide bonds in the heavy chain. IgG readily crosses the placenta and subclasses 1–3 are able to activate complement.

✱ **TABLE 1-1** Characteristics of Serum Immunoglobulins

	IgA	IgD	IgE	IgG	IgM
Molecular weight (Daltons)	160,000	180,000	190,000	150,000	970,000
Heavy chain class	α	δ	ε	γ	μ
Complement fixation	—	—	—	+	++
Placental transfer	—	—	—	+	—
Serum concentration (g/L)	2.5	0.03	0.00005	10	1.5

IgM is the first antibody produced in a primary immune response and is mainly found in the blood and lymph. IgM is bound to the surface of naive B lymphocytes along with IgD. Five monomers of IgM are linked by "J" chains to form a pentamer with 10 antigen-binding sites. The pentameric structure of IgM makes it especially effective in activating complement. Although some IgM may be produced in secondary immune responses, other isotypes such as IgG are more predominant. Table 1-1 ✱ summarizes the physical characteristics of each of the five isotype classes of immunoglobulins.[7]

☑ CHECKPOINT 1-5

Which immunoglobulin is best noted for its ability to cross the placenta?

A. IgA
B. IgD
C. IgE
D. IgG
E. IgM

ANTIGEN–ANTIBODY INTERACTIONS

Once an antibody has been formed against an antigen, the antigen's chemical composition plays the biggest role in the formation of an immune complex in that it determines the type of **noncovalent bonds** (a type of bonding that occurs through decentralized electromagnetic intereactions) that can form. In some reactions, antibody prefers to bind to its corresponding antigen because the resulting complex has less free energy than the two uncombined agents. Released energy appears as heat, and the reaction is called **exothermic**. This type of reaction is enhanced at lower temperatures, such as room temperature (71.6° F [22° C]) or even refrigerated temperatures (39.2° F [4° C]). IgM class antibodies preferentially react at these temperatures.[8] Some reactions between antigen and antibody require an increase of free energy. This increase in energy comes from the environment, and the reaction is called **endothermic**. This type of reaction in immunohematological terms occurs at 98.6° F (37° C). IgG class antibodies preferentially react at temperatures closer to body temperature.[8]

Observation of the temperatures at which particular classes of antibody prefer to react may lead to the mistaken conclusion that all IgM class antibodies are clinically insignificant and that only IgG class antibodies are clinically significant. Actually, the nature of the bond and the chemical composition of the binding site determine whether an antibody is cold- or warm-reacting. Each type of noncovalent bond has different thermodynamic properties. Carbohydrate antigens (i.e., ABO, M, N, Lewis, etc.) are less complex in structure and tend to form hydrogen bonds when combined with antibody, making bonding with this type of antigen exothermic, or preferring to occur at a lower temperature. Hydrophilic bonds tend to form with protein antigens (i.e., Rh, Kidd, Kell, etc.). These reactions are endothermic and therefore enhanced at higher reaction temperatures.[9]

The strength of the bonds between an antigen and an antibody, or the sum of attractive and repulsive forces between antigen and antibody, are referred to as antibody *affinity*.[10] Once antigen and antibody bind, the formed immune complex is not static. The antibody may dissociate from the complex and reform with an antigen on a different red blood cell. This association and dissociation continues until equilibrium is reached, and follows the **law of mass action** (Figure 1-3 ▪).

The equilibrium constant (K) of an antigen–antibody interaction is a measure of antibody affinity. K can be considered an indicator of the "goodness of fit" an antibody has for its corresponding antigen, as well as an indicator of the type of bonding between the antigen and antibody. For example, if an antibody has a high attraction and low repulsion for its corresponding antigen, binding is likely to occur. If an antibody has a high repulsion and low attraction for its corresponding antigen, binding is less likely to occur.

☑ CHECKPOINT 1-6

Which of the following characteristics apply to exothermic antigen and antibody reactions?

A. Decreased free energy
B. Reaction temperature best at 98.6° F (37°C)
C. Typically IgG antibody
D. Typically ABO and Lewis blood group antigens

Affinity and Avidity

Affinity refers to the initial force of attraction between one binding site on an antibody molecule and the portion of an antigen molecule where an antibody binds and a complex is formed known as an **epitope** of the corresponding antigen, (otherwise known as monovalent binding). In comparison, multivalent binding, or the functional affinity constant, refers to the binding of one or more antigen-binding sites on an antibody molecule to more than one antigenic determinant on a single carrier (e.g., red blood cell). This functional affinity constant is an indication of the avidity of an antibody and results in increased stability of a reaction. Antibody **avidity** is the sum of all attractive forces between antigens and antibodies, which keeps antigens and antibody molecules together once binding has occurred.[11] *In vivo*, avidity is more relevant than affinity because most antigens are multivalent. Increased avidity can compensate for decreased affinity (Figure 1-4 ▪).[12]

The binding of antigen and antibody is reversible.
Therefore both of the following reactions occur.

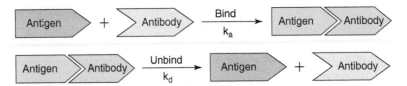

The relative rate of association is k_a. The relative rate of disassociation is k_d.
The amount of antigen/antibody complex will be highest when the two reactions
reach a state of balance: k_a equal to k_d.

How fast a state of balance is achieved is expressed mathematically
as the affinity constant (K_o).

K_o is proportional to the concentration of the antigen, the antibody and the antigen/
antibody complex according to the law of mass action, expressed mathematically as:

$$\frac{\text{Antigen antibody complex concentration}}{\text{Antigen concentration} * \text{Antibody concentration}} = K_o = \frac{k_a}{k_d}$$

K_o is different for each antigen/antibody pairing. K_o describes the goodness of fit of
the antigen and antibody. A large K_o means that antibody binds to antigen quickly
and that the antigen/antibody complex does not break apart easily. Speed of binding
is influenced by the degree of shape compatibility of the antigen and antibody.
Strength of binding is influenced by the type of chemical bond that occurs most often
between the antigen and antibody.

K_o is also affected by temperature, pH, and ionic strength.

In the laboratory, antigen concentration, antibody concentration, temperature, pH,
and ionic strength are controlled to try to achieve the fastest state of equilibrium and
therefore the most sensitive test for the presence of the antibody or antigen.

FIGURE 1-3   Law of Mass Action in Transfusion Medicine

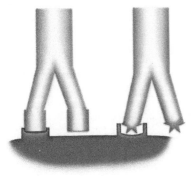

High affinity   Low affinity

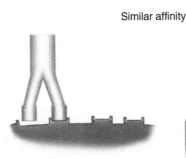

Similar affinity

Low avidity: IgG monomer has
capability to create maximum of 2
antigen/antibody complexes
between each IgG molecule and
red blood cell membrane

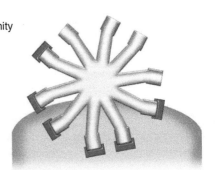

High avidity: IgM pentamer has capability
to create up to 10 antigen/antibody
complexes between each IgM molecule
and red blood cell membrane if the 3D
structure allows.

FIGURE 1-4   Affinity versus Avidity

Influences of Attraction

As previously stated, in order for antigen and antibody to bind and stay bound together, the goodness of fit must be high enough to allow the formation of multiple noncovalent bonds. Another factor to consider in the formation of immune complexes is the complementary nature between the antigen and the antibody. Characteristics such as size, shape, and charge affect the bonding capability between a specific antibody and antigen.

The basis of all blood bank testing is a reaction between an antigen (located on a red blood cell membrane) and an antibody (typically found in serum or plasma). This fairly simple premise can be used to perform a variety of tests (Table 1-2 ✶). Every test has a source of antigen or "cell reactant" and a source of antibody or "serum reactant." Generally, one reactant is *known* and the other is *unknown*, or the answer we are seeking. Antigen–antibody reactions may or may not result in red blood cell aggregation or agglutination. In general terms, when obtained in a blood bank test agglutination suggests that the antigen or antibody being sought (depending on the test being conducted) is present. No agglutination indicates the absence of the antigen or antibody being sought.

For example, ABO (Chapter 4) forward grouping uses *known* commercial antisera (anti-A and anti-B) to determine what antigens are found on a patient's red blood cells. If agglutination is detected, the antigen is present on the patient's red blood cells. If no agglutination is detected, the patient's red blood cells lack the antigen. In antibody detection testing (Chapter 8), commercial reagent red blood cells with *known* antigen phenotypes are tested with patient serum to determine if unexpected antibodies are present. If antibodies are detected, further testing is performed to determine the antibody specificity.

☑ CHECKPOINT 1-7

Which of the following characteristics best describes avidity?

A. Initial force of attraction between one binding site on an antibody and a single epitope on its corresponding antigen

B. Sum of attractive forces between antigens and antibodies

C. More relevant *in vivo* than affinity because most antigens are multivalent

D. Sum of attractive and repulsive forces between antigens and antibodies

---

Agglutination

As previously eluded to, agglutination is the visible endpoint of antigen–antibody reactions for blood bank testing. In some tests, antibody directly bridges the gap between adjacent cells; in others, antibody molecules attach to but do not agglutinate the red blood cells, and an additional step is needed to induce visible agglutination.[13] Detection of agglutination, or lack of agglutination, provides information to aid in the selection of the safest blood components for transfusion. **Agglutination** is defined as the "aggregation of particulate matter caused by combination with a specific antibody."[11]

Agglutination is a reversible reaction between antigen and antibody, and is thought to be a two-step process. The first step involves initial binding of antibody with antigen, also known as *sensitization*. In the second step, aggregates develop through lattice formation, which allows agglutination to be seen. Various factors can affect both steps and be manipulated to enhance or weaken reactions.[14]

Step One: Sensitization

The first step, **sensitization**, occurs when antigen and antibody come together to form an immune complex (Figure 1-5 ■). Binding between antigen and antibody only occurs if the size, shape, and charge of both molecules are complementary in nature. If conditions enhance these attractive influences, several noncovalent bonds will form simultaneously.[15] Noncovalent bonds are weak and reversible interactions that occur over short distances. Bonds of this type include electrostatic, hydrogen, hydrophobic (nonpolar), and van der Waals forces. The strength of a bond is critically dependent on the distance between the interacting groups, namely, the antigen and antibody.[16] The distance between antigen and antibody must be close for noncovalent bonds to occur. Optimum binding distance varies depending on the type of bond involved. The physical conditions of a test system—temperature, incubation time, pH, ionic strength, and antigen–antibody concentration—as identified and described next, can be altered to enhance or inhibit sensitization.

Temperature

Temperature affects the equilibrium constant as well as the rate or speed of reaction.[9] Most blood group antibodies react optimally at either "cold" temperatures (39.2–77° F [4–25° C]) or "warm" temperatures (86–98.6° F [30–37° C]). Most clinically significant antibodies tend to react at warm temperatures and are generally IgG class antibodies, whereas most IgM class antibodies prefer to react at cold temperatures. While many cold reactive antibodies can be considered clinically insignificant because they do not cause destruction of transfused cells *in vivo*, making this broad generalization can be dangerous. For example, ABO antibodies are clinically significant even

---

✶ **TABLE 1-2** Common Blood Bank Tests

Test	Test Reactants
ABO/D forward grouping (covered in detail in Chapters 4 and 5)	Patient red blood cells (the unknown) + known commercial antisera (anti-A, anti-B, anti-D)
ABO reverse grouping (covered in detail in Chapter 4)	Commercial red blood cells with known ABO antigenic makeup (A₁ cells, B cells) + patient serum (the unknown)
Antibody screen (covered in detail in Chapter 8)	Commercial red blood cells with known antigenic determinants + patient serum (the unknown)
Crossmatch (covered in detail in Chapter 7)	Donor red blood cells + patient serum

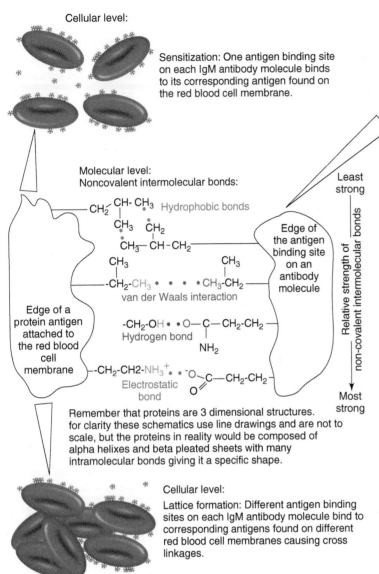

Cellular level:

Sensitization: One antigen binding site on each IgM antibody molecule binds to its corresponding antigen found on the red blood cell membrane.

Atomic level:
van der Waals interaction:

Molecular level:
Noncovalent intermolecular bonds:

Hydrophobic bonds

Edge of the antigen binding site on an antibody molecule

van der Waals interaction

Edge of a protein antigen attached to the red blood cell membrane

Hydrogen bond

Electrostatic bond

Remember that proteins are 3 dimensional structures. for clarity these schematics use line drawings and are not to scale, but the proteins in reality would be composed of alpha helixes and beta pleated sheets with many intramolecular bonds giving it a specific shape.

Least strong

Relative strength of non-covalent intermolecular bonds

Most strong

Hydrophobic bonds occur between non-polar hydrophobic groups immersed in water. Non-polar means there is an equal distribution of electrons and therefore charge across the structure of the molecule. Hydrocarbons in the middle of protein molecules are hydrophobic groups. Blood is an aqueous environment.
When a hydrophobic bond occurs between an antigen and antibody, a water molecule is excluded.
With numerous bonds occurring, the sum of hydrophobic bonds may contribute up to half the total strength of the bond between antigen and antibody.

van der Waals' interactions occur when electrons shift within an overall neutral molecule making each end have a slight temporary positive or negative charge. The charged ends are called dipoles. A weak bond can occur when a slightly positive charged end is near a slightly negative charged end. This type of bond accounts for a limited amount of the total interaction between antigen and antibody.

Hydrogen bonds occur when the electrons of two electronegative atoms are shared with the same hydrogen atom. The hydrogen atom is covalently bonded to an electronegative atom in the same molecule: this gives the hydrogen molecule a positive charge. The positively charged hydrogen is attracted to negatively charged atom on a different molecule. Common example is a hydrogen atom forming the bridge between two oxygen atoms, one on the same molecule via a covalent bond and one on a near by molecule via a hydrogen bond.

Electrostatic or ionic bonds occur between a negatively charged molecule and a positively charged molecule.

Cellular level:

Lattice formation: Different antigen binding sites on each IgM antibody molecule bind to corresponding antigens found on different red blood cell membranes causing cross linkages.

■ FIGURE 1-5   Bonds Resulting in Agglutination

though most are IgM. A better explanation for why ABO antibodies are IgM class is because the antigens are carbohydrate structures.[17]

Incubation Time
Adequate time is needed for antigen–antibody reactions to reach equilibrium. The amount of time needed for equilibrium to be reached varies with each procedure. The saline test or tube testing without enhancement reagents requires 30–60 minutes for detection of most clinically significant antibodies. The addition of enhancement reagents to the test system can decrease incubation time to as short as 10–15 minutes.

pH
Optimal pH has not been determined for immunohematologic testing, but it is generally believed that testing should be performed at the physiologic pH range of 6.8–7.2. Some examples of anti-M have been shown to react preferentially at a lower pH, but antibody detection errors have been known to occur when acidic saline is used in

test systems for routine testing.[18] For most routine testing, a pH of 7.0 should be used.

Ionic Strength
Saline present in the immunohematologic test system causes a shielding effect around red blood cells due to the clustering of Na^+ and Cl^- ions. Red blood cells carry a net negative charge on their membrane, thus attracting the Na^+ ions. This partial neutralization of opposite charges between antigen and antibody can hinder association.[17] The rate of interaction between antigens and antibodies is increased when ionic strength of the test system is decreased.

Antigen–Antibody Concentration
Optimal concentrations of antigen and antibody are necessary for antigen–antibody binding to take place. Antigen excess reduces the number of antibody molecules that bind on each red blood cell, limiting their ability to cause agglutination.[19] Antigen excess can lead to a false-negative reaction in immunohematology testing. Increasing

the antibody concentration in a test system is an easy way to increase the probability of collision with the corresponding antigen. Therefore, most test systems require a 2:1 ratio of plasma/antibody to cells/antigen.

Physical means of bringing red blood cells together, such as centrifugation, is another technique used to enhance lattice formation.

☑ CHECKPOINT 1-8

Which characteristics apply to the first step of agglutination (sensitization)?

A. Lattice formation
B. Incubation time required to reach immune complex equilibrium
C. IgG antibodies react best at cold temperatures (39.2–77° F [4–25° C])
D. Attachment of antibody to antigen

☑ CHECKPOINT 1-9

Which of the following characteristics apply to the second step of agglutination?

A. Antibodies cross-link between red blood cell antigens
B. Results in visible agglutination of red blood cells
C. Enhanced by addition of high ionic strength solution
D. IgM antibodies more efficient at lattice formation than IgG

Step Two: Lattice Formation

Lattice formation is the second step of the agglutination process (Figure 1-5). During this stage, antibody cross-links form between red blood cells, creating a lattice that allows visualization of antigen and antibody reactions. This stage is dependent upon many factors, including the ionic strength of the test system, pH, and temperature. For lattice formation to occur, an antibody must be able to bind to an epitope on each of two different red blood cells. IgG class antibodies are often not able to produce visible agglutination because of their small size and physical properties. In immunohematology testing an antibody of animal origin that reacts with human IgG antibodies is added. This antibody bridges the gap between red blood cells and a lattice forms (Chapter 3).

A large part of the second stage of agglutination is involved in overcoming the forces that keep red blood cells apart. While the net negative charge of red blood cell membranes can affect sensitization, it has an even bigger effect on lattice formation. Red blood cells possess a net negative charge and naturally repel each other. The force of repulsion between red blood cells in physiologic saline is called the **zeta potential**. **Cations** or positively charged particles from saline are attracted to the negatively charged membranes and form a stable cloud around the red blood cells. Molecules of similar charge repel each other, and this causes red blood cells to remain distant from each other. IgM molecules are big and can bridge the distance between red blood cells despite this natural repulsion. On the other hand, the smaller IgG molecules are unable to span the distance between repulsed red blood cells, making lattice formation impossible in most cases, unless the additional antihuman IgG antibody is added.

Decreasing the ionic strength of the test system through the use of different enhancement techniques can help overcome the net negative charge of red blood cell membranes. Decreasing the ionic strength of the entire test system by using low-ionic strength solution (LISS) is one method of enhancement. Using enzymes to decrease surface charge by cleaving chemical groups is also effective. Other methods can increase the viscosity of the test system, making it harder for the red blood cells to push away from each other. Viscous reagents include albumin that reduces the hydration layer around cells and macromolecules that increase the extracellular colloid osmotic pressure, which may influence the shape of red blood cells and allow them to get closer together.

CASE IN POINT (continued)

LC became increasingly anemic during her first 2 weeks in the hospital. She was dizzy and easily winded during her early physical therapy appointments. Her physician ordered transfusion of 2 additional units of red blood cells at which time a blood sample was sent to the blood bank for pretransfusion testing.

The laboratorian on duty tested LC's serum (the unknown) with a set of commercially prepared red blood cells; each vial of cells having a known antigenic makeup (this test is known as an antibody detection or antibody screen test and utilizes the indirect antiglobulin technique) (Chapter 3). This test was performed to look for unexpected red blood cell antibodies in LC's serum. During testing, the laboratorian added two drops of patient serum and one drop of reagent red blood cells suspended in normal saline into each test tube, thereby yielding the correct ratio of antibody to antigen. However, the laboratorian got distracted and forgot to add an enhancement reagent. She incubated the mixture at 98.6° F (37° C) for 15 minutes and looked for agglutination after she centrifuged the test tubes. She observed no agglutination at this juncture. After completing a washing step, she added antihuman globulin (AHG) reagent to each tube, centrifuged the mixture, and once again observed for agglutination. She still did not see agglutination in any of the test tubes. At this point the laboratorian determined that no unexpected red blood cell antibodies were present in LC's serum.

2. How did the laboratorian affect the test when she did not add an enhancement reagent and what effect might this have on the results?

RESPONSES TO ANTIGEN PRESENCE

There are three different types of responses that the body may participate in when it comes in contact with antigens: (1) innate immune response; (2) generation of antibody diversity; and (3) primary and secondary immune responses. A description of each response type follows.

Innate Immune Response

When a microorganism is able to penetrate the body's skin or mucosal defenses for the first time, the macrophages and neutrophils of the innate immune system provide the first line of defense against these invaders. Macrophages have receptors on their cell surfaces for common constituents of bacterial, viral, fungal, or parasitic surfaces that allow the macrophages to bind to the microorganism and engulf it. The now activated macrophages secrete biologically active molecules, specifically **cytokines** and **chemokines**. Cytokines are proteins released by cells that affect the behavior of other cells. Chemokines are small proteins that attract and cause the migration of cells with specific chemokine receptors such as neutrophils and monocytes from the bloodstream to the site of infection. The cytokines and chemokines initiate the process of inflammation.

Traditionally, four Latin words have been used to define inflammation: *calor* (heat), *dolor* (pain), *rubor* (redness), and *tumor* (swelling). The cytokines released by the macrophages increase blood vessel permeability, hence accounting for the localized heat, redness, and swelling. The migration of cells attracted by chemokines to the site of infection often results in pain. These additional cells augment the efforts of the front-line macrophages to kill the invading microorganisms. **Complement**, a system that consists of plasma proteins that interact with pathogens and mark them for destruction, is activated early in infection. The innate immune response, while important for prevention of pathogens growing freely in the body, does not have the important feature of memory.

Memory in the immune response allows the host to respond faster to subsequent antigen exposures. The property of memory is one important feature of the adaptive immune system. Another important feature of the adaptive immune system is the ability to respond to an essentially infinite variety of antigens, that is, the lymphocytes that mature in the bone marrow and the thymus carry antigen receptors with millions of different specificities.

☑ CHECKPOINT 1-10

In an innate immune response, which substances are released by activated macrophages?

A. Immunoglobulins
B. Cytokines
C. Chemokines
D. Memory cells

Generation of Antibody Diversity

When naive lymphocytes enter the bloodstream, only those that encounter an antigen to which their receptor binds will be stimulated to proliferate and differentiate into effector cells. Upon binding of antigen to their receptors, the lymphocyte is activated, divides and produces many identical offspring, or clones (Figure 1-6 ■). This theory was proposed by Macfarlane Burnet in the 1950s as the **clonal**

selection theory.[20] He also proposed that developing lymphocytes that are potentially self-reactive are eliminated prior to release into the bloodstream, a process known as **clonal deletion** (Figure 1-6). For his work, Burnet was awarded the Nobel Prize in Physiology or Medicine along with Peter Medawar in 1960.

For many years after this important discovery, scientists were unable to determine how antigen receptors with a nearly infinite number of specificities could be encoded by a finite number of genes. While it was known that humans and other vertebrates synthesize millions of antibody molecules prior to lymphocyte exposure to antigen, it was uncertain whether the genetic diversity that is required for all of these molecules is carried in the germline cells or is acquired during development and therefore present in somatic cells only. In the 1970s, experiments by Susumu Tonegawa and colleagues answered this question. They demonstrated that the germline genome of the immunoglobulin light chain carries multiple copies of different "V" or variable gene segments as well as multiple copies of different "J" or joining gene segments. A complete variable region is generated by random joining between these two types of segments (Figure 1-7 ■). They also determined that the heavy chain germline genome also contains numerous "D" or diversity segments. The various combinations of these segments can give rise to an incredibly diverse repertoire of antibodies. Finally, somatic hypermutation introduces point mutations into the rearranged gene segments when the B cells encounter antigen, which creates further diversity. Tonegawa was awarded the Nobel Prize in 1987 for this work.[21]

☑ CHECKPOINT 1-11

The type of cell involved in the generation of antibody diversity is:

A. Macrophage
B. Monocyte
C. Lymphocyte
D. Neutrophil

Primary and Secondary Immune Responses

The primary antibody response to a protein antigen is accomplished by B cells with the help of antigen-specific T cells. When a naive B cell leaves the bone marrow, it has membrane bound IgM and IgD antibody, but has yet to encounter antigen or to undergo somatic hypermutation. The naive B cell will bind the appropriate antigen once encountered via its membrane-bound antibody (receptor). The complex is internalized by endocytosis and the resulting endosome fuses with proteolytic enzyme-containing lysozomes. The antigen is degraded into fragments, complexed with major histocompatibility complex (MHC) Class II proteins, and the complex is expressed on the cell surface.

The expression of MHC–antigen fragment complex on the B-cell surface is necessary for interaction with an activated T-cell that recognizes the MHC–antigen complex. Signals that result from

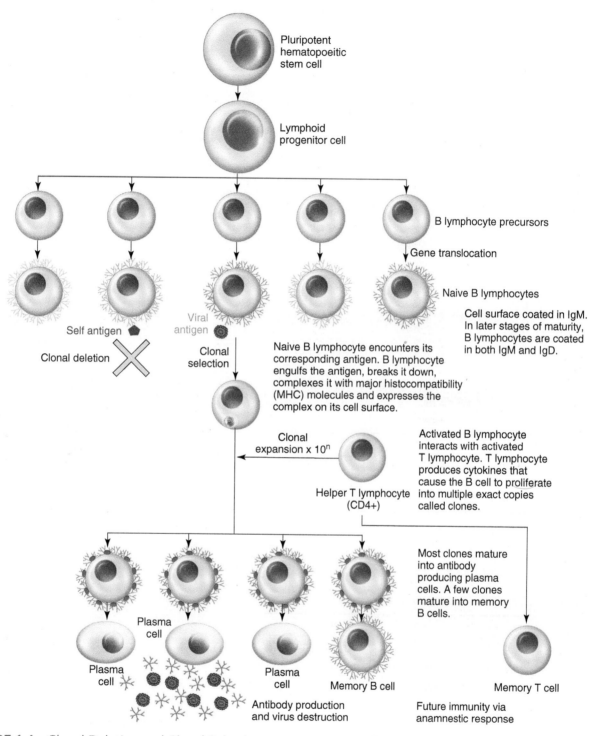

Pluripotent
hematopoeitic
stem cell

Lymphoid
progenitor cell

B lymphocyte precursors

Gene translocation

Naive B lymphocytes

Cell surface coated in IgM.
In later stages of maturity,
B lymphocytes are coated
in both IgM and IgD.

Self antigen

Clonal deletion

Viral
antigen

Clonal
selection

Naive B lymphocyte encounters its
corresponding antigen. B lymphocyte
engulfs the antigen, breaks it down,
complexes it with major histocompatibility
(MHC) molecules and expresses the
complex on its cell surface.

Clonal
expansion x 10ⁿ

Helper T lymphocyte
(CD4+)

Activated B lymphocyte
interacts with activated
T lymphocyte. T lymphocyte
produces cytokines that
cause the B cell to proliferate
into multiple exact copies
called clones.

Most clones mature
into antibody
producing plasma
cells. A few clones
mature into memory
B cells.

Plasma
cell

Plasma
cell

Plasma
cell

Plasma
cell

Memory B cell

Memory T cell

Antibody production
and virus destruction

Future immunity via
anamnestic response

FIGURE 1-6   Clonal Deletion and Clonal Selection

the binding of the activated T cell stimulate the B cell to divide, with the subsequent formation of a B-cell clone. These activated, dividing B cells have a number of different fates. Some will differentiate into plasma cells that secrete IgM antibodies, which comprise the majority of the antibodies in a primary immune response. Some of the cells will undergo isotype switching, meaning the constant region of the heavy chain of the antibody molecule is changed (usually from μ to γ or from an IgM to an IgG). The cells will also undergo somatic hypermutation, with some of the mutations resulting in antibodies of increased affinity for the antigen. These members of the clone will receive signals that will allow them to continue to proliferate and clonally expand. Some of the cells will differentiate to antibody-secreting plasma cells of the new isotype, whereas others will differentiate to memory cells that express the B cell receptor of the new isotype and

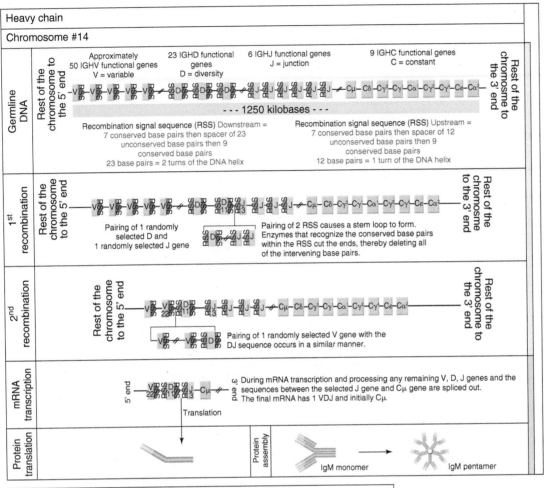

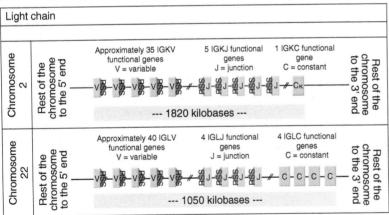

■ FIGURE 1-7   Immunoglobulin Chain Somatic Recombination

increased affinity. Thus memory cells have a higher affinity for antigen than the original naive lymphocyte.

A secondary or **anamnestic** immune response occurs upon re-exposure to an antigen. Due to their higher affinity for antigen, the memory B cells are able to respond to smaller amounts of antigen and are quickly driven to proliferate by interaction with antigen-specific T cells. The secondary response is characterized by rapid and vigorous differentiation of the B cells into plasma cells and the resulting production of high quantities of highly specific antibodies. The antibodies of the secondary immune response are primarily IgG (Figure 1-8 ■).

☑ CHECKPOINT 1-12

The class of antibody with the highest concentration in the primary immune response is:

A. IgA

B. IgD

C. IgE

D. IgG

E. IgM

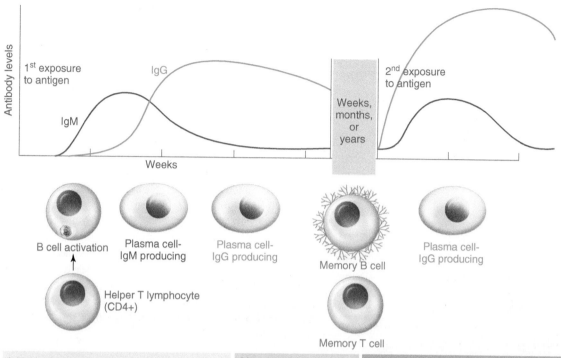

Initial immune response:

Naive B lymphocyte is activated after exposure to corresponding antigen.

T lymphocyte exposed to antigen secretes cytokines.

B lymphocyte proliferates into IgM producing plasma cell clones.

Isotype switching results in a later rise of IgG producing plasma cell clones.

Memory B cells are produced from activated B lymphocytes and remain primarily in the bone marrow.
Memory T cells are produced from activated T lymphocytes and remain primarily in lymphoid organs.

Secondary immune response:

Memory B lymphocyte exposed to its corresponding antigen and in the presence of activated T lymphocyte, rapidly differentiates into IgG producing plasma cell clones.

Memory T lymphocyte exposed to its corresponding antigen quickly differentiate into active T lymphocytes and mount cellular based immune response. For example: Cytotoxic T cells release cytotoxic substances. Helper T cells release cytokines that stimulate activation of B cells and T cells.

■ **FIGURE 1-8**   Primary and Secondary Immune Responses

COMPLEMENT

Complement is an important concept associated with antigen–antibody interactions, and therefore a thorough discussion of these important points follows:

- Role of complement in antigen–antibody interactions
- Complement cascade
- Three activation pathways
- Membrane attack complex
- Complement regulation
- Complement components related to blood group serology
- Effects of storage and anticoagulants
- Complement fixation tests

Role of Complement in Antigen–Antibody Interactions

Some antigen–antibody complexes activate complement, which in turn can lead to **hemolysis** or red blood cell lysis. Hemolysis can occur *in vivo*, meaning in the patient's body, or *in vitro*, meaning in

a test system in the laboratory. Complement activation requires two IgG molecules or one IgM molecule complexed with an antigen. An example of blood group antibodies able to activate complement are the naturally occurring antibodies anti-A and anti-B (IgM and/or IgG class). IgM class antibodies are typically very efficient at activating complement. If complement is activated in the vasculature and continues to the formation of the membrane attack complex, **intravascular** (pertaining to the vasculature) hemolysis may result.

IgG class antibodies are generally less efficient at activating complement but may cause **extravascular** hemolysis or destruction of the red blood cells outside the circulation. **Alloantibodies** formed as a response to transfusion or pregnancy may activate the complement cascade to C3b production before regulatory proteins stop the cascade (e.g., IgG antibodies to Rh, Kell, and Duffy system antigens). Cells coated with C3b usually have normal survival in the circulation. However, cells coated with both C3b and IgG are efficiently removed from circulation and eventually destroyed by reticuloendothelial system (RES) cells.

People who have problems regulating complement deposition on self red blood cells have increased red blood cell destruction, as in the case of autoimmune hemolytic anemias (AIHAs). Complement components as well as IgG are often found on red blood cells of patients with AIHAs, and these patients often suffer from the effects of severe red blood cell destruction (Chapter 15).

Overview of the Complement Cascade

The complement system consists of approximately 30 serum proteins, which act in a cascading manner. Many of the proteins in this system are **zymogens**, meaning they remain inactive until they are acted upon by another protein. The product of one reaction becomes the catalyst for the next step in the cascade, resulting in a tremendous amplification of a localized event.[22]

Complement is part of the innate immune system, requiring no previous exposure to work. The job of the complement system is to promote acute inflammatory events, to cause opsonization, and to kill invading microorganisms or altered host cells. The complement system causes cell destruction either directly through the formation of the membrane attack complex, or indirectly through C3b attachment. The function of C3b is to promote attachment to effector cells, as well as promote inflammation.[23] C3b binds rapidly to nonself particles such as microorganisms or immune complexes, while self cells are protected by surface molecules that limit C3b deposition. Normally, complement can distinguish self from nonself despite being part of the innate system. However, complement can sometimes initiate events which harm the host.

The complement system has three pathways by which it can be activated: the **classical pathway** (in which the presence of an antigen–antibody complex activates complement), the **alternative pathway** (in which activation complement part of the body's natural defense system and thus specific antibody presence is not required), and a pathway that is not antibody-dependent known as the **lectin- or mannose-binding pathway** (Figure 1-9 ■). The classical pathway is linked to the adaptive immune system, while the alternative pathway is linked to the innate system. All three pathways lead to formation of an enzyme that catalyzes the proteolytic cleavage of C3 into C3a and C3b called **C3 convertase**, the pivotal step in the process of complement activation.[24]

Activation of the Classical Pathway

Activation of the classical pathway involves what is known as a recognition unit and an activation phase.

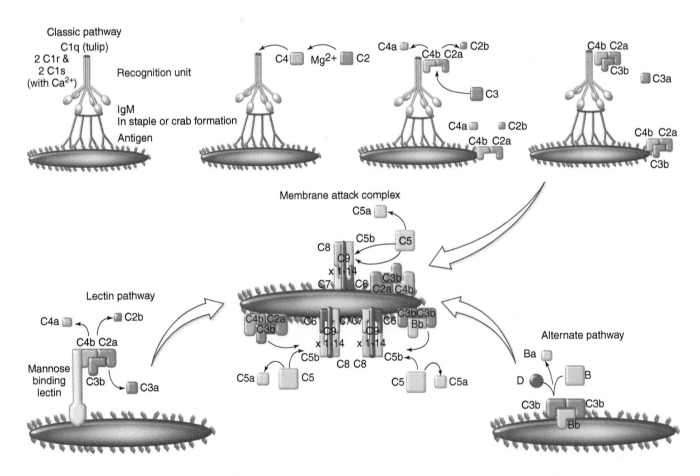

■ FIGURE 1-9   Complement Cascade

Recognition Unit

C1, called the recognition unit, is comprised of one C1q molecule and two molecules each of C1r and C1s. The C1 unit may thus be referred to as $C1qC1r_2C1s_2$. C1q, shaped like six tulips held in a bunch, starts the sequence by binding with a constant region of one IgM molecule or two IgG molecules (IgG1, IgG2, or IgG3) complexed with an antigen. Of the three IgG subclasses, IgG3 is the most effective at activating the recognition unit. In addition, IgM is extremely efficient at binding complement as it contains 10 potential C1q binding sites because of its structure. When IgM is complexed with an antigen, it is often flexed into a "staple" or "crab" configuration, which exposes a large number of C1q binding sites, further enhancing the activation of the classical pathway.[25] C1 is a Ca^{2+}-dependent complex and without it, the complex would dissociate. The C1r and C1s molecules are associated with the "stems" of C1q. When C1q binds to its target, the stems move and activate C1r and C1s.

Activation Phase

Next is the classical activation phase, the phase responsible for C3 convertase production. C1s cleaves C4 into two fragments: C4b and C4a. C4a, the smaller fragment, is a weak anaphylatoxin. Most of the C4b is inactivated in the fluid phase, but some may attach to cell surfaces and act as a binding site for C2. C2 binds to the attached C4b in the presence of Mg^{2+}, and is cleaved by C1s into C2a and C2b. C2a remains bound, making C4b2a or C3 convertase. C3 convertase acts on C3 to cleave it into C3a, an anaphylatoxin that floats off into the fluid phase, and C3b. If C3b is bound close enough to C4b2a, there is further complement activation. One C3 convertase (C4b2a) can convert 200 C3 molecules.[26] C3b is highly labile and has a short lifespan.

☑ CHECKPOINT 1-14

Which complement pathway requires an activation phase?

A. Classical pathway
B. Lectin pathway
C. Alternate pathway
D. All of the above

Activation of the Alternative Pathway

The alternative pathway is usually triggered by something other than an immunoglobulin complexed with an antigen. This pathway primarily responds to charged and neutral sugar targets such as fungal cell walls, endotoxins, or membranes of microorganisms. The alternative pathway is often called the **amplification loop**. A small amount of C3b is continuously produced through a process called *spontaneous tickover activation*.[27] Whether or not the reactions are ratcheted up is determined by the location of C3b generation and regulated by Factors I and H. If C3b is activated near a surface that does not protect C3b from degradation, production of more C3b will be amplified by Factors B and D.

Activation of the Lectin Pathway

The lectin pathway is homologous to the classical pathway, but is activated in an antibody-independent fashion. Mannose-binding lectin (MBL), a molecule belonging to the same family as C1q, binds to

bacteria and interacts with proteins similar in structure to C1r and C1s to activate the classical pathway.

☑ CHECKPOINT 1-15

Match the three different complement pathways on the left with their unique characteristics on the right.

_____ 1. Mannose-binding lectin
_____ 2. Initiated by bacterial membranes
_____ 3. Antibody complexed to antigen
_____ 4. Amplification loop
_____ 5. $C1qC1r_2C1s_2$

A. Classical pathway
B. Alternate pathway
C. Lectin-binding pathway.

Membrane Attack Complex

The **membrane attack complex (MAC)** consists of C5b and C6-C9. Once C3b is produced, it binds to C4b2a to form C4b2a3b, or **C5 convertase** (an enzyme in the complement cascade that catalyzes the proteolytic cleavage of C5 into C5a and C5b). Activation of the complement cascade often stops here because only C3b can bind C5 and C3b is rapidly converted to the inactive form iC3b. A large amount of C3b is needed to bind with C5. If C3b does not react with C4b2a before it inactivates, bound C3b can act as a focus for further complement activation by the alternative pathway, and it can also act as an opsonin.[28]

If conditions are favorable, C4b2a3b cleaves C5 and releases C5a, a potent anaphylatoxin, into the environment, leaving C5b bound. Next, C6 and C7 bind to C5b, inserting into the lipid bilayer of the red blood cell and creating a structure resembling a rod. C8 binding follows and creates a small pore. After the addition of up to 14 monomers of C9, a tubular structure is formed that allows water and solutes to pass freely through the membrane. Sodium and water move into the cell causing swelling and lysis. Some lysis can occur when C8 forms the small pore, but the majority of damage is due to C9 binding (the structure formed is the MAC).

Regulation of the Complement System

The classical pathway is regulated by two mechanisms in the fluid phase (Figure 1-10 ■). The first involves a protein called C1 inhibitor, which binds to and inhibits C1r, as well as inactivating C1r and C1s. The second mechanism blocks formation of C3 convertase. Factor I and C4 binding protein (C4bp) both **catabolize**, or break down, C4b. C4bp also promotes dissociation of C2a from C4b2a, whereas Factor I can cleave bound C3b into C3c. Once C3 is inactivated, it can no longer bind C5, stopping the formation of MAC. Factor I and its cofactor H are also regulators of the alternative system (Table 1-3 ✷).

The classical pathway is regulated on cell surfaces with complement control proteins, or CCPs. CCPs work by inhibiting binding of C2 to C4b (DAF or CR1), disassociating C2a from C4b, known as "decay acceleration" (DAF or CR1), and promoting catabolism of

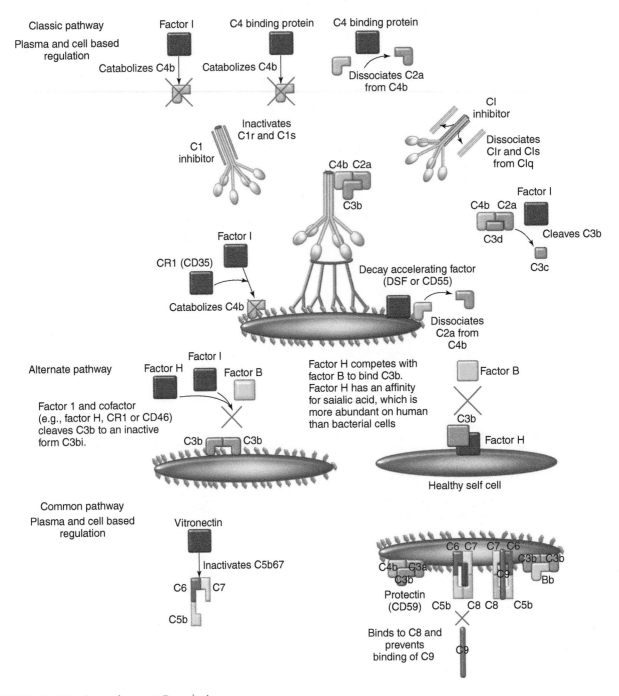

FIGURE 1-10 Complement Regulation

C4b by Factor I (CR1). Because of the lytic nature of complement, it is important to regulate the formation of the MAC. In the fluid phase, C5b67 can insert into other cell membranes, but it can be inactivated in this phase by vitronectin, a protein present in plasma. Also, if C8 binds to a fluid phase C5b67, it cannot insert into a cell membrane. Protectin (CD59), a widely distributed cell membrane protein anchored by a glycophospholipid, binds to C8 and blocks insertion of C9 into cell membranes. Similar to CD59 but weaker in activity is the homologus restriction factor (HRF), which is distributed on red blood cells and platelets.[29]

☑ **CHECKPOINT 1-16**

Which of the following substances are involved in the regulation of the classical complement pathway in the fluid phase?

A. C1 inhibitor
B. CCPs
C. Factor I
D. C4 binding protein

✳ **TABLE 1-3** Complement Regulators

Regulatory Molecule	Location	Target Molecule(s)	Mode(s) of Action
C1 inhibitor (C1INH)	Plasma	C1q, C1s, C1qrs, MASP-1, and MASP-2	– Binds to C1r and C1s, thereby removing C1r and C1s from C1qrs complex in the classic pathway – Inactivates MASP-1 and MASP-2 in lectin pathway – Combined action prevents splitting of C4 and C2 by C1qrs or mannose-binding lectin (MBL) complexes
C4-binding protein (C4BP)	Plasma	C4b	– Binds to C4b, both soluble and cell bound – This prevents binding of C2b – Therefore prevents formation of C3 convertase – Removes C4b from C4b2a when attaches to cell-bound C4b – This stops the classical pathway activation
Complement receptor 1 (CR1) (CD35)	Cell membrane	C3b and C4b	– Removes Bb and 2b from C3 convertase (C4b2a) – Thereby inactivating C3 convertase – Binds C3b and C4b as cofactor in Factor I regulation
Complement S protein* (vitronectin)	Plasma	C7, C8, C9, and C5b67	– Binds to C7, C8, and/or C9 – Blocks C5b67 binding to cell membrane – Therefore prevents C9 polymerization
Decay-accelerating factor (DAF) (CD55)	Cell membrane	C3b and C4b	– Removes Bb and 2b from C3 convertase (C4b2a) – Thereby inactivates C3 convertase – Binds C3b and C4b as cofactor in Factor I regulation
Factor I	Plasma	C3b and C4b	– With cofactors, splits and therefore inactivates cell-bound and soluble (plasma) C3b and C4b – Cell-bound C3b is split into C3f (released into plasma) and iC3b (which remains cell bound but is inactive) – iC3b is further split by Factor I and CR1 into C3c and C3dg
Factor H	Plasma	C3b	– Binds soluble C3b, preventing up-regulation of complement cascade – Binds C3b as cofactor in Factor I regulation – Binds to cell-bound C3bBb complex and removes Bb – Thereby inactivates C3 convertase activity via the alternative pathway
Membrane cofactor protein (MCP) (CD46)	Cell membrane	C3b and C4b	– Binds C3b and C4b as cofactor in Factor I regulation
Membrane inhibitor of reactive lysis (MIRL) (protectin) (CD59)	Cell membrane	C5678	– Binds to C8 portion of C5678 – Therefore limits binding of C9 and progression to the membrane attack complex

CD, cluster of differentiation; MASP, mannose-associated serine protease.

*Can also be called S protein. Note that S protein is a different molecule from Protein S, which is a regulatory molecule in the coagulation cascade.

Source: Based on data from Stevens CD. *Clinical immunology and serology: a laboratory perspective*: 2nd ed. Philedelphia (PA): F.A. Davis Company; 2003, and *Initiation and Regulation of Complement during Hemolytic Transfusion Reactions*, by Stowell et. al., *Clinical and Developmental Immunology*, Hindawi Publishing Corporation.

CASE IN POINT *(continued)*

LC noticed that her urine was red within hours of receiving her second blood transfusion. An investigation revealed that the laboratorian that performed the pretransfusion testing missed a clinically significant red blood cell antibody. The antibody was present on the transfused red blood cells. The antibodies in LC's plasma attached to form an antigen–antibody complex that was able to activate complement and lyse the donor red blood cells.

3. By which pathway was the complement cascade activated?
4. List the steps that likely occurred between recognition of the antigen–antibody complex and lysis of the red blood cells.

Complement Components and Blood Group Serology

The complement system plays a role in blood group serological testing. For example, Chido/Rogers antigens are found on the C4d fragment of C4b and C4a, respectively. They are plasma antigens that are adsorbed onto red blood cells. The different antigens arise from polymorphism of the C4 gene. Antibodies to either antigen do not cause red blood cell destruction and are not considered clinically significant.[30] DAF or CD55 carries the Cromer blood group system; however, antibodies to Cromer system antigens have not been shown to cause red blood cell destruction.[31] It is likely that as research continues in the area of complement and blood group serology, additional antigen specificities will be assigned to complement components.

Complement Storage and Effects of Anticoagulants

Complement is inactivated by heating serum at 132.8° F (56° C) for 30 minutes. Heat treatment inactivates the C1 and C2 components. Complement also degrades upon room temperature or refrigerated storage.[32] Samples for complement testing should be tested within a few hours of collection or frozen if the assay cannot be run within 24 hours.

Complement activation can occur in refrigerated storage temperatures, causing nonspecific binding of complement components. False-positive reactions may be obtained when using polyspecific or C3d antihuman globulin to perform direct antiglobulin testing (DAT) on a serum specimen that has been refrigerated. An EDTA tube is the preferred specimen for DAT testing to ensure any complement detected on red blood cells was attached *in vivo* rather than as a consequence of activation during storage.

Complement activity is inhibited by anticoagulants. The anticoagulant ethylenediaminetetraacetic acid (EDTA) chelates Ca^{2+}, which stabilizes the recognition unit, and Mg^{2+}, which is necessary in the activation phase of both the classical and alternative pathways. The anticoagulant sodium citrate is a weaker chelator of calcium. Any substance that chelates Ca^{2+} and/or Mg^{2+} inhibits complement activity. Heparin can also inhibit complement activity *in vitro*. Heparin works by inhibiting C1 from cleaving C4.

Complement Fixation Testing

Complement fixation testing may be performed to detect and/or determine the amount of antigen or antibody present in a sample (Figure 1-11 ■). Antigen–antibody reactions lead to the formation of immune complexes, and complement can become fixed via the classical pathway.[33]

To perform complement fixation testing, doubling dilutions are made of the patient's serum, and a fixed amount of antigen is added to each tube. If the corresponding antibody is present, immune complexes will form. Next, complement is added, and if immune complexes are present, complement becomes fixed and is consumed by the test system. Then indicator cells (red blood cells) are added along with a small amount of red blood cell agglutinating antibody. If any complement is left in the system, the red blood cells will be lysed. If the complement was consumed in the second step, no lysis will be detected. Controls are a very important component of this test procedure and should include testing of antibody alone and antigen alone. This ensures that neither the antibody nor antigen can fix complement by itself.

☑ CHECKPOINT 1-17

Which of the following may cause a false-positive test for complement with the direct antiglobulin test (DAT)?

A. Heating serum at 132.8° F (56° C) for 30 minutes
B. Prolonged storage
C. Refrigerated patient specimens
D. Patient specimen collected in EDTA

☑ CHECKPOINT 1-18

Which of the statements apply to the complement fixation test?

A. Fixed amount of antigen is added to patient serum
B. Doubling dilutions of patient serum is required
C. Add complement prior to addition of antigen
D. Controls need only include testing for antibody alone

Review of the Main Points

- When the immune system encounters a foreign substance or antigen for the first time, the innate immune system responds quickly to rid the host of the offending organism or toxin. The adaptive immune system also responds, but takes longer.
- The adaptive immune response is also known as acquired immunity and is able to respond to a limitless variety of antigens. The adaptive immune system has the additional feature of memory.
- Antibodies are the soluble excreted form of the B cell receptor immunoglobulins.
- Plasma cells, which are terminally differentiated B lymphocytes, produce antibodies.
- Antibodies bind to their specific antigens and accomplish removal of the antigen either by neutralization, opsonization, or activation of complement.

- Once an antibody has been formed against an antigen, the antigen's chemical composition plays the biggest role in the formation of an immune complex in that it determines the type of noncovalent bonds that can form.
- Factors that affect the physical conditions of a test system designed to detect antigen–antibody complexes can be altered to increase or decrease a test's sensitivity during the sensitization step, and include temperature, incubation time, pH, ionic strength, and antigen–antibody concentration.
- The association and dissociation of antigen and antibody in a test system continues until equilibrium is reached and follows the law of mass action. The equilibrium constant (K) of an antigen–antibody interaction is a measure of antibody affinity. K can be considered an indicator of the "goodness of fit" an antibody has for its corresponding antigen, as well as an

Serial dilution of test serum:

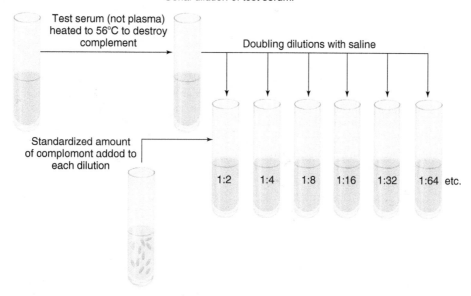

Positive and negative reaction in test system:

Using a known antigen and looking for corresponding antibody in the test serum

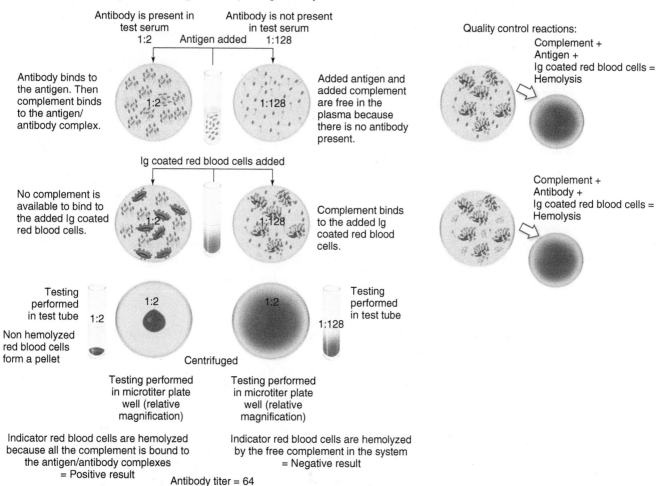

FIGURE 1-11 Complement Fixation Test

indicator of the type of bonding between the antigen and antibody.

- Agglutination is the aggregation of particulate matter caused by combination with a specific antibody and is the endpoint of antigen–antibody reactions for blood bank testing. Agglutination is a reversible reaction between antigen and antibody and is thought to be a two-step process. The first step involves initial binding of antibody with antigen, also known as sensitization. During sensitization, antibody binds to antigen on a red blood cell membrane, but agglutination is not observable. Sensitization occurs when random collisions between antigens and antibodies cause complexes to form. Noncovalent bonds occur during sensitization. These bonds are weak and reversible interactions that occur over short distances. Bonds of this type include electrostatic, hydrogen, hydrophobic (nonpolar), and van der Waals forces. Lattice formation is the second step of the agglutination process. During this stage, cross-linkages form between red blood cells and allow visualization of antigen and antibody reactions. This stage is dependent upon many factors, including the ionic strength of the test system, pH, and temperature.

- Two important concepts associated with antigen–antibody interactions are affinity and avidity. Affinity refers to the initial force of attraction between one binding site on an antibody molecule and a single epitope on the corresponding antigen, otherwise known as monovalent binding. Antibody avidity is the sum of all attractive forces between antigens and antibodies, which keeps antigens and antibody molecules together once binding has occurred.

- The job of the complement system is to promote acute inflammatory events, to cause opsonization, and to kill invading microorganisms or altered host cells. Hemolysis is the destruction of red blood cells with release of intracellular hemoglobin and is caused by the activation of the complement system.

- The complement system causes cell destruction either directly through the formation of the membrane attack complex or indirectly through C3b attachment. The complement system has three pathways by which it can be activated. The pathways are the classical pathway, the alternative pathway, and the lectin- or mannose-binding pathway.

- C1, called the recognition unit of the classical pathway, is comprised of one C1q molecule and two molecules each of C1r and C1s (C1qC1r$_2$C1s$_2$). C1q, shaped like six tulips held in a bunch, starts the sequence by binding with a constant region of one IgM molecule or two IgG molecules (IgG1, IgG2, or IgG3) complexed with an antigen.

- The alternative pathway is usually triggered by something other than an immunoglobulin complexed with an antigen. This pathway primarily responds to charged and neutral sugar targets such as fungal cell walls, endotoxins, or membranes of microorganisms.

- The lectin pathway is homologous to the classical pathway, but is activated in an antibody-independent fashion. Mannose-binding lectin (MBL), a molecule belonging to the same family as C1q, binds to bacteria and interacts with proteins similar in structure to C1r and C1s to activate the classical pathway.

- The membrane attack complex (MAC) consists of C5b and C6-C9. The MAC forms a tubular structure that allows water and solutes to pass freely through the membrane. Sodium and water move into the cell, causing swelling and lysis.

- The classical pathway is regulated by C1 inhibitor, Factor I, and C4 binding protein in the fluid phase. The classical pathway is regulated on cell surfaces with complement control proteins, or CCPs. Because of the lytic nature of complement, especially with the formation of the MAC, it is important to regulate the formation of this structure. Vitronectin, protectin (CD59), and homologous restriction factor all are responsible for the regulation of the MAC.

- Complement activity has been found to be inhibited by the use of anticoagulants. EDTA chelates Ca^{2+}, which stabilizes the recognition unit, as well as Mg^{2+}, which is necessary in the activation phase of both the classical and alternative pathways. Heparin works by inhibiting C1 from cleaving C4. Complement is inactivated by heating serum at 132.8° F (56° C) for 30 minutes. Heat treatment inactivates the C1 and C2 components. Complement also degrades in serum upon storage.

- Complement fixation testing may be performed to detect and/or determine the amount of antigen or antibody present in a sample. Antigen–antibody reactions lead to the formation of immune complexes, and complement can become fixed via the classical pathway.

Review Questions

1. Match the term with its corresponding definition. (Objective #1)

_____ A. Plasma cells

_____ B. Innate immunity

_____ C. Anamnestic

_____ D. Antigen

_____ E. Clonal selection theory

1. The immune response that occurs upon repeated exposure to the same antigen.

2. The binding of antigen to lymphocytes, resulting in activated cells that may result in clones.

3. Any substance that elicits an immune response.

4. A producer of soluble antibodies.

5. The body's natural defense system.

6. Developing lymphocytes that are potentially self-reactive eliminated prior to release into the bloodstream.

2. For a substance to act as an antigen and produce an immune response, the substance must have which characteristics? (Objective #5)

A. Foreign

B. Structurally complex

C. Agglutinate with an antibody

D. Chemical complexity

3. The purpose of B lymphocytes is to: (Objective #5)

    A. Secrete antibody

    B. Engulf foreign antigens

    C. Secrete antigen

    D. Alter microorganisms in preparation for phagocytosis

4. What role do immunoglobulins play in the process of neutralization? (Objective #5)

    A. They are responsible for activating complement.

    B. They prevent entry of foreigners into cells.

    C. They bind to foreigners in preparation for digestion.

    D. They trigger the production of plasma cells.

5. In terms of size, the largest class of immunoglobulins is: (Objective #8)

    A. IgM

    B. IgG

    C. IgE

    D. IgD

    E. IgA

6. This immunoglobulin class accompanies IgM by binding to the surface of naive lymphocytes. (Objective #8)

    A. IgA

    B. IgD

    C. IgE

    D. IgG

7. Complement has been activated in a test. This activation may be detected by: (Objective #20)

    A. Agglutination at 98.7° F (37° C)

    B. Activation of the membrane attack complex

    C. Agglutination at room temperature

    D. Hemolysis in the tube

8. Characteristics of IgM antibodies include: (Objective #8)

    A. Able to cross the placental barrier

    B. Good complement activator

    C. Reacts best at cold temperatures (39.2–71.6° F [4–22° C])

    D. Antigen is usually carbohydrate

9. Which of the following factors affects the first step of agglutination (sensitization)? (Objective #12)

    A. pH

    B. Incubation time

    C. Incubation temperature

    D. Enhanced by addition of antihuman IgG

10. Which of the following represent noncovalent bonds involved in step one of agglutination? (Objective #10)

    A. Hydrogen bonds

    B. Van der Waals forces

    C. Hydrophilic bonds

    D. Electrostatic bonds

11. Which of the following immune complex characteristics applies to the affinity between antigen and antibody? (Objective #6)

    A. Monovalent binding

    B. Multivalent binding

    C. Force of attraction between single binding sites on antibody with antigen

    D. Sum of all attractive forces

12. Which of the following best describes the purpose of the complement membrane attack complex? (Objective #20)

    A. Required for lysis of red blood cells

    B. C5 convertase

    C. Major contributor to red blood cell damage is due to C9

    D. C6 and C7 bind to C5b, creating a rod through the red blood cell membrane

13. Which statement best differentiates between passive and adaptive immunity? (Objective #4)

    A. The process of passive immunity occurs within the body whereas adaptive immunity is transferred to the body from an outside source.

    B. Individuals are born with the ability to display passive immunity but not adaptive immunity.

    C. Individuals obtain passive immunity from outside the body whereas in adaptive immunity the body remembers first exposures to antigens without outside assistance.

14. Which of the following factors affects the strength of antigen and antibody reactions? (Objective #6)

    A. Concentration of red blood cell suspension (antigen)

    B. Incubation temperature

    C. Number of antigen sites on the red blood cell membrane

    D. Immunoglobulin class

15. Characteristics of the law of mass action that affect antigen and antibody reactions include: (Objective #9)

A. Concentration of antigen

B. Concentration of antibody

C. Valence of antibody

D. Antigen and antibody complementarity

16. Which of the following characteristics applies only to the classical complement pathway? (Objective #18)

A. Shaped like six tulips in a bunch

B. Binds with variable region of an IgM molecule

C. Binds with two IgG molecules

D. $C1qC1r_2C1s_2$

17. Which of the following phrases differentiates sensitization from lattice formation? (Objective #14)

A. Antibody bound to red blood cell antigen

B. Antibody bridges between red blood cells

C. Allows visualization of antigen–antibody reactions

D. Ionic strength of the test system

References

1. Janeway CA, Traver P, Walport M, Shlomchik MJ. Basic concepts in Immunology. In: *Immunobiology, the immune system in health and disease, 6th ed.* New York: Garland Science Publishing; 2005.
2. Stevens CD. Historical concepts and introduction to serologic testing. In: *Clinical Immunology and Serology, a laboratory perspective, 2nd ed.* Philadelphia (PA): F.A. Davis Company; 2003.
3. Edelman GM. Antibody structure and molecular immunology. *Science* 1973; 180: 830–840.
4. Stevens CD. *Clinical immunology and serology: a laboratory perspective, 2nd ed.* Philedelphia (PA): F.A. Davis Company; 2003. p. 46.
5. Merler E, Rosen FS. The Gamma Globulins: The structure and synthesis of the immunoglobulins. *NEJM* 1966; 275: 480–486.
6. Ohta Y, Flajnik M. IgD, like IgM is a primordial immunoglobulin class perpetuated in most jawed vertebrates. *Proc Nat Acad Sci* 2006; 103: 10723–10728.
7. Johansson, SGO. The discovery of immunoglobulin E. *Allergy and Asthma Proc* 2006; 27: S3–S6.
8. Klein HG, Anstee DJ. Blood transfusion in clinical medicine, 11th ed. Malden (MA): Blackwell Publishing; 2005. pp. 86–7.
9. Brecher, ME (ed). *Technical manual,* 15th ed. Bethesda (MD): AABB; 2005. p. 273.
10. Roitt I, Brostoff J, Male D. *Immunology,* 6th ed. London: Harcourt Publishers; 2001. p. 72.
11. Stevens CD. *Clinical immunology and serology: a laboratory perspective, 2nd ed.* Philedelphia (PA): F.A. Davis Company; 2003. p. 129.
12. Romans DG, Tilley CA, Dorrington KJ. Monogamous bivalency of IgG antibodies. I. Deficiency of branched ABHI-active oligosaccharide chains on red cells of infants causes the weak antiglobulin reaction in hemolytic disease of the newborn due to ABO incompatibility. *J Immunol* 1980; 124(6): 2807–11.
13. Brecher, ME (ed). *Technical manual,* 15th ed. Bethesda (MD): AABB; 2005. p. 271.
14. Brecher, ME (ed). *Technical manual,* 15th ed. Bethesda (MD): AABB; 2005. p. 272.
15. Roitt I, Brostoff J, Male D. *Immunology,* 5th ed. London: Mosby International Ltd; 1998. p. 107.
16. Roitt I, Brostoff J, Male D. *Immunology,* 5th ed. London: Mosby International Ltd; 1998. p. 108.
17. Brecher, ME, (ed). *Technical manual,* 15th ed. Bethesda (MD): AABB; 2005. p. 274.
18. Rolih S, Thomas R, Fisher F, Talbot J. Antibody detection errors due to acidic or unbuffered saline. *Immunohematol* 1993; 9(1): 15–8.
19. Brecher, ME, (ed). *Technical manual,* 15th ed. Bethesda (MD): AABB; 2005. p. 274–5.
20. Burnet FM. Clonal selection theory of acquired immunity. Nashville (TN): Vanderbilt University Press; 1959.
21. Tonegawa S. The Nobel Lectures in Immunology, The Nobel Prize for Physiology or Medicine 1987, Somatic generation of immune diversity. *Scand J Immunol* 1993; 38: 303–319.
22. Brecher, ME (ed). *Technical manual,* 15th ed. Bethesda (MD): AABB; 2005. p. 259.
23. Klein HG, Anstee DJ. *Blood transfusion in clinical medicine,* 11th ed. Malden (MA): Blackwell Publishing; 2005. p. 94.
24. Roitt I, Brostoff J, Male D. *Immunology,* 5th ed. London: Mosby International Ltd; 1998. pp. 44–5.
25. Roitt I, Brostoff J, Male D. *Immunology,* 6th ed. London: Harcourt; 2001. p. 59.
26. Brecher, ME (ed). *Technical manual,* 15th ed. Bethesda (MD): AABB; 2005. p. 261.
27. Roitt I, Brostoff J, Male D. *Immunology,* 5th ed. London: Mosby; 1998. p. 48.
28. Roitt I, Brostoff J, Male D. *Immunology,* 6th ed. London: Harcourt; 2001. pp. 54–5.
29. Roitt I, Brostoff J, Male D. *Immunology,* 6th ed. London: Harcourt; 2001. p. 58.
30. Klein HG, Anstee DJ. *Blood transfusion in clinical medicine,* 11th ed. Malden (MA): Blackwell Publishing; 2005. p. 230.
31. Chaplin, H. Review: the burgeoning history of the complement system 1888–2005. *Immunohematol* 2005; 21(3): 85–93.
32. Burtis CA, Ashwood ER, Bruns DE (eds). *Tietz Textbook for Clinical Chemistry and Molecular Diagnostics,* 4th ed. St. Louis (MO): Elsevier Saunders; 2006. p. 568.
33. Roitt I, Brostoff J, Male D. *Immunology,* 6th ed. London: Harcourt; 2001. pp. 417–20.

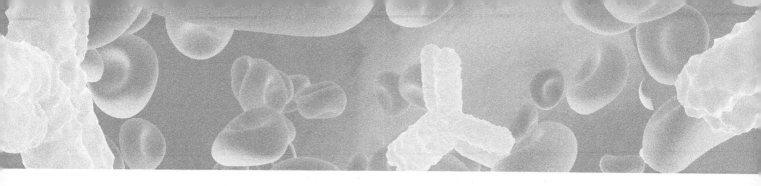

2 Immunogenetics
The Origin of Antigens

MARY F. SIGNAIGO

Chapter Objectives

Upon completion of this chapter, the student will be able to:

1. Describe the processes of mitosis and meiosis.
2. Define common genetic terms.
3. Apply common genetic terms to blood group inheritance using specific blood group system examples.
4. Describe the structure of the DNA molecule.
5. Describe the role of DNA in inheritance.
6. Differentiate the physical and chemical characteristics of DNA and RNA.
7. Give an example of each of the primary patterns of inheritance.
8. Describe the synthesis and localization of blood group antigens.
9. Discuss the differences between homozygous and heterozygous inheritance and expression of blood group antigens.
10. Differentiate between phenotype and genotype using examples.
11. Use a Punnett square to predict the phenotype and genotype of offspring when given the genotype of the parents.
12. Describe position effect and give an example from blood group genetics that demonstrates this phenomenon.
13. Discuss compatibility considerations for patients who have antibodies to high- and low-frequency antigens.
14. Describe and list the uses of polymerase chain reaction (PCR) technology.

Key Terms

Allele(s)
Amorphic(amorph)
Antithetical
Chromosome(s)
Cis
Co-dominant
Codon
DNA replication
Dominant
Dosage effect
Gene(s)
Genotype(s)
Haplotype(s)
Heterozygous
Homozygous
Karyotype(s)
Linkage
Locus (loci)
Meiosis
Mitosis
Pedigree chart
Phenotype(s)
Polymorphism
Punnett square
Recessive
Recombination
Trans
X-linked

CASE IN POINT

PH is a 28-year-old woman who has been married for 7 years. She is pregnant with the couple's third child. Her physician orders ABO/Rh and antibody screen testing at her first prenatal visit.

What's Ahead?

An understanding of how red blood cell antigens are inherited is critical in providing safe blood products for transfusion. This chapter addresses the following questions:

• What are the basic principles of inheritance?
• How are red blood cell antigens inherited and synthesized?
• What practical applications of genetic knowledge are routinely used in transfusion medicine?

BASIC PRINCIPLES

Genetics is the study of the inheritance of transmissible characteristics or traits, including red blood cell antigens. The roots of modern genetics can be traced to the observations of Gregor Mendel, a monk and scientist who made detailed studies of the nature of inheritance in plants. He observed that single traits are passed from generation to generation.[1]

The genetic material that determines each trait is found in the nucleus of cells. With a few exceptions—for example, mature red blood cells and mature platelets—each cell in the body has a nucleus that contains chromosomes. A **chromosome** is a linear thread of deoxyribonucleic acid (DNA). Figure 2-1 ▧ illustrates the structure of a chromosome. DNA contains the genetic instructions used in the synthesis, development, and functioning of all living organisms. A discussion of the relevant basic principles pertinent to blood banking (immunohematology) follows.

Structure of DNA

DNA usually exists in a coiled double strand. DNA is made up of nucleotides.[2] A nucleotide has a deoxyribose sugar, a phosphate group, and one of four bases. The four bases—cytosine, guanine, adenine, and thymine—bond to each other in specific pairs, resulting in the coiled double-strand structure. Adenine pairs with thymine (A-T) and cytosine pairs with guanine (C-G). Each half of the DNA strand has a 3' end and a 5' end, which are named based on the carbon atom in the sugar that is attached to the phosphate group. The 3' end of one strand of DNA pairs with the 5' end of the complementary strand. Figure 2-2 ▧ is a schematic showing the structure of DNA.

☑ CHECKPOINT 2-1

What does the acronym DNA mean?

Mitosis and Meiosis

Cells must undergo division to allow for growth and continual renewal and repair. **Mitosis** is somatic or nonsexual cell division, yielding two diploid daughter cells that contain the same number of chromosomes as the parent cell. Diploid refers to the fact that human cells, except for sexual cells, contain two sets of chromosomes. Figure 2-3 ▧ is a photograph of a normal set of human chromosomes known as a **karyotype**. All cells, except sex cells, undergo mitosis. Chromosomes within the nucleus are duplicated before cell division, in a process called **DNA replication**. The double-stranded DNA in the chromosome is unwound, separated, and then each strand acts as a model for the replication of the opposite strand. The new strand is assembled from nucleotides by the enzyme, DNA polymerase. The steps in mitosis are illustrated in Figure 2-4 ▧.

Meiosis is sexual cell division, yielding four daughter cells each containing half of the number of chromosomes found in the parent cell. The sex cells, either eggs or sperm, are haploid in humans, meaning that they contain one copy of each chromosome rather than two. The major steps in meiosis are illustrated in Figure 2-5 ▧.

While maintenance of the original cell's genome is of primary concern in cell division, mutations may occur when there is crossover, recombination, or nucleotide substitution. Mutations increase genetic variability because they have the potential to create new *phenotypes*. Some mutations will prove fatal to the organism and will not be passed down to future generations, but some mutations are either neutral or even give the organism a survival advantage. For example, Fy(a–b–) red blood cells are resistant to a strain of malaria and therefore this phenotype is rare in European ethnicities but relatively common in people of African ethnicity (Chapter 6). Similarly, sickle cell trait confers resistance to malaria and is more prevalent in ethnicities where malaria was historically endemic, both African and Mediterranean.

Crossover occurs when two genes are near each other on the chromosome. During meiosis the homologous chromosomes may become intertwined, break, exchange genetic material, and

▧ **FIGURE 2-1** Pair of Chromosomes
Humans have 23 matched pairs of chromosomes carrying specific genetic information. One-half of each pair is inherited from each parent.

Centromere

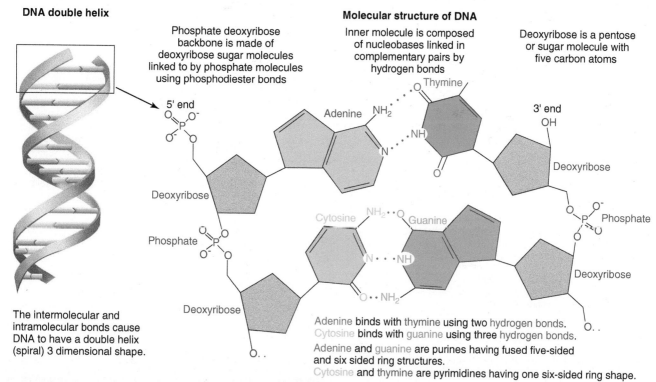

DNA double helix

The intermolecular and intramolecular bonds cause DNA to have a double helix (spiral) 3 dimensional shape.

Molecular structure of DNA

Phosphate deoxyribose backbone is made of deoxyribose sugar molecules linked to by phosphate molecules using phosphodiester bonds

Inner molecule is composed of nucleobases linked in complementary pairs by hydrogen bonds

Deoxyribose is a pentose or sugar molecule with five carbon atoms

Adenine binds with thymine using two hydrogen bonds.
Cytosine binds with guanine using three hydrogen bonds.
Adenine and guanine are purines having fused five-sided and six sided ring structures.
Cytosine and thymine are pyrimidines having one six-sided ring shape.

■ **FIGURE 2-2** Structure of Deoxyribonucleic Acid (DNA)

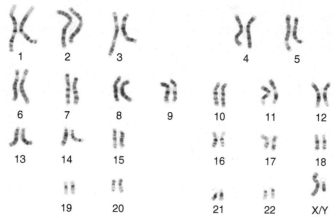

■ **FIGURE 2-3** Human Karyotype

Human cells have 46 chromosomes: two each of chromosomes 1–22, then a pair of X chromosomes if female or one X and one Y chromosome if male.

Source: National Cancer Institute.

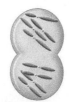
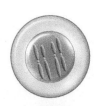

Parent cell

Two out of the 23 in total chromosome pairs shown. One of each pair is of maternal inheritance and the other is of paternal inheritance.

Chromosome duplication

One of the illustrated chromosomes has a central centromere with arms of relatively equal size. The other has an off-center centromere and arms of unequal size.

Sister chromatids separate

Cell division begins

Two identical daughter cells

■ **FIGURE 2-4** Mitosis

Mitosis is normal cell division, yielding two diploid daughter cells.

Parent cell	Chromosome duplication	First cell division begins	First cell division begins	End of first meiosis/ Beginning of second meiosis	Chromosomes divide	Four nonidentical daughter cells
Two out of the 23 in total chromosome pairs shown. One of each pair is of maternal inheritance and the other is of paternal inheritance.	One of the illustrated chromosomes has a central centomere with arms of relatively equal size. The other has an off-center centomere and arms of unequal size.	Homologous chromosomes pair up and crossover can occur.				

FIGURE 2-5 Meiosis
Meiosis is sexual cell division, yielding four haploid gamete cells.

repair. The new genetic material is called a **recombination** as it will contain bits of one gene from one chromosome with bits of the closely linked gene from the other chromosome. For example, less common antigens in the MNS blood group system result from recombination of the *GYA* and *GYB* genes (Chapter 6).[3] Some partial D phenotypes in the Rh blood group system (Chapter 5) are the result of recombination between the closely linked *RHD* and *RHCE* genes.[3]

Most common blood group antigens result from a single-nucleotide *polymorphism*, often called a SNP or "snip." SNPs are the result of a nucleotide substitution. The change in nucleotide results in an amino acid change in the protein blood group antigen. Table 2-1 ✳ lists some examples of nucleotide substitutions found in blood group systems.

✳ **TABLE 2-1** Examples of Single-Nucleotide Substitutions in Blood Group Systems

Blood Group System	Antigen	Nucleotide*	Amino Acid*
Duffy	Fy^a	125G	42Gly
	Fy^b	125A	42Asp
Kidd	Jk^a	838G	280Asp
	Jk^b	838A	280Asn
Kell	K	698T	193Met
	K	698C	193Thr
	Kp^a	961T/962G	281Trp
	Kp^b	961C/962G	281Arg
	Kp^c	961C/962A	281Gln
	Js^a	1910C	597Pro
	Js^b	1910T	597Leu

*The position number is followed by nucleotide or amino acid identification.

A, adenine; C, cytosine; G, guanine; T, thymine; Asn, asparagine; Asp, aspartic acid; Arg, arginine; Gln, glutamine; Gly, glycine; Leu, leucine; Met, methionine; Pro, proline; Thr, threonine; Trp, tryptophan.

☑ **CHECKPOINT 2-2**

List three types of genetic mutations.

DNA Translation

The genetic information carried by the DNA is transformed into an organism via DNA translation. The basic process is very similar regardless of the size or complexity of the organism. In the cell nucleus, the DNA is unwound and a complementary strand of messenger ribonucleic acid (mRNA) is produced. RNA is similar to DNA, but is usually single-stranded, contains ribose instead of deoxyribose as its sugar, and uses the base uracil instead of thymine. The mRNA is transported from the cell's nucleus to the cell's cytoplasm. In the cytoplasm the ribosomes translate the mRNA into proteins, which are composed of amino acids. A set of three base pairs, called a **codon**, will translate into a particular amino acid or a stop codon. Table 2-2 ✳ lists codon translations.

☑ **CHECKPOINT 2-3**

What is DNA transcribed into?

In a simple, single-cell organism such as a bacteria or a yeast, each cell may express all the same proteins. In a complex organism different cells with different functions will have different genes turned on or off. For example, a human's skin cells will express certain genes and will produce a different set of proteins than a B-lymphocyte from the same human, even though both cells' nuclei contain the same sets of chromosomes. Some proteins may be expressed on a variety of different cells, for example, human leukocyte antigens (HLAs), whereas other proteins will be very cell-specific, for example, the Kidd blood group antigens are expressed only on red blood and kidney cells.[4]

✶ TABLE 2-2 Codon Translations

Each RNA codon is followed by the corresponding amino acid translation.

AAA = Lys	ACA = Thr	AGA = Arg	AUA = Ile
AAC = Asn	ACC = Thr	AGC = Ser	AUC = Ile
AAG = Lys	ACG = Thr	AGG = Arg	AUG = Met
AAU = Asn	ACU = Thr	AGU = Ser	AUU = Ile
CAA = Gln	CCA = Pro	CGA = Arg	CUA = Leu
CAC = His	CCC = Pro	CGC = Arg	CUC = Leu
CAG = Gln	CCG = Pro	CGG = Arg	CUG = Leu
CAU = His	CCU = Pro	CGU = Arg	CUU = Leu
GAA = Glu	GCA = Ala	GGA = Gly	GUA = Val
GAC = Asp	GCC = Ala	GGC = Gly	GUC = Val
GAG = Glu	GCG = Ala	GGG = Gly	GUG = Val
GAU = Asp	GCU = Ala	GGU = Gly	GUU = Val
UAA = Stop	UCA = Ser	UGA = Stop	UUA = Leu
UAC = Tyr	UCC = Ser	UGC = Cys	UUC = Phe
UAG = Stop	UCG = Ser	UGG = Trp	UUG = Leu
UAU = Tyr	UCU = Ser	UGU = Cys	UUU = Phe

Ribonucleotide abbreviations: A, adenine; C, cytosine; G, guanine; U, uracil.

Amino acid abbreviations: Ala, alanine; Arg, argnine; Asn, asparagine; Asp, aspartic acid; Cys, cysteine; Gly, glutamine; Glu, glutamic acid; Gly, glycine; His, histidine; Ile, isoleucine; Leu, leucine; Lys, lysine; Met, methionine; Phe, phenylalanine; Pro, proline; Ser, serine; Thr, threonine; Trp, tryptophan; Tyr, tyrosine; Val, valine.

☑ CHECKPOINT 2-4

What is mRNA translated into?

Genes are made of DNA and are the basic unit of heredity. Each gene consists of a specific sequence of nucleotides occupying a specific location on a chromosome. The site of the gene on the chromosome is the **locus**.

An **allele** is one of two or more different forms of a gene at a specific locus on a chromosome. Antigens that represent different forms of a gene product from the same locus are called **antithetical**. Often, antithetical alleles are represented by related nomenclature to indicate their relationship. For example, in the Kidd blood group system, the *JKA* and *JKB* alleles are responsible for the expression of the Jk^a and Jk^b antigens, which are antithetical (Chapter 6).

Homozygous and Heterozygous Alleles

When alleles at a given locus on both chromosomes are identical they are **homozygous** (e.g., *JKA/JKA*). The alleles are **heterozygous** when they are nonidentical at a given locus (e.g., *JKA/JKB*).

There is often a difference in the amount of antigen expressed on the red blood cell membrane between a homozygous versus a heterozygous phenotype. This difference can be detected serologically by a stronger reaction between the specific antibody and the cell with a homozygous expression of the corresponding antigen. The serologic difference encountered with a heterozygous versus a homozygous antigen expression is termed **dosage effect.** An example of dosage effect would be in the case of the Duffy blood group system (Chapter 6). Dosage in this case is demonstrated when a person whose phenotype is Fy(a+b−) exhibits a stronger reaction with anti-Fy^a antiserum than a person whose phenotype is Fy(a+b+). Not all blood group systems demonstrate dosage.

CASE IN POINT *(continued)*

The physician receives the results of the laboratory work performed on PH. He notes that she is blood type O Rh(D) positive. Her antibody screen is positive and anti-c (pronounced "anti-little c") was identified in her blood.

1. What is the most likely method by which PH was sensitized (exposed) to the little-c antigen?
2. Big C and little c are antithetical alleles. Given the fact that Mary possesses an antibody to the little-c antigen, what is her probable genotype for these antigens?

Predicting Genotypes

One method used for predicting genotype frequencies of offspring is called a **Punnett square**. Figure 2-6 ■ illustrates an example of a Punnett square. A Punnett square shows the different ways that genes can separate and combine. One parent's possible genotype is listed on the left and the other parent's possible genotype is listed on the top of the square. The combinations of offspring are then determined for each intersecting row and column. Remember, an

Mom \ Dad	A	A
A	AA	AA
A	AA	AA

100% A offspring

Mom \ Dad	A	O
A	AA	AO
A	AA	AO

100% A offspring

Mom \ Dad	A	O
A	AA	AO
O	AO	OO

75% A and 25% O offspring

■ **FIGURE 2-6** Punnett Square Examples—ABO Blood Group System

Punnett squares are used to predict the genes inherited by offspring. In the ABO blood group system, genes inherited are either *A*, *B*, or *O*. *O* is a silent allele without phenotype expression. When a person is blood group A, their genotype may be *A/A* or *A/O*. If both parents are homozygous for *A* (*A/A*), then all offspring are homozygous for *A*. If one parent is heterozygous (*A/O*), then half the offspring are heterozygous and half are homozygous and if both of the parents are heterozygous, then one-fourth are homozygous for *A* (*A/A*), half are heterozygous (*A/O*), and one-fourth are homozygous for *O* (*O/O*).

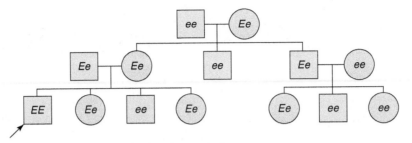

FIGURE 2-7 Pedigree Chart Example—Rh Blood Group System

The chart shows a pedigree for the E and e antigens. In a pedigree chart, each generation is shown on a horizontal band. This chart illustrates three generations. Females are represented by circles and males are represented by squares. A horizontal line indicates a random mating. The person whose phenotype or genotype prompted the family study is called the *propositus* and is identified by an arrow. There are common symbols that indicate consanguineous matings, miscarriages, stillbirths, identical or fraternal twins, and other family relationships, none of which are present in this family.

individual inherits one gene from each parent for each inherited characteristic, such as blood type, they display.

A **pedigree chart** records a family tree in which a trait is mapped through several generations. Figure 2-7 ■ is an example of a pedigree chart. Pedigree charts capture the information gained from a family study. Family studies may be used to determine the most likely pattern of inheritance when a new mutation is discovered.

As with other genetically inherited traits, there are often differences in phenotypic frequency of blood group antigens among different racial populations. For example, approximately 15% of Caucasians are Rh(D) negative, yet less than 1% of China's dominant ethnic group is Rh(D) negative (Chapter 5).[3]

CASE IN POINT (continued)

The physician requests that the father of the fetus be antigen-typed for both the big-C and little-c antigens.

3. Using a Punnett square, predict the chances the baby will possess the little-c antigen when the father is homozygous for the little-c antigen.

4. Using a Punnett square, predict the chances the baby will possess the little-c antigen when the father is heterozygous for the little-c antigen.

5. Why do you think the physician wants to know whether the father possesses these antigens?

BLOOD GROUP ANTIGENS

There are three key points regarding blood group antigen that are pertinent to blood bank (immunohematology) testing: (1) synthesis and localization, (2) patterns of inheritance, and (3) expression. A description of each concept follows.

Synthesis and Localization

Blood group antigen molecules are produced as a result of alleles at a specific gene locus. The production of a blood group antigen can be direct; the gene codes for a red blood cell membrane–associated protein. The antithetical blood group antigens are *polymorphisms*

(a concept described in more detail later in the chapter) found on that red blood cell membrane protein. Examples of protein blood group systems include Kell, Kidd, and Duffy.

Carbohydrate blood group antigens—for example, ABO and MNS—are produced indirectly by the allele. The allele codes for the presence or absence of a glycosyltransferase, which is an enzyme. Enzymes are proteins that catalyze a chemical reaction. The enzyme, if present, causes a carbohydrate molecule to attach to a protein or lipid on the red blood cell membrane, resulting in the carbohydrate blood group antigen.

☑ CHECKPOINT 2-5

List one example of a protein-based blood group system and one example of a carbohydrate-based blood group system.

Red blood cell antigens may be located almost entirely on the surface of the red blood cell or may be a structural part of the red blood cell membrane, with only a small portion exposed on the outer surface of the cell. Figure 2-8 ■ is a simplified schematic of the red blood cell membrane.

Patterns of Inheritance

A **dominant** gene expresses a trait that does not allow the expression of a trait encoded by an alternative allele at the same locus on the other chromosome. Figure 2-9 ■ is a pedigree chart of a dominant gene. A **recessive** gene does not express itself in the presence of its dominant allele. A recessive trait is only apparent if both alleles are recessive. Figure 2-10 ■ is a pedigree chart of a recessive gene. Blood group antigens, as a rule, are expressed as **co-dominant** traits. Figure 2-11 ■ is a pedigree chart of a co-dominant gene. A co-dominant gene expresses a trait regardless of whether or not an alternative allele at the same locus is also expressed on the other chromosome. For example, if a person is genetically *JKA/JKB*, then his or her red blood cells will carry both JK antigens and will phenotype as JK(a+b+).

An **X-linked** gene is on the X chromosome. In males who inherit an X and a Y chromosome, the antigen will be expressed based on the allele on the X chromosome because the Y chromosome does

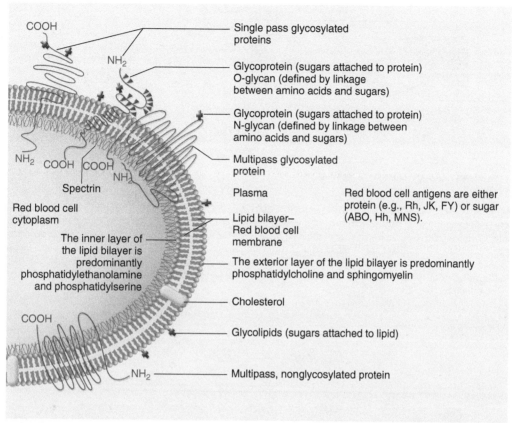

☩ Chains of various sugars (oligosaccharide) attached
via N-linkage (N-glycan).
N-linked sugars are attached to the three amino acid
sequences (1) ASN (2) any aa (3) either SER or THR.
ASN = asparagine; aa = amino acid; SER = serine;
THR = threonine

▼ Chains of various sugars (oligosaccharide)
attached via O-linkage (O-glycans).
O-linked sugars are attached to either
SER or THR.

Proteins can interact with one another to form larger structures within the membrane.
For example the protein cytoskeleton of the red blood cell is made up of two macromolecules:
–Ankyrin associating with Band 3 and RHAG
–Band 4.1 associating with glycophorin C, glycophorin D, RHD, RHCE, KX, FY, adducin, and dematin
Other membrane proteins function as transport or adhesion molecules.

■ **FIGURE 2-8** Simplified Schematic of the Red Blood Cell Membrane
The diagram does not illustrate the three-dimensional structures of the molecules. Only a few representative proteins, carbohydrates, and lipids are included. Not drawn to scale.

not carry corresponding alleles. In a pedigree, an X-linked trait will exhibit a recognizable pattern of inheritance because females carry two X chromosomes and males carry one X and one Y. Figure 2-12 ■ is a pedigree chart of an X-linked gene. The only blood group system genes found on the X chromosome are *Xg* and *XK*.[4]

Interaction among alleles or the products of different genes may modify the expression of a trait. One example is positional effect, for example, the weakening of the D antigen expression when the C allele is present in the **trans** position, meaning on the opposite paired chromosome (*Dce/Ce*). The term **cis** is used to describe two or more alleles present on the same chromosome. For example, with the genotype *DCe/ce*, the D and C alleles are in the cis position.

Linkage is the tendency for genes that are close together on the same chromosome to be inherited as a unit. These gene units are called **haplotypes**.[5] Linkage can affect gene frequency in the population due to the fact that the genes are inherited together rather than

individually. The HLA (human leukocyte antigen) genes are linked and are inherited as haplotypes (Chapter 18).

☑ **CHECKPOINT 2-6**

Define genetic linkage and give one example.

The null phenotype is the inheritance of genes that code for no expression of the usual blood group antigens for that system. It may be due to various reasons such as an **amorphic** gene in the homozygous state or interaction between two unrelated genes. An amorphic gene does not express a phenotype and can be called the silent gene. Examples of amorphic genes in blood group systems include *O*, *h*, and *JK* (Chapter 4 and Chapter 6). When an unrelated gene affects the expression of a gene, it can be called a modifier, inhibitor, or

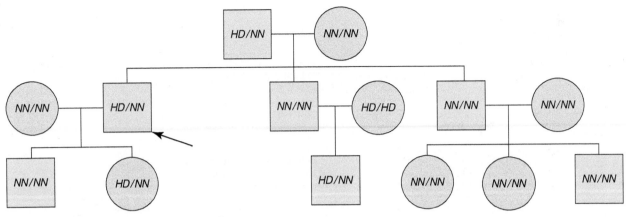

HD = one of the alleles causing Huntington's disease.
NN = normal allele

FIGURE 2-9 Dominant Pedigree Example—Huntington's Disease

Huntington's disease is an example of an autosomal-dominant disease in humans. In the first generation shown, an affected male mates with an unaffected female, producing three sons. Because the affected male is heterozygous for the Huntington's gene, approximately one-half his offspring are likely to be affected. The eldest son is affected and the younger two are not. The affected son mates with an unaffected female, producing an unaffected son and an affected daughter. The middle son mates with an affected female, producing an affected son. Because the affected female is homozygous for the Huntington's gene, all her offspring would be affected. The youngest son mates with an unaffected female, producing three unaffected children.

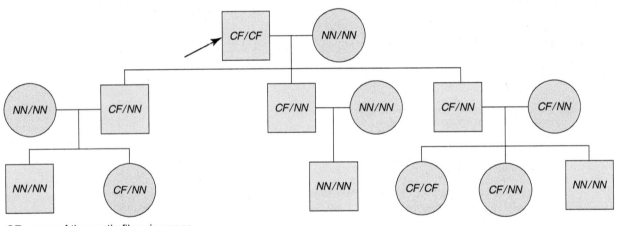

CF = one of the cystic fibrosis genes
NN = normal gene

FIGURE 2-10 Recessive Pedigree Example—Cystic Fibrosis

Cystic fibrosis is an autosomal-recessive disease in humans. In the first generation, an affected male mates with an unaffected noncarrier female. They produce three sons, all of whom are unaffected carriers. The eldest son mates with an unaffected noncarrier female. Neither of their children is affected, but their daughter is a carrier. The middle son mates with an unaffected female. Their child is unaffected and is not a carrier. The youngest son mates with an unaffected carrier female. Their offspring will have a 25% chance of being affected and a 50% chance of being a carrier. They produce an affected daughter, an unaffected carrier daughter, and an unaffected noncarrier son.

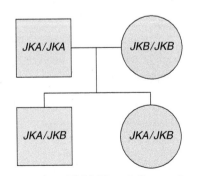

FIGURE 2-11 Co-Dominant Pedigree Example—Kidd Blood Group System

Homozygous father will phenotype as Jk(a+b−). Homozygous mother will phenotype as Jk(a−b+). Both children are heterozygous and will phenotype as Jk(a+b+)

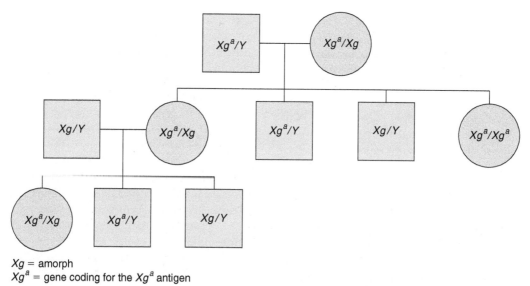

Xg = amorph
Xg^a = gene coding for the *Xg^a* antigen

 FIGURE 2-12 X-linked Pedigree Example—Xg Blood Group System

The Xg blood group system is inherited in an X-linked dominant fashion because the antithetical gene to Xgᵃ is an amorph. The illustrated geno-types produce the following phenotypes:

$$Xg^a/Y = Xg^a(+)$$
$$Xg^a/Xg = Xg^a(+)$$
$$Xg/Y = Xg^a(-)$$
$$Xg^a/Xg^a = Xg^a(+)$$

regulator gene. Examples in blood group systems include the *RHAG* allele that results in the Rh$_{mod}$ phenotype[4] and the *In(Jk)* gene that inhibits expression of Kidd blood group antigens.[3]

Expression

The **genotype** is the actual genetic makeup and may be inferred by the phenotype. The **phenotype** is the observable expression of inherited traits. Recessive genes will not be observed in the phenotype, but are present in the genotype. Blood group antigen typing using antiserum identifies a phenotype. A positive reaction with antiserum determines the presence of the antigen. For example, if we test a person's red blood cells with anti-A and it causes the red blood cells to clump or agglutinate, then that person has A antigens and their phenotype is Group A. A negative reaction determines the absence of the antigen.

CASE IN POINT *(continued)*

The father of the fetus is tested for the big-C and little-c antigens. He is positive for both, phenotype of C+c+.

6. What are the potential genotypes of the fetus?
7. What are the potential phenotypes of the fetus?

    Polymorphism refers to a genetic system that expresses two or more phenotypes.[5] The Rh system is polymorphic due to the number of alleles possible at the RHD and especially RHCE loci (Chapter 5). The frequency of a phenotype is dependent on the polymorphism of the blood group system. The more polymorphic

the system, the less likely it is to find two identical individuals. The HLA system is highly polymorphic, making finding suitable donors for transplantation a challenge (Chapter 18). Due to polymorphism, both the blood group and HLA systems are useful in parentage testing (Chapter 19).

PRACTICAL APPLICATIONS

The basic principles of genetics covered in this chapter have several practical applications in the areas of available blood bank (immunohematology) tests involving population genetics and genetic testing methods. A discussion of each of these aspects follows.

Population Genetics

There are three immunohematology tests, each addressed in the sections that follow, that involve population genetics: paternity testing, transfusion, and determining high- and low-frequency antigens.

Paternity Testing

Analysis of the genes inherited from each parent can be used to calculate the likelihood that a particular man is the biological father of a child (Chapter 19).

Transfusion

Knowledge of gene frequencies in the population for a particular antigen can help determine the number of compatible units to be found in an inventory of blood. The gene frequency is used in the Hardy-Weinberg equation to calculate how many donor units need to be screened in order to realistically find the required number of compatible units (Chapter 8).

High- and Low-Frequency Antigens

The Hardy-Weinberg equation is helpful for the majority of common antibodies where the antigen frequency in the population is midrange. However, it is not particularly helpful when dealing with high- or low-frequency antigens.

High-frequency red blood cell antigens are present in 98–99% of the population. For example, the k antigen is present in 99.8% of the Caucasian population (Chapter 6). A person that is negative for a high-frequency antigen has a great risk of exposure and subsequent antibody formation with blood transfusion or pregnancy. If an antibody is developed, the likelihood of finding antigen-negative, compatible blood is minimal. Family members rather than unrelated donors may be the best source of compatible blood.

At the other end of the spectrum are low-frequency red blood cell antigens, which are found in less than 1% of the population. For example, the Kpᵃ antigen has a frequency of 2% in Caucasian populations but is even less common in other ethnicities. The likelihood of someone developing an antibody to low-frequency antigens is minimal due the low number of positive donors. If a person develops an antibody to a low-frequency antigen, antigen-negative, compatible blood would be easy to find. Generally speaking, all units tested are likely to be antigen negative.

☑ CHECKPOINT 2-7

What is the definition of a low frequency blood group antigen?

Genetic Testing Methods

The Human Genome Project resulted in the determination of over 99% of the nucleotide sequences in the human genome.[6] This effort improved DNA-sequencing technology and provided a complete blueprint of the proteins that are relevant in transfusion medicine. DNA sequencing may be performed using laser detection of fluorescent-labeled sequencing products, capillary electrophoresis, or mass spectrometry. Three of these methods—polymerase chain reaction, DNA microarray, and restriction fragment-length polymorphism analysis—are described in the following sections.

Polymerase Chain Reaction

Knowledge of a gene sequence allows for synthesis of DNA using polymerase chain reaction (PCR) technology, which rapidly and precisely amplifies a defined segment of DNA several million times.[7] Very small amounts of DNA, as little as the amount from a single cell, can be tested because of the amplification steps. The high sensitivity is valuable for early detection of transfusion-transmitted diseases and eliminates the reliance on seroconversion, which can occur much later. For example, nucleic amplitude testing (NAT) for hepatitis C is estimated to detect infection in a donor 47–58 days sooner than testing for the antibody to hepatitis C (Chapter 9).[8,9] Sequence-specific PCR in which alleles are distinguished is used in HLA typing (Chapter 18).

DNA Microarray

A technique used to analyze the differential expression of multiple genes is DNA microarray or gene chip.[10,11] In this technique, known DNA molecules are spotted or synthesized on a small area of a solid support, usually a glass slide. DNA, often generated by PCR, is then incubated on the slide with fluorescent markers that are only incorporated if an exact match occurs. The result is a picture of gene expression on the microarray. Microarrays can be used for genotyping for blood group antigens.

Restriction Fragment Length Polymorphism Analysis

Different strains of bacteria produce a restriction endonuclease. This enzyme recognizes a single specific nucleotide sequence and cleaves the DNA strand wherever the sequence occurs, generating a number of DNA fragments. These DNA fragments can be isolated and identified. Restriction fragment length polymorphism (RFLP) analysis has been used in gene mapping, parentage testing, and forensic science.[12]

Review of the Main Points

- Human cells carry 46 chromosomes consisting of 23 pairs of chromosomes: two copies of chromosomes 1–22 plus two sex chromosomes.
- Mitosis is the process of cell division where two daughter cells with the same DNA are produced; in humans the daughter cells contain a diploid number of chromosomes.
- Mitosis is used for growth and cell replacement.
- Meiosis is the process of cell division to produce sex cells (sperm and eggs) that each has a haploid number or one set of chromosomes.
- Human and other mammalian chromosomes are composed of deoxyribonucleic acid (DNA).

- DNA carries the genetic code of the organism.
- Some viruses use ribonucleic acid (RNA) rather than DNA to carry their genetic code.
- In human cells, DNA is transcribed to mRNA that is translated into protein; the resulting proteins build the cell.
- Mendelian inheritance patterns include dominant, recessive, co-dominant, and X-linked.
- Most red blood cell antigen alleles show co-dominant inheritance.
- Red blood cell antigens are either proteins coded for directly by DNA or are carbohydrates that result from a specific glycosyltransferase that is coded directly by DNA.

- Dosage effect refers to the situation where homozygous versus heterozygous expression of a blood group antigen alters the number of antigens to the degree that the corresponding antiserum shows a difference in strength of reaction.
- Blood group antigen phenotypes are determined by serologic testing with commercial antisera.
- Blood group antigen genotype can be inferred by family studies or can be tested for using various DNA typing methodologies, such as DNA microarray testing.
- A Punnett square can be used to predict genotype frequencies in offspring.

- A pedigree chart is used to map a specific trait through several generations.
- Population genetics and the Hardy-Weinberg equation can be used to estimate the number of donors that would need to be tested to find compatible blood for a recipient with an antibody.
- Polymerase chain reaction (PCR) methods are frequently used in transfusion-transmissible disease testing of donated blood.
- Restriction fragment length polymorphism (RFLP) methods are used in gene mapping, parentage testing, and forensic science.

Review Questions

1. Match the characteristics with the appropriate cellular division process: (Objective #1)

____Somatic cell division   a. Mitosis

____Daughter cells are haploid   b. Meiosis

____Sexual reproduction

____Daughter cells have two sets of chromosomes

2. A DNA nucleotide consists of: (Objective #4)

A. Deoxyribose sugar, phosphate group, four bases

B. Deoxyribose sugar, phosphate group, one of four bases

C. Ribose sugar, potassium group, one of four bases

D. Ribose sugar, phosphate group, one of four bases

3. Most common blood group antigens are formed as a result of: (Objective # 3)

A. Genetic mutations

B. Recombinations

C. Crossovers

D. Single-nucleotide substitutions

4. Select the characteristics that differentiate RNA from DNA: (Objective #6)

A. RNA is single-stranded.

B. RNA contains a thymine base.

C. RNA contains a ribose sugar.

D. RNA is transcribed to mRNA.

5. Which of the following blood group phenotypes result in a homozygous expression of the Jk^b antigen? (Objective #9)

A. Jk(a + b−)

B. Jk(a − b+)

C. Jk(a + b+)

D. Jk(a − b−)

6. The synthesis of a carbohydrate blood group antigen occurs as a result of: (Objective #8)

A. A mutated protein that attaches a carbohydrate group to the red blood cell membrane.

B. A direct expression of the gene on the red blood cell surface.

C. An enzymatic reaction that causes a carbohydrate molecule to attach to the red blood cell membrane.

D. Attachment of a red blood cell membrane associated protein.

7. The most common inheritance pattern for blood group antigens is: (Objective #7)

A. Autosomal dominant

B. Autosomal recessive

C. Autosomal co-dominant

D. Sex-linked

8. A maternal ABO blood group genotype is determined to be AA and the paternal genotype is BO. What percentage of their offspring is expected to be blood type A? (Objective #11)

A. 25%

B. 50%

C. 75%

D. 100%

9. An antibody to a high-incidence antigen is identified in a patient. Which of the following donors could best serve as a source of compatible blood? (Objective #13)

A. Sibling

B. Community donor

C. Friend

D. None of the above

10. The advantages of using polymerase chain reaction (PCR) technology for DNA amplification include: (Objective #14)

A. Small sample size requirement

B. High sensitivity

C. High specificity

D. Enzymatic recognition of DNA sequence

References

1. Mendel G. Versuche über Plflanzhybriden. Verhandlungen des naturforschenden Vereines in Brünn, Bd. IV für das Jahr 1965, Abhandlungen, 3–47. English translation: Blumberg RB (ed) [Internet]. MendelWeb; [cited 2010 Mar 12]. Available from: http://www.mendelweb.org/Mendel.html

2. Watson JD, Crick FHC. Molecular structure of nucleic acids. *Nature* 1953; 171(4356): 737–8.

3. Roback JD, Combs MR, Grossman BJ, Hillyer CD (eds). *Technical manual, 16th ed.* Bethesda (MD): AABB Press; 2008.

4. Reid ME, Lomas-Francis C. *The blood group antigen facts book,* 2nd ed. San Diego (CA): Elsevier Academic Press; 2004.

5. Blaney KD, Howard PR. *Basic and applied concepts of immunohematology.* Philadelphia (PA): Mosby Elsevier; 2000.

6. International human genome sequencing consortium. Finishing the euchromatic sequence of the human genome. *Nature* 2004; 431(7011): 931–45.

7. Mullis KB, Faloona FA. Specific synthesis of DNA in vitro via a polymerase-catalyzed chain reaction. *Methods Enzymol* 1987; 155: 335–50.

8. O'Brien SF, Ye QL, Fan W, Scalia V, Kleinman SH, Vamvakas EC. Current incidence and estimated residual risk of transfusion-transmitted infections in donations made to Canadian Blood Services. *Transfusion* 2007; 47(10): 316–25.

9. Chiavetta JA, Escobar M, Newman A, He Y, Driezen P, Deeks S, Hone D, O'Brien S, Sher G. Incidence and estimated rates of residual risk for HIV, hepatitis C, hepatitis B and human T-cell lymphotopic viruses in blood donors in Canada, 1990–2000. *CMAJ* 2003; 169(8): 767–73.

10. Karpasitou K, Drago F, Crespiatico L, Paccapelo C, Truglio F, Frison S, Scalamogna M, Poli F. Blood group genotyping for Jk^a/Jk^b, Fy^a/Fy^b, S/s, K/k, Kp^a/Kp^b, Js^a/Js^b, Co^a/Co^b, and Lu^a/Lu^b with microarray beads. *Transfusion* 2008; 48(3): 505–12.

11. Hasmi G, Shariff T, Seul M, Vissavajjhala P, Hue-Roye K, Charles-Pierre D, Lomas-Francis C, Chaudhuri A, Reid ME. A flexible array format for large-scale, rapid blood group DNA typing. *Transfusion* 2005; 45(8): 680–8.

12. Gill P, Jeffreys AJ, Werrett DJ. Forensic application of DNA "fingerprints." *Nature* 1985; 18(6046): 577–9.

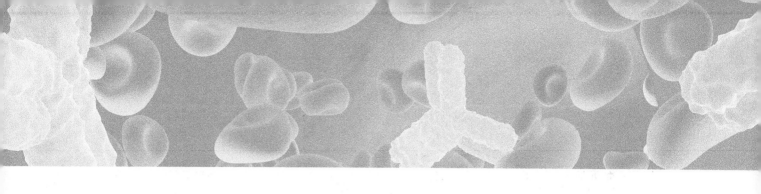

3 Blood Bank Applications of Antigen–Antibody Reactions

BRENDA COLLEEN BARNES

Chapter Objectives

Upon completion of this chapter, the student will be able to:

1. Summarize each of the key historical events that contributed to the development and understanding of the antihuman globulin (AHG) technique.
2. Summarize the purpose and theory of the antiglobulin technique.
3. Review the functions, characteristics, and structure of immunoglobulins.
4. Compare and contrast the two classes of immunoglobulins that are associated with blood bank testing: IgM and IgG.
5. Summarize the principle, purpose, and associated theory behind each of the following tests that utilize the AHG technique:
   a. Direct antiglobulin test (DAT)
   b. Indirect antiglobulin test (IAT)
6. Examine DAT and IAT test results and:
   a. Interpret the results
   b. Correlate the results with disease states
7. Compare and contrast DAT and IAT testing.
8. Compare and contrast the reagents used in the AHG technique.
9. Summarize the factors that affect the AHG technique.
10. Identify and explain the sources of error that can cause false-negative results when performing an AHG technique.
11. Identify and explain the sources of error that can cause false-positive results when performing an AHG technique.
12. Describe the mode of action for each of the following types of enhancement media used in the IAT:
    a. Low ionic strength solution (LISS)
    b. Albumin
    c. Polyethylene glycol (PEG)
13. State the name of the traditional method of detecting antigen–antibody reactions.

(continued)

Chapter Objectives (continued)

14. Identify and describe the three phases associated with tube testing.
15. State and briefly describe the alternative methods of detecting antigen–antibody reactions covered in this chapter.

Key Terms

Allotype(s)
Antihuman globulin (AHG) technique
Check cells
Direct antiglobulin test (DAT)

Indirect antiglobulin test (IAT)
Monospecific AHG
Polyspecific AHG
Valency

 ## CASE IN POINT

BW is a 54-year-old male in good health who is seeing his physician for a routine physical examination. His physician noted a slightly enlarged spleen and decided to order some laboratory tests to determine the cause of the splenomegaly. The patient's significant laboratory results are as follows:

Test	Patient Value	Normal Range
Hemoglobin	11.9 g/dL (119 g/L)	13.5–17.5 g/dL (135–175 g/L)
Platelet Count	$580 \times 10^3/\mu L$ ($580 \times 10^9/L$)	$150–450 \times 10^3/\mu L$ ($150–450 \times 10^9/L$)
Reticulocyte	3.6% (0.036)	0.6–1.9% (0.006–0.019)
LD	252 U/L	<194 U/L
Bilirubin, Total	1.5 mg/dL (26 μmol/L)	0.2–1.2 mg/dL (3–21 μmol/L)
Bilirubin, Direct	0.1 mg/dL (2 μmol/L)	0.1–0.4 mg/dL (2–7 μmol/L)
Haptoglobin	<30.0 mg/dL (<3.00 μmol/L)	44–215 mg/dL (4.4–21.50 μmol/L)
Occult Blood, Stool	Negative	Negative

The physician suspects the patient has hemolytic anemia and refers him to a hematologist for follow-up.

What's Ahead?

For all practical purposes, every blood bank test performed in a typical clinical laboratory is designed to detect targeted antigen–antibody reactions. With minimal exception, such tests incorporate the use of a multistep technique using *antihuman globulin* (abbreviated as AHG, which consists of a commercially produced antibody targeted against immunoglobulin, complement, or both that is harvested from rabbits or other appropriate animals). This technique is used for numerous purposes including but not limited to detect and identify unexpected antibodies (Chapter 8) and to predict the success of transfusion prior to administration (typically referred to as *compatibility testing* or *crossmatch testing*, as described in Chapter 7).

It is important to note here that oftentimes in blood bank literature the terms *technique* and *tests* are intertwined as they relate to AHG. In an attempt to clarify confusion, this chapter refers to AHG in a global sense as a technique (except where noted) and the specific procedures that are followed to detect antigen–antibody reactions as tests. General descriptions of these specific procedures are woven into this chapter and are not designed to be step-by-step guides. Readers interested in further exploration of these procedures for specific steps are encouraged to seek assistance from other sources including but not limited to actual blood bank laboratory procedure manuals.

The purpose of this chapter is to provide the reader with some historical perspective and review of immunoglobulin followed by a detailed examination of the antihuman globulin (AHG) technique and associated topics by answering the following questions:

- What historical events led to the development and understanding of the AHG technique?
- What is the theory behind the antihuman globulin (AHG) technique?
- What are the differences between the various AHG reagents and when is each utilized in testing?
- What is the difference between indirect antiglobulin testing (IAT) and direct antiglobulin testing (DAT)?
- What is the purpose of the antibody screen test?
- What are the three phases of IAT testing and what is the purpose of each phase?
- What is the importance of using enhancement reagents in IAT testing?
- What is the purpose of check cells in the AHG technique?
- What factors affect the AHG phase of the antibody screen test?
- What are some alternative methods, other than traditional tube testing, of detecting antigen–antibody reactions?

HISTORICAL BACKGROUND

The ABO system (Chapter 4), discovered by Landsteiner in 1900, was the first blood group system, and undoubtedly the most important to be discovered. In 1927, the M, N, and P_1 antigens (Chapter 6) were discovered through the use of serum from rabbits immunized with human red blood cells. These early discovered antigens are all carbohydrate based, and were discovered because IgM is the predominant class of antibody made in response to them. IgM antibodies are able to cause agglutination at room temperature. IgG class immunoglobulins may cause sensitization but rarely produce agglutination at room temperature. Early discoveries in the world of transfusion medicine were limited to IgM antibodies until a technique to assist IgG antibodies to agglutinate red blood cells was discovered.

The **antihuman globulin (AHG) technique** was developed by Coombs, Mourant, and Race in 1945. Upon noticing that red blood cells can combine with antibodies but not produce agglutination *in vitro*, Coombs and associates used a reagent with specificity for human proteins or globulins, called antihuman globulin, to agglutinate sensitized red blood cells. The AHG test is used to detect IgG antibodies and complement proteins attached *in vitro* or *in vivo*. After the development of the AHG test, rapid advancement in the field of transfusion medicine occurred. The Kell system (Chapter 6) was discovered in 1946, just a few weeks after the introduction of the antiglobulin test.[1] The AHG test was an important part of a number of significant discoveries about blood groups, antibody-induced hemolytic anemia (Chapter 15), and hemolytic disease of the newborn and fetus (Chapter 14). The development of the AHG test rates with the discovery of the ABO blood group system was vitally important to establishing the transfusion medicine field.[2]

☑ CHECKPOINT 3-1

The detection of IgG class antibodies became possible after the development of _____, which led to rapid advancements in transfusion medicine.

IMMUNOGLOBULIN REVIEW

Immunoglobulins have two functions: to combine with antigens and to mediate various biological effects by binding to host tissues, to various cells of the immune system, to some phagocytic cells, and to the first component of the classical complement system.[3] The ability to recognize antigens is a product of the adaptive immune system. Antibodies themselves are present in plasma and tissue fluid, with some carried on the surface of B cells and some free in the blood and lymph.

Immunoglobulins (Chapter 1) are proteins composed of two heavy chains and two light chains. There are five isotypes, with IgM and IgG being the types tested for in transfusion medicine. Immunoglobulins bind with their corresponding antigens via the variable region of the protein. The constant region is responsible for binding to cells or to complement.

When the body first encounters a foreign antigen, a primary immune response is stimulated. After this initial exposure there is a period of time lasting approximately 5–7 days called the *lag phase*, where circulating antibody is not detectable. Antibody levels slowly rise, plateau, and then decline during the log phase. IgM is the first class of immunoglobulin to be produced. One of the residual effects of the primary response is the retention of memory B cells. When antigen is encountered the second time, antibody levels are detectable within 1–2 days of exposure, with higher levels of antibody produced that are sustained longer. In this situation, IgG is the primary class of antibody produced, although IgM is present at a reduced level.

IgM

IgM is the first immunoglobulin class produced in a primary immune response. The structure of the secreted form of IgM is five basic immunoglobulin molecules held together with a joining (J) chain, forming a pentamer structure (Figure 3-1 ■). This pentamer structure gives IgM a **valency** of 10, meaning the molecule has 10 potential antigen-binding sites. When the multiple binding sites on an IgM molecule react with antigen, the antibody often adopts a staple- or crab-like structure. IgM is considered a direct agglutinate, or complete antibody, because it can bind to multiple red blood cells and agglutinate them without the addition of antihuman globulin. It

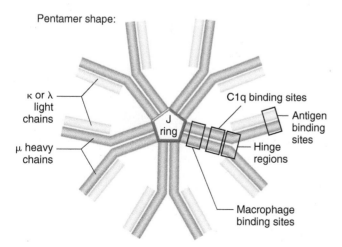

Pentamer shape:

κ or λ light chains
μ heavy chains
J ring
C1q binding sites
Antigen binding sites
Hinge regions
Macrophage binding sites

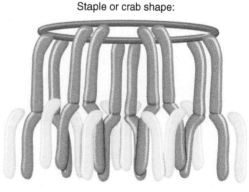

Staple or crab shape:

■ **FIGURE 3-1**   IgM Structure

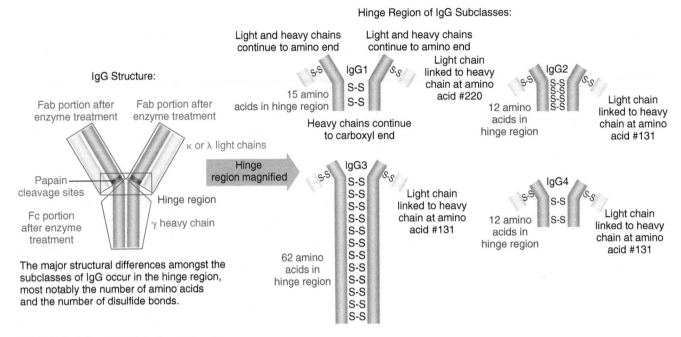

FIGURE 3-2 IgG Subclass Structure

is also very efficient at complement activation, needing only one IgM molecule to initiate the process. IgM comprises approximately 10% of the immunoglobulins in the plasma (Table 3-1 ✳).[2]

IgG

IgG is the most abundant class of immunoglobulins, comprising approximately 75% of the total plasma immunoglobulin (Table 3-1).[2] It is present in the plasma as a monomer, making it a bivalent antibody molecule, capable of binding to two antigen sites that are very close together. IgG molecules are smaller by nature than IgM and thus often not well detectable in nonenhanced testing environments (this concept is further explained later in this chapter). IgG is the predominant class of antibody produced in a secondary immune response.

There are four subclasses of IgG that differ slightly in structure (Figure 3-2 ■) and function. IgG1 and IgG3 strongly activate complement. IgG2 weakly activates complement whereas IgG4 does not activate it at all. IgG1 and IgG3 are readily recognized and bound by macrophages, initiating a series of responses. Recognition occurs less with IgG2 and probably not at all with IgG4. All four subclasses have the ability to cross the placental barrier, although IgG1 crosses best and IgG2 crosses poorly or not at all. Variants within immunoglobulin classes are known as **allotypes** and are the result of inheritance of different alleles. Immunoglobulin allotypes occur mostly as variants

✳ **TABLE 3-1** Comparison of IgM and IgG

Characteristic	IgM	IgG
Heavy chain composition	Mu (μ)	Gamma (γ)
Light chain composition	Kappa (κ) or lambda (λ)	Kappa (κ) or lambda (λ)
J chain	Yes	No
Molecular weight (daltons)	900,000	150,000
Valence	10	2
% Total serum concentration	5–10%	75–80%
Serum half-life	5–6 days	23 days *IgG3—7 days
Ability to cross placenta	No	Yes
Complement activation	Yes; very efficient	Yes; not as efficient *IgG4—No
Optimal temperature for reaction in *in vitro* tests	Room temperature or below	98.6°F (37°C)
Agglutination in immediate spin testing	Yes	No
Agglutination in antiglobulin tests	No	Yes

of heavy chain regions. For example, there is a variant of IgG3 known as G3m.[4]

ANTIGLOBULIN TECHNIQUE

The AHG technique is most often used to demonstrate *in vitro* reactions between red blood cells and corresponding IgG antibodies by using an **indirect antiglobulin test (IAT)** method. In this method, a source of antigen (that is red blood cells) is combined with a source of antibody (serum or plasma) and allowed to interact. Since this step is necessary for interactions to occur, it is referred to as an "indirect" technique. If the corresponding antibodies are present, they sensitize but do not agglutinate the red blood cells. The **direct antiglobulin test (DAT)** detects red blood cells that have been sensitized *in vivo* and therefore antibodies when present are on the red blood cell (RBC) surface. Thus, this case is considered as a direct technique. In both tests, AHG is added to the test system and forms a "bridge" when antigen–antibody complexes are present that spans the distance between coated IgG molecules and thus allows for visualization (seen as *agglutination*) that might otherwise be missed. Note that in both IAT and DAT, the "T" stands for test. These represent the two categories of the antiglobulin technique. The use of "technique" versus "test" in the subsequent sections is made based on the content and context being presented.

ANTIHUMAN GLOBULIN REAGENTS

Monospecific AHG contains either anti-IgG or anti-C3d, whereas **polyspecific AHG** contains both. AHG reagents can be made by injecting an animal with a specific human protein and then harvesting the antibody that the animal makes in response. Today, there are also clonal AHG reagents that are made by developing a cell line that will produce an antibody to a specific human protein. Table 3-2 ✱ lists some of the advantages and disadvantages of monoclonal reagents.

AHG reagents must contain anti-IgG when used for antibody detection (Chapter 8) and pretransfusion compatibility testing (Chapter 7). Anti-IgG is preferred over polyspecific AHG for antibody detection to avoid detecting clinically insignificant cold-reactive antibodies that bind complement. Anti-IgG reagents are usually directed to react with gamma heavy chains, although unless specifically labeled as "heavy-chain-specific," they may react with other immunoglobulin classes due to light chain reactivity.

Polyspecific AHG is the reagent of choice when performing DAT on adults as either IgG or complement coating the cells has clinical significance. If positive, a DAT using monospecific AHG reagents is usually performed to determine if IgG, complement, or both are present. Anticomplement reagents detect membrane-bound complement components, usually C3b and/or C3d.

CASE IN POINT *(continued)*

BW sees a hematologist who reviews his peripheral smear (differential). The hematologist notes slight polychromasia with a few spherocytes but no schistocytes. He orders another CBC, a direct antiglobulin test (DAT), and an antibody screen (IAT).

1. Diagnostically, what is the difference between the DAT and IAT tests?

INDIRECT ANTIGLOBULIN TEST

The indirect antiglobulin test (IAT) is one of the two categories of the antiglobulin technique. Although from a strictly "technical" standpoint this is a technique, in the spirit of tradition, IAT is called a test in many settings. For the purposes of this section the terms *technique* and *test* will be used as appropriate for the context. IAT consists of a two-step method to determine if antibody reacts with antigen *in vitro*, and is a very versatile test within the blood bank laboratory (Table 3-3 ✱). As previously noted, in IAT testing, a source of antigen and a source of antibody are added to the test tubes. Three phases of testing are performed. After each phase, the test tubes are examined for visualization in the form of agglutination that indicates the presence of antigen–antibody reactions. During the first step, antibody binds to red blood

✱ **TABLE 3-2** Monoclonal Reagent Advantages and Disadvantages

Advantages	Disadvantages
Unlimited production Small variation between batches	Specificity may be relative because an antigenic determinant may be shared by several antigens
No human or animal source materials No contaminating antibodies	Antibody with single specificity may not react with all antigens because antigen may not express every epitope

✱ **TABLE 3-3** Indirect Antiglobulin Test (IAT) Uses

Test	Function
Antibody screen	Detects antibodies to red blood cell antigens
Antibody identification	Identifies the specificity of red blood cell antibodies
Crossmatch	Determines serologic compatibility between donor and patient prior to transfusion
Antigen typing	Identifies a specific antigen on a patient or donor's red blood cells

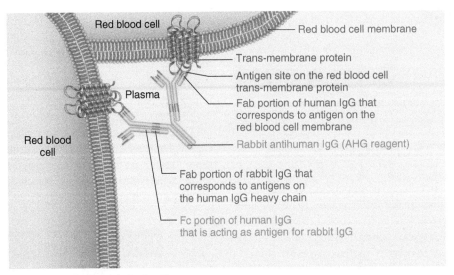

Red blood cell

Red blood cell membrane

Trans-membrane protein

Antigen site on the red blood cell trans-membrane protein

Plasma

Fab portion of human IgG that corresponds to antigen on the red blood cell membrane

Red blood cell

Rabbit antihuman IgG (AHG reagent)

Fab portion of rabbit IgG that corresponds to antigens on the human IgG heavy chain

Fc portion of human IgG that is acting as antigen for rabbit IgG

FIGURE 3-3   Positive Indirect Antiglobulin Test

cell antigens during incubation, in other words, sensitization occurs. In the second step AHG attaches to the IgG coating the red blood cells, causing a lattice to form, making agglutination visible (Figure 3-3 ■). Please note that there are specific tests that incorporate the indirect antiglobulin technique. Among such tests is the antibody screen test, which serves as an appropriate representative test to describe antihuman globulin test phases, as noted next.

ANTIBODY SCREEN TEST

The antibody screen test is performed to determine if a patient has unexpected antibodies in his or her plasma and utilizes the indirect antiglobulin technique. Commercial red blood cells with known antigenic determinants (which are determined by the manufacturer) provide the known source of antigen and patient plasma provides the unknown antibody, if present. Tube testing is the traditional method for performing an antibody screen test and the subsequent test details are based on this methodology. This test usually involves three phases and a step designed to ensure that the AHG phase worked properly, each of which is described in the following sections.

Immediate Spin Phase

After commercial red blood cells and patient plasma (or serum depending on the testing facility protocol) are combined following the test procedure, the test tubes are then centrifuged, forcing antigens and antibodies to come into contact with each other if they are present. At the completion of the centrifugation phase, a button of red blood cells forms at the bottom of each tube. The laboratorian gently dislodges the red blood cell button and examines it for agglutination (also referred to as clumping) and/or hemolysis. Any agglutination seen is graded (Table 3-4 ✳). This phase of testing is known as immediate spin (IS; conducted at room temperature) because no additional reagents or incubation phases are used. The primary purpose of this phase of testing is to detect antibodies that react at room temperature, typically antibodies of the IgM class.

It is important to note that determination of an individual's blood type is made via immediate spin (room temperature) testing (blood type testing is covered in later chapters of this text). In some settings, it is presumed that most room temperature reactive antibodies are not clinically significant and thus this phase of testing may not be performed. If, however, there are problems in determining a person's blood type and an IgM unexpected antibody is suspected, IS phase testing may be included in an effort to identify the IgM antibody and subsequently help resolve the discrepancy. IS phase testing may also be included in compatibility/crossmatch testing between patient plasma and donor red blood cells and is designed to detect ABO incompatibility. This testing is known as an IS crossmatch (Chapter 7).

Incubation Phase

Once the immediate spin phase of testing is completed, an appropriate enhancement reagent (common enhancement reagents are described in detail later in this chapter) is typically added to the test tubes. After thorough mixing, the tubes are incubated at 98.6° F (37° C) for a designated amount of time, usually 10–30 minutes depending on the enhancement reagent used. After incubation, the test tubes are centrifuged and examined for agglutination. The purpose of this phase of testing is to create an enhanced environment for antigen–IgG antibody reactions to occur. These reactions may appear weak to strong in terms of visual agglutination. Oftentimes weak reactions at this phase of testing are enhanced further after the next phase of testing AHG and become even stronger. It is interesting to note that typically IgM antibodies that were present at the IS phase of testing often disappear because the testing environment is too warm for their survival.

Antihuman Globulin (AHG) Phase

The purpose of the AHG test phase is to provide further enhancement to the test environment necessary for the visualization of antigen–antibody reactions. Prior to adding AHG reagent to the test tubes, the red blood cells must be washed with saline. This is accomplished by resuspending the red blood cell button, adding saline in a forcible stream from a wash bottle to each test tube until it is $2/3$ to $3/4$ full. The tubes are then centrifuged. During centrifugation, the cells will be forced to the bottom of the tube and form a button. After centrifugation, the supernatant is removed. This process is repeated three

✱ **TABLE 3-4** Grading of Agglutination

	Description	
Grade	Tube Test	Gel Test
4+	Single clump of cells, clear background	Single layer of cells at the top of the gel column, no cells trailing down into the column
3+	Large clump of cells plus some small clumps, clear background	Majority of cells trapped at the top of the gel column with some cells or agglutinates trailing down through the top half of the column
2+	Medium and small clumps of cells, background may be cloudy	Cells and agglutinates distributed through the column
1+	Small clumps of cells, cloudy background	Small agglutinates mostly in the bottom half of the gel column, may be a cell pellet at the bottom.
W	Cell clumps seen under the microscope but not macroscopically	Most cells at the bottom of the gel column with a few trailing up into the column
H	Hemolysis: Cherry red color before cell button is disturbed and cell button is smaller or may have disappeared entirely	No cells in the gel layer; hazy red background to the gel
MF	Two cell populations: easiest to see in a 4+MF reaction, where there is a large single clump of cells against a background of free cells	Layer of agglutinated cells at or near the top of the gel column and a pellet of cells at the bottom
Neg	No agglutination; free flowing cells	Pellet of cells at the bottom of the gel column

to four times. After the last wash, all remaining saline is removed from the cells, resulting in what blood bankers often refer to as a "dry button." The washing process may be performed manually or by automated cell washers. Once the washing step is complete, AHG reagent is added to the dry button. The tubes are then mixed, centrifuged, and examined for agglutination. AHG provides a "bridge" that spans the distance between the small coated IgG red blood cells when present and thus connects these cells allowing for visualization in the form of agglutination to occur.

☑ CHECKPOINT 3-3

In the antibody screen test, which phase of testing detects mainly IgM antibodies?

A. Immediate spin (IS) phase
B. Incubation phase
C. Antihuman globulin (AHG) phase
D. All of the above

Check Cells

Check cells (also known as *Coombs control cells*, named after the AHG technique developer of the same name) are IgG-sensitized or complement-coated red blood cells. IgG sensitized cells are prepared by coating D positive cells with human anti-D (Chapter 5). In tube testing, the appropriate check cells must be added to all of the tubes that did not exhibit agglutination. The tubes are then centrifuged, and the cell button is resuspended and examined for agglutination. Agglutination must be present at this time or the negative AHG test result is invalid and the test must be repeated.

If an AHG test is negative, free or unbound AHG should be available in the test tube. This free AHG should cause agglutination of the check cells (Figure 3-4 ■). Agglutination after the addition of

check cells verifies that adequate washing was performed, AHG was added, and the AHG reagent was working properly. Complement-coated red blood cells are used as controls for AHG antisera directed against complement components (Box 3-1).

The most common cause for the check cells not reacting is improper washing. Inadequate washing allows unbound antibody or complement to remain in the test tube, which can then bind to (and neutralize) the AHG reagent, making it unavailable to cause agglutination with sensitized check cells. One important point to remember is while the use of check cells detects some errors in the

BOX 3-1   Check Cells: Description, Action, and Interpretation of Negative Results

Description:
- Red cells coated with human IgG or complement
- Added to all negative reactions in tube-based AHG testing

Action:
- Validates the test because free AHG binds with IgG or complement on the check cells
- Causes agglutination or a positive reaction after centrifugation
- If check cells are negative, the test must be repeated

If negative results obtained (i.e., no agglutination is seen after addition of check cells):
- AHG was not added
- Inactive AHG reagent
- AHG reagent was neutralized, usually due to inadequate washing

Valid Negative
Indirect Antiglobulin Test

1. Plasma and cells incubated

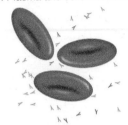

Antibody does not attach to red blood cells because corresponding antigen is not present.

2. Wash cell suspension.
3. Add anti-IgG reagent.
4. Centrifuge.

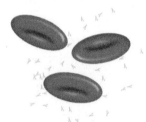

No agglutination.

5. Add check cells.
6. Centrifuge.

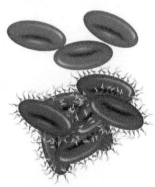

Anti-IgG binds to check cells, which are Rh(D) positive cells sensitized with anti-D. Check cells are agglutinated and antigen negative cells are not resulting in a 2+ grade positive reaction.

7. Report as negative.

False Negative
Indirect Antiglobulin Test

1. Plasma and cells incubated

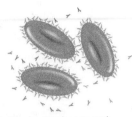

Antibody attaches to red blood cells because corresponding antigen is on the membrane

2. Wash cell suspension.
3. Add anti-IgG reagent.
4. Centrifuge.

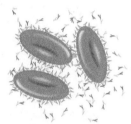

Wash was not successful. No agglutination because anti-IgG binds to free antibody instead of antibody sensitizing red blood cells.

5. Add check cells.
6. Centrifuge.

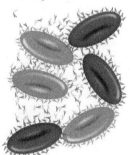

Anti-IgG cannot bind with check cells because it is already bound to free antibody. No agglutination is seen indicating an invalid result.

7. Repeat test from the beginning.

Positive
Indirect Antiglobulin Test

1. Antibody binds to antigen on the red blood cell membrane.
2. Excess antibody washed away.
3. Anti-IgG reagent is added.
4. Centrifugation brings sensitized red blood cells close enough together for lattice formation to occur.
5. Agglutination is seen when the indirect antiglobulin test is read.
6. Check cell addition is not required.
7. Report as positive.

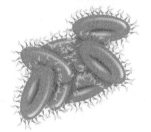

■ **FIGURE 3-4**   Check Cell Reactions

system, their use does not detect all potential failures of the AHG test. A false-negative AHG test with a positive check cell reaction can occur if plasma is not added at the beginning of the procedure, if the centrifuge is not working properly, or if the wrong concentration of test red blood cells was used.

☑ CHECKPOINT 3-4

What are check cells (Coombs control cells), and how are they prepared?

Enhancement Reagents

Enhancement reagents are added to an antibody test system to increase the rate and sensitivity of antibody attachment to red blood cell antigens and thereby reduce the incubation period. Enhancement reagents can affect either the first or second stage of agglutination. There is no one perfect method for antibody detection and identification testing, but knowledge of how different enhancement reagents work allows selection of the best method for each individual antibody case. The most common types of enhancement reagents are described next.

Albumin

Bovine serum albumin (BSA) is typically added before the incubation phase of the AHG technique. It works by influencing the second stage of agglutination or lattice formation by reducing the zeta potential. This disperses the charges in the test system and allows red blood cells to approach each other closer, increasing the chances of agglutination. The exact effect of BSA is not clearly understood, but it may affect the degree of water hydration of the RBC membrane itself. BSA works well in enhancing Rh system antibodies, but is not sensitive enough to dependably detect antibodies to other blood group systems. BSA was the first enhancement reagent used in transfusion medicine but is not in routine use today due to its long incubation period and its decreased sensitivity compared to other enhancements.

Low Ionic Strength Solution

Low ionic strength solution (LISS) reduces the ionic strength of the test system. Decreasing the ionic strength lowers the zeta potential, which helps to increase the rate of antibody uptake during the sensitization phase. Like BSA, LISS is typically added to the test system prior to the incubation phase. LISS is economical and offers good test system sensitivity, but may also enhance cold autoantibodies. It is important to follow the manufacturer's instructions when using any reagent. For example, using increased amounts of plasma to enhance weakly reactive antibodies is not recommended with LISS because altering the plasma to cell ratio changes the ionic strength of the test system, thus decreasing sensitivity. It has also been reported that some weakly reactive examples of anti-K may be missed in LISS testing systems.[5]

Polyethylene Glycol

Polyethylene glycol (PEG) is a linear polymer that works by removing water from the test system, concentrating any antibodies present and allowing a greater chance for antigen–antibody collisions. Decreased water in the environment also works to accelerate antibody uptake. PEG offers increased sensitivity for clinically significant antibodies over LISS and BSA, while diminishing the enhancement of IgM, cold-reactive antibodies. PEG can cause nonspecific aggregation of red blood cells and because of this the incubation phase is not performed. PEG can enhance warm autoantibodies, which may complicate detection of alloantibodies. PEG may not be appropriate for use in patients with elevated protein levels as protein precipitation can occur, causing false-negative reaction when antibody is present on the RBCs. Increasing the number of washes following incubation prior to the addition of AHG reagent may prevent this problem.

☑ CHECKPOINT 3-5

Which enhancement reagent increases antigen–antibody binding by removing water from the test system?

FACTORS AFFECTING THE AHG PHASE OF THE ANTIBODY SCREEN

The number of IgG molecules that will sensitize a red blood cell and the rate at which sensitization occurs *in vitro* can be influenced by several factors including temperature, ionic strength, plasma-to-cell ratio, incubation time, and pH.

Temperature

Antibody screens must include an incubation phase.[6] The optimal reaction temperature for IgG antibodies is 98.6° F (37° C). The immediate spin (IS) phase, which occurs at room temperature (RT), is often omitted to limit detection of insignificant cold antibodies, which are frequently IgM.

Ionic Strength

A decrease in the ionic strength enhances antibody uptake on the red blood cells. The use of enhancement reagents, such as LISS or PEG, helps to decrease the ionic strength of the test system. Normally, sodium and chloride ions cluster around and partially neutralize opposite charges on antigens and antibodies, causing a shielding effect which can hinder antigen–antibody interactions. If the ionic strength of the test system is decreased, the length of incubation time can be decreased because the shielding effect is minimized and antigen and antibody can interact at a faster rate.

Plasma-to-Cell Ratio

For tube testing, the most commonly used ratio is two drops of plasma and one drop of 5% suspension of red blood cells. If an antibody appears to be weakly reactive, the amount of plasma can be increased to add more antibody and increase the sensitivity of the test system. If there is a limited amount of specimen available, reducing the concentration of cells from 5% to 2–3% also doubles the plasma-to-cell ratio without using additional plasma. Caution must be taken when increasing the plasma to cell ratio of the test system because doing so affects the ionic strength. Therefore, if LISS is used, the procedure must be modified to maintain the appropriate plasma-to-LISS ratio.[5]

Incubation Time

If antigen and antibody are allowed limited contact time in the test system, it is likely that not enough cells will become sensitized, leading to a false-negative test result. In contrast, if the test system is allowed to incubate too long, bound antibody may dissociate, also decreasing the strength of the reaction. The incubation time of a test system is influenced by the nature of the reagent being used. Saline, which refers to an antibody screen using no enhancement reagent, or albumin test systems generally require incubation of 30–60 minutes. If PEG or LISS are used, incubation time is decreased considerably and can cause problems if the incubation is extended past the manufacturers' recommended length of time. The manufacturer's instructions must be followed for all reagents.

pH

The saline used for washing should be fresh or should be buffered at a pH of around 7.0. Decreased pH caused by long-term storage in plastic containers may increase antibody elution during the washing process. Some monoclonal antibodies have very narrow pH ranges for optimal reactivity, which can be crucial when using monoclonal AHG. Acidifying the test system may enhance the detection of some examples of anti-M, as detailed in Chapter 6.[5]

☑ CHECKPOINT 3-6

List five factors that affect the AHG phase of the antibody screening test.

The laboratorian is about to start testing BW's DAT with polyspecific AHG reagent. As stated earlier, the blood bank has a clot tube and hematology has an EDTA anticoagulated tube on the patient.

2. Which specimen should be used for testing and why?
3. The tube tested with polyspecific AHG looks like this. How should these results be interpreted?

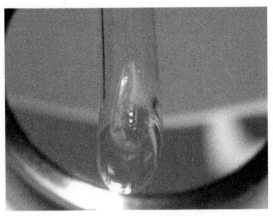

Source: Stephanie Codina.

4. What is coating BW's cells?
5. What should be done next?

DIRECT ANTIGLOBULIN TEST

The direct antiglobulin test (DAT) differs from IAT (Table 3-5 ✳) because it detects red blood cells sensitized with antibody or complement *in vivo*. In this case, DAT is both a technique and the name of the associated test and thus the terms may be used interchangeably at times. In traditional tube testing only the AHG phase of testing, complete with the addition of check cells when appropriate, is performed. IS and the incubation phases are not performed because this test does not involve adding sources of antigen and antibody to each other and allowing reactions to take place if present. In the DAT, if there is a reaction, it has already taken place. Thus a DAT is performed for the purpose of visualization (via agglutination) of antigen–antibody reactions when present.

✳ **TABLE 3-5** Comparison of IAT and DAT

IAT		DAT	
Detect *in vitro* sensitization of red blood cells with antibody		Detect *in vivo* sensitization of red blood cells with antibody, complement, or both	
Procedure Step	**Purpose**	**Procedure Step**	**Purpose**
Antibody and red blood cell incubated	Allow attachment of antibody to corresponding red blood cell antigen	Red blood cells washed	Removes any unbound antibody
Red blood cells washed	Removes any unbound antibody	AHG, usually combination of anti-IgG and anti-C3d, added, followed by centrifugation	Anti-IgG and/or anti-C3d bind to any antibody or complement that is attached to the red blood cell, causing agglutination
AHG, usually anti-IgG, added, followed by centrifugation	Anti-IgG binds to any antibody that is bound to the red blood cell, causing agglutination		

✳ **TABLE 3-6** Direct Antiglobulin Test (DAT) Uses

DAT Used to Help Diagnose	
Disease	DAT Detects
Autoimmune hemolytic anemia (AIHA)	Patient autoantibody
Hemolytic disease of the newborn and fetus (HDNF)	Maternal antibody
Drug-related hemolytic anemia	Drug/antidrug complex
Hemolytic transfusion reaction	Recipient antibody

✳ **TABLE 3-7** Causes of False AHG Test Results

Affecting Both IAT and DAT	
False Negative	False Positive
Inadequate washing	Dirty glassware
Interruption in testing	Contaminated saline or AHG
Deteriorated or neutralized AHG or AHG not added	Cells agglutinating prior to AHG addition
Improper concentration of RBC	Improper reading technique
Improper centrifugation	Improper centrifugation
Affecting IAT	
Plasma not added	Preservative-dependent antibody in LISS reagent
Inadequate incubation	Cells with positive DAT
Affecting DAT	
Deterioration of complement	Clotted or refrigerated specimen

The DAT is not usually included in routine pretransfusion testing today, but it is an important test in the diagnosis of certain clinical conditions (Table 3-6 ✳). A positive DAT may indicate potential immune-mediated red blood cell destruction. If IgG attaches to patient red cells *in vivo*, Fc receptors on macrophages and other cells can bind to antibody-coated cells and clear them from circulation through the reticuloendothelial (RES) system.

The complement cascade may be activated but not progress all the way to the membrane attack complex (Chapter 1), which results in red blood cells coated with complement, most notably C3b and C3d. Like IgG-coated cells, C3b-coated cells can be cleared from the circulation because phagocytic cells have receptors for C3b. The significance of bound IgG and/or complement should be assessed in relation to the patient's medical history and clinical condition.

The preferred sample for DAT testing is an EDTA (ethylenediaminetetraacetic acid) tube. Complement can attach nonspecifically to red blood cells when serum samples are stored, but EDTA negates the *in vitro* activation of the complement pathway. When using an EDTA sample, any complement components detected on red blood cells will have been bound *in vivo*, making their significance clear.

Although each blood bank has its own protocol regarding initial and follow-up direct antiglobulin testing, it is common practice to perform the initial DAT test using polyspecific AHG reagent. If agglutination occurs with the polyspecific reagent, the test is interpreted as "positive." At this juncture, the patient's cells are tested with monoclonal reagents anti-IgG and anti-C3d to determine the cause of initial agglutination. A positive anti-IgG result requires additional work-up, among which includes identification of the causative IgG antibody (Chapter 8).

☑ CHECKPOINT 3-7

What type of AHG reagent should be used to perform the initial DAT on a patient specimen?

SOURCES OF ERROR

Both false-positive and false-negative reactions may occur in AHG testing, in either the IAT or DAT (Table 3-7 ✳).

False-Negative Reactions

A false-negative reaction is a test result where no agglutination is observed when it should have been observed. In tube testing, the most common cause for a false-negative reaction is the failure to wash red blood cells adequately. Unbound globulins, if not washed away, may neutralize the AHG reagent when added, resulting in a negative reaction even if the red blood cells are sensitized.

If AHG is not added immediately after washing, the antibody may elute off the red blood cell. This may result in either too little IgG on cells to be detected or neutralization of the AHG by antibody that has eluted from the cells. Also, agglutination weakens with time, which may cause a very weakly reactive antibody to be overlooked.

Loss of AHG reagent reactivity may occur due to bacterial contamination or improper storage. AHG reagent can also be neutralized if the dropper becomes contaminated or the wrong dropper is placed into a bottle of AHG reagent.

Proper centrifugation is a critical step in both IAT and DAT tests by tube or gel. Undercentrifugation provides suboptimal conditions for agglutination. Overcentrifugation of a tube test packs red blood cells so tightly that when reading, the excessive agitation required may break up fragile agglutinates, causing a weak reaction to be missed. In gel testing, centrifugation is the pivotal step in visualizing the reaction as this is when the free or agglutinated cells move into the gel matrix.

The concentration of red cells used is also important. Manufacturer's instructions should always be followed, as the appropriate concentration may vary. For example, antibody detection tests using the gel system require a red blood cell concentration of 0.8%, whereas most tube-based systems require a red blood cell concentration of 2–5%. If too many cells are in the system, the number of antibodies attached to any one red blood cell is decreased and agglutination may not occur. If too few cells are sensitized, it can be difficult to observe agglutination and a weak reaction may be overlooked. Antibody concentration is also important. Collection of samples from infusion lines should be avoided if possible, as dilution with the infusing solution may reduce any antibody present to a nondetectable level.

False-Positive Reactions

A false-positive reaction is a test result in which agglutination is observed when it should not have been.

Samples collected in EDTA, acid–citrate–dextrose (ACD), or citrate–phosphate–dextrose (CPD) are preferred for DAT testing. Using a refrigerated or clotted specimen may detect *in vitro* complement attachment. Complement components, primarily C4, may bind to cells from clotted serum patient samples or CPDA-1 donor segments during storage at 39.2° F (4° C). Occasionally samples stored at higher temperatures may be affected. The use of tubes containing silicone gel can cause complement to attach to red blood cells. Dextrose-containing solutions can also cause complement attachment, therefore specimens should not be collected from infusion lines.

A cold reactive autoantibody may cause cells to agglutinate spontaneously. The agglutination may be falsely attributed to AHG attachment. Cells should be observed before the addition of AHG; agglutination present in the tube before the addition of AHG reagent invalidates the test.

Particles or contaminates in glassware may cause clumping of red blood cells, which may be interpreted as agglutination. Fibrin or precipitates may produce cell clumps, which can be mistaken for agglutination. In tube testing, red blood cells packed too tightly due to overcentrifugation may be mistaken for agglutination and interpreted as positive.

Cells that are DAT positive (*in vivo* sensitization) will cause a positive result in any IAT test. In antigen typing tests that use an IAT phase, any *in vivo*–bound IgG must be removed from the red blood cells prior to testing. Reagents used to remove IgG from red blood cells include chloroquine and EDTA-glycine. Care must be taken to choose the right reagent for the test being performed, as these reagents may also destroy certain red blood cell antigens (Chapter 8).

☑ CHECKPOINT 3-8

In the antiglobulin technique, why must the AHG reagent be added immediately after washing the red blood cells?

CASE IN POINT (continued)

The laboratory received two specimens drawn from BW. The first specimen was collected in an EDTA anticoagulated tube and is sent to hematology for CBC testing. The second specimen was drawn in a clot tube (no anticoagulant) and is sent to the blood bank for DAT and IAT testing. The laboratorian (a.k.a. blood bank tech) sets up his antibody screen using the gel method. She pipettes reagent red blood cells (screening cells) and patient serum in the gel microtubes, then places the gel cards in the heat block to incubate for 15 minutes per laboratory procedure. Unfortunately, the blood bank tech gets extremely busy tending to a bleeding patient and no one is able to pull BW's gel cards out of the heating block when the timer sounds. When the workload finally slows down, the tech returns to her bench. BW's gel cards are still in the heat block, but the tech does not know how long they have been there.

6. The tech decides that the increased incubation time will improve sensitization and proceeds with testing. Did she make the correct choice? Why or why not?
7. The antibody screen results are as follows. How would this test be interpreted?

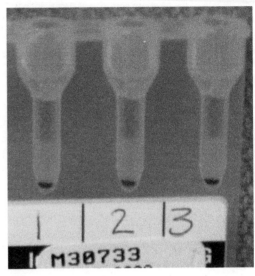

Source: Stephanie Codina.

ALTERNATIVE METHODS OF DETECTING ANTIGEN–ANTIBODY REACTIONS

Alternative methods to traditional tube testing have been developed for detection of antigen–antibody interactions. Many of these methods can be automated.

Gel

The gel technique is an alternative method offering sensitivity equivalent to the polyethylene glycol test tube method. Testing is performed in a microtubule filled with dextran acrylamide gel (Figure 3-5 ■). The principle of the gel technique is molecular sieving. In antibody detection and identification testing, patient plasma and reagent red blood cells suspended in LISS are added to the reaction chambers of the gel card (six reaction chambers per gel card), which is then incubated at 98.6° F (37° C). Sensitization of the cells should occur if antibody is present. The gel card is then

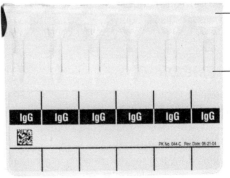

Reaction chamber
Add reactants—plasma/serum and/or red blood cells

Gel and reagent
After centrifugation step—agglutinates or free cells will be trapped in different layers depending on size

■ FIGURE 3-5 Gel Card

Source: Lisa Denesiuk and Peter Verboom.

Positive reaction:

Negative reaction:

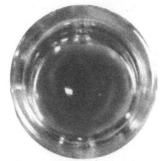

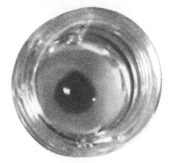

Diffuse coating of red blood cells
in the microtiter plate well.

Red blood cell pellet
in the microtiter plate well.

FIGURE 3-6 Positive and Negative Reaction by Solid Phase

Source: Lisa Denesiuk.

slowly centrifuged for 10 minutes. The red blood cells are forced into the gel microtubule, which contains anti-IgG. In a positive reaction, the sensitized cells will react with the anti-IgG and agglutinate; the agglutinated cells become trapped near the top or throughout the gel depending on the size of the agglutinates. Negative tests will be seen as a pellet of red blood cells at the bottom of the microtubule, since all of the nonsensitized, nonagglutinated cells will pass through the gel. Advantages of the gel technique include the elimination of both the washing phase and the addition of IgG-coated red blood cells. The reaction endpoints are stable over time and can be reviewed later if desired. Gel methodology may be used for ABO/Rh typing, other RBC phenotyping such as in the Rh system, IAT antibody screens or identification, crossmatching, and direct antiglobulin tests. This technique has been adapted for automation.

Solid Phase

In solid-phase methodology, red blood cell antigens are coated to the bottom of microtiter plate wells. In antibody detection and identification testing, patient plasma is added along with LISS. The test is incubated at 98.6° F (37° C) and any antibody, if present, will react with the antigens that coat the well. Unbound antibody is washed away,

indicator cells coated with antihuman IgG are added, the plates are centrifuged, and then they are read. In a positive reaction, the indicator cells react with patient antibody bound to the red blood cell antigens coating the microtiter well, appearing as a diffuse pattern (Figure 3-6 ■). In a negative reaction where no sensitization occurred, the indicator cells form a pellet at the bottom of the well. This methodology is best suited to antibody detection and identification and is very sensitive. Automation is also available with this technique.

Other Methodologies

Enzyme-linked immunosorbent assays (ELISA) and flow cytometry methods can be used to detect antigen–antibody interactions, as well as quantify the amount of antibody or antigen present in a sample. The use of these techniques may become more widespread as research with both of these tests continues.

☑ CHECKPOINT 3-9

Which alternative method does not require a washing phase and the addition of IgG-coated red blood cells?

Review of the Main Points

- Immunoglobulins combine with antigens and mediate various biological effects.
- Secreted IgM is a pentamer joined with a J chain.
- Secreted IgG is a monomer.
- There are four subclasses of IgG, each with slightly different structure and function.
- IgM is the predominant class of immunoglobulin produced in a primary immune response.
- IgG is the predominant class of immunoglobulin produced in a secondary immune response.
- Antihuman globulin (AHG) is antibody against human IgG and/or complement components.
- Polyspecific AHG reagent contains both anti-IgG and anti-C3b.
- Monospecific AHG reagents contain either anti-IgG or anti-complement.

- AHG reagents are produced either via cell culture, which results in a monoclonal antibody, or by injecting human IgG or complement into an animal, which results in polyclonal antibodies.
- Check cells are required to validate negative tube testing AHG results.
- Indirect antiglobulin test (IAT) is used to demonstrate *in vitro* attachment of antibody to red blood cell antigen.
- Direct antiglobulin test (DAT) is used to demonstrate *in vivo* attachment of antibody or complement to the red blood cell.
- Enhancement reagents may be used in the IAT to reduce the incubation time or to increase the test sensitivity.
- Alternatives to tube testing include gel, solid phase, ELISA, and flow cytometry.

Review Questions

1. Select the characteristics that are associated with antibodies of the IgM class: (Objective #3)

   A. Produced in the primary immune response

   B. 10 antigen-binding sites

   C. React best at room temperature

   D. Can cross the placenta

2. Which of the following methods detects *in vivo* sensitization of red blood cells with antibody? (Objective #5)

   A. Indirect antiglobulin test

   B. Direct antiglobulin test

   C. Polyspecific antihuman globulin

   D. Enzyme treatment

3. The DAT and IAT methods are similar in that they both: (Objective #7)

   A. Require the addition of check cells to confirm test validity

   B. Detect *in vitro* sensitization of red blood cells with antibody

   C. Require enhancement media for maximal binding

   D. Require the use of AHG reagent

4. In the antibody screening procedure, IgG antibody is detected at the _____ phase of testing. (Objective #5)

   A. Immediate spin

   B. AHG

   C. Coombs control

   D. Check cell

5. Upon the addition of check cells in the direct antiglobulin test, no agglutination is seen in the test tube. The test is interpreted as: (Objective #6)

   A. Positive for IgG antibody

   B. Negative for IgG antibody

   C. Valid

   D. Invalid

6. Nonspecific aggregation of red blood cells occurs at 98.6°F (37°C) with which of the following enhancement reagents? (Objective #12)

   A. LISS

   B. Albumin

   C. Ficin

   D. PEG

7. Select the factors that can affect the AHG phase of the antibody screen test: (Objective #9)

   A. Ionic strength

   B. Incubation time

   C. Use of check cells

   D. Temperature

8. The solid phase methodology for antigen–antibody interactions is based on which of the following principles? (Objective #15)

   A. Antibody binds to red blood cell antigens that are coated to the bottom of microtiter plate test wells.

   B. Antibody and antigen form visible agglutination complexes in a test tube upon centrifugation.

   C. Antigen–antibody complexes become trapped in a microtubule filled with dextran acrylamide gel.

   D. Antigen and antibody interactions in a sample are detected and quantified.

9. False-positive reactions in the indirect antiglobulin test include: (Objective #11)

   A. Failure to add test plasma

   B. Contaminated saline

   C. Excessive centrifugation

   D. Neutralized AHG reagent

10. When the body first encounters a foreign antigen, the period of time when there is no detectable antibody is referred to as: (Objective #3)

    A. Lag phase

    B. Log phase

    C. Plateau phase

    D. Decline phase

11. Choose the appropriate immunoglobulin: (Objective #4)

    1. _____ Crosses the placenta   a. IgM

    2. _____ Pentamer structure   b. IgM

    3. _____ Has two binding sites

    4. _____ Has four subclasses

    5. _____ Direct agglutinate

12. In the gel test, a negative reaction is demonstrated by: (Objective #15)

    i. A single layer of cells at the top of the gel column

    ii. Cells and agglutinates distributed through the column

    iii. No cells in the gel layer, hazy red background to the gel

    iv. Pellet of cells at the bottom of the gel column

13. A DAT is performed on a newborn cord blood specimen. A 2+ agglutination is observed upon the addition of AHG reagent. What clinical situation is most likely occurring? (Objective #6)

    A. Hemolytic transfusion reaction

    B. Hemolytic disease of the newborn

    C. Autoimmune hemolytic anemia

    D. Drug-induced anemia

14. Clinically significant antibodies are detected at which phase(s) of testing? (Objective #14)

    A. Immediate spin (IS) phase

    B. Incubation phase

    C. AHG phase

    D. Coombs control phase

15. Which anticoagulant is preferred for DAT testing? (Objective #5)

    A. Ammonium oxalate

    B. EDTA

    C. Heparin

    D. No anticoagulant

References

1. Westoff CE, Reid ME. Review: the Kell, Duffy, and Kidd blood group systems. *Immunohemtol* 2004; 20: 37–49.
2. Issitt PD, Anstee DJ. *Applied blood group serology*, 4th ed. Durham (NC): Montgomery Scientific Publications; 1998.
3. Roitt I, Brostoff J, Male D. *Immunology*, 6th ed. London: Harcourt Publishers Limited; 2001.
4. Roitt I, Brostoff J, Male D. *Immunology*, 6th ed. London: Harcourt Publishers Limited; 2001.
5. Brecher, ME, editor. *Technical manual*, 15th ed. Bethesda (MD): AABB; 2005. p. 343.
6. Silva MA, editor. *Standards for blood banks and transfusion services*, 24th ed. Bethesda, MD: *AABB*, 2006.

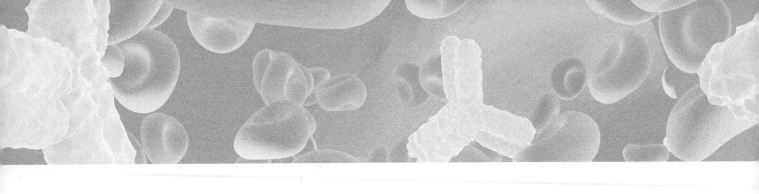

4

ABO and Hh Blood Group Systems

LISA DENESIUK

Chapter Objectives

Upon completion of this chapter, the student will be able to:

1. Identify the chromosome where the ABO and Hh blood group system genes reside.
2. Identify the biochemical structures that define the ABO and Hh blood group system antigens.
3. Describe some common genetic differences responsible for the phenotypes in the ABO and Hh blood group systems.
4. Identify the biochemical structures of the ABO and Hh blood group system antigens and explain the differences found among various cells and fluids.
5. List antigen frequencies for the four blood types in the ABO blood group system.
6. Identify phenotype given the genotype for *ABO*, *Hh*, and *Sese* genes.
7. Identify ethnic differences of ABO and Hh phenotype frequencies.
8. Describe the genetic and antigenic differences between ABO secretors and non-secretors.
9. State the genetic basis for Bombay and para-Bombay phenotypes.
10. List the common and rare subgroups in the ABO blood group system and expected serological findings.
11. Describe the theory for the serological test that can be used to identify secretors and nonsecretors.
12. Explain the genetic theories for cis-AB.
13. Describe the main characteristics of antibodies in the ABO and Hh blood group systems.
14. Describe the tests that are performed to determine an ABO blood type.
15. Identify serological and clinical findings associated with ABO testing discrepancies.
16. Propose and discuss common resolution strategies for ABO discrepancies.
17. Describe the causes of polyagglutination.
18. Describe the role that the ABO blood group system plays in transfusion, transplantation, and disease.

Key Terms

ABO discrepancy
  (discrepancies)
Absorption
Autoabsorption
Cold autoagglutinin(s)
Cryptantigen(s)
Forward group (grouping)
Hemagglutination
Immunodominant sugar(s)

Intravascular hemolysis
Lectin(s)
Naturally occurring antibody
  (antibodies)
Nonsecretor(s)
Polyagglutination
Reverse group (grouping)
Rouleaux
Secretor(s)

CASE IN POINT

GB is a 72-year-old woman who is admitted to the hospital the night before a scheduled hip replacement surgery. She is in relatively good health and has no significant medical history. She has four children; the last was born via C-section 40 years ago. The nurse orders her preoperative laboratory work per hospital protocol and the tests include a complete blood count (CBC), prothrombin time (PT)/International normalized ration (INR), and (blood) type and crossmatch (Chapter 7) for 2 units of packed red blood cells (Chapter 11). The samples are properly labeled and sent to the laboratory for testing.

What's Ahead?

The discovery of the ABO blood group system marks the start of modern transfusion medicine. Although physicians attempted to perform transfusions previously, without knowledge of the ABO system most of these patients died. The ABO blood group system is the most critical consideration in choosing the right donor units to transfuse to a patient. An ABO-incompatible transfusion can cause death.

This chapter addresses the following questions:

- What is the genetic and biochemical basis of the ABO and Hh blood group systems?
- What tests are used in determining an ABO group?
- What role does the ABO blood group system play in transfusion, transplantation, and disease?

HISTORICAL BACKGROUND

The ABO blood group system was first described by Karl Landsteiner in an article published in 1901.[1] Like many great scientific breakthroughs, his experiment was simple and elegant. He obtained blood from his coworkers and then mixed serum and cells from different individuals. He observed three different patterns of *agglutination* (cells sticking together) that he named A, B, and C. The pattern that he described as C we now call O. The AB blood group was described the next year by Decastello and Sturli.[2] Agglutination is still one of the standard detection methods that we use today in transfusion medicine.

GENETICS AND BIOCHEMISTRY

Due to the complexity of the genetics and biochemistry associated with the ABO and Hh blood group systems, this section is presented in subsections, beginning with a brief genetics review.

Brief Genetics Review

DNA constitutes the building blocks of life (Chapter 2). DNA is used as the template to make messenger ribonucleic acid (mRNA). In turn, mRNAs are used as templates by transfer RNA (tRNA) to make proteins. These proteins either make up structural components of an organism directly or cause chemical reactions that result in the additional substances necessary to form an organism. Figure 4-1 summarizes the flow of genetic information.

ABO Genetics

This section describes the important aspects associated with ABO genetics. Topics covered in this discussion include chromosomes and alleles, the amorphic gene known as O, ABO gene products, Hh genes, and ABO phenotypes.

Chromosomes and Alleles

The gene for the ABO blood group system resides on chromosome 9.[3] There are three possibilities or alleles for the gene: *A*, *B*, or *O*.

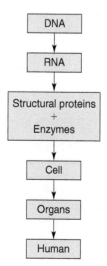

■ **FIGURE 4-1** Flow of Genetic Information

Since every person has two copies of chromosome 9, every person has two *ABO* genes—one inherited from their mother and one from their father. In total, there are six combinations of alleles possible. Table 4-1 ✱ lists the allele combinations and their corresponding phenotype. The *ABO* genes are said to be co-dominant, like most blood group system genes. This means that if the gene is present, the gene product (a protein or enzyme) is made. One gene does not suppress the other gene in a co-dominant system. A Punnett square can be used to identify the phenotype of possible offspring (Chapter 2).

Amorphic Gene

The *O* gene is an amorph, meaning no functional gene product (protein or enzyme) is produced from this sequence of DNA. Therefore, although *ABO* genes are called co-dominant, the phenotype of a person who is group A can result from one of two allelic combinations: *AA* or *AO*. Similarly, people who are genetically *BB* or *BO* will both type as group B. The co-dominant nature of the *ABO* genes is apparent when both the *A* and *B* genes are present as these people type as group AB, proving that one gene does not suppress the other gene.

ABO Gene Products

Genes code only for proteins. ABO antigens are not proteins; they are carbohydrates.[4] The *A* gene does not code for the A antigen itself but rather for an enzyme that makes the A antigen. Likewise, the *B* gene codes for the production of an enzyme that makes the B antigen. Figure 4-2 ■ illustrates the flow of genetic information in the ABO blood group system.

Hh Genes and ABO Phenotypes

The H antigen is the precursor substance or building block for both A and B antigens. However, the Hh system is separate from the ABO system and the *ABO* and *Hh* genes are inherited independently of one another. The *Hh* genes are found on chromosome 19.[5] The *H* gene is also called *FUT1* for fucosyltransferase I (the action of the enzyme produced). The H antigen, being the precursor substance to the A and B antigens, is of course another carbohydrate.

Like the *O* gene, the *h* gene is an amorph and therefore the sequence of DNA called the *h* gene does not code for a functional product. Only one copy of the *H* gene is needed to make the H antigen. If a person has two copies of the *h* gene (*hh*), neither the enzyme nor the H antigen is made. Since H antigen is necessary as the basic structure for making both the A and B antigens, without any H antigen there is no A or B antigen on the red blood cells, regardless of which ABO genes are present. The phenotypes, resulting from the

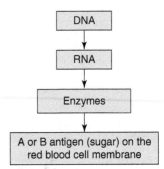

■ FIGURE 4-2   Flow of Genetic Information in the ABO Blood Group System

genotype *hh*, are called the Bombay and para-Bombay phenotypes. These phenotypes are very rare, occurring in less than 0.1% of the population worldwide. There is a slightly higher prevalence in people of Japanese or Indian heritage.[6]

☑ CHECKPOINT 4-1

Which gene in the ABO blood group system is an amorph and which gene in the Hh blood group system is an amorph?

Advanced Concepts in ABO Genetics

In 1990, Yamamoto and colleagues published the DNA sequence of the *A* gene that results in the enzyme for A antigen production.[7] In 1995, the same laboratory published the entire *A* gene sequence, which was named A101. The substitutions and deletions that make all the other *ABO* genes are described in relation to A101.

There are only seven nucleotide differences between the *A* and *B* genes. The enzyme products, coded for by the *A* and *B* genes, differ from each other by only four amino acids.[8] In fact, the amino acid identity at only two of the four positions (positions 266 and 268) appears to be responsible for the differences in the enzymes' specificities. The *O* gene has a single nucleotide deletion of guanine at position 261.[9] This frame shift mutation in the *O* gene results in a premature stop codon, which in turn produces a nonfunctional enzyme.

Biochemistry of ABO and Hh Antigens

The red blood cell membrane is a lipid bilayer, which has carbohydrates (sugars), lipids (fats including cholesterol), and proteins both running through it and attached to it. ABO antigens reside on sugar molecules that are attached to the outside of the red blood cell membrane.

Immunodominant Sugars

The difference between the A antigen and the B antigen is one sugar molecule. A sugar that makes one antigen different from another antigen is called the **immunodominant sugar**. Table 4-2 ✱ lists the immunodominant sugar for the H, A, and B antigens. The immunodominant sugars for the ABO blood group are attached at the end of the carbohydrate precursor substance, which is the H antigen.

The *H* gene codes for the enzyme α-1,2-L-fucosyltransferase, which adds L-fucose to a precursor carbohydrate chain, called

---

✱ **TABLE 4-1**   ABO Genotypes and Corresponding Phenotypes

Genotype	Phenotype
AA	A
AO	
BB	B
BO	
OO	O
AB	AB

✳ **TABLE 4-2** Immundominant Sugars of the ABO and Hh Blood Group Systems

Antigen	Immunodominant Sugar	Enzyme that Adds the Sugar
H	L-Fucose	α-1,2-L-fucosyltransferase
A	N-acetyl-D-galactosamine	α-1,3-N-acetyl-galactosaminyltransferase
B	D-galactose	α-1,3-D-galactosyltransferase

paragloboside, to form the H antigen. The enzyme coded for by the *A* gene is called α-1,3-N-acetyl-galactosaminyltransferase. This enzyme attaches an N-acetyl-D-galactosamine to the H antigen. Therefore, the immunodominant sugar of the A antigen is N-acetyl-D-galactosamine. For the B antigen, the immunodominant sugar D-galactose is attached to the H antigen by the enzyme, α-1,3-D-galactosyltransferase. Both enzymes coded for by the *A* and *B* genes can only add their sugar onto the H antigen and not on the precursor substance for the H antigen. Table 4-3 ✳ summarizes the genes, enzymes, and antigens of each phenotype.

☑ CHECKPOINT 4-2

What is the immunodominant sugar of the A antigen?

Type 1 and Type 2 Carbohydrate Chains
There are two major forms of the ABH precursor substance, called type 1 and type 2.[10] Type 1 precursor substances make up the majority of precursor substances found in the gut lining, plasma, and secretions such as urine, milk, and saliva. The A, B, and H antigens on the red blood cells and some in the saliva are made from type 2 precursor substances. The difference between the two types is the attachment or linkage of the last galactose sugar molecule on the precursor substance. ABO and Hh blood group system carbohydrate chains are composed of hexoses, which are sugar molecules with six carbon atoms. Figure 4-3 ▣ illustrates the basic composition of a hexose molecule. The linkage describes which carbon atoms are involved in binding the two sugar molecules together, in this case the last

two sugars on the precursor molecule. Type 2 precursor substances have a β 1–4 linkage, which connects carbon one on the last sugar to the third carbon on the next to the last sugar, and type 1 substances have a β 1–3 linkage. Figure 4-4 ▣ illustrates the linkage of type 1 and type 2 substances.

ABO Antigens on the Red Blood Cell Membrane
On the red blood cell, most of the carbohydrate/sugar molecules that carry the A, B, or H antigens are attached to a protein. This biochemical combination is called a glycoprotein. There are small amounts of A, B, or H antigens that occur on the red blood cell membrane in the form of a glycolipid (carbohydrate/sugar attached to a fat) or a glycosphingolipid (carbohydrate/sugar attached to a ceramide molecule).[10] Ceramide is a specific type of lipid made up of a sphingosine and a fatty acid. Figure 4-5 ▣ is a simplified view of ABO antigen attachment. ABO and H antigens are also found on the membrane of epithelial and endothelial cells.

☑ CHECKPOINT 4-3

What biochemical structure most commonly carries the ABO and Hh antigens on the red blood cell membrane?

▣ **FIGURE 4-3** Basic Hexose Molecule

✳ **TABLE 4-3** Genes, Enzymes, Antigens, and Phenotypes of the ABO and Hh Blood Group Systems

Genes Present	Enzyme(s) Made	Antigens Present on Red Blood Cell Membrane	Phenotype
H and *A*	α-1,2-L-fucosyltransferase α-1,3-N-acetyl-galactosaminyltransferase	H and A	A
H and *B*	α-1,2-L-fucosyltransferase α-1,3-D-galactosyltransferase	H and B	B
H and *O*	α-1,2-L-fucosyltransferase	H	O
H, *A*, and *B*	α-1,2-L-fucosyltransferase α-1,3-N-acetyl-galactosaminyltransferase α-1,3-D-galactosyltransferase	H, A, B	AB
hh and *A*, *B*, or *O*	Depending on ABO genes inherited, may make α-1,3-N-acetyl-galactosaminyltransferase and/or α-1,3-D-galactosyltransferase, but the enzyme has no H antigen to act upon	No H No or little ABO	Bombay or para-Bombay

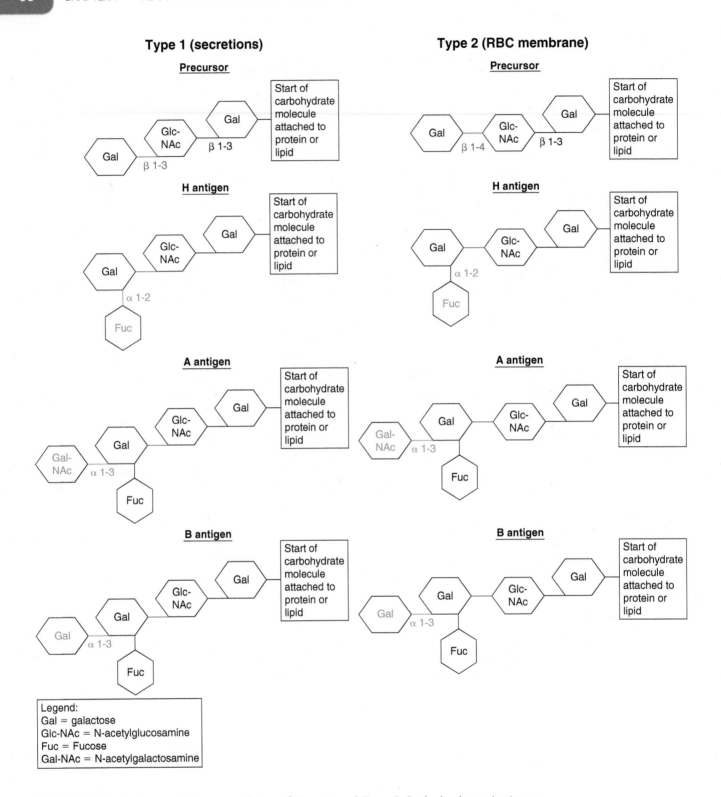

FIGURE 4-4   Schematic Representation of Type 1 and Type 2 Carbohydrate Antigens

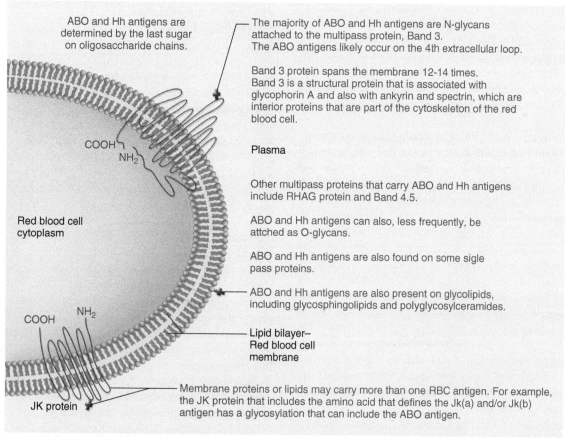

ABO and Hh antigens are determined by the last sugar on oligosaccharide chains.

The majority of ABO and Hh antigens are N-glycans attached to the multipass protein, Band 3.
The ABO antigens likely occur on the 4th extracellular loop.

Band 3 protein spans the membrane 12-14 times.
Band 3 is a structural protein that is associated with glycophorin A and also with ankyrin and spectrin, which are interior proteins that are part of the cytoskeleton of the red blood cell.

COOH
NH₂

Plasma

Other multipass proteins that carry ABO and Hh antigens include RHAG protein and Band 4.5.

ABO and Hh antigens can also, less frequently, be attached as O-glycans.

Red blood cell cytoplasm

ABO and Hh antigens are also found on some sigle pass proteins.

ABO and Hh antigens are also present on glycolipids, including glycosphingolipids and polyglycosylceramides.

COOH   NH₂

Lipid bilayer–
Red blood cell membrane

Membrane proteins or lipids may carry more than one RBC antigen. For example, the JK protein that includes the amino acid that defines the Jk(a) and/or Jk(b) antigen has a glycosylation that can include the ABO antigen.

JK protein

FIGURE 4-5   Simplified Schematic of ABO Attachment to a Red Blood Cell Membrane

ABO Antigen Frequency

The most common ABO blood group is group O. However, like all genetically determined traits, there are differences among people of different racial ancestry. Table 4-4 ✱ summarizes the incidence of ABO groups among ethnic ancestry common in the United States.[11]

ABO Subgroups

Genetic variations in the *ABO* gene are known as subgroups. Individuals more commonly have variations in the *A* gene than the *B* gene. Both variations are described here.

A₁, A₂, and anti-A₁

Genetic variations in the *ABO* gene can produce subgroups of A, B, and AB. The most common subgroups of A are the A_1 and A_2 antigens. About 80% of group A and AB people have the A_1 gene. Most of the other 20% are A_2 or A_2B. Both A_1 and A_2

antigens have the same immunodominant sugar: N-acetyl-D-galactosamine. And both A_1 and A_2 genes code for a transferase, α-1,3-N-acetyl-galactosaminyltransferase. However, the enzyme coded for by the A_1 gene is better at converting H substance to A antigen. Therefore, A_1 red blood cells have more A antigen than A_2 red blood cells (10.5×10^5/red blood cell versus 2.21×10^5/red blood cell).[10] There are also qualitative differences in the A antigen made by A_1 and A_2 patient/donors.[12] This is demonstrated by the fact that about 1–2% of A_2 and 20–25% of A_2B patient/donors make anti-A_1.[12] Anti-A_1, similar to other ABO antibodies, is a *naturally occurring antibody* (a concept that is described in detail later in this chapter) that is IgM in nature, reacting best at temperatures less than 98.6° F (37° C). It is generally considered clinically insignificant. However, some patients will make an anti-A_1 that reacts at 98.6° F and reduces the lifespan of transfused cells. If the recipient's anti-A_1 reacts at 98.6° F, only A_2 or group O cells should be transfused.

Other Subgroups of A

Genetic differences can also result in other subgroups of A. Some of these subgroups of A are A_3, A_x, A_{el}, and A_m. All of these subgroups result in a weaker expression of the A antigen than seen with A_1 or A_2 patient/donors and all occur infrequently.[13] Figure 4-6 ▪ illustrates

✱ **TABLE 4-4** Incidence of ABO Groups in Select Populations

ABO Group	European	African	Asian	Hispanic
O	44	49	43	55
A	43	27	27	28
B	9	20	25	13
AB	4	4	5	4

$$A_1 > A_2 > A_3 > A_x > A_m > A_{el}$$

Most ·············· Least

▪ **FIGURE 4-6**   Relative Amount of A Antigen on Common and Uncommon Red Blood Cells

the differences in amount of A antigen on different red blood cells. Historically, the A subgroups were divided based on their detection with human anti-A, anti-A,B, and anti-H. Monoclonal antibody activity does not always correlate with the historic divisions. Manufacturers will report in their direction circular or package insert how the clones that they have used typically react with A subgroups. Subgroup A_3 is noted for giving a mixed field reaction pattern with human source anti-A.

It is rarely necessary to identify to which A subgroup a recipient belongs. Identifying an anti-A_1 in a patient that is A_1 negative is usually sufficient. Patients with unresolved ABO discrepancies will be transfused with group O blood whether the cause of the ABO discrepancy is a weak A subgroup or something else.

It is important to identify donors as a weak subgroup of A. Donors with a very weak A antigen expression may be mistyped as group O. The small amount of A antigen on their red blood cells can result in *intravascular hemolysis* (a process that is discussed in detail later in this chapter) if transfused to a group O patient who has strong anti-A activity. Subgroups of A donors will usually have an ABO discrepancy in their ABO grouping results; the reaction with A_1 reverse cells is commonly absent or less strong than in group O donors. The presence of the A antigen can usually be demonstrated by **absorption** (a process by which unwanted antibodies are removed from red blood cells) and elution (Chapter 8) of anti-A. Other methods that may be required to resolve the discrepancy include molecular analysis, saliva studies, or family studies.

Weak subgroups of A can be identified by molecular analysis, as many of the mutations that result in these phenotypes have been categorized. Alternatively, the subgroup of A can be identified by the:

- Strength of reaction with human source anti-A, anti-B, and anti-A,B.
- Reaction or nonreaction with specific anti-A clones.
- Strength of reaction with anti-H **lectin** (a plant extract, made in this case from *Ulex europaeus*, that binds to specific red blood cell membrane carbohydrates).
- Presence or absence of anti-A_1.
- Presence or absence of A and H in the saliva of secretors.
- Presence or absence of detectable plasma α-1,3-N-acetyl-galacto-saminyltransferase activity.

> ### ☑ CHECKPOINT 4-4
>
> Which subgroup of A is noted for displaying mixed field agglutination with human anti-A?

Subgroups of B

Subgroups of B are extremely rare. The subgroups of B have been divided in a fashion similar to the weak subgroups of A: B_3, B_x, B_{el}, and B_m. These divisions historically have been based on the pattern of reactivity with human source anti-B and anti-A,B. Some of the mutations that result in these subgroups have been discovered. The subgroups of B can also be identified by serologic and chemical analysis, similar to that used for A subgroups. Sometimes patient/donors with a very weak subgroup of B will produce a weak anti-B.[14]

Secretors and Nonsecretors

Some individuals produce A, B, and/or H antigens in various body fluids, as described next.

ABO Antigens in Secretions

A, B, and/or H antigens can be found in various fluids in about 80% of the general population. Table 4-5 ✱ lists fluids that contain ABO and H antigens. The people who have ABO antigens in their fluids are called **secretors** and they have inherited at least one secretor (*Se*) gene. The *Se* gene codes for an α-1,2-L-fucosyltransferase that is similar to the enzyme coded for by the *H* gene. The difference is that the enzyme coded for by the *Se* gene prefers to act on Type 1 precursor substance whereas the enzyme coded for by the *H* gene acts primarily on Type 2 precursor substance. Since Type 2 precursor substance is on the red blood cell membrane, the *H* gene is eventually responsible for ABO antigen expression on the red blood cell membrane. Since type 1 precursor substance is in fluids, the *Se* gene is eventually responsible for ABO antigen production in fluids.

The *Se* gene is on chromosome 19, close to the *H* gene.[15] The *Se* gene is also called *FUT2*. The *se* gene, like the *h* gene, is an amorph. People who are *sese* do not produce any A, B, or H antigen in their secretions and are called **nonsecretors**. The 20% of the population that are genetically *sese* do not produce a functional fucosyltransferase. The type 1 precursor substance secreted into their fluids is not converted to H substance and therefore cannot be converted into A or B antigens, regardless of their ABO genotype.

The A, B, and/or H antigens found in secretions are primarily glycoproteins, except for A, B, and/or H antigens found in milk and urine, which can exist as oligosaccharides (small chains made of sugar molecules only that are not attached to either proteins or lipids).[10] The A, B, and/or H antigens found in plasma are either glycoproteins or glycosphingolipids. These plasma antigens can absorb onto platelets and lymphocytes. Platelets also possess A, B, and/or H antigens that are part of their cell membrane.[13] Granulocytes and monocytes do not possess A, B, or H antigens.

> ### ☑ CHECKPOINT 4-5
>
> What is the frequency of secretors in the world's population?

✱ **TABLE 4-5** Fluids that Contain A, B, and H Antigens

Fluid	A, B, and/or H present
Plasma	In all people except those with Bombay phenotype
Amniotic fluid Bile Digestive juices Milk Saliva Tears Urine	Only if person is a secretor (80% of the population)
Pleural Peritoneal Pericardial Ovarian cyst	Only in pathological fluids, such as produced by a tumor

Laboratory Determination of Secretor Status

The presence of Lewis antigens can help determine whether the person is a secretor or nonsecretor because the genetic combinations at the *Se* and *Le* loci together determine the Lewis phenotype (Chapter 6). The presence or absence of A, B, H, Le[a], and/or Le[b] antigens in saliva can be determined using an inhibition test.[13]

In the inhibition test, saliva is collected from the patient/donor and incubated with reagent anti-A, anti-B, anti-H, anti-Le[a], and anti-Le[b], each in a separate tube. If the corresponding antigen is present in the saliva, it will bind to the antibody in the antiserum. Then the incubated saliva/antiserum mixture is tested with reagent cells positive for the corresponding antigen. If antigen was present in the saliva, it will have bound to the antibody and the antibody will not be free to react with the reagent antigen positive cells.

For example, saliva from a group B secretor contains group B antigen. When the saliva is mixed with human source, reagent anti-B, the B antigen in the saliva binds to the anti-B. When reagent B cells are typed using the saliva/antiserum mixture, a negative result occurs. The reagent anti-B is bound to the B antigen in the saliva and therefore the anti-B is not able to attach to the B antigen on the reagent cells. The secretor's saliva has inhibited the anti-B that is in the anti-B reagent. This test result, interpreted as B antigen, is present in the saliva or the patient/donor is positive for secretor status.

Interpretation of inhibition tests can appear confusing because a "positive" result (presence of the antigen in the saliva) is the outcome of a negative result in the test tube. Proper controls must be run to ensure that the procedure worked as expected, the antisera worked as expected, and dilution did not cause any of the negative test tube results.

Bombay and Para-Bombay Phenotypes

The Bombay phenotype results from *hh* and *sese* genotypes.[15] These people lack H substance both on their red blood cells and in their secretions. Their red blood cells and secretions also lack A and/or B antigens, regardless of their ABO genotype, because there is no H substance to be converted to A and/or B antigen. The red blood cells of the Bombay phenotype appear to be group O in routine ABO testing. Antibody testing with their plasma or serum is what differentiates a common group O from a Bombay phenotype. People of the Bombay phenotype produce an anti-H that reacts with all red blood cells except those of the Bombay phenotype. Therefore, the plasma from a person with the Bombay phenotype will react with antibody screening cells, which are typically ABO type O.

There are some people who appear to be Bombay phenotype but who have very small amounts of A and/or B antigen on their red blood cells. They are said to have the para-Bombay phenotype. It was discovered that their genotype is *hh* but that they possess at least one *Se* gene.[16] The *Se* gene produces a fucosyltransferase that acts on type 1 precursor substance in fluids and secretions. The type 1 H substance formed by the *Se* gene can then be converted into A and/or B antigen depending on which ABO genes are inherited. People with the para-Bombay phenotype have H, A, and/or B antigens in their secretions and plasma. Sometimes a small amount of A, B, and/or H antigen will absorb from the plasma onto the red blood cell membrane, resulting in the very weak expression of A or B antigen on their red blood cells. Generally, the A, B, and/or H antigen from their red blood cells can only be detected by absorption/elution studies. The red blood cell membrane of para-Bombay individuals does not possess intrinsic A, B, or H antigens because the type 2 precursor substance on their red blood cells remains unconverted, due to the lack of an *H* gene. Table 4-6 ✳ lists the phenotypes of common gene combinations of *ABO*, *Hh*, and *Se*. Table 4-7 ✳ lists the phenotypes of uncommon gene combinations.

Cis-AB

Another very rare genotype in the ABO blood group system is cis-AB. Usual AB patient/donors have an *A* gene on one chromosome 9 and a *B* gene on the other. In cis-AB patient/donors, both the *A* and *B* genes are on the same chromosome 9 and an *O* gene is on the other. Cis-AB may be caused by a mutation that produces an enzyme that attaches both the A and B immunodominant sugars to H substance.[17] Alternatively, a cis-AB child may come from an AB parent with an *A* gene on one chromosome and a *B* gene on the other, but in whom a crossover event occurred in the parent's chromosomes during meiosis.[18] The crossover event results in both the *A* and *B* genes being on one chromosome 9 that is passed to the child and no *ABO* gene being on the other chromosome 9.

Some cis-AB patient/donors are indistinguishable from usual AB patient/donors in the laboratory, in which case they are only discovered through family studies. An example where family studies may be undertaken is when a cord sample is tested and the baby is group O, although the mother is group AB. On the other hand, some cis-AB patient/donors are discovered because their test results produce an ABO discrepancy. These cis-AB patient/donors have weakened expression of the A and/or B antigen on their cells. If the B antigen

✳ **TABLE 4-6** Common Gene Combinations of *ABO*, *Hh*, and *Sese*

Genotype			Antigens in Secretions	Antigens on Red Blood Cell	Phenotype
HH or Hh	SeSe or Sese	AA or AO	A and H	A and H	A secretor
		BB or BO	B and H	B and H	B secretor
		OO	H	H	O secretor
		AB	A, B, and H	A, B, and H	AB secretor
HH or Hh	sese	AA or AO	None	A and H	A nonsecretor
		BB or BO	None	B and H	B nonsecretor
		OO	None	H	O nonsecretor
		AB	None	A, B, and H	AB nonsecretor

✳ **TABLE 4-7** Uncommon Gene Combinations of *ABO*, *Hh*, and *Sese*

Genotype			Antigens in Secretions	Antigens on RBC	Phenotype
hh	*sese*	Any ABO combination	None	None	O_h (Bombay)
hh	*SeSe* or *Sese*	*AA* or *AO*	A and H	None (or very small amount absorbed from plasma)	A_h (para-Bombay)
		BB or *BO*	B and H		B_h (para-Bombay)
		OO	H		O_h (para-Bombay)
		AB	A, B, and H		AB_h (para-Bombay)

expression is very weak, the patient/donor may produce a weak anti-B in their plasma. This anti-B typically reacts with all normal B cells but does not react with cells from other cis-AB people.

ABO AND Hh ANTIBODIES

Antibodies are made against foreign antigens (Chapter 1). In most blood group systems, antibodies may be formed after the person is exposed to red blood cells that carry antigens different from their own antigens. This exposure happens either through pregnancy, transfusion, or transplantation. Thus, healthy individuals typically make antibodies against the antigens they lack. The antibodies and associated concepts connected with the ABO/Hh blood group systems are described next.

Naturally Occurring Antibodies

In the ABO blood group system, unlike most other blood group systems, everyone develops antibodies to the antigens that are not on their own red blood cells. Antibodies that develop without any apparent stimulus are called **naturally occurring antibodies**. Babies are not born with ABO antibodies. The antibodies tend to develop at about 3–4 months of age. Many common bacteria that colonize the human gastrointestinal tract have carbohydrates that have the same or very similar structure to the human ABO antigens. It is believed, but has not been proven, that we make ABO antibodies in response to these antigens. Whatever the cause, healthy humans have antibodies in their plasma to any ABO antigen that is lacking on their own red blood cells. Therefore group A people have anti-B, group B people have anti-A, group O people have both anti-A and anti-B, and group AB people have neither anti-A or anti-B. Group O people also make a third antibody that reacts with either A or B antigens. This antibody is called anti-A,B. Table 4-8 ✳ lists the antigens and antibodies in common ABO groups.

Immunoglobulin Class

Most ABO antibodies are IgM. Like all IgM antibodies, they react best at colder temperatures. However, they have a large thermal range and will react at body temperature. IgM antibodies can bind complement. When this occurs, the cascade progresses all the way to the membrane attack complex, resulting in red blood cell lysis (Chapter 1). ABO antibodies can also be IgG and IgA. IgG ABO antibodies are especially prevalent in group O people.[10]

Intravascular Hemolysis

ABO antibodies, when presented with red blood cells that have the corresponding antigen, initiate the complement cascade, which progresses all the way to the membrane attack complex. The membrane attack complex creates a hole in the red blood cell membrane, allowing hemoglobin to escape. This destruction of red blood cells occurs inside the veins and arteries and is called **intravascular hemolysis**. The presence of free hemoglobin and the release of the red blood cell contents in the circulation cause the severe consequences seen in ABO-incompatible transfusion reactions, namely, shock, disseminated intravascular coagulation (DIC), and kidney failure. These conditions are the direct cause of patient death associated with ABO-incompatible transfusions.[13]

Anti-H and Anti-IH

Patient/donors of the Bombay phenotype lack H substance both on their red blood cells and in their secretions. They will make a naturally occurring anti-H, as well as anti-A, anti-B, and anti-A,B. The

✳ **TABLE 4-8** Antigens and Antibodies in Common ABO Groups

ABO Group	Antigens Present on Red Blood Cell	Antibodies Present in Plasma
A	A	Anti-B
B	B	Anti-A
O	Neither A or B	Anti-A, anti-B, and anti-A,B
AB	Both A and B	Neither anti-A or anti-B

anti-H made by people of the Bombay phenotype is an IgM antibody that reacts strongly at 98.6° F (37° C). Like ABO antibodies, this anti-H can cause intravascular hemolysis. In the laboratory, patient/donor RBCs of the Bombay phenotype will look like group O in ABO forward testing, but their plasma will react strongly with all group O cells (e.g., screening, panel, and donor cells). An *autocontrol* (a test that consists of testing patient cells with patient plasma designed to detect antibodies against self, also known as *autoantibodies*; see Chapter 8 for more details) will be negative and their cells will not react with anti-H lectin. The only red blood cells that will be compatible in laboratory testing and that can be transfused are cells from the very rare donors possessing the Bombay phenotype.

Patient/donors of the para-Bombay phenotype have H substance in their secretions due to the presence of at least one *Se* gene. Therefore, they do not usually make the potent anti-H found in patient/donors of the Bombay phenotype. They do usually make a combination antibody known as anti-IH (see Chapter 6 for information on the I blood group system). Anti-IH is generally a weaker, cold reactive antibody that is not usually clinically significant. Occasionally they can also make a weak, clinically insignificant anti-H.[14]

Anti-H and/or anti-IH can also be found in the plasma of some patient/donors of the A_1 phenotype. A_1 red blood cells have the least amount of II substance because the majority of H antigen has been converted to A antigen.[13] Figure 4-7 illustrates the relative amount of H antigen found on various red blood cells. The anti-H or anti-IH produced by A_1 patient/donors is not usually reactive at 98.6° F (37° C) and therefore is not clinically significant. Suspect anti-IH or anti-H if all group O cells (e.g., screen and panel cells) are reactive but group A cells (e.g., crossmatched donor units) are nonreactive. Anti-IH will exhibit weaker or no reaction with cord red blood cells, which exhibit the i antigen and are very little or no I antigen. Anti-IH will react strongly with O cord red blood cells, but weakly or not at all with A cord red blood cells.

Anti-IH can also be a nuisance cold autoantibody. It reacts best at low temperatures, but some examples have a high enough thermal range to cause problems in laboratory testing at room temperature or even 98.6° F (37° C). Although anti-IH causes problems in the laboratory, it generally does not have any effect on the patient.

LABORATORY TESTING

In order to understand laboratory testing associated with antigen–antibody reactions (including ABO and beyond), an introduction to test terminology is appropriate. To perform such tests, there must be a source of antigen and a source of antibody. Antigen sources include patient cells, commercially prepared reagent cells, donor cells, and cells retrieved in the birthing process from the umbilical cord. Antibody sources may be patient plasma (or serum) or commercially prepared reagent antisera. It is important to point out here that the use of plasma versus serum for ABO testing varies based on the specific policies and procedures being followed. Historically serum was the specimen of choice but due to the possibility of components in serum

clustering and mimicking agglutination, plasma has gained popularity for blood bank testing. For the purposes of the remainder of this chapter the terms plasma and serum will be used appropriately based on context.

With minimal exception and depending on the test being performed, either the source of antigen or antibody is considered as the "known" because its makeup is known. The "known" source of antigen or antibody is used to determine whether the corresponding antigen or antibody to that "known" is present (the part of the test called the "unknown"). Sources of antigen and antibody that are obtained from commercial suppliers may be called "known" reagents/cells, commercial reagents/cells, reverse cells, commercial antiserum/sera, or reagent(s).

Specific to ABO testing, it is also important to point out here that terms describing an ABO test include *ABO typing*, *ABO group/grouping*, and *ABO blood type*. These terms may be used interchangeably both in the literature and the blood bank setting. For the purposes of this text, these terms will be used as appropriate to the content context.

The presence of both ABO antigen and antibody is very useful in the laboratory because it gives us a built-in double-check for our ABO group/type. In adults, ABO testing consists of two components: testing for antigen(s) on the person's red blood cells and antibody(ies) in the person's plasma.[13] Antigen is identified by combining the unknown (patient or donor) red blood cells with known antibody (anti-A or anti-B). The results of this testing is called a **forward group (grouping)**. The presence of antibody is identified by combining the unknown (patient or donor) plasma with known ABO red blood cells (A_1 or B). This results in a **reverse group (grouping)**. A positive test, seen as agglutination, indicates the presence of the corresponding antigen or antibody. A negative test or no agglutination indicates the absence of the corresponding antigen or antibody. Although the actual blood type assigned to a patient technically relates to the antigens present on patient red blood cells, the results of the forward and reverse ABO grouping should always correlate. Performing both components of the test (forward and reverse testing/typing) serves as a double-check in the ABO testing. Table 4-9 lists the usual ABO test result patterns.

Typically the result of each component of ABO testing is recorded on a sheet (usually by paper or electronically). An example of how to read such reaction sheets follows. The first horizontal row in Table 4-9 consists of the expected reactions of an ABO group A individual. The far left column is titled "anti-A," meaning that this 'known' commercial reagent (antisera) was used to detect the presence of A antigen (noted by the + sign indicating that agglutination occurred) on the 'unknown' red blood cells being tested. Since this component of the ABO test is designed to detect antigen, it is part of the ABO forward grouping. Likewise, the column titled "A_1 cells" refers to the 'known' commercial red blood cells used to test for the presence of anti-A antibody which in this case was negative (noted by the symbol 0, indicating that agglutination did *not* occur). Since this

O>A_2>B>A_2B>A_1>A_1B> weaker subgroups of A or AB> para-Bombay>Bombay
Most ·········· Least ······· None

FIGURE 4-7 Relative Amount of H Antigen on Common and Uncommon Red Blood Cells

✳ **TABLE 4-9** Usual ABO Test Results

Forward Group Unknown cells tested with commercial sera		Reverse Group Unknown plasma tested with commercial cells		
Anti-A	Anti-B	A₁ cells	B cells	Interpretation
+	0	0	+	A
0	+	+	0	B
0	0	+	+	O
+	+	0	0	AB

component of the test is designed to detect antibodies in the plasma being tested, it is part of the ABO reverse grouping.

An **ABO discrepancy** occurs when the results of the forward and reverse grouping do not correlate. In these cases, further testing is required before the ABO group can be reported. ABO discrepancies are described in more detail later in this chapter.

It is important to note here that tests for the H antigen as well as H antibody are not routinely performed. Examination for Hh blood group system components occurs only when indicated.

☑ **CHECKPOINT 4-7**

What are the two components of an ABO grouping and how is each component performed?

CASE IN POINT *(continued)*

You review patient GB's historical blood bank data and determine that she has never had a blood type performed at your hospital in the past.

1. What will be your next step?

Methodologies

The ABO test is easy to perform. Plasma or antiserum is combined with red blood cells, mixed, centrifuged (the term *spin* may also be used to indicate centrifugation), and read for agglutination. If the antigen on the red blood cells is the same as the antibody specificity in the plasma, then the cells clump together. This is called **hemagglutination**. The hemagglutination may be visualized in several ways. Traditional testing, which is still widely used, is done in a test tube. The strength of the hemagglutination is graded based on the size and number of clumps seen. Some automated test systems utilize hemagglutination but perform the test in the wells of a microtiter plate rather than in test tubes. Gel columns may also be used to visualize the agglutination in either manual or automated systems[19] (Chapters 3 and 7).

ABO Discrepancies

ABO discrepancies are categorized into four groups: missing or weak reaction in the forward group, missing or weak reaction in the reverse group, unexpected positive in the forward group, and unexpected positive in the reverse group. Detecting mixed field agglutination or obtaining different results with current testing as compared to historical testing are also considered discrepancies. Table 4-10 ✳ lists some ABO discrepancies that might be encountered. Table 4-11 ✳ consists of the major categories and associated possible causes of ABO discrepancies. Further discussion of ABO discrepancies is detailed in the following sections.

Identifying the Problem

The strength of the reactions observed will usually identify the most promising resolution strategy. Weaker reactions are more likely to be aberrant than stronger reactions. If the reaction strength does not provide a clue, then investigate the more common causes of discrepancies before the very rare. For each category, described separately in the following sections, it is important to remember that it is possible for more than one discrepancy to occur in a single sample.

Missing or Weak Reaction in the Forward Group

Missing or weak reactions in the forward group may indicate that the patient/donor is a subgroup of A or B. Subgroups of A are fairly common, but subgroups of B are rare. ABO subgroups are genetically

---

✳ **TABLE 4-10** ABO Discrepancy Examples

Forward Group		Reverse Group		
Anti-A	Anti-B	A₁ Cells	B Cells	Interpretation
4+	0	0	0	Likely: group A with a missing anti-B Alternate: group AB with a missing B antigen
1+	4+	4+	0	Likely: group B with an extra reaction with anti-A
1+	4+	2+	0	Likely: group B with an extra reaction with anti-A Alternate: group AB with a weakly reactive A antigen and an extra reaction with A cells
0	4+	4+	2+	Likely: group B with an extra reaction with B cells
0	0	0	4+	Likely: group A with missing A antigen reaction Alternate: group O with missing anti-A reaction
0	0	0	0	Likely: group O with missing antibody reactions Alternate: group AB with missing antigen reactions
4+	0	1+	4+	Likely: group A with extra reaction with A cells
4+	4+	2+	2+	Likely: group AB with extra reactions with A and B cells
2+	2+	4+	4+	Likely: group O with extra reactions with anti-A and anti-B

✳ **TABLE 4-11** Causes of ABO Discrepancies

ABO Discrepancy Suspected	Possible Causes
Missing or weak reaction in the forward group	• ABO subgroup • Diseases that alter the ABO antigen expression (e.g., leukemia, Hodgkin's lymphoma) • Transfusion or transplantation • Excessive soluble ABO antigens in patient/donor's plasma
Missing or weak reaction in the reverse group	• Age (neonates or elderly) • Hypogammaglobulinemia (either primary disease or secondary to leukemia/lymphoma) • Agammaglobulinemia or other congenital immunodeficiencies • Patients on immunosuppressive therapy • Transplantation • Patients whose antibodies have been diluted by plasma exchange therapy • ABO subgroup
Unexpected positive reaction in the forward group	• Panagglutinating cells due to changes in red blood cell membrane or interference from plasma proteins • Wharton's jelly in cord samples • Acquired B antigen • B(A) phenomenon • Transplantation
Unexpected positive reaction in the reverse group	• ABO subgroup • Cold reactive autoantibody or alloantibody • Antibody to reagent • Excess serum protein due to multiple myeloma, Waldstrom's macroglobulinemia, or other diseases • Treatment with plasma expanders such as dextran • Passive ABO antibodies (e.g., transfusion of IVIG, maternal transfer of antibodies to child)
Mixed field agglutination in the forward group	• Recent transfusion • Transplantation • Feto–maternal hemorrhage • ABO subgroup, notably A_3 • Chimerism (twins or dispermy)
Different current ABO group from historic ABO group	• Patient/sample identification error during collection • Patient is victim or perpetrator of identity theft • Sample mix-up during testing • Patient has received an ABO nonidentical bone marrow transplant

determined. The very rare cis-AB genotype may also result in weak expression of ABO antigens. Leukemia and other malignancies may result in alteration of the A or B antigen on the red blood cells. The altered antigens do not react normally with routine antisera, resulting in a missing or weak reaction. Transfusion or transplantation with non-ABO identical cells may result either in mixed field agglutination or a weakened reaction in the forward group. Some people may have excessive amounts on soluble A and/or B antigen in their plasma. If plasma suspended cells are used in the testing, the soluble antigens can neutralize the reagent antiserum, resulting in a false-negative reaction.

Whenever there is a suspected problem in the forward group, repeating the testing using red blood cells that have been washed and then suspended in saline is a good first step. If a subgroup of A is suspected, the patient/donor cells may be tested with anti-A_1 lectin (*Dolichos biflorus*).

There are several methods that can be used to enhance the detection of a weak ABO antigen, independent of the cause which is typically inherited or acquired. Table 4-12 ✳ is an example of a testing algorithm for resolving a discrepancy with a weak or missing reaction in the forward group. As always, manufacturer's instructions should be consulted for limitations or controls that should be used, related to any change from the usual method. The forward group can be incubated at room temperature or at 39.2° F (4° C), if an albumin or autocontrol

is included. Enzyme treatment of the patient/donor cells may resolve the discrepancy. To ensure that any reaction is due to ABO antigens, group O cells should be enzyme treated and tested with the antisera at the same time as the patient/donor cells. Additionally, an autocontrol using enzyme-treated cells should be run in parallel. Absorption/elution methods may be used. The absorption method should be done at a low temperature (e.g., 39.2° F) because ABO antibodies react best at this temperature. Suitable elution methods include heat, Lui freeze–thaw, or one of the acid elution kits, if the manufacturer states that the method is suitable for detecting ABO antibodies.

Saliva may be tested for A, B, H, and Lewis antigens by an inhibition test. This may provide useful information in resolving an ABO discrepancy if the person is a secretor. Measuring the transferase activity responsible for H, A, or B antigen expression can help identify ABO subgroups. Finally, genetic analysis can be used to identify the absence of common ABO genes and/or the presence of mutations known to result in ABO subgroups.

Missing or Weak Reaction in the Reverse Group

Discrepant results in the reverse group are more common than in the forward group. Missing or unexpectedly weak reactions are due to low antibody levels related to age, disease, or transplantation. ABO antibodies can be enhanced by lowering the testing temperature,

✱ **TABLE 4-12** Example Testing Algorithm for Resolution of Suspected Weak/Missing Forward Group Using Tube Testing

Step 1	Repeat testing using saline-washed red blood cells.
Step 2	Check specimen labeling.
	Check for transcription and/or interpretation errors.
	Check equipment and reagent quality control results.
	Obtain patient diagnosis and transfusion/transplantation history.
Step 3	If discrepancy not resolved:
	Incubate at room temperature for 15 minutes. Respin (that is, repeat centrifugation step) and reread.
Step 4	If discrepancy not resolved:
	Incubate at 39.2° F (4° C) for 15 minutes. Respin and reread. Include appropriate controls.
Step 5	If discrepancy not resolved:
	Enzyme-treat patient/donor cells and appropriate control cells. Repeat testing using enzyme-treated cells.
Step 6	If discrepancy not resolved and patient has not been transfused:
	Perform absorption/elution studies.
Step 7	If discrepancy not resolved:
	Consider if discrepancy may be in reverse group.
	Consider performing secretor, transferase, or genetic studies based on test availability and value of the information that may be obtained.
	If transfusion required before discrepancy is resolved or if discrepancy is not resolved:
	Issue only group O red blood cell units.

increasing the ratio of serum/cells, increasing the incubation time, or enzyme-treating the cells. Table 4-13 ✱ is an example of a testing algorithm for resolving a discrepancy with a weak or missing reaction in the reverse group.

The usual first step when a missing reaction in the reverse group is suspected is to check the patient's age. If the patient is younger than 4 months of age, the reverse group should not be tested and the ABO group should be interpreted based on the forward group alone. Elderly patients may also exhibit decreased antibody concentration. Similarly, certain diseases such as agammaglobulinemia, hypogammaglobulinemia, and some leukemias and lymphomas may decrease ABO antibody production. However, in adult patients the ABO blood group should not be based solely on the forward grouping. All

attempts should be made to enhance ABO antibodies to a detectable level. If the antibodies cannot be detected even with enhancement techniques, then the ABO group remains discrepant.

Transfusion and transplantation histories are also important in resolving ABO discrepancies. ABO antibodies may be diluted to a nondetectable level in a patient who has recently received therapeutic plasma exchange therapy. Patients who are on aggressive immunosuppressant therapy can have decreased expression of their ABO antibodies. Patients who have had a nonidentical ABO bone marrow transplant will exhibit various ABO discrepancies depending on their stage of engraftment. ABO-incompatible heart transplants are being performed during the neonatal period. These babies do not produce the antibody corresponding to the ABO antigens on the transplanted

✱ **TABLE 4-13** Example Testing Algorithm for Resolution of Suspected Weak/Missing Reverse Group Using Tube Testing

Step 1	Check patient's age. If <4 months old, interpret group based on forward group. If ≥4 months old, proceed with resolution.
Step 2	Repeat testing.
	Check specimen labeling.
	Check for transcription and/or interpretation errors.
	Check equipment and reagent quality control results.
	Obtain patient diagnosis and transfusion/transplantation history.
Step 3	If discrepancy not resolved:
	Incubate at room temperature for 15 minutes. Respin and reread.
Step 4	If discrepancy not resolved:
	Incubate at 39.2° F (4° C) for 15 minutes. Respin and reread. Include appropriate controls.
Step 5	If discrepancy not resolved:
	Enzyme-treat reverse grouping cells and appropriate control cells. Repeat testing using enzyme-treated cells.
Step 6	If discrepancy not resolved:
	Consider if discrepancy may be in forward group.
	If transfusion required before discrepancy is resolved or if discrepancy is not resolved:
	Issue only group O red blood cell units.

heart even when the antigen is absent from their red blood cells.[20] ABO-incompatible heart transplants cannot be performed in patients who have already formed ABO antibodies.

Decreasing the testing temperature and/or increasing the serum-to-cell ratio are easy techniques that are often performed near the beginning of an investigation into a suspected missing or weak reverse reaction. Remember that most ABO antibodies are IgM and that IgM antibodies are generally cold-reactive. In tube testing, adding two additional drops of patient/donor plasma can sometimes enhance a weak reaction. This should only be done, like any variation from routine testing, after consulting the manufacturer's instructions—in this case, the manufacturer of the reverse grouping cells. Initially, the reverse group can be incubated for 15–30 minutes at room temperature (68–75.2° F [20–24° C]). Additional controls are not usually required for this modification. If the room temperature incubation does not resolve the discrepancy, the testing temperature can be lowered to 39.2° F (4° C). When testing at 39.2° F, group O cells and an autocontrol should also be tested. This will help identify if an additional reaction is truly due to an enhanced ABO antibody or due to another cold-reactive antibody. Table 4-14 ✳ lists interpretation of various result patterns possible when incubation at 39.2° F is performed.

Enzyme treatment of the reverse grouping cells can sometimes help enhance a weakly reactive ABO antibody (Chapter 8). Enzyme treatment may be done using ficin, papain, or bromelin. To ensure that any reactivity observed is due to an ABO antibody, controls of group O and autologous cells ("self" red blood cells; in this case refers to patient red blood cells) should be enzyme-treated and tested at the same time.

Unexpected Positive Reaction in the Forward Group
Unexpected positive reactions in the forward group can be due to substances in the plasma if the testing is done using unwashed cells. Wharton's jelly is a gelatinous, intercellular substance in umbilical cords, rich in hyaluronic acid. Samples obtained by stripping the cord are often contaminated with Wharton's jelly, causing nonspecific agglutination in ABO tests. Cells from cord samples should always be washed prior to testing. When there is particularly heavy contamination with Wharton's jelly, washing the cells with 98.6° F (37° C) saline will often solve the problem. If the cells still demonstrate a *panagglutinating pattern* (positive with inert control, anti-A and anti-B), a capillary sample should be collected from the newborn and tested.

Additional substances in the plasma that may cause false-positive reactions in the forward group include strong *cold autoagglutinins*

(cold-reacting antibodies), Ph-dependent autoantibody, antibody to a constituent of the antiserum, infused high-molecular weight substances, and abnormal proteins that cause *rouleaux* (clumping of red blood cells resembling a "stack of coins" that may be interpreted as agglutination but is really due to protein abnormalities or as a result of select intravenous fluid infusion). All of these discrepancies are usually resolved by repeating the tests using washed, saline-suspended cells. Table 4-15 ✳ is an example of a testing algorithm for resolving a discrepancy with an unexpected positive reaction in the forward group. Many of these substances also cause false-positive reactions in the reverse group and have been discussed previously. Patient/donors may have antibodies against a constituent of the antiserum, including preservatives (both forward tests will usually be falsely positive) and dye (usually only one of the forward tests is falsely positive). Depending on the ABO group of the donor/patient, the forward or reverse group results may include a true positive and a false positive. Autoantibodies that react at the same pH as the antiserum may cause a false-positive reaction.

Differences in the red blood cell membrane from the norm may also cause unexpected reactions in the forward group. Some patient/donors may have acquired or inherited changes to the red blood cell membrane that causes their cells to agglutinate with all plasma. This is called **polyagglutination**. Polyagglutination is the result of exposure of an antigen on the red blood cell membrane that is usually hidden. These antigens are called **cryptantigens**. Most normal adult plasma contains naturally occurring antibodies against various cryptantigens. Today, polyagglutination is rarely discovered on routine ABO testing because clonal rather than human source antisera are used. It should be suspected when a patient experiences a hemolytic transfusion reaction with no explanation (no antibodies are found in the patient's plasma directed against antigens on the donor cells). Patients with polyagglutinating cells generally do not have the corresponding antibody in their plasma. However, the normal human plasma in the transfused unit will contain antibody against the patient's exposed cryptantigen and can cause extravascular or intravascular hemolysis.[14]

Polyagglutinating cells will usually react negatively in an autocontrol and when tested with plasma or serum from cord samples. If the autocontrol is positive, the cells may be heavily coated with antibody, causing nonspecific agglutination. Polyagglutinating cells can be classified using lectins. Most causes are acquired and are due to bacterial infections. Table 4-16 ✳ lists causes and types of polyagglutination. Letters, such as T or Tx, are the names given to identify

✳ **TABLE 4-14** Interpretation of 39.2° F (4° C) Reverse ABO Group Results

Reverse Group	Group O Cells	Autocontrol	Action
Matches forward group results	0	0	Interpret ABO group
Does not match forward group results	Any result	Any result	Do not interpret ABO group
Any result	+	Any result	Cold-reactive antibody other than ABO present. Identify the cold-reactive antibody and repeat ABO-reverse group using cells that are negative for the corresponding antigen.
Any result	Any result	+	*Cold autoagglutinin* (antibodies that react at room temperature, aka "cold"-reacting). Do not interpret ABO group.

★ **TABLE 4-15** Example Testing Algorithm for Resolution of Unexpected Positive Result in the Forward Group Using Tube Testing

Step 1	Repeat testing using washed, saline-suspended cells.
Step 2	If discrepancy is not resolved:
	Check specimen labeling.
	Check for transcription and/or interpretation errors.
	Check equipment and reagent quality control results.
	Obtain patient diagnosis and transfusion/transplantation history.
Step 3	Perform an autocontrol.
Step 4	If autocontrol is negative, the cells may be polyagglutinating.
	Identification of polyagglutination includes:
	• Investigating history of recent bacterial infections.
	• Testing cells with group AB cord serum.
	• Testing cells with a lectin panel.
	• Other tests as appropriate depending on the suspected type of polyagglutination.
Step 5	If B(A) phenotype is suspected, repeat testing with other anti-A reagent(s).
Step 6	If autocontrol is positive, the cells may be agglutinating due to antibody coating the cells. Remove the antibody using an appropriate elution technique and test the treated cells.
Step 7	If discrepancy not resolved, consider if discrepancy may be in reverse group.
	If transfusion required before discrepancy is resolved or if discrepancy is not resolved:
	Issue only group O red blood cell units.

some types of polyagglutination. Sometimes the letters refer to the cryptantigen exposed and sometimes they do not. In fact, in the case of Tx, the antigen has not yet been fully described. Due to these differences, the types of polyagglutination listed in Table 4-16 consist of the names with no further description.

Bacterially induced polyagglutination is a transient condition, whereas genetically coded membrane changes resulting in polyagglutination are permanent. Healthy blood donors may have one of the inherited forms of polyagglutination, all of which are rare. Additionally, there have been reports of blood donors exhibiting one of the acquired forms of polyagglutination. There is one form of polyagglutination that is caused by a mutation in the bone marrow. Rather than an inherited mutation, the mutation occurs later in life and results in a clone that produces red blood cells with the altered membrane. Other clones produce normal red blood cells, so there is often a mixed population of cells. This is a persistent condition.

In most acquired forms of polyagglutination, enzymes produced by the bacteria, virus, or parasite remove carbohydrates from the normal red blood cell membrane, exposing carbohydrates that are usually hidden.

Acquired B occurs in group A_1 patient/donors and is usually associated with conditions of the gastrointestinal tract that lead to septicemia. In acquired B, the bacterial enzyme removes an acetyl group from the A antigen. The resulting carbohydrate is very similar in structure to the B antigen and it cross-reacts with human anti-B and at least one

monoclonal anti-B.[21] Manufacturers that use the implicated clone, ES4, have lowered the pH of their reagent to avoid detection of the acquired B antigen. The ABO discrepancy can be resolved by testing with a clonal anti-B reagent that does not detect the acquired B antigen. Before the advent of clonal reagents, acquired B was investigated by a variety of methods that replace the acetyl group onto the A antigen or that otherwise inactivate the acquired B antigen.

The use of clonal reagents has decreased the detection of polyagglutinating cells, but has resulted in the detection of "new" phenotypes. An example of this is the B(A) phenotype, in which some group B patient/donor RBCs react weakly with monoclonal anti-A made from the MHO4 clone.[22] Most B(A) people have greater than the usual amount of the enzyme that produces the B antigen. The enzymes responsible for formation of the A and B antigens use the same substrate and are very similar. Approximately 1/100 B persons has a minor mutation, which causes their B enzyme to be slightly more similar to the A enzyme. This can result in a small amount of A-like antigens being made by the B-specific enzyme. These people still make anti-A and must be transfused with B blood products. Their RBCs can be safely given to other B patients, however. The A(B) phenotype has also been described, although much less commonly and some cases may actually be acquired B antigens in patients with gastrointestinal disease.

Unexpected Positive Reactions in the Reverse Group

Unexpected positive reactions in the reverse group may be due to the presence of non-ABO antibodies in the patient/donor plasma that are cross-reacting in the ABO test. The antibodies could be **cold autoagglutinins**, an alloantibody that reacts at room temperature to an antigen present on the reverse cell(s), or, rarely, an antibody to one of the constituents of the reverse cells' suspension medium.

A positive reaction with A_1 cells in a suspected group A or AB person could indicate that the person is a subgroup of A with an anti-A_1. Patient/donors who are weak subgroups of A or B or who are cis-AB may produce unexpected ABO antibodies. Additionally,

★ **TABLE 4-16** Causes and Types of Polyagglutination

Cause	Type(s) of Polyagglutination
Bacterially acquired (transient)	T, Th, Tk, Tx, acquired B, possible VA
Inherited (permanent)	Cad, hemoglobin M-Hyde Park, HEMPAS, NOR
Somatic mutation (persistent)	Tn

✳ **TABLE 4-17** Example Testing Algorithm for Resolution of Suspected Anti-A_1

Step 1	Initial results: forward group looks like group A or AB. Reverse results: positive reaction with A_1 cells. (In group A people the reaction is usually less strong than with the B reverse cells.)
Step 2	If not recently transfused, type the patient/donor's cells with *Dolichos biflorus*.
Step 3	If patient/donor types A_1 negative or cannot be A_1 typed, test the patient/donor plasma against 3 A_1 positive cells, 3 A_1 negative cells, and 3 group O cells.
Step 4	If anti-A_1 is identified, repeat the reverse grouping using group A cells that are A_1 negative. (Note this has usually already been done as part of the identification procedure for anti-A_1 as in step 3.)
Step 5	If discrepancy not resolved: Consider if discrepancy may be caused by an antibody other than anti-A_1. Consider if discrepancy may be in forward group. If transfusion required before discrepancy is resolved or if discrepancy is not resolved: Issue only group O red blood cell units.

the expression of their A and/or B antigens is weakened. Cis-AB and weak subgroups of A or B, except A_2, are very rare.

Alternatively, the positive reactions may be due to substances in the patient/donor plasma that are causing nonspecific agglutination of the red blood cells. The nonspecific agglutination is called **rouleaux** (from the French word for cylinder) and the red blood cells resemble stacks of coins that have been knocked over. Rouleaux can be caused by diseases that greatly increase serum protein concentrations, such as multiple myeloma and Waldenström's macroglobulinemia or by the transfusion of high-molecular-weight substances, such as dextran.

The ABO test cannot differentiate between naturally occurring and passively acquired antibodies. ABO antibodies may be passively acquired by transfusion of intravenous immune globulin or, less frequently, by ABO nonidentical plasma or platelet transfusions. ABO antibodies detected in neonates less than 4 months old will almost always be maternal IgG antibodies that have crossed the placenta and have not yet been cleared from the baby's circulation.

To confirm anti-A_1 in a person who has not been recently transfused, type the patient/donor cells with anti-A_1 lectin (*Dolichos biflorus*). Table 4-17 ✳ is an example of a testing algorithm for resolving a discrepancy suspected of being an anti-A_1. If the patient's red blood cells are A_1 positive, then the reaction is not due to anti-A_1. If the patient is A_1 negative or cannot be typed due to recent transfusion, test the patient/donor plasma against three examples each of A_1 positive, A_1 negative, and group O cells. An autologous control should also be run. An anti-A_1 should react with all three A_1 positive cells but not with any of the A_1 negative or group O cells. Reactions with A_1 negative and/or group O cells indicate that an antibody other than anti-A_1 is causing the discrepancy or there may be a combination of an anti-A_1 and another room temperature–reactive antibody. Table 4-18 ✳ summarizes the reaction patterns that may occur.

Cold-reactive alloantibodies can be identified by testing panels of cells with known phenotypes using the patient/donor's plasma and the same technique as the ABO testing (e.g., tube testing at room temperature with no additives). To confirm that the identified antibody was the cause of the ABO discrepancy, the reverse cell(s) should be *phenotyped* (i.e., tested for in this case by combining the reagent reverse cells [the unknown] with known commercial antiserum for the corresponding antigen). If the reverse cell(s) are negative for the corresponding antigen, then the alloantibody, while present, may not have caused the ABO discrepancy.

As the last step in the resolution of the discrepancy, the patient/donor's plasma should be tested against A or B cells that are negative for the corresponding antigen to the alloantibody. *Alloantibodies* (antibodies that are produced after red blood cell exposure, typically via pregnancy, transfusion reaction, or transplantation) that cause problems in ABO typing include anti-P1 and anti-M (Chapter 6). Rarely, an antibody to a low-incidence antigen can be the problem. The panel cell testing (Chapter 8) will usually be completely negative in the case of an antibody to a low-incidence antigen, whereas the panel results for Anti-P1 or Anti-M would have positive reactions with several cells. If an ABO discrepancy is due to an antibody to a low-incidence antigen is suspected, a viable course of action would be to test several different examples of A or B cells. If all the cells except the original A or B cells test negative, then the original A or B cells may be positive for a low-incidence antigen. The patient/donor's antibody can be identified by setting up examples of cells that are known to be positive for low-incidence antigens, if available. Often this is done by a referral laboratory. Also contact the manufacturer of the reverse cells, as they may choose to not use that donor in the future for reverse grouping cells.

Cold-reactive autoagglutinins and cold-reactive alloantibodies can sometimes be neutralized in the ABO testing by prewarming the plasma and cells before combining them. Rather than centrifuging the tests, which would expose the antibody–cell combination to room temperature, allow the cells to settle to the bottom of the tube

✳ **TABLE 4-18** Plasma Reaction Pattern in the Identification of anti-A_1

A_1 Positive Cells	A_1 Negative Cells	O Cells	Interpretation
+	0	0	Anti-A_1
Some or all +	+ or 0	Some or all +	Antibody other than anti-A_1 alone or in combination with anti-A_1
0	+ or 0	Some or all +	Antibody other than anti-A_1
0	0	0	Likely an antibody to a low-incidence antigen

by incubating at 98.6° F (37° C) for 1 hour. The agglutination seen may not be as strong as when the test is centrifuged; therefore, weakly reactive ABO antibodies may not be detected. If prewarming does not work and the patient has not been recently transfused, a cold **autoabsorption** can be performed to remove the autoagglutinin from the plasma. The absorbed plasma is then used in the ABO test. Cold agglutinins that can interfere in ABO testing include anti-I and anti-IH.

If rouleaux is suspected, a saline replacement technique can be used to disperse the nonspecific agglutination. Box 4-1 lists some instances where rouleaux may be present. In this technique, plasma and cells are allowed to react. The combination is centrifuged and the plasma carefully removed. Saline is added equal to the amount of plasma removed and the cells are resuspended in the saline before being centrifuged again. True agglutination should remain but agglutination due to excess protein or other high-molecular-weight substances should disappear.

In rare cases, patients/donors develop an antibody to one of the chemicals that is in the solution in which the reverse cells are suspended. Often the same diluent is used for other blood bank tests (specifically antibody screening and panel cells), causing false-positive results in these tests. The autocontrol and serologic crossmatch with donor cells will be negative. Repeating the testing using washed screening and panel cells will resolve the ABO discrepancy and will allow underlying alloantibodies to be detected.

Table 4-19 ✷ is an example of a testing algorithm for resolving a discrepancy with an unexpected positive reaction in the reverse group.

BOX 4-1   Clues to Presence of Rouleaux

Suspect rouleaux if all transfusion medicine tests that use the patient's plasma are positive:

- For example, in tube testing: reverse ABO group, immediate spin crossmatch but not the indirect antiglobulin (IAT) phase of antibody screens or crossmatches.

And one or more of the following:

- Patient has multiple myeloma or Waldenström's macroglobulinemia or other disease that results in high serum protein concentrations or the presence of abnormal serum proteins.
- Microscopically, the agglutination looks like stacks of coins. This is more easily seen on a fixed slide prepared for a white blood cell differential than in the transfusion medicine test tube.
- On some automated hematology instruments, rouleaux or cold agglutinins will cause an abnormally high MCHC.
- Patient has received a plasma volume expander that contains high-molecular-weight substances (e.g., dextran).

☑ CHECKPOINT 4-8

When is saline replacement performed?

CASE IN POINT (continued)

You are performing the type and crossmatch on GB's blood and begin with the ABO typing. You set up your testing per laboratory protocol and obtain the following results:

Patient cells (unknown) + Reagent antisera as noted below (known)			Patient plasma (unknown) + Reagent cells as noted below (known)	
Anti-A	Anti-B	Anti-D**	A₁ Cells	B Cells
4+	0	4+	1+	4+

**This test is performed to determine the presence or absence of the D antigen and to determine the "positive" or "negative" component of a complete blood type (see Chapter 5).

2. How should these results be interpreted?
3. What is the next logical step you should take?

Mixed-Field Agglutination

Mixed field agglutination is seen when a sample has two different cell populations. The most common cause of mixed field agglutination occurs when a nongroup O patient has received an emergency transfusion of group O cells. In order to avoid the chance of intravascular hemolysis, only group O red blood cells are transfused in emergency situations when testing on a current sample is not complete. Group O cells are also used for intrauterine transfusions and exchange transfusions. Feto–maternal bleeding causes exchange of cells between mother and child. If mother and baby have different ABO groups and the bleed is large, it can cause a mixed field agglutination pattern, particularly in samples from the newborn. In all these cases, the mixed-field reaction is transient and will disappear once the transfused cells die.

ABO nonidentical bone marrow or hematopoietic progenitor cell transplantation can also result in two cell populations. This is usually transient but persists in a subgroup of patients. Other causes of mixed-field agglutination in the ABO forward group include weak ABO subgroups, chimerism, and mosaicism. Chimerism occurs when fraternal twins exchange blood-forming cells *in utero* or when two different populations of cells (donor and recipient) reside together in the bone marrow after transplantation. Mosaicism occurs when two sperm fertilize one egg (dispermy). Mixed-field agglutination due to chimerism or mosaicism exists throughout the patient/donor's life. In addition, antigens on both cell populations are considered self by the person's immune system and therefore no corresponding ABO antibodies are made.

★ **TABLE 4-19** Example Testing Algorithm for Resolution of Unexpected Positive Result in Reverse Group Using Tube Testing

Step 1	Repeat testing.
	Check specimen labeling.
	Check for transcription and/or interpretation errors.
	Check equipment and reagent quality control results.
	Obtain patient diagnosis and transfusion/transplantation history.
Step 2	If anti-A_1 is suspected, follow steps to identify anti-A_1.
Step 3	If discrepancy is not resolved and rouleaux is suspected, repeat reverse group using a saline replacement technique.
Step 4	If discrepancy is not resolved, repeat reverse group using a prewarm technique.
Step 5	If discrepancy is not resolved and alloantibody is suspected, identify alloantibody by testing screening and panel cells at room temperature.
	If alloantibody is identified, type reverse cell(s) for the corresponding antigen and repeat the reverse group using cells that are negative for the corresponding antigen.
Step 6	If discrepancy does not appear to be due to blood group antibody, repeat reverse group using washed reagent cells.
Step 7	If discrepancy not resolved:
	Consider if discrepancy may be in forward group.
	If transfusion required before discrepancy is resolved or if discrepancy is not resolved:
	Issue only group O red blood cell units.

CASE IN POINT *(continued)*

You determine that the patient's antibody screen is negative, repeat the ABO testing on GB's sample, and rule out all technical errors and reagent problems. Your repeat ABO results match the original results:

Anti-A	Anti-B	Anti-D**	A_1 Cell	B Cell
4+	0	4+	1+	4+

**This test is performed to determine the presence or absence of the D antigen and to determine the "positive" or "negative" component of a complete blood type (see Chapter 5).

4. Into which category of ABO discrepancy does this sample likely fit?
   (a) Missing or weak reaction in the reverse group
   (b) Missing or weak reaction in the forward group
   (c) Unexpected positive reaction in the reverse group
   (d) Unexpected positive reaction in the forward group

5. What are some possible causes for these results?

Technical Errors

No matter which type of discrepancy is discovered, a good first step in the resolution is to repeat the testing. This will resolve many technical errors such as forgetting to add plasma or antiserum, over- or under-centrifuging, making the cell suspension too heavy or too light, and recording or interpreting the results incorrectly. It is unlikely, but not impossible, that the same technical error would occur twice in a row.

As previously alluded to, if the testing is done using serum, red blood cells may stick to small fibrin clots that are present.

This may be misinterpreted as agglutination. Although serum was commonly used in the past, most laboratories today use plasma for blood bank testing. This is especially true if the testing is automated.

An ABO discrepancy, especially between current and historical results, can also be a warning that a specimen has been mislabeled. Drawing and testing a new sample can shed light on what may have occurred. If testing of a new sample shows that a specimen mix-up likely occurred, it is important to remember to redraw and/or retest other samples that were collected at the same time as the original ABO sample. These specimens could be part of the label or sample switch that is not apparent until testing is repeated on new specimens, especially when there are no previous results available for comparison.

It is also good laboratory practice to check the reagent control results when a discrepancy occurs. Decreasing strength of reaction over time could indicate a contaminated or expired reagent. Also check the expiration date and appearance of reagents. Signs of contamination can include cloudiness, changes in color, or hemolysis. Similar ABO discrepancies on sequential samples may indicate an equipment problem, for example, centrifuge overdue for calibration. Perform appropriate tests to identify the problem and take the steps to repair and revalidate the equipment.

Resolution Strategies

Common causes and resolution strategies were discussed earlier by category. There are a few global rules to keep in mind:

1. Always check the manufacturer's instructions when using commercial reagents and cells. Some resolution strategies may not be appropriate with all testing methodologies.
2. Run appropriate controls.
3. Always follow your laboratory's operating procedure. The order of steps will vary from laboratory to laboratory.

Although example testing algorithms are available in various textbooks or generic procedures, each laboratory must consider the characteristics that make them unique when writing their own procedure. This can include their initial methodology, their patient or donor population, and the techniques, reagents, and expertise available to them. For example, the ABO discrepancy resolution procedure for a large donor center that tests healthy donors by automated gel testing will be different from the procedure used by a hospital laboratory that tests mostly oncology/hematology patients by a manual tube method.

CASE IN POINT (continued)

You test the patient's red blood cells against the A_1 lectin (*Dolichos biflorus*) and do not see agglutination. Next, you test the patient's plasma against three different lot numbers of A_1, A_2, and group O commercial cells and obtain the following results:

	A_1 Cell	A_2 Cell	O Cell
Lot 1	1+	0	0
Lot 2	1+	0	0
Lot 3	1+	0	0

6. Given these results, what type is the patient and what is the most likely cause of the ABO discrepancy?
7. What ABO type(s) of blood should be prepared and tested (called *compatibility testing* or *crossmatching*; Chapter 7) for the patient and why?

Unresolved Discrepancies

Sometimes an ABO discrepancy will not be resolved with additional testing. Even deciding whether it is likely the forward or reverse grouping (or both) that is discrepant can remain a mystery in some patients. In order to avoid the chance of an acute hemolytic transfusion reaction, most laboratories will transfuse only group O red blood cell units and group AB plasma products to patients who have an unresolved ABO typing discrepancy. Group O red blood cells have neither A nor B antigens; therefore they can be transfused to a patient of any ABO blood type (except Bombay). Similarly, group AB plasma lacks both anti-A and anti-B and therefore can be transfused to a patient of any ABO blood group. Blood components from donors with unresolved ABO discrepancies are likely to be diverted for nontransfusion purposes.

☑ CHECKPOINT 4-9

What type of red blood cells should be transfused to a patient with an unresolved ABO discrepancy? What type of plasma should be transfused to a patient with an unresolved ABO discrepancy?

CASE IN POINT (continued)

GB undergoes her hip replacement surgery and is transfused 3 units of group O packed red blood cells during the procedure. Three days after her surgery she is still very tired and experiences shortness of breath and dizziness during physical therapy. Her physician notes that her morning hemoglobin was 7.8 g/dL (78 g/L) and decides to transfuse 1 additional unit of red blood cells to help alleviate symptoms. Her pre-op crossmatch sample has expired so a new sample is sent to the blood bank for testing. Her ABO results are as follows:

Anti-A	Anti-B	Anti-D	A_1 Cell	B Cell
2+MF	0	4+	1+	3+

8. What is the most likely cause of the mixed-field result with anti-A?
9. What type of red blood cells should be given?

TRANSPLANTS AND THE ABO BLOOD GROUP SYSTEM

The ABO blood group plays a critical role in a variety of successful transplants, such as blood (transfusion), kidney, liver, and heart (except in newborns). However, ABO compatibility is not necessary in hematopoietic progenitor cell (HPC) transplants, sometimes referred to as stem cell transplants. These transplants include bone marrow and cells collected by *apheresis* (a process by which whole blood is removed from a donor, the desired component is harvested for future use, and the remainder of the blood is returned to the donor) such as peripheral blood stem cells and cells collected from cord blood. Patients receiving nonidentical ABO HPC transplants will switch their ABO group from their own genetic type to the donor type over time. This will cause various types of ABO discrepancies.

Although ABO-incompatible HPC transplants can be successful, these patients are at increased risk for hemolysis of patient or donor red blood cells or delayed engraftment of donor red blood cells.[13] Neutrophil and platelet engraftment are not affected by ABO incompatibility. If the recipient has antibodies to the donor's red blood cell antigens, the mismatch is said to be a major ABO incompatibility. Any donor red blood cells present in the HPC would be rapidly hemolyzed if they were not removed during processing of the product. The recipient's antibody may be made for 3 or 4 months after transplantation and may cause delay of red blood cell engraftment for 40 days or longer. Hemolysis of the engrafted donor red blood cells will occur until the recipient's antibodies are no longer present.

A minor ABO incompatibility is present when the donor has antibodies to the recipient's red blood cell antigens. The donor plasma can be removed along with the antibody to the recipient's red blood cells. However, about 10–15% of patients will have hemolysis of the recipient's red blood cells beginning around day 7 and lasting about 2 weeks, due to donor lymphocytes making ABO antibodies. The direct antiglobulin test (DAT) is positive and an elution will recover the anti-A and/or anti-B. The recipient may have free hemoglobin in the plasma or urine. Another 30% of patients may be DAT positive without evidence of gross hemolysis. A recipient and donor may have both a major and minor incompatibility, such as an A recipient receiving a B bone marrow product.

Transfusion of transplant recipients can be divided into three stages: before transplantation, after transplantation but before complete engraftment, and after complete engraftment. A process that involves gamma or electron treatment of cellular blood products, known as *irradiation*, coupled with the removal of the majority of white blood cells results in a product called *irradiated, leukoreduced cellular blood product*. This type of product, compatible with the recipient's ABO type, is given to such patients during preparation for transplantation to reduce the possibility of a condition known as *graft versus host disease* (a condition in which grafted tissue attacks host tissue. After the patient has been transplanted until the recipient's red blood cells are no longer detectable (forward type is now the donor's), the patient's DAT is negative and the recipient's antibodies are no longer found (reverse type has also become the donor's), blood products must be compatible with both the donor and the recipient. Some centers give all transplant patients in this stage O red blood cells and AB plasma products. Table 4-20 ✳ illustrates another option for selecting products. Once the forward and reverse ABO groups are both consistent with the donor's type, blood products compatible with the donor's ABO type are utilized, as engraftment is complete. Irradiated, leukoreduced products are used throughout the transplantation process to prevent transfusion-associated graft versus host disease or production of new human leukocyte antigen alloantibodies.

Processing of the HPCs and transfusion of blood products that are compatible with both recipient and donor types reduce the risks of delayed engraftment and hemolysis. Transfusion of blood components that are not identical to the patient's ABO group can result in mixed-field agglutination in the forward group and weaker reactions in the reverse group. As the HPC engraftment progresses, any ABO-incompatible antibodies will begin to disappear from the patient's plasma. This may present as missing or weak reactions in the reverse group alone or in combination with unusual reactions in the forward group.

Once the incompatible ABO antibodies are gone, red blood cells of the donor's ABO group will become detectable. This may be seen as mixed-field agglutination or a weaker reaction in the forward group. In the long term there will be differences between current ABO typing and historical (pretransplant) ABO typing results. Laboratory professionals who work in facilities that do not perform HPC transplants should still be aware of the effect of ABO nonidentical transplants because patients may return to their communities and their community hospitals for supportive care post-transplant. Patients who have had HPC transplants are at risk for graft versus host disease and should receive irradiated cellular blood components.

☑ CHECKPOINT 4-10

What type of mismatch is present if group O donor hematopoietic progenitor cells are transplanted to a group A recipient?

ABO HEMOLYTIC DISEASE OF THE FETUS AND NEWBORN

Hemolytic disease of the fetus and newborn (HDFN) is caused by maternal IgG antibodies crossing the placenta and causing hemolysis of the baby's cells with the corresponding antigen (Chapter 14). ABO HDFN is a relatively common cause of jaundice in the

---

✳ **TABLE 4-20** Selection of Blood Products in Patients with ABO Mismatched Allogeneic Human Progenitor Cell Transplant

Type of Mismatch	Recipient/ Donor ABO Type	Transfuse		
		Red Blood Cells	Platelets (in order of choice)	Plasma
Minor	A / O	O	A > AB > B > O	A, AB
Minor	B / O	O	B > AB > A > O	B, AB
Minor	AB / O	O	AB > A > B > O	AB
Minor	AB / A	A	AB > A > B > O	AB
Minor	AB / B	B	AB > B > A > O	AB
Major	O / A	O	A > AB > B > O	A, AB
Major	O / B	O	B > AB > A > O	B, AB
Major	O / AB	O	AB > A > B > O	AB
Major	A / AB	A	AB > A > B > O	AB
Major	B / AB	B	AB > B > A > O	AB
Major and minor	A / B	O	AB > A > B > O	AB
Major and minor	B / A	O	AB > B > A > O	AB

newborn. Luckily, the jaundice is rarely severe enough to require aggressive medical intervention, unlike HDFN that is caused by Rh antibodies (Chapter 5). ABO HDFN occurs most commonly when the mother is group O because group O people make more IgG ABO antibodies. However, any combination of ABO groups where the mother makes an antibody that is on the baby's cells can result in HDFN.

TRANSFUSION REACTIONS AND ABO BLOOD GROUP SYSTEM

The three leading causes of transfusion-associated deaths are transfusion-related acute lung injury, immediate hemolytic transfusion reactions, and bacterial contamination[23] (Chapter 12). Transfusion of ABO-incompatible red blood cells is the most common cause of immediate hemolytic transfusion reactions. Transfusion of ABO-incompatible blood may occur as a result of errors in specimen collection and labeling, testing, and reporting of ABO results; labeling of blood components; and/or identification of the patient prior to administration of the blood product.

Symptoms of an immediate hemolytic transfusion reaction include fever, chills, pain at the intravenous site, back pain, anxiety, hypotension, hemoglobinuria, renal failure, and disseminated intravascular coagulation (DIC). The symptoms are caused by the interaction of ABO antibodies with the corresponding antigens on the transfused red blood cells, which leads to activation of the complement cascade, activation of the coagulation cascade, and release of cytokines.

Most of the immediate testing done when a suspected transfusion reaction has occurred is performed in order to rule out an immediate hemolytic transfusion reaction. This includes identification checks of the patient, donor unit, and samples; examination of the post-transfusion plasma for visible hemolysis; repeat ABO testing; and performance of a direct antiglobulin test (DAT). If the investigation indicates that an ABO-incompatible transfusion has occurred, the patient should be monitored closely so aggressive therapy to combat shock, kidney failure, and DIC can be initiated as required.

Review of the Main Points

- ABO genes are co-dominant.
- O, h, and se genes are amorphs.
- A, B, H, and Se genes code for enzymes that attach immunodominant sugars to precursor substances.
- Immunodominant sugar for H is L-fucose, for A is N-acetyl-galactosamine, and B is D-galactose.
- H antigen is the precursor for A and B antigens.
- Enzyme coded for by H acts on type 2 precursor substance on red blood cells and enzyme coded for by Se acts on type 1 precursor substance in secretions.
- Eighty percent of people have at least one Se gene. They are called secretors and ABO antigens are present in their secretions.
- Bombay phenotype is caused by hh and sese genotype. No H and therefore no ABO antigens are produced.
- People with Bombay phenotype make a naturally occurring, hemolytic anti-H.
- Para-Bombay phenotype is caused by hh and Sese or SeSe genotype. Their red blood cells lack H and ABO antigens but their secretions have the antigens.
- ABO antigens on red blood cells exist as glycoproteins, glycolipids, and glycosphingolipids. ABO antigens in secretions exist as glycoproteins, glycolipids, and oligosaccharides.
- ABO antigen frequency is approximately 45% group O, 40% group A, 10 % group B, and 5% group AB.
- A_1 and A_2 are the common subgroups of A.
- Approximately 20% of group A and AB people are A_2. A_2 and A_2B people can make an anti-A_1.

- There are rare weaker subgroups of A and weak subgroups of B.
- ABO antibodies are naturally occurring IgM and IgG.
- ABO antibodies bind complement and cause intravascular hemolysis.
- The ABO blood group test consists of a forward and reverse group. Forward group identifies the ABO antigen on patient/donor cells using known (commercial) antisera. Reverse group identifies the ABO antibodies in the patient/donor plasma using known (commercial) cells.
- An ABO discrepancy occurs when the forward and reverse grouping results do not correlate. Further investigation must be performed before the ABO blood group is interpreted.
- ABO discrepancies fall into four categories:
    1. Weak or missing reaction in the forward grouping
    2. Weak or missing reaction in the reverse grouping
    3. Unexpected positive reaction in the forward grouping
    4. Unexpected positive reaction in the reverse grouping.
- ABO blood group system compatibility is critical for many transplant procedures, not including hematopoietic progenitor cell transplants.
- Patients who have received an ABO nonidentical hematopoietic progenitor cell transplant can change ABO types.
- ABO antibodies can cause hemolytic disease of the fetus and newborn.
- ABO-incompatible blood transfusions result in immediate hemolytic transfusion reactions, which can be fatal.

Review Questions

1. The immunodominant sugar for blood type B is _____. (Objective #2)

   A. N-acetyl-D-galactosamine

   B. L-fucose

   C. D-galactose

   D. All of the above

2. The H gene codes for _____, which adds L-fucose to a precursor carbohydrate chain to form the H antigen. (Objective #2)

   A. α-1,2-L-fucosyltransferase

   B. α-1,3-N-acetyl-galactosaminyltransferase

   C. α-1,3-D-galactosyl transferase

   D. α-1,3-N-acetyl-glucosamine

3. The frequency of blood type AB in the general population is: (Objective #5)

   A. 10%

   B. 7%

   C. 4%

   D. 1%

4. Weak subgroups of A can be identified through all of the following *except:* (Objective #10)

   A. Strength of reaction with anti-H lectin

   B. Presence or absence of anti-A_1

   C. Strength of reaction with human source anti-A, anti-B, and anti-A,B

   D. Absence of Lewis substance in the saliva of secretors

5. Characteristics of antibodies of the ABO blood group system include all of the following *except:* (Objective #13)

   A. Naturally occurring

   B. Present at birth

   C. Mainly IgM class

   D. Activate complement

6. The genotype of a para-Bombay individual is: (Objective #9)

   A. *hh, Sese*

   B. *HH, Sese*

   C. *hh, sese*

   D. *Hh, Sese*

7. The following reactions were observed in an ABO typing test: (Objective #16)

Forward Group		Reverse Group	
Anti-A	Anti-B	A1 cells	B cells
0	4+	0	0

   Before reporting blood typing results, the laboratorian should:

   A. Perform the saline replacement test

   B. Type the patient red blood cells with *Dolichos biflorus*

   C. Wash patient red blood cells four times and repeat

   D. Incubate reverse typing for 15 minutes at 39.2° F (4° C)

8. Causes of unexpected positive reactions in the forward grouping include: (Objective #15)

   A. Contamination with Wharton's jelly

   B. Presence of cold autoantibody

   C. Subgroup of A

   D. Age of the patient

9. Which of the following statements is true regarding ABO-*incompatible* hematopoietic progenitor cell (HPC) transplants? (Objective #18)

   A. Results in immediate engraftment of donor red blood cells to the recipient

   B. Causes various types of ABO discrepancies

   C. Causes red blood cell hemolysis

   D. Are usually fatal

10. The forward grouping test identifies which of the following red blood cell antigens? (Objective #14)

    A. A

    B. B

    C. A and B

    D. A, B, and H

11. Which of the following statements is true regarding the characteristics of the Bombay and para-Bombay phenotypes? (Objective #7)

    A. Occurs in 1% of the population and most frequently in Indian and Japanese ethnicities.

    B. Occurs in 1% of the population and least often in Indian and Japanese ethnicities.

    C. Occurs in 0.1% of the population and most frequently in Indian and Chinese ethnicities.

    D. Occurs in 0.1% of the population and most frequently in Indian and Japanese ethnicities.

12. The genetic difference between the most common gene responsible for group O and the *A101* gene is: (Objective #3)

    A. Deletion of cytosine at position 261

    B. Deletion of guanine at position 261

    C. Addition of cytosine at position 261

    D. Addition of guanine at position 261

13. Which of the following statements is true regarding poly-agglutination? (Objective #17)

    A. Tx is a bacterially acquired and transient cause of polyagglutination.

    B. Tn is a bacterially acquired and transient cause of polyagglutination.

    C. Hemoglobin M-Hyde Park is an inherited and transient cause of polyagglutination.

    D. Hemoglobin S is an inherited and permanent cause of polyagglutination.

14. The B phenotype within the United States is: (Objective #7)

    A. More common in people of European and African descent than those of Hispanic descent

    B. More common in people of Hispanic and African descent than those of Asian descent

    C. More common in people of Asian and African descent than those of European descent

    D. More common in people of Europeon and Hispanic descent than in those of African descent

15. If a cis-AB male and a group O female have a baby, the baby's phenotype could be which of the following? (Objective #12)

    A. A, B, O, or AB

    B. A, B, or AB

    C. A or B

    D. AB or O

References

1. Landsteiner K. Über aggluntinationserscheinugen normalen menschlichen blutes. [Agglutination phenomena in normal human blood.] *Wien Klin Wochenschr* 1901; 14: 1132–4.

2. von Decastello A, Stürli A. Über die isoaggluntinie im serum gesunder und kranker menschen. [Concerning isoagglutinins in serum of healthy and sick humans.] *München Med Wochenschr* 1902; 26: 1090–5.

3. Westerveld A, Jongsma AP, Meera Khan P, van Someren H, Bootsma D. Assignment of the AK1:Np:ABO linkage group to human chromosome 9. (Abstract) *Proc Natl Acad Sci USA* 1976; 73: 895–9.

4. Morgan WTJ, Watkins WM. Unravelling the biochemical basis of blood group ABO and Lewis antigenic specificity. *Glycoconj J* 2000; 17: 501–30.

5. Larsen RD, Ernst LK, Nair RP, Lowe JB. Molecular cloning, sequence and expression of a human GDP-L-fucose: β-D-galactoside 2-α-L-fucosyltransferase cDNA that can form the H blood group antigen. *Proc Natl Acad Sci USA* 1990; 87: 6674–8.

6. Reid ME, Lomas-Francis C. *The Blood Group Antigen Facts Book*, 2nd ed., New York: Elsevier Academic Press; 2004.

7. Yamamoto F, Marken J, Tsuji T, White T, Clausen H, Hakomori S. Cloning and characterization of DNA complementary to human UDP-GalNAc:Fuc α1 → 2Galα1 → 3GalNAc transferase (Histo-blood group A transferase) mRNA. *J Biol Chem* 1990; 265: 1146–51.

8. Yamamoto F, Hakomori S. Sugar-nucleotide donor specificity of histo-blood group A and B transferases is based on amino acid substitutions. *J Biol Chem* 1990; 31: 19257–62.

9. Yamamoto F, Clausen H, White T, Marken J, Hakomori S. Molecular genetic basis of the histo-blood group ABO system. *Nature* 1990; 345: 229–33.

10. Geoff Daniels. *Human Blood Groups*, 2nd ed. Malden (MA): Blackwell Science; 2002.

11. Garratty G, Glynn SA, McEntire R for the Retrovirus Epidemiology Donor Study. ABO and Rh (D) phenotype frequencies of different racial/ethnic groups in the United States. *Transfusion* 2004; 44: 703–6.

12. Clausen H, Levery SB, Nudelman E, Tsuchiya S, Hakomori S. Repetitive A epitope (type 3 chain A) defined by blood group A1-specific monoclonal antibody TH-1: chemical basis of qualitative A1 and A2 distinction. *Proc Natl Acad Sci USA* 1985; 82: 1199–1203.

13. Roback JD, et al. *Technical Manual*, 16th ed. Bethesda (MD): AABB; 2008.

14. Harmening D. *Modern blood banking and transfusion practices*, 5th ed. Philadelphia (PA): F.A. Davis; 2005.

15. Oriol R, Danilovs J, Hawkins BR. A new genetic model proposing that the *Se* gene is a structural gene closely linked to the *H* gene. *Am J Hum Genet* 1981; 33: 421–31.

16. Kelly RH, Ernst LK, Larsen RD, Bryant JG, Robinson JS, Lowe JB. Molecular basis for H blood group deficiency in Bombay (O_h) and para-Bombay individuals. *Proc Natl Acad Sci USA* 1994; 91: 5843–7.

17. Yoshida A, Yamaguchi H, Okubo Y. Genetic mechanisms of cis-AB inheritance. II. Cases associated with structural mutation of blood group glycosyltransferase. *Am J Hum Genet* 1980; 32: 645–50.

18. Yoshida A, Yamaguchi H, Okubo Y. Genetic mechanisms of cis-AB inheritance. I. A case associated with unequal chromosomal crossing over. *Am J Hum Genet* 1980; 32: 332–8.

19. Lapierre Y, Rigal D, Adam J, Josef D, Meyer F, Greber S, Drot C. The gel test: a new way to detect red cell antigen–antibody reactions. *Transfusion* 1990; 30: 109–13.

20. Obhrai JS, Lakkis FG. Transplantation tolerance: Babies take the first step. *Nat Med* 2004; 10: 1165–6.

21. Beck ML, Kowalski MA, Kirkegaard JR, Korth JL. Unexpected activity with monoclonal anti-B reagents [Letter]. *Immunohematology* 1992; 8: 22.

22. Beck ML, Yates AD, Hardman J, Kowalski MA. Identification of a subset of group B donors reactive with monoclonal anti-A reagent. *Am J Clin Pathol* 1989; 92: 625–9.

23. US Food and Drug Administration [Internet]. FDA's safety surveillance system for blood and blood products. Presentation by Robert Wise, Office of biostatistics and epidemiology, CBER, FDA to the Advisory Committee on Blood Safety and Availability, 2005. [updated 16 May 2005; cited 12 Dec 2006]. Available from: www.hhs.gov/bloodsafety/presentations/Wise.pdf

Additional Resources

1. Chester MA, Olsson ML. The ABO blood group gene: A locus of considerable genetic diversity. *Transfus Med Review* 2001; 15: 177–200.

2. Garratty G. In vitro reactions with red blood cells that are not due to blood group antibodies: A review. *Immunohematology* 1998; 14: 1–11.

3. Lee AH, Reid ME. ABO blood group system: a review of molecular aspects. *Immunohematology* 2000; 16: 1–6.

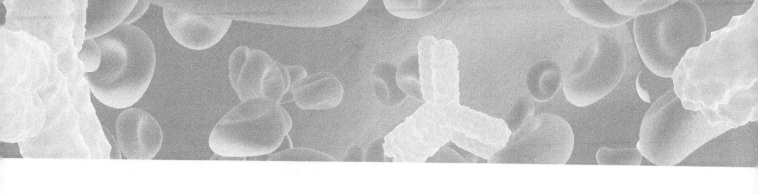

5

Rh, RHAG, and LW Blood Group Systems

KAREN McCLURE

Chapter Objectives

Upon completion of this chapter, the student will be able to:

1. List the three major allele groups in the Rh system.
2. Recognize other unusual Rh phenotypes and rare alleles: C^w, f (ce), Ce, G, Rh null.
3. Describe the biochemistry of the Rh system antigens.
4. Describe the genetics of the Rh system.
5. Explain the relationship of the RHAG and Rh blood group systems.
6. Describe the different genetic mutations resulting in deletions and Rh_{null}.
7. Compare and contrast the Fisher-Race, Wiener, Rosenfield, and ISBT nomenclature systems.
8. Convert members of the Rh blood group system between the Fisher-Race and Wiener nomenclature systems.
9. Convert between the genotypes and phenotypes of the Rh blood group system.
10. Identify the variations of the D antigen.
11. Compare and contrast the theories on weak and partial D expression.
12. Describe the role of Rh-associated glycoprotein in Rh antigen expression.
13. Recognize the sources of possible error in determining Rh status and identify appropriate corrective action(s).
14. Describe the purpose and use of Rh control.
15. Compare different types of Rh antisera.
16. Describe the Rh system antibodies, including reactivity patterns and characteristics.
17. Discuss the role of Rh system antibodies in hemolytic disease of the fetus and newborn (HDFN).
18. Discuss the role of the Rh system antibodies in transfusion reactions.
19. Estimate the most probable genotype of an individual, given the reactions with Rh antisera.
20. Briefly discuss the history of the Rh and LW systems.

Key Terms

Cell culture(s)
Exon
Hybridoma
Ion channel(s)
Monoclonal
Nonglycosylated
Nucleotide(s)
Syntenic

CASE IN POINT

TT is a 6-month-old child who was diagnosed with sickle cell disease during his routine newborn screening. His pediatrician believes the child will need routine blood transfusions. He orders an Rh phenotype and requests that all subsequent blood transfusions be phenotypically matched for the Rh antigens. A blood sample is collected, properly labeled, and submitted to the transfusion medicine laboratory for testing.

What's Ahead?

The Rh blood group system is the second most important in terms of immunogencity, rivaled only by the ABO system. In European and American transfusion services, "Rh typing" for the D antigen combined with ABO grouping is the most basic of transfusion medicine tests. This chapter addresses the following questions regarding the Rh and related blood group systems:

- What events led to the discovery of the D antigens, and LW antigens?
- What is the current genetic model for the Rh blood group system?
- What is the relationship between the Rh and RHAG blood group systems?
- What are the older genetic theories for the Rh blood group system and how are they used in the modern transfusion service?
- What are the characteristics of Rh and LW antigens and antibodies?
- What tests are used for Rh blood group system antigen typing?
- What is the clinical significance of Rh blood group system antibodies?
- How is immunization to the D antigen prevented?

HISTORICAL BACKGROUND

In 1941, Landsteiner and Wiener discovered an antibody produced by rabbits and guinea pigs when they were exposed to rhesus monkey red blood cells.[1] These researchers went on to describe an antibody that reacted with 85% of the human red blood cells against which it was tested. Early speculation was that this antibody was the same one that Levine and Stetson had identified as causing hemolytic disease of the fetus and newborn (HDFN) in 1939.[2] Their case involved a woman who delivered a child affected by HDFN (Chapter 14). Post-delivery, she received a transfusion of blood from her husband and experienced a hemolytic transfusion reaction (Chapter 12). Levine and Stetson hypothesized that there was a "factor" in the husband's blood that was passed to the child; the mother was reacting to this "factor," therefore leading to both problems observed. We now know they hypothesized correctly.

The antibody was termed anti-D, named after the rhesus monkey in which it was first thought to be discovered. However, the antibody associated with the monkeys was really anti-LW and not anti-D, but this discovery was not to be made until many years later. The antibody formed by the rabbits and guinea pigs was then renamed anti-LW after the researchers Landsteiner and Wiener and the antibody described by Levine and Stetson in the HDFN and hemolytic transfusion reaction case kept the name anti-D.

☑ CHECKPOINT 5-1

What was the *original name* of the antibody made by rabbits when exposed to rhesus monkey red blood cells?

What is the *current name* of the antibody made by rabbits when exposed to rhesus monkey red blood cells?

Research into the Rh blood group system has discovered a wonderfully complex genetic interplay resulting in more than 50 known antigens, including low incidence, high incidence, compound, and the five common antigens: D, C, c, E, and e.

RHD and *RHCE* Genes

In 1986, Tippett postulated that Rh genetic expression was controlled by two closely linked genes called *RHD* and *RHCE*.[3] In 1991, Southern blot testing confirmed that the Rh locus of D-positive individuals is composed of two different but related genes.[4] Molecular analysis has helped to explain the genetic control of the expression of the Rh antigens and also to support Tippett's theory. However, it is important to note that prior to Tippett's theory, two other mechanisms of Rh inheritance were proposed: one by Fisher and Race and the other by Wiener.[5, 6] These theories gave rise to Rh terminology still in use today.

The two *Rh* genes are located on chromosome 1.[7] The *RHD* gene codes for the D antigen only. There is a small piece of almost identical DNA code on either side of the *RHD* gene; these are called rhesus boxes. If the *RHD* gene and therefore the D antigen are present, the individual is called Rh positive or, more correctly, D positive; if the D antigen is absent the individual is called D negative. There is no d antigen, unlike the allelic pairs of C/e and E/e. To express the absence of the D antigen, a lowercase *d* is used in some terminologies. Therefore, the "*d*" allele can be considered an amorph. The absence of the D antigen occurs most commonly when the *RHD* gene is deleted. However, nonfunctional, mutated, or partial *RHD* alleles, which result in a Rh(D)-negative phenotype, have also been described.[8]

The *RHCE* gene codes for the RHCE protein that carries both the C/c and E/e antigens. There are multiple alleles of the *RHCE* gene, including *RHCE*, *RHcE*, *RHCe*, and *RHce*. The *RHD* and *RHCE* genes are very similar in structure, sharing about 97% of the same DNA sequence. Many of the different Rh antigens are caused by point mutations in the genes. Some less common Rh antigens result from recombination of the RHD and RHCE genes, which can occur because of the close proximity of the *RHD* and *RHCE* loci to each other.

CASE IN POINT (continued)

The venous blood sample from TT arrives in the laboratory with a request for Rh phenotype. The laboratorian notes that the baby's cord blood typed as group O at the time of birth.

1. What antigens are generally tested for when an Rh phenotype is ordered?
2. Would the laboratorian test for the d antigen? Why or why not?

☑ CHECKPOINT 5-2

What genes control the expression of the Rh antigens? List the alleles of the RHCE gene.

RhD and RhCE Proteins

The isolation and identification of Rh polypeptides was published in 1982.[9, 10] The common Rh blood group antigens are only found on the red blood cell membrane. However, other human tissues express structurally similar proteins.

The Rh proteins are **nonglycosylated**, unlike the ABO (Chapter 4) or MNS (Chapter 6) blood group antigens. Nonglycosylated means that no carbohydrate molecule, often called a sugar molecule, is attached to the protein. The proteins, like their genes, are very similar, differing by only a few amino acids. Both proteins are 417 amino acids long.[11] The difference between the RhD and RhCE proteins are the 33–35 amino acids, depending on the Rh phenotype. The D antigen has no corresponding "d" antigen. What is called "d" or "D negative" results from the lack of the D antigen, as the *RHD* gene is missing in these Rh- or D-negative people. The C and c antigens (proteins) differ from each other only by four amino acids and the E and e antigens by just a few amino acids as well. One critical amino acid change between the C and c protein (and the E and e protein) extends on the outside of the RBC membrane and causes the body to recognize the C versus the c antigen and the E versus the e antigen (Table 5-1 ✱).

✱ **TABLE 5-1** Amino Acid Changes Resulting in Cc and Ee Antigens

Antigen	Amino Acid	Position
C	Serine	103
C	Proline	103
E	Proline	226
E	Alanine	226

The RhD and RhCE proteins each pass through the membrane 12 times.[12] Figure 5-1 ■ shows a schematic of the transmembrane Rh and Rh-associated proteins. The Rh proteins likely play a structural role in the red blood cell membrane. Individuals who lack all Rh antigens, which is called the Rh$_{null}$ phenotype, have a compensated hemolytic anemia due to changes in the membrane structure that shorten survival of the red blood cells. Morphologically, the Rh$_{null}$ red blood cells are abnormal, appearing as stomatocytes.

The structure of the RhD and RhCE proteins suggest that they may also be **ion channels**. Ion channels form pores that establish and control the small voltage gradient that exists across the lipid bilayer of the red blood cell, thus allowing the flow of ions down their electrochemical gradient.[13] Proteins structurally similar to the Rh proteins act as ammonia transporters both in human tissues other than the red blood cell and in other organisms.[14] The red blood cell RhD and RhCE proteins do not transport ammonia but may act as another type of ion channel, although their exact function is still being investigated.[15]

☑ CHECKPOINT 5-3

What is the proposed function of the Rh proteins?

Rh Associated Glycoprotein (RhAG)

A third protein important for Rh antigen expression is the Rh-associated glycoprotein (RhAG). Despite the role it plays in Rh antigen expression, RhAG is not part of the Rh blood group system, but is a separate blood group system called RHAG.[16] The protein carries no Rh antigens and is coded for by a gene located on chromosome 6. As of 2010, there are two antigens recognized as being part of the RHAG system: Duclos and Ol^a.[16] Additionally, a third antigen called Duclos-like has been provisionally assigned to the RHAG blood group system. RhAG shares 40% homology with RHD and RHCE proteins.

In the absence of RhAG, multiple molecular defects in the red blood cell membrane occur. These defects include the absence of RHCE and RHD proteins, absent LW glycoproteins, and deficiency of CD47 and glycophorin B. Regulator-type RH$_{null}$ individuals have been found to harbor mutations in the *RHAG* gene, which cause nonsense, missense, and splice mutations.[17]

☑ CHECKPOINT 5-4

What non-Rh system gene is required for normal expression of Rh antigens?

Other Genetic Relationships

There are several disease-causing genes located on chromosome 1 that show linkage with the *RH* gene, but the only blood group system gene that is linked is *SC*, which determines antigens in the Scianna blood group system. The *RH* and *FY* genes are **syntenic**, which means on the same chromosome but not linked.

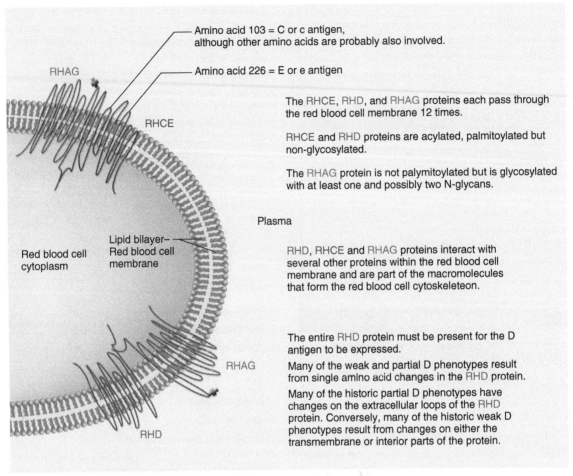

Amino acid 103 = C or c antigen, although other amino acids are probably also involved.

Amino acid 226 = E or e antigen

RHAG

RHCE

The RHCE, RHD, and RHAG proteins each pass through the red blood cell membrane 12 times.

RHCE and RHD proteins are acylated, palmitoylated but non-glycosylated.

The RHAG protein is not palymitoylated but is glycosylated with at least one and possibly two N-glycans.

Plasma

Red blood cell cytoplasm

Lipid bilayer– Red blood cell membrane

RHD, RHCE and RHAG proteins interact with several other proteins within the red blood cell membrane and are part of the macromolecules that form the red blood cell cytoskeleteon.

RHAG

The entire RHD protein must be present for the D antigen to be expressed.

Many of the weak and partial D phenotypes result from single amino acid changes in the RHD protein.

Many of the historic partial D phenotypes have changes on the extracellular loops of the RHD protein. Conversely, many of the historic weak D phenotypes result from changes on either the transmembrane or interior parts of the protein.

RHD

■ **FIGURE 5-1**   Simple Schematic of the Rh and Rh-Associated Proteins

NOMENCLATURE

While the Fisher-Race and Wiener genetic theories postulating either three or one gene have been shown to be incorrect,[4] the related terminology is still used. Table 5-2 ✳ compares the Fisher-Race, Wiener, Rosenfield, and the International Society of Blood Transfusion (ISBT) terminology for the Rh system. Each of the systems is described in the following paragraphs.

✳ **TABLE 5-2** Rh System Terminology Comparison

ISBT		Fisher-Race	Wiener	Rosenfield
Numerical	Symbol			
004001	D	D	Rh_0	Rh1
004002	C	C	rh′	Rh2
004003	E	E	rh″	Rh3
004004	C	c	hr′	Rh4
004005	E	e	hr″	Rh5
004006	f(ce)	ce	hr	Rh 6
004007	Ce	Ce	rh_i	Rh7
004008	C^w	C^w	rh^{w1}	Rh8
004009	C^x	C^x	rh^x	Rh9
004010	$V(ce^s)$	ce^s	hr^v	Rh10

Fisher–Race Terminology

Fisher and Race suggested that there were three closely linked sets of alleles within the Rh system.[5] Gene products are defined as the letters D and d, C and c, and E and e, with the "d" antigen representing an amorph. The Rh phenotype in Fisher-Race terminology is expressed as the presence or absence of D, C, c, and E, e antigens.

Wiener Terminology

Alexander Wiener postulated that individuals inherit Rh antigens as a product of a single gene at a single locus.[6] However, this single gene coded for an agglutinogen composed of multiple antigens. Major antigens were designated as Rh_0(D), rh′(C), rh″(E), hr′(c), and hr″ (e). There is also a shorthand method for indicating groups of Rh antigens found on the red blood cell. The most commonly used are $R_0 = Dce$, r = dce, $R_1 = DCe$, $R_2 = DcE$, $R_z = DCE$, r′ = dCe, r″ = dcE, and $r^y = dCE$.

☑ **CHECKPOINT 5-5**

In Wiener terminology, what is the name of the antigen that is called c in Fisher-Race terminology?

Rosenfield Terminology

In 1962, Rosenfield and his colleagues proposed a numerical model for the Rh blood group system.[18] Their impetus was the evolving complexity of the Rh system and the inadequacies of the systems in use at that time to include the new findings. The alphanumeric system provided a way to address the new antigens identified by assigning letters to the blood group and numbers to the specific antigen in the order in which they were discovered. In writing, if the red blood cells were positive for the specified antigen, the corresponding number would be included after the letter identifying the blood group system. If the red blood cells tested negative for a specific antigen, the corresponding number would be written with a minus sign in front. For example, Rh: 1,2,3,4,–5 would identify a phenotype where the cells tested positive for D, C, c, and E but negative for e.

International Society of Blood Transfusion

In 1980, the International Society of Blood Transfusion (ISBT) formed a working group to standardize nomenclature of blood group systems. The system developed is based on genetic classification. There is both an alphanumeric and strictly numeric system. The numeric system is designed for use in computer systems where letters might interfere with data manipulation. Each blood group system is numbered and given an alphabetical designation. Then each antigen within the system is sequentially numbered. The Rh system is designated either 004 or RH, and the D antigen would be RH1 or in computer code would be 004001.

Terminology Associated with the Designation of "D"

Historically, the terms D antigen and Rh factor and anti-D were used to designate the various forms of "D". Since D antigen and anti-D are part of the Rh system and the term D antigen is synonymous with the term Rh factor, more recent designations of D as Rh(D) and Rh_0(D) evolved, particularly when referring to D antigen, D antibody, and result interpretation. Thus, the new designation for the term D positive is Rh(D)/Rh_0(D) positive; D negative is Rh(D)/Rh_0(D) negative; and anti-D is anti-Rh(D)/Rh_0(D). References to variations of Rh(D)/Rh_0(D), for example weak D, remain as is except when notating result interpretation such as weak Rh_0(D) positive. The old terminology may still be used in other instances, such as on reagent vials. Because each terminology has its place in modern transfusion services and the goal here is to expose readers to all three terminologies, D and Rh(D) are used interchangeably in the rest of the chapter. D is an important concept in the Perinatal and Neonatal Transfusion Issues chapter (Chapter 14) and thus the Rh_0(D) is used that chapter.

PHENOTYPES AND GENOTYPES

The D antigen is routinely tested for in all blood donors and recipients in most countries. In some cases the Rh phenotype as defined by testing with anti-D, anti-C, anti-E, anti-c, and anti-e is performed. The genotype can only be determined either by molecular testing or by phenotyping in a family study. For example, a person phenotypes as D positive, C positive, c positive, E negative, or e positive with Rh antisera. Based on the gene frequencies given in Table 5-3 ✶, the most likely genotype is DCe/dce (R_1r). However, the patient could also be DCe/Dce (R_1R_0) or Dce/dCe (R_0r'). Table 5-4 ✶ is a more comprehensive list of Rh phenotypes and the most likely genotypes.

☑ CHECKPOINT 5-6

If an individual's red blood cells react with antisera for the D, c, E, and e antigens, what is his or her most probable genotype?

CASE IN POINT (continued)

The laboratorian tests TT's red blood cells against reagent antisera and obtains the following results:

Anti-D	Anti-C	Anti-c	Anti-E	Anti-e
4+	3+	3+	0	4+

3. What is the patient's Rh phenotype?
4. What is the most probable genotype associated with this phenotype?

✶ **TABLE 5-3** Routinely Encountered Rh Phenotypes

Nomenclature System			Frequency	
Fisher-Race	Wiener	Rosenfield	White	Black
DCe/dce	R_1r	Rh: 1,2,–3,4,5	31%	9%
DCe/DCe	R_1R_1	Rh: 1,2,–3,–4,5	18%	3%
dce/dce	Rr	Rh: –1,–2,–3, 4,5	15%	5%
DCe/DcE	R_1R_2	Rh: 1,2,3,4,5	12%	4%
DcE/dce	R_2r	Rh: 1,–2,3,4,5	10%	6%
DcE/DcE	R_2R_2	Rh: 1,–2,3,4,–5	2%	1%

✶ **TABLE 5-4** Rh Phenotypes and Genotypes

Reactions with Antisera							
D	C	E	c	e	Phenotype	Most Probable Genotype*	Shorthand Notation
+	+	+	+	+	DCEce	DCe/DcE	R_1R_2
+	+	+	+	0	DCEc	DcE/DCE	R_2R_z
+	+	+	0	+	DCEe	DCe/DCE	R_1R_z
+	+	0	+	+	DCce	DCe/dce	R_1r
+	0	+	+	+	DEce	DcE/dce	R_2r
0	+	+	+	+	CEce	dCe/dcE	r′r″
0	0	+	+	+	Ece	dcE/dce	r″r
0	0	0	+	+	ce	dce/dce	rr
+	0	0	+	+	Dce	Dce/dce	R_0r
+	+	+	0	0	DCE	DCE/DCE	R_zR_z
+	0	+	+	0	DcE	DcE/DcE	R_2R_2
0	+	0	+	+	Cce	dCe/dce	r′r

*European ethnicity

D ANTIGEN

The D antigen is very immunogenic as evidenced by the high rate of hemolytic disease of the fetus and newborn (HDFN) due to anti-D that was observed before Rh immune globulin prophylaxis became available. Rh(D)-negative recipients should receive red blood cells containing products that lack the D antigen to avoid immunization. By contrast, Rh(D)-positive individuals may receive either Rh(D)-positive or Rh(D)-negative blood products. The D antigen is expressed only on red blood cells, not on platelets, white blood, or tissue cells. The Rh(D) type is recorded on blood products such as platelets because red blood cells may be present in the product.

The number of D antigen sites on each red blood cell varies among individuals.[19] Among the more commonly encountered Rh phenotypes, the R_2R_2 phenotype possesses the most D antigen sites, with 16,000–33,000 sites per red blood cell. The Rh phenotype demonstrating the greatest number overall is the unusual D– – cell, with 100,000–200,000 D antigen sites. Red blood cells with the phenotype D– –, pronounced "D dash dash," do not possess the antigens CcEe.

☑ CHECKPOINT 5-7

What is the phenotype of the red blood cells that has the most D antigen sites?

Weakened Expression of D

The majority of Rh(D)-positive red blood cells give easily readable, macroscopic reactions when tested with anti-D. However, some individuals' cells may appear to be Rh(D) negative with some anti-D reagents and positive with others. Alternately, some individuals type as Rh(D) negative unless the Rh typing is taken through the antiglobulin phase of testing (Chapter 3). The first description of red blood cells that did not react with anti-D until the antiglobulin phase was reported by Stratton in 1946.[20] Originally given the title D^u, these cells are now referred to as weak D. There are three different mechanisms, discussed in the subsequent sections, by which D antigen expression could be reduced so that it is not detected by all anti-D reagents: (1) C in trans position to D; (2) weak D, gene variation resulting in fewer number of D antigen sites on the red blood cells; and (3) partial D, gene variation resulting in the D antigen missing one or more epitopes.

C in Trans Position to D

The *RHC* gene inherited in the trans position or on the opposite chromosome to the *RHD* gene has a suppressive effect on D antigen expression. An example of D and C being in trans position would be the genotype Dce/dCe. The D antigen produced is functionally normal, but decreased in number. These individuals do not produce anti-D. *RHC* gene in the cis position or on the same chromosome as the *RHD* gene has no suppressive affect.

Weak D

Individuals with this type of D antigen expression result from the inheritance of an *RHD* gene that codes for a reduced number of D antigens expressed. Most weak D phenotypes appear to be the product of genetic mutations that alter the Rh protein that are either inside the lipid bilayer or facing the interior of the red blood cell. Weak D is found most among people of African ethnicity and is rarely found in people of European ethnicity. The most common form of weak D identified in people of European ethnicity is weak D, type 1.

Partial D

When it was discovered that some individuals who appeared D positive could produce anti-D that reacted with most D-positive red blood cells but not their own, the idea of the D antigen being composed of multiple epitopes was born. The partial-D or D-mosaic individuals were first described in the 1950s.[21] Whether someone with a partial-D phenotype types as Rh(D) positive or negative with modern reagents depends on the particular clone or clones used in the reagent.

Molecular studies have shown that most partial-D phenotypes are due to an exchange of genetic information between *RHD* and *RHCE* genes. These may come in the form of the transfer of an entire **exon** or a partial exchange of a single **nucleotide** all the way to multiple exchanges.[22] An exon is a sequence of DNA that codes for a protein. Nucleotides are the molecules that, when present in aggregate, make up DNA. Generally, these genetic mutations appear to alter the Rh protein where it loops outside the red blood cell membrane. The most common partial-D type in people of European ethnicity is partial D, type VI. Because historic weak and partial D both result from genetic variation, some have suggested that using the term "aberrant or variant D" might be more accurate.[23]

Weak D Test

Despite the differences between historic reagents and current clonal reagents, the weak D test is still defined as an Rh(D) typing taken through an antiglobulin test phase (Chapter 3). Weak D tests must be performed on all donors. If a donor types as either D positive or weak D positive, the unit is labeled as Rh(D) positive; only when the D and weak D tests are negative is the unit given the Rh(D)-negative designation.

☑ CHECKPOINT 5-8

If a blood donor types positive with the weak D test, should the unit be labeled as Rh(D) positive or Rh(D) negative?

On the other hand, the determination of weak D status in the case of the recipient is not so clear. Some transfusion services will label a recipient Rh(D) negative if immediate spin typing for the antigen is negative. Other services will type the recipient using the weak D test as well and if positive will designate the recipient as Rh(D) positive, reasoning that the majority of weak D individuals do not produce anti-D. The decision to screen or not to screen for the weak D phenotype in transfusion recipients is established by each individual transfusion service.

Rh ANTISERA

There are three concepts associated with Rh antisera that are worthy of discussion here: clonal antisera, high- and low-protein human antisera, and the Rh control and weak D test. Each of these concepts along with sources of error are described in the following sections.

Clonal Antisera

Historically, reagent antisera, including anti-D, were made from the plasma of people who had formed the antibody of interest. Some antisera are still made this way, but clonal antisera are replacing human source antisera in many cases. Clonal antisera are made from **cell culture**, which is a cell line that is capable of growing outside a body in a liquid medium. These are often derived from cancer cells or they may be a **hybridoma**, which are two or more cell types merged into a new cell. For example, a human plasma cell that produces anti-D may be combined with a mouse cancer cell that is capable of growing in cell culture. The anti-D produced is **monoclonal** because all of the cells in the cell culture, which are called *clones*, produce the same anti-D that the parent plasma cell produced. Reagent anti-D is usually a blend of monoclonal antibodies so that the reagent can detect more than one epitope of the D antigen. This ensures that more partial-D phenotypes are identified, which is especially important when typing donors. Clonal reagent anti-D may be IgG or IgM or may be a blend of both. Rh antisera are used with tube, microplate, and gel methodologies (Chapter 3).

High- and Low-Protein Human Antisera

In the past anti-D and other Rh reagents made from human plasma were divided into high-protein and low-protein formulations. The low protein forms were sometimes called saline antisera. The low-protein formulations used either an IgG anti-D that had been chemically modified to permit a wider span of the IgG or an IgM anti-D. This allowed the anti-D to cause visible agglutination of Rh(D)-positive cells without the need for the antiglobulin phase of testing. Low-protein medium, including modern monoclonal blend reagents, do not require a specific control.

The other way that anti-D reagents were historically formulated to allow agglutination without the antiglobulin phase was to add 20–24% protein, generally albumin, and sometimes other macromolecules. This would help the red blood cells come close enough together for the IgG anti-D to span the distance between them and cause agglutination. However, any cells coated with IgG would also agglutinate. Therefore, it was important to use a control to identify potential false-positive reactions. The control usually contained everything that was in reagent antisera except the anti-D. Alternately, 20–24% albumin would be used. When using high-protein anti-D, the Rh type is only valid if the control gives a negative reaction.

Rh Control and Weak D Test

Controls are used when an Rh typing test is taken through an antiglobulin phase, including when a weak D test is performed, even when using a low-protein or clonal reagent. Cells that are already coated with IgG can give a false-positive reaction in the antiglobulin phase.

Sources of Error

As with all antisera, it is important to follow the manufacturer's directions. False-negative reactions can occur in weak D testing if the test is incubated longer than recommended. False-positive results can occur in either the immediate spin or antiglobulin phase, if

★ TABLE 5-5 Sources of Error in Rh Typing

Possible Reasons for False-Positive Reactions
Contaminated reagents
Abnormal proteins in patient/donor plasma causing rouleaux
Use of wrong antiserum
Failure to follow manufacturer's directions
Cold agglutinins, either autoagglutinins or alloagglutinins, in patient/donor's plasma
Possible Reasons for False-Negative Reactions
Failure to add antiserum
Use of wrong antiserum
Red blood cell suspension too heavy
Patient/donor red blood cells with a variant Rh antigen that does not react with the antiserum
Failure to follow manufacturer's directions

cold-reacting autoantibodies are present, or if there are abnormal concentrations of serum protein leading to rouleaux. These problems are observed when using cells suspended in human plasma; using washed patient red blood cells will eliminate the above problems. Table 5-5 ★ contains a list of sources of error in Rh typing.

> ### ☑ CHECKPOINT 5-9
>
> What type of reaction may occur if the red blood cell suspension used for Rh typing is too heavy?

OTHER Rh ANTIGENS

As of 2010, there are 50 known antigens assigned to the Rh system. Anti-D, anti-C, anti-c, anti-C^W, anti-E, and anti-e are the most frequently encountered Rh antibodies in the transfusion service. Antibodies to the other Rh system antigens are rarely encountered. For the purposes of this text, five Rh antigens other than D are described: C/c and E/e, G, C^W, f(ce), and Ce.

C/c and E/e

The C, c and E, e antigens are co-dominate alleles, thus if the gene is present for the antigen it will be expressed on the red blood cells. The C/c antigens arise from a single amino acid difference at position 103, whereas the E/e antigens are different at position 226. These antigens are less immunogenic than the D antigen. The immunogenicity of the common Rh antigens in order of ability to stimulate an antibody response is D > c > E > C > e.

G

If serine is at position 103 on the Rh polypeptide, then G antigen results; this expression may be coded for by either the *RHD* or *RHCE* gene.[24] Therefore, the G antigen is almost always found on red blood cells that also have the D and/or C antigen. The designation r^G is used to indicate individuals who are Rh(G+D−C−), which is a rare phenotype.

The G antigen was discovered when a Rh(D) negative individual appeared to produce anti-D when transfused with Rh(D−C+)-positive red blood cells. Anti-G initially will appear to be a combination of anti-C and anti-D; however, the serologist will be unable to demonstrate separate anti-D and anti-C specificity. Anti-G is generally identified by using an adsorption/elution method (Chapter 8) with two separate sets of red blood cells, chosen to have phenotypes that will demonstrate separate anti-D, anti-C, and/or anti-G specificities.

For transfusion purposes, it is not necessary to differentiate between anti-G and a combination of anti-C and anti-D because the vast majority of Rh(D–C–) red blood cells are also Rh(G–). Some serologists believe it is important to distinguish between anti-D, anti-C, and anti-G in the case of obstetric patients to determine if Rh immunoglobulin should be given.[25] Absorption and elution studies may be performed to identify which antibody or combination of antibodies are present.

C^w

Initially it was thought that the C^w antigen was an allele of the C/c locus.[26] It was later demonstrated that C^w may be present in the presence or absence of the C and c antigens. C^w is antithetical to the high-incidence antigen MAR. The C^w antigen is found in about 2% of people of European ethnicity and is very rare in people of African ethnicity. The development of anti-C^w occurs after exposure, through pregnancy or transfusion, to red blood cells carrying the antigen. The antibody may exhibit *dosage* (a phenomenon in which antibodies react stronger with cells carrying a double dose of the corresponding antigen [homozygous cells] than with cells carrying a single dose [heterozygous cells]) during *in vitro* testing.

f (ce)

When both c and e antigens are present on the red blood cell and the respective genes are in the cis position or on the same chromosome, the f antigen is expressed. Therefore, red blood cells of the Dce/dCE genotype will have the f antigen, while red blood cells of the DcE/dCe will be f negative, even though both cells have the same phenotype testing results of positive with anti-D, anti-C, anti-c, anti-E, and anti-e. Anti-f can cause transfusion reactions and HDFN.

Ce

When C and e are found in the cis position the Ce antigen is also present. In older literature the Ce antigen may be called rh$_i$. An apparent anti-C will actually turn out to be anti-Ce. Anti-Ce will only react with DCe or dCe red blood cells and only weakly or not at all with DCE or Dce cells. Historically, when producing human source reagent antisera it was important for manufacturers to ensure that anti-Ce was not the primary antibody in an anti-C reagent.

Rh ANTIBODIES

Most Rh antibodies are of the immunoglobulin class IgG. Generally they are detected after incubation at 98.7° F (37° C), but some may not react until the antiglobulin phase of testing. Reactivity of Rh antibodies is enhanced when incubated with enzyme-treated red blood cells.

Alloantibodies

Rh antibodies are red blood cell stimulated; the patient must be exposed to the antigen before the antibody will be formed. Exposure to red blood cells can occur during pregnancy or through transfusion of blood products that contain red blood cells, which include granulocyte and platelet components in addition to red blood cell components. Many Rh antigens are very immunogenic, with the Rh(D) antigen being the most immunogenic. It is often quoted that as little as 0.1 mL of Rh(D)-positive blood can stimulate production of anti-D in an Rh(D)-negative recipient. This figure results from early studies where red blood cells were injected into volunteers.[27]

Once Rh antibodies are formed they tend to remain in circulation for long periods of time and are detected by routine antibody screening methods. These antibodies do not bind complement but cause extravascular hemolysis when the IgG-coated red blood cells are removed from circulation.

Individuals who develop one Rh antibody are more prone to develop other Rh system antibodies. This phenomenon is particularly true in the case of R$_1$R$_1$ (DCe/DCe) individuals who have developed anti-E. Oftentimes, although not always readily detected, these individuals will also develop anti-c.

☑ CHECKPOINT 5-10

Antibodies in the Rh blood group system may cause what condition associated with transfusion reactions?

Autoantibodies

Sometimes developing autoantibodies have apparent Rh specificity, either specific to a common Rh antigen or more often to a high-incidence Rh antigen. The latter, broad specificity may be determined by testing the autoantibody against rare Rh$_{null}$ or Rh-deletion red blood cells. The autoantibody, if it has an Rh specificity, will demonstrate a weaker reaction than when tested with red blood cells having normal Rh antigen expression. Sometimes an autoantibody will not react with the Rh$_{null}$ or Rh-deletion red blood cells.

There is controversy over whether to transfuse antigen-negative blood to patients whose autoantibody demonstrates an apparent specificity to a known blood group antigen. Transfusion of antigen-positive red blood cells when the patient has a clinically significant alloantibody is a proven risk. Therefore, if the compatible blood is of a rare type, such as Rh$_{null}$, it is generally believed that these donor units should be saved for transfusion to patients who have the corresponding alloantibody.

Unlike patients with alloantibodies, many patients with an autoantibody showing specificity to a common red blood cell antigen appear to show no difference in red blood cell survival whether antigen-positive or antigen-negative cells are transfused. Rather, the red blood cell survival may mimic the patient's own red blood cell survival; patients experiencing rapid hemolysis as a symptom of warm autoimmune hemolytic anemia (Chapter 15) are more likely to have poor transfusion outcomes whereas more stable patients achieve a longer-lasting benefit from the transfusion. In other patients, red blood cells negative for the antigen corresponding to the autoantibody appear to remain in circulation longer.

The risk of alloimmunization should also be taken into consideration. Sometimes antigen frequencies predict that donor red blood cells negative for the antigen corresponding to the alloantibody put the patient at higher risk for developing an alloantibody. For example, a patient with an apparent alloanti-e may be E negative (about 70% of people overall are E negative, with differences among ethnicities). Donor red blood cells that are e negative will be E positive, unless they are of a rare deletion phenotype. Therefore, transfusion with e-negative red blood cells would put the patient at a higher risk for developing an anti-E. Patients with autoantibodies have an increased tendency to produce alloantibodies (Chapter 15). This well-documented observation, combined with the difficulties in identifying an alloantibody in the presence of an autoantibody, lead some laboratories to choose donor units that are similar to the patient's phenotype for transfusion over donor units that are negative for the antigen corresponding to the autoantibody.

As with all transfusions, the various risks and benefits general to transfusion and specific to the patient should be considered by the attending physician and discussed with the patient when making treatment decisions. Consultation between clinical and laboratory professionals can be valuable in cases of warm autoimmune hemolytic anemia because the laboratory results as well as the clinical picture can be complex.

CASE IN POINT (continued)

No other testing is requested at this time, but TT may require future transfusion.

5. If the physician were to request a blood transfusion, what antigen(s) should the donor red blood cells lack?

6. Why is the physician requesting that all transfused red blood cells be Rh matched?

Rh-IMMUNE GLOBULIN (RhIg)

The Rh system was discovered during an investigation into a case of HDFN. HDFN (Chapter 14) caused by Rh antibodies can be severe. Rh antigens are well developed on the fetus red blood cells even before birth and Rh antibodies are IgG, which are able to cross the placenta. The D antigen may be present as early as at 8 weeks' gestation.

In the late 1960s, the development of Rh-immunoglobulin (RhIg) almost eliminated Rh immunization of pregnant patients.[28] RhIg is a purified concentrate of human anti-D, which is given to Rh(D)-negative pregnant patients to prevent allogenic production of anti-D. The mechanism of action of RhIg is still unknown. It is likely that a combination of actions prevents the formation of an anti-D. Some of the popular theories include a feedback loop that inhibits plasma cells from developing into anti-D producing-cells and the removal of anti-D-coated cells before the mother's immune system

mounts a response. RhIg prevents immunization against the D antigen only and not against the other Rh antigens.

Rh-DELETION PHENOTYPES

Although rare, some individuals either only inherit part of the traditional Rh-associated genes and thus are missing components (called *partial deletions*), do not inherit Rh genes at all (known as Rh_{null}), or they inherit Rh genes but are unable to express them at the normal level (a phenomenon known as Rh_{mod}). These three scenarios are collectively called Rh-deletion phenotypes, each of which is described next.

Partial Deletions

Very rare people may lack C/c or E/e or both antigens on their red blood cells. These phenotypes are denoted with dashes where the C/c or E/e would be; for example, someone of the phenotype DC– would lack the E/e antigen. Sometimes other high-incidence Rh antigens will also be lacking; for example, Rh18 or the Hr antigen is often lacking in people with CE deletions. The D– – phenotype is noted for having the strongest expression of Rh(D) antigen. Patients with Rh deletions are often not recognized until they form broadly reacting Rh antibodies following pregnancy or transfusion. Blood with similar deletions, either from family members or via rare donor files, is required for future transfusions to prevent hemolytic transfusion reactions.

Rh_{null}

Rare individuals who lack all Rh antigens are said to suffer from Rh_{null} syndrome. There are two different genetic means by which this syndrome may develop. The regulator type arises from a mutation in the *RHAG* gene. The amorphic type arises from a mutation in the *RHCE* genes and deletion of the *RHD* genes but with a normal *RHAG* gene.[29]

Individuals who are Rh_{null} may experience hemolytic anemia that is caused by a defective red blood cell membrane leading to stomatocyte formation. The morphological weakness is due to the fact that Rh antigens are part of the lipoprotein structure forming the RBC membrane. However, Rh_{null} individuals seldom require transfusion because their anemia is usually compensated. Characteristics of the Rh_{null} phenotype are found in Table 5-6 ✱. Transfusion of an Rh_{null} patient requires Rh_{null} blood, available only through rare donor files.

✱ **TABLE 5-6** Characteristics of the Rh_{null} Syndrome

Rh_{null} Syndrome
Compensated hemolytic anemia
Slight-to-moderate decreased hemoglobin/hematocrit
Reticulocytosis
Stomatocytosis
Decreased haptoglobin
Increased hemoglobin F
Absence of FY5 antigen

☑ CHECKPOINT 5-11

If a person's red blood cells are missing all the Rh antigens, what is his or her phenotype?

LW^aLW^a or LW^aLW LW^aLW^b LW^bLW^b or LW^bLW $LWLW$

LW(a + b −)   LW(a + b +)   LW(a − b +)   LW(a − b −)

FIGURE 5-2   LW Genotypes and Phenotypes

Rh$_{mod}$

Parents or offspring of people with the regulator type of Rh$_{null}$ may have overall depression of Rh antigens known as Rh$_{mod}$. Since these individuals have only partial expression of Rh antigens, they exhibit characteristics similar to individuals who are Rh$_{null}$. Generally, the symptoms exhibited are less severe than those seen in the Rh$_{null}$ individual.[30] Rh$_{mod}$ cells, like Rh$_{null}$ cells, may have decreased S, s, and U antigen expression (Chapter 6). Unlike Rh$_{null}$ cells, Rh$_{mod}$ cells do not completely lack FY5, LW, or Rh antigens.

LW BLOOD GROUP SYSTEM

The LW antigen was originally thought to be the D antigen; testing on a woman who was Rh(D) positive but LW negative demonstrated that the Rh and LW systems are separate.[31] It was decided at that time to rename the antibody anti-LW in honor of Landsteiner and Wiener's pioneering work with the Rh system. LW^a, LW^b, and LW are the three alleles that compose the LW system. The LW gene is a silent allele and when individuals are LW/LW they do not express LW antigens on the surface of their red blood cells. Figure 5-2 demonstrates the expressed phenotypes and their associated potential genotypes.

The majority of Rh(D)-positive red blood cells will react strongly with anti-LW; however, Rh(D)-negative red blood cells may be nonreactive or react only weakly. Rh$_{null}$ cells will not react with anti-LW. Anti-LW will react with cord blood cells regardless of Rh(D) type. Anti-LW can be erroneously identified as anti-D if the antibody is not reacting with Rh(D)-negative red blood cells. However, testing with enzyme-treated cells will differentiate an anti-D, which will have enhanced reactivity, from an anti-LW, which will have no reactivity as enzymes destroy the LW antigens.

Review of the Main Points

- Rh antigen expression relies on two genes closely linked on chromosome 1 called *RHD* and *RHCE* as well as the *RHAG* gene located on chromosome 6.
- *RHD* and *RHCE* are the genes of the Rh blood group system. *RHAG* is the only gene in the RHAG blood group system.
- The Fisher-Race and Wiener models of genetic expression have been shown to be incorrect; however, the nomenclature established by these earlier theories are still in use today.
- The most commonly encountered Rh antibodies are to the antigens D, C, E, c, and e.
- The D antigen is second in immunogenicity only to the ABO antigens.
- When Rh(D) typing is taken to the indirect antiglobulin phase, the test is called weak D testing.
- Donors who are weak D positive are classified as Rh(D) positive.
- Today clonal Rh antisera are most often used to type for Rh antigens.
- There are three different mechanisms by which the Rh(D) antigen expression can be weakened:
  - C in trans position to D.
  - Weak D due to decreased number of D antigens on each red blood cell.
  - Partial D or the loss of part of the D antigen.
- The G antigen is usually found on D- and/or C-positive red blood cells.
- C^w antigen is found in 2% of people of European ethnicity but rarely in people of African ethnicity.
- The f antigen is found when c and e antigens are in the cis position.
- Rh antibodies are known to cause extravascular transfusion reactions and hemolytic disease of the fetus and newborn.

Review Questions

1. The *RHD* and *RHCE* genes are located on which chromosome? (Objective #4)

   A. 1

   B. 5

   C. 8

   D. 10

2. The presence of the _____ antigen on the surface of the red blood cell membrane designates a person as Rh positive. (Objective #3)

   A. Rh

   B. D

   C. d

   D. CE

3. Which of the following genetic circumstances results in the absence of the D antigen? (Objective #4)

   A. Deletion of RHD

   B. Mutated RHD alleles

   C. Partial RHD alleles

   D. Partial RHCE alleles

4. How do Rh proteins differ from ABO blood group antigens? (Objective #3)

   A. Rh proteins are not an integral part of the red blood cell membrane.

   B. Rh proteins are not present at birth.

   C. Rh proteins are found in most body fluids.

   D. Rh proteins do not contain a carbohydrate group.

5. The Rh null phenotype is associated with: (Objective #2)

   A. Hemolytic anemia

   B. The presence of stomatocytes on the peripheral blood smear

   C. Blood clotting abnormalities

   D. Weak expression of Rh antigens

6. How is Rh-associated glycoprotein (RhAG) distinguished from Rh protein? (Objective #12)

   A. Their genes are found on different chromosomes.

   B. Their blood group systems are different.

   C. RhAG protein contains no Rh antigen.

   D. Absence of RhAG protein does not result in RBC membrane defects.

7. Cells that do *not* have the RhAG protein will also lack: (Objective #5)

   A. RHCE and RHD proteins

   B. LW glycoproteins

   C. CD47

   D. Glycophorin B

8. Which blood group system is linked with the RH gene? (Objective #4)

   A. Duffy

   B. Scianna

   C. Kidd

   D. Lewis

9. The terminology that describes the inheritance of the Rh antigens through a single gene at a single locus was developed by: (Objective #7)

   A. Weiner

   B. Fisher-Race

   C. Rosenfield

   D. Tippett

10. Matching. Convert Fisher-Race to Wiener nomenclature: (Objective #8)

    _____ dce/dce   A. R1r

    _____ DCe/DcE   B. rr

    _____ DCe/dce   C. R1R2

    _____ DcE/dce   D. R2r

11. Which of the following phenotypes will react with anti-f? (Objective #16)

    A. DCe/DcE

    B. dce/dce

    C. DcE/dCE

    D. Dce/Dce

12. What is the most probable genotype for a patient's red blood cells that demonstrates the following results with reagent antisera? (Objective #19)

Antisera	Result
D	3+
C	3+
E	0
c	0
e	3+

    A. R2R2

    B. R1R1

    C. R1r

    D. RzR1

13. A patient's red blood cell phenotype is R1r . The Rosenfield nomenclature should be interpreted as: (Objective #7)

   A. Rh: −1, 2, −3, 4, 5

   B. Rh: 1, −2, −3, 4, 5

   C. Rh: 1, −2, 3, 4, 5

   D. Rh: 1, 2, −3, 4, 5

14. Explanations for the weak D phenotype include which of the following: (Objective #11)

   A. Reduced number of antigen sites

   B. Suppression of the RHD gene through a position effect

   C. Missing epitope

   D. Inheritance of Rh null gene

15. Which of the following Rh antisera requires the use of a negative control?(Objective #15)

   A. Low-protein anti-D

   B. High-protein anti-D

   C. Monoclonal anti-D

   D. Polyclonal anti-D

16. Match the sources of error in the Rh typing test: (Objective #13)

   _____ Rouleaux   A. False-positive reaction

   _____ RBC suspension too heavy   B. False-negative reaction

   _____ Failure to add antiserum

   _____ Autoagglutinins

17. Persons with the weak D phenotype are considered to be: (Objective #10)

   A. Rh positive

   B. Rh negative

   C. Rh null

   D. Neither Rh positive or Rh negative

18. Select the characteristics of Rh blood group system antibodies. (Objective #16)

   A. Naturally occurring

   B. Cross the placenta

   C. Strongly immunogenic

   D. Deteriorate rapidly

19. _____ is a substance that prevents the allogeneic production of anti-D in pregnant women. (Objective #17)

   A. Rh-immunoglobulin (RhIg)

   B. Antihuman globulin (AHG)

   C. Monoclonalglobulin (MHG)

   D. 22% albumin

20. The high-incidence Rh antigen that is missing in an individual who has a CE deletion is: (Objective #6)

   A. e

   B. Rh6

   C. Rh18

   D. F

References

1. Landsteiner K, Wiener AS. Studies on agglutinogen (Rh) in human blood reacting with anti-rhesus sera and with human isoantibodies. *J Exp Med* 1941; 74(4): 309–20.

2. Levine P, Stetson RE. Landmark article July 8, 1939. An unusual case of intragroup agglutination. *JAMA* 1984; 251(10): 1316–7.

3. Tippett P. A speculative model for the Rh blood groups. *Ann Hum Genet* 1986; 50 (Pt 3): 241–7.

4. Colin Y, Chérif-Zahar B, Le Van Kim C, Raynal V, Van Huffel V, Cartron JP. Genetic basis of the RhD-positive and RhD-negative blood group polymorphisms as determined by Southern analysis. *Blood* 1991; 78(10): 2747–52.

5. Race R, Sanger R. Fisher's contribution to Rh. *Vox Sang* 1982; 43(6): 354–6.

6. Wiener A. Genetic theory of the Rh blood types. *Proc Soc Exp Biol* 1943; 53: 167–70.

7. Chérif-Zahar B, Mattéi MG, Le Van Kim C, Bailly P, Cartron JP, Colin Y. Localization of the human Rh blood group gene structure to chromosome region 1p34.3-1p36.1 by in situ hybridization. *Hum Genet* 1991; 86(4): 398–400.

8. Roback JD, editor. *Technical Manual*, 16th ed. Bethesda (MD): AABB; 2008.

9. Moore S, Woodrow CF, McClelland DB. Isolation of membrane components associated with human red cell antigens Rh(D), (c), (E) and Fyª. *Nature* 1982; 295(5849): 529–31.

10. Gahmberg CG. Molecular identification of the human Rh₀ (D) antigen. *FEBS Lett* 1982; 140(1): 93–7.

11. Chérif-Zahar B, Bloy C, Le Van Kim C, Blanchard D, Bailly P, Hermand P, Salmon C, Cartron JP, Colin Y. Molecular cloning and protein structure of a human blood group Rh polypeptide. *Proc Natl Aca Sci USA* 1990; 87(16): 6243–7.

12. Eyers SAC, Ridgwell K, Mawby WJ, Tanner MJA. Topology and organization of human Rh (rhesus) blood group-related polypeptides. *J Biol Chem* 1994; 269(9): 6417–23.

13. Purves D, Fitzpatrick D, Hall WC, LaMantia A-S, McNamara JO, Williams SM, editors. *Neuroscience,* 4th ed. Sunderland (MA): Sinauer Associates; 2007.

14. Marini A, Urrestarazu A, Beauwens R, André B. The Rh (rhesus) blood group polypeptides are related to NH₄ transporters. *Trends Biochem Sci* 1997; 22(12): 460–1.

15. Conroy MJ, Bullough PA, Merrick M, Avent ND. Modeling the human rhesus proteins: implications for structure and function. *Transfusion* 2005; 131(4): 543–53.

16. The international blood group reference laboratory [Internet]. Names for RHAG (ISBT 030) Blood Group Alleles- draft. Bristol, England: [updated 2010 June 14; cited 2010 July 5]. Available from: http://ibgrl.blood.co.uk/ISBTPages/AlleleTerminology/030%20RHAG%20alleles%20final%20Oct%2009.pdf

17. Avent ND. Molecular biology of the Rh blood group system. *Journal of Ped Hem Onc* 2001; 23(6): 394–402.

18. Rosenfeld RE, Allen FH, Swisher SN, Kochwa S. A review of Rh serology and presentation of a new terminology. *Transfusion* 1962; 2(5): 287–311.

19. Hughes-Jones NC, Gardner B, Lincoln PJ. Observations on the number of available c, D, and E antigen sites on red cells. *Vox Sang* 1971; 21(3): 210–6.

20. Stratton F. A new Rh allelomorph. *Nature* 1946; 158(4001): 25–6.

21. Argall CI, Ball JM, Trentelman E. Presence of anti-D antibody in the serum of a Du patient. *J Lab Clin Med* 1953; 41(6): 895–8.

22. Huang C, Liu P, Cheng J. Molecular biology and genetics of the Rh blood group system. *Semin Hematol* 2000; 37(2): 150–65.

23. Daniels G. *Human blood groups*, 2nd ed. Malden (MA): Blackwell Science; 2002.

24. Issitt P and Anstee D. *Applied blood group serology*, 4th ed. Durham (NC): Montgomery Scientific Press, 1998.

25. Shirey RS, Mirabella DC, Lumadue JA, Ness PM. Differentiation of anti-D, -C, and -G: clinical relevance in alloimmunized pregnancies. *Transfusion* 1997; 37(5): 493–6.

26. Callender ST, Race RR. A serological and genetical study of multiple anti-bodies formed in response to blood transfusion by a patient with lupus erythematosus diffusus. *Ann Eugen* 1946; 13: 102–17.

27. Zipursky A, Israels LG. The pathogenesis and prevention of Rh immunization. *CMAJ* 1967; 97(21): 1245–57.

28. Queenan JT. *Modern Management of the Rh Problem,* 2nd ed. New York: Harper and Row; 1977.

29. Schmidt P, Vos GH. Multiple phenotypic abnormalities associated with Rh null (---/---). *Vox Sang* 1967; 13(1): 18–20.

30. Chown B, Lewis M, Lowen B. An unlinked modifier of Rh blood groups: effects when heterozygous and when homozygous. *Am J Hum Genet* 1972; 24(6): 623–37.

31. Rosenfield RE, Haber GV, Schroeder R, Ballard R. Problems in Rh typing as revealed by a single Negro family. *Am J Hum Genet* 1960; 12(2): 147–59.

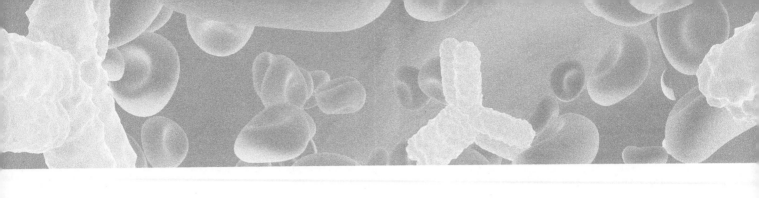

6

Other Blood Group Systems

MARGARET A. SPRUELL

Chapter Objectives

Upon completion of this chapter, the student will be able to:

1. Discuss the history and nomenclature of other blood group systems including ISBT terminology.
2. Identify the chromosomes where the genes for other blood group systems reside.
3. Differentiate homozygosity and heterozygosity of other blood group genes and the respective antigen phenotypes that are produced.
4. List antigen frequencies for other blood group systems.
5. Discuss the concept of dosage in antigen expression.
6. Describe the null phenotypes in other blood groups, including their clinical significance.
7. Differentiate the following characteristics for other blood group systems: antibody class, mode of reactivity, ability to bind complement, effect of enzymes, incidence of hemolytic transfusion reaction, and incidence of hemolytic disease of the newborn.
8. Discuss how antigen profiles of other blood groups can be used to rule out or confirm the presence of unexpected antibodies.
9. Identify diseases and clinically significant situations that are associated with other blood group system antigens and antibodies.
10. Explain delayed hemolytic transfusion reactions (DHTR) and associated clinical findings.
11. Discuss the significance of the Mcleod phenotype.
12. Describe the interaction of the H, Lewis (Le), and secretor genes (Se) in the development of the Lewis blood group system antigens (Lewis phenotype).
13. Given a genotype, predict the presence or absence of Lewis antigens in the plasma and on the red blood cell surface.
14. Name the other blood group system antigens whose reactivity can be altered by chemical treatment.
15. List the different antigen-altering reagents that can be used to change the reactivity of other blood group system antigens and antibodies.
16. Explain the characteristics and significance of the I blood group system.
17. Discuss the Bg blood group system antigens and antibodies.
18. Describe the Sid blood group, including clinical significance and tests that are used to identify antigen and antibody presence.

Key Terms

Antigen profile(s)
Antigram(s)
Antithetical
Blood group system(s)
Bromelin
Chronic granulomatous
 disease (CGD)
Cold autoagglutinin(s)
Crossmatch compatible
Crossmatch incompatible
Dithiothreitol (DTT)
Donath-Landsteiner test
Extravascular hemolysis
Ficin
Glycoprotein(s)

Hemolytic disease of the fetus
 and newborn (HDFN)
Hemolytic transfusion
 reaction(s)
Human leukocyte antigen(s)
 (HLA)
McLeod phenotype
Null phenotype
Papain
Paroxysmal cold
 hemoglobinuria (PCH)
Paroxysmal nocturnal
 hemoglobinuria (PNH)
Trypsin

CASE IN POINT

FH is a 77-year-old female with hereditary hemorrhagic telangiectasia. She requires frequent blood transfusions due to anemia caused by constant occult GI blood loss and has been receiving them at your hospital every 2–3 weeks for several years. She has a known history of multiple antibodies that include anti-E, anti-K, anti-Jk^a, anti-Fy^a, anti-M, and anti-Le^a, which make her blood bank work-up difficult. You have just received a call from the Outpatient Transfusion Department indicating that FH will be transfused 2 units in the morning and she is on her way to the laboratory to have a specimen collected for blood bank testing that consists of a blood type, antibody screen, antibody identification if warranted, and preparation of blood for possible transfusion (a test known as crossmatch or compatibility testing; see Chapter 7).

What's Ahead?

Many antigens are known to be on human red blood cells besides those in the ABO and Rh blood group systems. New antigens were usually discovered when an antibody was detected in either human or animal serum that did not match previous reaction patterns. For instance, after the ABO antigens were described, an antibody was found in the serum of rabbits injected with human red blood cells that reacted with eight of every 10 samples no matter what the ABO of the red blood cells; it was designated anti-M.

This chapter presents information on blood group systems other than ABO (Chapter 4) and Rh (Chapter 5) and answers the following questions:

- How is the nomenclature of blood groups determined?
- How do genetics play a role in the development of these blood group systems?
- How can antigen sites be altered in *in vitro* testing to assist the immunohematologist in determining the identification of corresponding antibodies?
- In general terms, what is the clinical significance associated with these other blood group systems?
- What are the members, characteristics, and clinical significance, when present, of the other blood group systems?

HISTORICAL BACKGROUND AND NOMENCLATURE

Usually the name of the antibody producer or the person whose red blood cells expressed the corresponding antigen was used to name the new antigen. For example, anti-K1, previously called anti-Kell, was named after Mrs. Kellacher, the patient in whose serum it was first discovered. As each new antibody pattern was evaluated and testing of families could be done, some antigens were shown to be related. The first antigen sometimes was given the designation "a," the related, second antigen the designation "b." The antigens shown to be related by serological testing and family inheritance studies and distinct from all previous antigens were placed in **blood group systems**. More recent biochemical and genetic studies have confirmed the serologic and family studies as well as determined new blood group systems.

Since 1980, the International Society of Blood Transfusion (ISBT) has organized the human red blood cell antigens using uniform classification and terminology.[1] Related antigens are placed in a blood group system once the genetic basis is confirmed. Antigens where the genetic basis is still unknown are placed in collections. Each group or collection of antigens has a name and the individual antigens have a numeric designation based on the chronological order in which they became a part of the group (e.g., M is MNS1).

QUICK GENETICS REVIEW

Knowledge of some genetic terms is essential to understanding red blood cell antigens and antibodies. The result obtained from testing red blood cells with known reagent antisera is the phenotype. For example, a person has the Fy (a+b+) phenotype if their red blood cells agglutinate with both anti-Fy^a and anti-Fy^b antisera. See Table 6-1 ✳ for the phenotype frequencies of the antigens shown on antigen profile sheets. From the phenotype results we can estimate a probable genotype; genetic testing or family phenotype studies would be required if there was a need to confirm the genotype.

✳ **TABLE 6-1** Phenotype Frequency

Blood Group System	Phenotype	Frequency (%) European Ethnicity	African Ethnicity
Kell	K−k+	91	98
	K+k+	9	2
	K+k−	<1	Rare
	Kp(a−b+)	98	100
	Kp(a+b+)	2	Rare
	Kp(a+b−)	Rare	0
	Js(a−b+)	100	80
	Js(a+b+)	Rare	19
	Js(a+b−)	0	1
Duffy	Fy(a+b+)	49	1
	Fy(a−b+)	34	22
	Fy(a+b−)	17	1
	Fy(a−b−)	Rare	68
Kidd	Jk(a+b+)	49	34
	Jk(a+b−)	28	57
	Jk(a−b+)	23	9
✳	Jk(a−b−)	Rare	Rare
Lewis	Le(a−b+)	72	55
	Le(a+b−)	22	23
	Le(a−b−)	6	22
P	P₁+	79	94
	P₁−	21	6
MNS	M+N+	50	44
	M+N−	28	26
	M−N+	22	30
	S−s+	45	69
	S+s+	44	28
	S+s−	11	3
	S−s−U−	0	<1
Lutheran	Lu(a−b+)	92	Similar
	Lu(a+b+)	7	
	Lu(a+b−)	<1	
	Lu(a−b−)	Rare	

- The phenotypes listed here are those of antigens commonly found on reagent red blood cell sheets provided by commercial manufacturers known as *antigrams*, a concept described in detail later in this chapter.
- The blood group systems are usually listed on antigrams in the following order: Rh, Kell, Duffy, Kidd, and then followed by the blood group systems where the antibodies are variable in their clinical significance.
- Rh phenotype frequencies are listed in Chapter 5.
- Anti-K is the most commonly encountered, clinically significant antibody outside the ABO and Rh blood group system.
- Antibodies within the Duffy and Kidd blood groups systems are almost always clinically significant.
- The most common phenotype among people of European ancestry is listed first.

Alternative genes that may be at a single locus on paired chromosomes are alleles and are designated by italics (e.g., *FYA* and *FYB*). When a locus can have different alleles, the corresponding antigens are called **antithetical**. The red blood cell antigens that result from the gene presence are designated without italics, Fyᵃ and Fyᵇ. If both alleles at a locus are the same, the person is said to be homozygous for the allele, genotype is *FYA/FYA*, and the antigen expression on their red blood cells can be considered to be of double dose, phenotype is Fy (a+b−). If different alleles are present at that locus, the person is said to be heterozygous, genotype is *FYA/FYB*, and each antigen expression is single dose, phenotype is Fy (a+b+).

Most blood group system genes are *co-dominant*, which means that the antigen will be expressed when the gene is present and one gene does not suppress another. For example, when a person inherits a *Fya* and *Fyb* gene, both Fyᵃ and Fyᵇ antigens will be expressed on their red blood cell membrane, resulting in the phenotype Fy(a+b+). If a red blood cell has no detectable antigens in a system, it is said to demonstrate the **null phenotype**. For example, the null phenotype in the Duffy system is produced by inheriting two *FY* genes. No Duffy protein is produced either on red blood cells or other tissue cells; therefore, these cells lack the Fyᵃ, Fyᵇ, and high-incidence Fy3 antigens. Please see Table 6-2 ✳ for chromosome information about the presently defined blood group systems.

ANTIGEN-ALTERING REAGENTS

Antibodies may be detected by a variety of techniques (Chapter 8). Chemical treatment of reagent red blood cells can aid in patient antibody identification by creating either an enhancement or reduction of agglutination reaction, resulting in a more obvious pattern of reactivity. Use of these reagents may be especially helpful when dealing with a patient who has produced multiple antibodies. The most common chemical used in North America is the enzyme **ficin**. It removes some structures from the red blood cell membrane, thus destroying the related antigens (e.g., M, N, Fyᵃ, and Fyᵇ). At the same time, other antigen expression is enhanced and thus more easily detected (e.g., Jkᵃ, Jkᵇ, and Rh antigens). Other, less commonly used enzymes include **papain**, **trypsin**, and **bromelin**. The reducing agent **dithiothreitol (DTT)**, which breaks disulfide bonds, will destroy antigens that rely on such a bond to maintain their structure, such as the Kell system antigens. Antigens may also be destroyed by reagents used primarily for other purposes, such as chloroquin diphospate and EDTA-glycine.

☑ **CHECKPOINT 6-1**

How does the chemical treatment of reagent red blood cells assist with the identification of unexpected antibodies?

Clinically significant antibodies are defined as those that can cause shortened survival of transfused red blood cells, which may result in a **hemolytic transfusion reaction** (an adverse reaction to transfused cells in which recipient antibody typically destroys transfused red blood cells, causing them to hemolyze) or fetal or neonatal red blood cells in a condition called **hemolytic disease of the fetus and newborn (HDFN)**, a condition in which antibodies in maternal circulation target and attach to corresponding antigens on fetal

✳ **TABLE 6-2** ISBT Blood Group System Information[2]

Assigned Number	Name	Symbol	Gene(s)	Chromosome
001	ABO	ABO	ABO	9
002	MNS	MNS	GYPA, GYB, GYE	4
003	P	P1		22
004	Rh	RH	RHD, RHCE	1
005	Lutheran	LU	LU	19
006	Kell	KEL	KEL	7
007	Lewis	LE	FUT3	19
008	Duffy	FY	DARC	1
009	Kidd	JK	SLC14A1	18
010	Diego	DI	SLC4A1	17
011	Yt	YT	ACHE	7
012	Xg	XG	XG, MIC2	X
013	Scianna	SC	ERMAP	1
014	Dombrock	DO	DO	12
015	Colton	CO	AQP1	7
016	Landsteiner-Wiener	LW	ICAM4	19
017	Chido/Rodgers	CH/RG	C4A, C4B	6
018	Hh	H	FUT1	19
019	Kx	XK	XK	X
020	Gerbich	GE	GYPC	2
021	Cromer	CROM	DAF	1
022	Knops	KN	CR1	1
023	Indian	IN	CD44	11
024	Ok	OK	BSG	19
024	Raph	MER2	CD151	11
026	John Milton hagen	JMH	SEMA7A	15
027	I	I	GCNT2	6
028	Globoside	GLOB	B3GALT3	3
029	Gill	GIL	AQP3	9
030	Rh-associated glycoprotein	RHAG	RHAG	6

red blood cells. Survival of antigen-positive red blood cells is more commonly shortened by antibodies reacting at body temperature, which are generally IgG, than by those reacting at lower temperatures, which are generally IgM. The ability of an antibody to bind complement usually means that the length of survival of antigen-positive cells will be shortened even more. HDFN can occur only if the maternal antibody is IgG that can cross the placenta and the fetal or neonatal red blood cells express the corresponding antigen (Chapter 14). See Table 6-3 ✳ for characteristics of the most commonly encountered antibodies.

BLOOD GROUP SYSTEMS ON STANDARD ANTIGEN PROFILES AND RELATED SYSTEMS

The United States Food and Drug Administration (FDA) requires that antigens corresponding to the commonly encountered antibodies be shown on red blood cell **antigen profiles**, defined as grids that indicate the antigen makeup of commercial red blood cells used for antibody detection or identification.[3] Manufacturers of commercial red blood cells typically provide a paper **antigram**, a chart that includes the antigen profile grids and other pertinent information with each group of red cells (known as a kit or panel) sold. Antigrams are also commonly referred to as *panel sheets* or *profile sheets*. The required antigens requiring manufacturer-provided profiles are M, N, S, s, P_1, K, k, Le^a, Le^b, Fy^a, Fy^b, Jk^a, Jk^b, and several Rh antigens (Chapter 5). A few other antigens, such as Lu^a, Lu^b, and Xg^a, are commonly also included on the antigram. Many other antibody specificities and the red blood cell antigens with which they react have been determined.[1] Reagent red blood cells are not routinely typed for all these other antigens because the corresponding antibody is rarely encountered. Most of these antigens are of high or low incidence, which explains the rarity of the corresponding antibody. Those antigens not of high or low incidence but for which the corresponding antibody is rare probably have low immunogenicity. If a red blood cell used on a commercial panel is known to lack an antigen of high incidence or to express an antigen of low incidence, this information is also provided.

✳ **TABLE 6-3** Characteristics of Most Commonly Encountered Antibodies

Blood Group System	Antibody	IgM	IgG	Antigen Present on Fetal Red Blood Cells
Kell	Anti-K	Rare	Usual	Yes
	Anti-k	No	Usual	Yes
	Anti-Kp^a	No	Usual	Yes
	Anti-Kp^b	No	Usual	Yes
	Anti-Js^a	No	Usual	Yes
	Anti-Js^b	No	Usual	Yes
Duffy	Anti-Fy^a	No	Usual	Yes
	Anti-Fy^b	No	Usual	Yes
Kidd	Anti-Jk^a	No	Usual	Yes
	Anti-Jk^b	No	Usual	Yes
Lewis	Anti-Le^a	Usual	Rare	No
	Anti-Le^b	Usual	Rare	No
P1	Anti-P$_1$	Usual	Rare	Weak
MNS	Anti-M	Usual	Rare	Yes
	Anti-N	Usual	Rare	Yes
	Anti-S	Rare	Usual	Yes
	Anti-s	Rare	Usual	Yes
	Anti-U	No	Usual	Yes
Lutheran	Anti-Lu^a	Some	Some	Weak
	Anti-Lu^b	Rare	Usual	Weak

MNS Blood Group System

MNS is a complex blood group system with over 40 known antigens. The antigens of this system are found on **glycoproteins**, which are also called glycophorins and are composed of carbohydrates, specifically glycol, attached to proteins. The *GYPA* gene controls production of the M and N antigens found on glycophorin A; the *GYPB* gene controls production of the S, s, and U antigens found on glycophorin B. Glycophorins A and B transverse the red blood cell membrane with the common MNS antigens existing on the outside of the membrane. Refer to Figure 6-1 ■. The amino acid sequence of these glycophorins is numbered, with 1 as farthest from the red blood cell membrane. Single amino acid substitutions differentiate the M from N and S from s antigens. The U antigen is a high-incidence antigen located on

glycophorin B. The amino acid sequences of common MNS antigens are in Table 6-4 ✳. Known high- and low-frequency antigens of the MNS system are in Table 6-5 ✳.

There are very rare people who do not have normal glycophorin A; this is called the En(a–) phenotype. The null phenotype in the MNS system is called M^k; these red blood cells lack both glycophorin A and B and therefore are type M–N–S–s–U–.

Treatment of the red blood cells with enzymes, most commonly ficin, removes the portion of glycoprotein that contains M and N, but cannot be relied upon to consistently remove S or s antigens.

Anti-M and anti-N are usually IgM, and therefore react best at room temperature. Reactivity of anti-M may be enhanced by slight acidification (pH 6.5) of the test sample. Anti-N is generally

✳ **TABLE 6-4** Amino Acid Variation of MNS Antigens Most Commonly Encountered in Antibody Investigations

Antigen	Amino Acid Location	Amino Acid(s)	Frequency (%) European Ethnicity	African Ethnicity
M	GYPA 1-5	Ser-Ser-Thr-Thr-Gly	78	74
N	GYPA 1-5	Leu-Ser-Thr-Thr-Glu	72	75
S	GYPB 29	Met	55	31
S	GYPB 29	Thr	89	93

- Ser, serine; Thr, threonine; Gly, glycine; Leu, leucine; Glu, glutamic acid, Met methionine
- Most of the other antigens in the MNS system are either high- or low-frequency antigens.
- M^e is another MNS antigen. It is a common amino acid sequence within the M and He antigens and therefore is neither of high nor low frequency (M antigen having a frequency of approximately 75%). However, anti-M^e is not a commonly identified antibody.

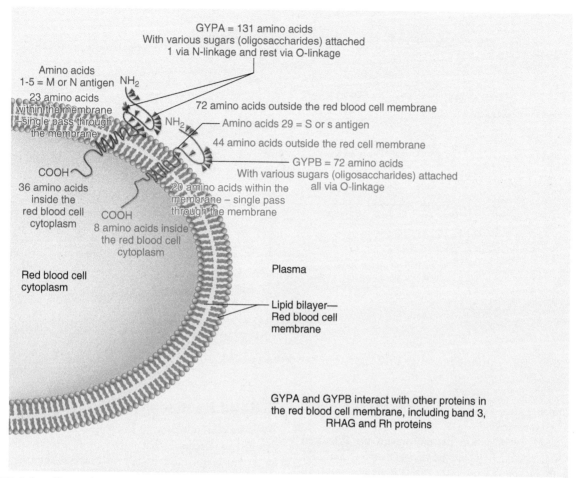

FIGURE 6-1   Glycophorin A and Glycophorin B

considered clinically insignificant, whereas anti-M is a rare cause of HDFN but almost never causes hemolytic transfusion reactions. Anti-M may be more likely to have clinical significance if it has an IgG component or is reactive at 98.7° F (37° C). MNS antigens are well developed at birth. Anti-S, anti-s, and anti-U are usually IgG, are clinically significant, and are best detected in antiglobulin tests.

☑ CHECKPOINT 6-2

On which glycoprotein is the M and N antigen produced?
On which glycoprotein is S and s antigen produced?

P and Globoside Blood Group Systems

The expression of the P_1 antigen is fully expressed by the age of 7 and varies from person to person. This can result in panel reactivity of varying strength and may be misinterpreted as the presence of multiple antibodies rather than just anti-P_1. P_1 is the only antigen in the P system.

Soluble P_1 antigen, usually from pigeon egg white, is available as a reagent that can be used to aid in antibody identification by inhibiting or neutralizing anti-P_1. Anti-P_1 is almost always IgM and is not clinically significant; therefore, it is often considered a nuisance antibody. Elimination of the immediate spin phase of testing, use of monospecific anti-IgG in indirect antiglobulin testing, and use of

✱ **TABLE 6-5** High- and Low-Frequency Antigens of the MNS System

Frequency	Antigens
High	U, En^a, ENKT, "N," ENP, ENEH, ENAV
Low	He, Mi^a, M^c, Vw, Mur, M^g, Vr, Mt^a, St^a, Ri^a, Cl^a, Ny^a, HUT, Hil, M^v, Far, s^D, Mit, Dantu, Hop, Nob, Or, DANE, TSEN, MINY, MUT, SAT, ERIK, Os^a, HAG, MARS

High- and low-frequency antigens in the MNS system are either the result of single amino acid substitutions or are combinations of glycoprophorin A and B amino acid sequences that result from genetic recombination of the *GYA* and *GYB* genes.

Source: Based on data from Daniels, G. *Human Blood Groups*, 2nd ed, Antigens of the MNS System, Table 3, Wiley-Blackwell Publishing.

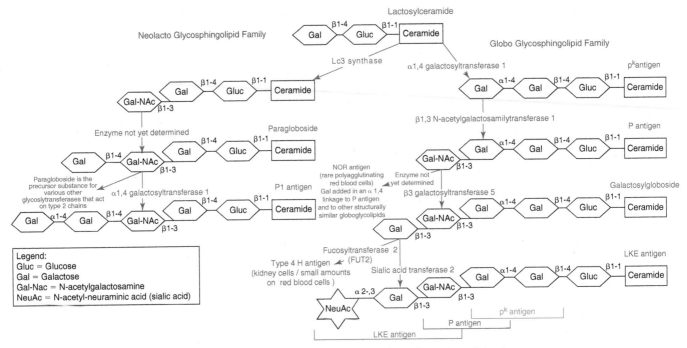

FIGURE 6-2 Biosynthetic Pathway of Globoside- and Paragloboside-Related Antigens

non-tube techniques such as gel have reduced the number of anti-P_1 detected during routine testing.

The Globoside blood group system contains the P antigen and the globoside blood group collection contains the P^k and LKE antigens. The P^k antigen is a precursor to the P antigen and both are present on the red blood cells of almost everyone. Figure 6-2 illustrates a pathway of production of these antigens. There are rare people of the p phenotype, whose red blood cells do not have P_1, P^k, or P. Other people lack the P antigen only. Naturally occurring IgM antibodies may be made against any of these antigens when they are absent. Thus people of the p phenotype produce an antibody called anti-PP_1P^k, which is directed at P_1, P^k, and P antigens. These antibodies usually bind complement and are clinically significant.

With use of rare P-negative red blood cells, it has been shown that the biphasic IgG hemolysin of **paroxysmal cold hemoglobinuria (PCH)**, a rare autoimmune disease that results in acquired hemolytic anemia, can have autoanti-P specificity. The routine test for PCH is the **Donath Landsteiner test**, which mimics the temperature changes that occur as blood flows into and out of the extremities of the body. The temperature changes are a critical factor in the pathogenesis of PCH as the causative antibody attaches to red blood cells at colder temperatures, such as when the blood is in the extremities, but only initiates complement activation leading to hemolysis once the red blood cell is warmed to 98.7° F (37° C) as happens when the blood flows back to the body's core.

The genetic basis of the high-incidence LKE antigen has not been determined. Anti-LKE is a very rare antibody that has not been reported to cause either transfusion reactions or HDFN.

☑ **CHECKPOINT 6-3**

What type of reactivity does a biphasic hemolysin exhibit?

Kell and Kx Blood Group Systems

There are currently over 30 antigens in the Kell blood group system. The FDA requires that antigen profiles include the phenotype for K and k, but most usually also include information on Kp^a, Kp^b, Js^a, and Js^b. Refer to Tables 6-6 * and 6-7 * for a list of Kell blood group system antigens. Kx is a high-frequency antigen and is the only known antigen in the Kx blood group system. Refer to Figure 6-3 , a simplified schematic of the glycoproteins carrying the antigens of the Kell and Kx blood group systems. The antigens of the Kell system are found on a glycoprotein that passes through the red blood cell membrane once. The presence or absence of Kell antigens on this glycoprotein is determined by a single gene called *KEL*, located on chromosome 7.

After D, the K antigen is the most immunogenic. Transfusion with K-positive red blood cells results in production of IgG anti-K about 10% of the time.[4] Antibodies in the Kell blood group system can cause hemolytic transfusion reactions. The antigens of the Kell system are fully developed at birth. Anti-K can cause severe HDFN attributed more to suppression of *erythropoiesis* (production of red blood cells) than fetal red blood cell destruction.[4] Therefore, the titer of anti-K does not correlate with the severity of the fetus or neonate's anemia.[5] Anti-K may rarely be detected as an IgM antibody in association with bacterial infections.[6]

The k, Kp^b, and Js^b antigens are all high-incidence antigens, present in over 99% of the population. Kp^a, which is allelic to Kp^b and Js^a, which is allelic to Js^b, are both low-incidence antigens. However, there are ethnic differences in the frequency of these low-incidence antigens, with Kp^a being more common in people of European ethnicity, with a frequency of 2%, and Js^b being more common in people of African ethnicity, with a frequency of 20%. Kell system antigens are destroyed by treatment with 0.2M DTT.

✳ **TABLE 6-6** Allelic Pairs of the Kell System

Alleles	Amino Acid Location	Antigen	Amino Acid	Frequency (%)	
				European Ethnicity	African Ethnicity
K / k	193	K	Met	9	2
		k	Thr	99.8	100
Kp^a / Kp^b / Kp^c	281	Kp^a	Trp	2	<0.01
		Kp^b	Arg	100	100
		Kp^c	Gln	<0.01	<0.01
Js^a / Js^b	597	Js^a	Pro	0.01	20
		Js^b	Leu	100	99

• Met, methionine; Thr, threonine; Trp, tyrosine; Arg, arginine; Gln, glutamine; Pro, proline; Leu, leucine

The other allelic pairs of the Kell blood group system that are rarely encountered in antibody investigations are
• K11 (high frequency) and K17 (low frequency)
• K14 (high frequency) and K24 (low frequency)

Source: Based on data from Daniels, G. *Human Blood Groups*, 2nd ed., Antigens of Kell and Kx systems, Table 7.1, Wiley-Blackwell Publishing.

✳ **TABLE 6-7** High- and Low-Frequency Antigens of the Kell System

Frequency	Antigens
High	k, Kp^b, Js^b, Ku, K11, K12, K13, K14, k-like, K18, K19, Km, K22, TOU, RAZ
Low	Kp^c, Ul^a, K17, K23, K24, VLAN

High- and low-frequency antigens in the Kell system all result from single amino acid substitutions.

Source: Based on data from Daniels, G. *Human Blood Groups*, 2nd ed., Antigens of Kell and Kx systems, Table 7.1, Wiley-Blackwell Publishing.

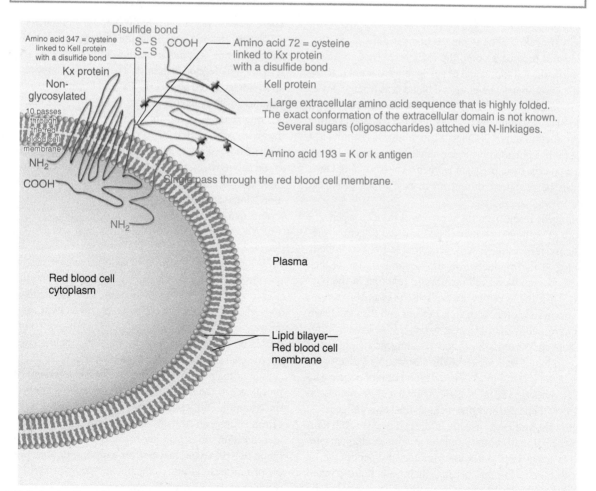

✳ **FIGURE 6-3** Kell and Kx Glycoproteins

There are people whose red blood cells do not have any Kell system antigens due to inheritance of a double dose of the silent allele K^o. The antibody they produce is known as anti-Ku, which reacts with all cells except K^o.

A gene, *XK*, carried on the X chromosome results in production of the high-incidence antigen Kx. Although the *XK* and *KEL* genes are not linked and in fact are on separate chromosomes, their protein products are linked. Deletion of the *XK* gene or inheritance of a nonfunctional *XK* gene results in the **McLeod phenotype**. Because the gene is X-linked, the McLeod phenotype appears only in males; females can be carriers. The McLeod phenotype is very rare and is often associated with a hereditary form of **chronic granulomatous disease (CGD)**, defined as an X-linked hereditary condition in which significant phagocyte biochemical changes occur resulting in affected patients being much more susceptible to severe bacterial infections. This association was explained when it was discovered that the gene for CGD is also X-linked and located very close to the *XK* gene. Therefore, a deletion or mutation in one of these genes will often, but not always, result in deletion or loss of function of both genes. Red blood cells of the McLeod phenotype lack Kx, lack the high-incidence Kell antigen known as Km, and have depressed expression of the other Kell system antigens. Once transfused, patients with the McLeod phenotype may produce anti-KL, a mixture of anti-Kx and anti-Km.

Lewis Blood Group System

Lewis antigens are not intrinsic to the red blood cell membrane but are absorbed from the plasma onto the red blood cell. This action begins after birth; the full expression of Lewis antigens is not reached until around 7 years of age. Therefore, red blood cells from neonates and children should not be phenotyped for Lewis antigens. Transfused red blood cells acquire the Lewis type of the recipient. During pregnancy production of Lewis antigens can diminish, resulting in a transitory Le (a–b–) phenotype; Lewis phenotyping should also not be performed on cells from pregnant women. Corresponding Lewis antibodies can be produced during pregnancy, which disappear postdelivery.

Lewis antigens result from the presence of the Lewis gene, *Le* or *FUT3*, with or without a secretor gene, *Se*. If the *Le* gene is present, an L-fucosyl transferase enzyme acts on type 1 chains in body fluids, resulting in the production of the Le^a antigen. Le^a is then adsorbed onto the red blood cell membrane, resulting in the phenotype Le(a+b–). If the secretor gene, *Se*, is also present, the secretor transferase enzyme adds fucose to type 1 chains and then the Lewis transferase enzyme adds another fucose to this H type 1 chain, forming the Le^b antigen. When both Le^a and Le^b antigens are present in body fluids, red blood cells preferentially adsorb only Le^b antigens and the phenotype is Le(a–b+). The red blood cells of people who do not have *Le* genes type Le (a–b–). See Figure 6-4 ■ for an illustration of the biosynthetic pathway that includes the Lewis antigens.

The Lewis antibodies are usually IgM, react best at room temperature, and occasionally bind complement, with resultant *in vitro* hemolysis. No Lewis antibodies are produced by people whose red blood cells type Le (a–b+) because their body fluids contain both Lewis structures. Anti-Le^b can be produced by people of the Le(a+b–) phenotype and anti-Le^a and/or anti-Le^b by those of the Le(a–b–) phenotype. Neither antibody causes HDFN because the Lewis antigens are not developed at birth. Anti-Le^a rarely causes hemolytic transfusion reactions and anti-Le^b is considered clinically insignificant. During *in vitro* testing an anti-Le^b by itself or in combination with an anti-Le^a may cause most cells to react, raising a concern that other, clinically significant antibodies may be masked. In these cases, Lewis antibodies can be neutralized by saliva containing Lewis substance. This will also confirm that the antibodies are Lewis and not an antibody to a high-incidence antigen.

Anti-Le^{bH} can be produced by people whose red blood cells lack Le^b and have small amounts of the H antigen (Chapter 4), such as people with the A_1 Le (a–b–) phenotype. This antibody reacts well with group O red blood cells such as those used in antibody detection and identification, but will not usually react with group A cells, allowing crossmatch-compatible cells to be easily found.

☑ **CHECKPOINT 6-4**

How does the production of Lewis antigens differ from most other blood group antigens?

Duffy Blood Group System

There are six antigens in the Duffy blood group system, with the commonly encountered ones being the allelic pair, Fy^a and Fy^b. The other antigens are of high incidence in most populations. The Duffy antigens are well developed at birth. They have been reported to weaken upon storage of red blood cells. Fy^a and Fy^b antigens are destroyed by treatment with ficin enzyme, but Fy3 and Fy5 are not. The Fy4 antigen might not exist; the antibody has only been reported once and the results obtained at the time varied among testing laboratories. With no other samples to test in the intervening years, doubt has been raised about whether the original antibody really was to an antigen in the Duffy system. Fy6 is an antigen that has only been identified with monoclonal antibodies; as far as we know, a human has never made an anti-Fy6.

A weak expression of the Fy^b antigen, which is called Fy^x, is detected only by adsorption and elution techniques using anti-Fy^b. Fy^x occurs in people of European ethnicity. Conversely, the Fy (a–b–) phenotype is more common in people of African ethnicity, occurring in about 70% of this population. Besides lacking both the Fy^a and Fy^b antigens, cells of the Fy (a–b–) phenotype also lack the Fy3 antigen. In African populations, the Fy (a–b–) phenotype is usually caused by homozygous inheritance of the silent *FY* gene. The phenotype changes the red blood cell membrane, resulting in increased resistance to malarial infections by *Plasmodium vivax*. Because of the prevalence of the *FY* gene in black populations, the genetics behind the common Duffy phenotypes may differ between people of African and European ethnicity. This can have consequences for antibody identification investigations because the commercial reagent red blood cells on a panel may be from a black or nonblack donor. In people of European ethnicity, the phenotype Fy (a–b+) is usually the result of inheriting two *FYB* genes and the cells have a double dose of

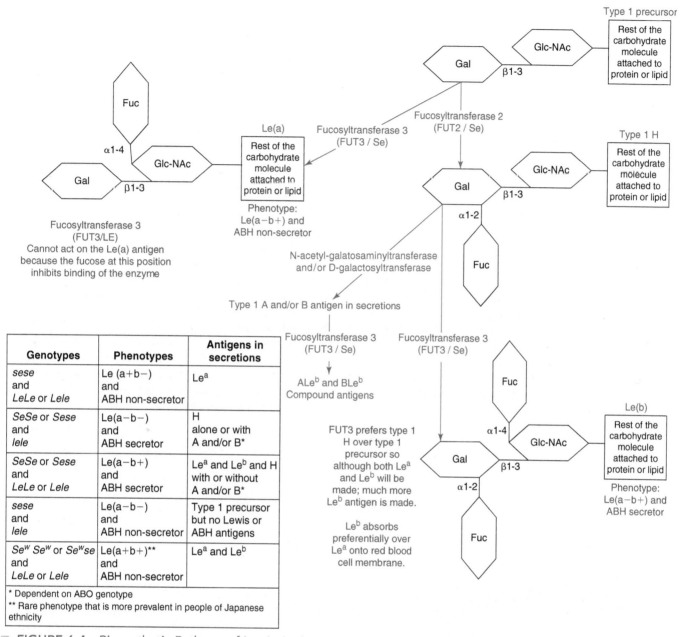

Genotypes	Phenotypes	Antigens in secretions
sese and *LeLe* or *Lele*	Le (a+b−) and ABH non-secretor	Le^a
SeSe or *Sese* and *lele*	Le(a−b−) and ABH secretor	H alone or with A and/or B*
SeSe or *Sese* and *LeLe* or *Lele*	Le(a−b+) and ABH secretor	Le^a and Le^b and H with or without A and/or B*
sese and *lele*	Le(a−b−) and ABH non-secretor	Type 1 precursor but no Lewis or ABH antigens
Se^w Se^w or *Se^{w}se* and *LeLe* or *Lele*	Le(a+b+)** and ABH non-secretor	Le^a and Le^b

* Dependent on ABO genotype
** Rare phenotype that is more prevalent in people of Japanese ethnicity

FIGURE 6-4 Biosynthetic Pathway of Lewis Antigens

Fy^b antigen. However, in people of African ethnicity, the Fy(a−b+) phenotype may just as likely result from inheriting one *FYB* gene and one silent *FY* gene, in which case the cells only have a single dose of antigen. A similar situation exists for the Fy (a+b−) phenotype. See Table 6-8 ✳ for a list of Duffy antigens. Figure 6-5 ▣ is a simplified schematic of the Duffy glycoprotein.

The Duffy antibodies are IgG and do not bind complement. Anti-Fy^a and anti-Fy^b rarely cause HDFN, but may cause hemolytic transfusion reactions. The transfusion reactions are usually of the delayed type, resulting in destruction of red blood cells outside of the blood vessel by antibodies that do not bind complement, a process known as **extravascular hemolysis**. The hemolysis is usually mild, but severe reactions have been reported.

☑ **CHECKPOINT 6-5**

Which phenotype provides resistance to *Plasmodium vivax* malaria?

Kidd Blood Group System

The glycoprotein carrying the Kidd blood group system antigens transports urea across the red blood cell membrane. Figure 6-6 ▣ is a simplified schematic of the Kidd glycoprotein.

There are three antigens in the Kidd system: Jk^a, Jk^b, and the high-incidence antigen, Jk3. The Kidd antigens are fully developed at birth.

★ TABLE 6-8 Antigens of the Duffy System

Antigen	Protein Structure	Frequency (%)	
		European Ethnicity	African Ethnicity
Fya	Gly at amino acid #42	66	10
Fyb	Asp at amino acid #42	83	23
Fy3	Missing from Fy(a–b–) cells	100	32
Fy4	Unconfirmed antigen	N/A	N/A
Fy5	Missing from both Fy(a–b–) and Rh null cells	> 99.9	32
Fy6	Amino acids 19–25 Gln-Leu-Asp-Phe-Glu-Leu-Val	100	32

Gly, glycine; Asp, aspartic acid; Gln, glutamine; Leu, leucine; Phe, phenylalanine; Glu, glutamic acid; Val, valine.

Source: Based on data from Daniels, G. *Human Blood Groups*, 2nd ed., Antigens of the Duffy system, Table 8.1, Wiley-Blackwell Publishing.

Enzyme treatment generally enhances Kidd antigen expression. The Jk (a–b–) null phenotype is rare. The Jk3 antigen is also absent from the red blood cells when two silent *JK* genes are inherited. The *JK* gene, although rare, is more common in people of Polynesian ethnicity. These patients may produce an anti-Jk3, which reacts with all cells except those of the Jk(a–b–) phenotype. Even more rare are people with phenotypically Jk (a–b–) cells, believed to be caused by inheritance of a dominant inhibitor gene. The site of the dominant inhibitor gene, *In (Jk)*, has not been discovered but it does not reside at the same site as the *Jk* genes. People with this inheritance pattern do not make an anti-Jk3;

absorption and elution studies (Chapter 8) can demonstrate that the red blood cell membranes express small quantities of the Jk3 antigen and the other Kidd antigens, depending on the Kidd genes inherited.

Anti-Jkª may cause HDFN, but anti-Jkᵇ and anti-Jk3 rarely do. Anti-Jkª and anti-Jkᵇ are notorious for causing delayed hemolytic transfusion reactions. The reasons for this are two-fold. First, the antibodies can drop below serologically detectable levels within months of production. Second, the IgG antibodies of the Kidd blood group system are very good at binding complement. Therefore, a patient who previously developed, for example, an anti-Jkª may now

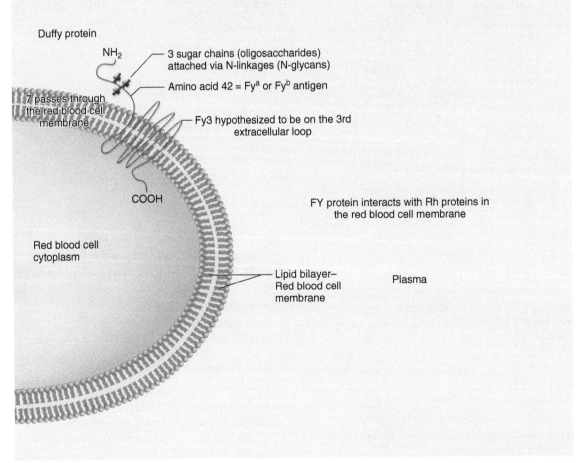

FIGURE 6-5 Duffy Glycoprotein

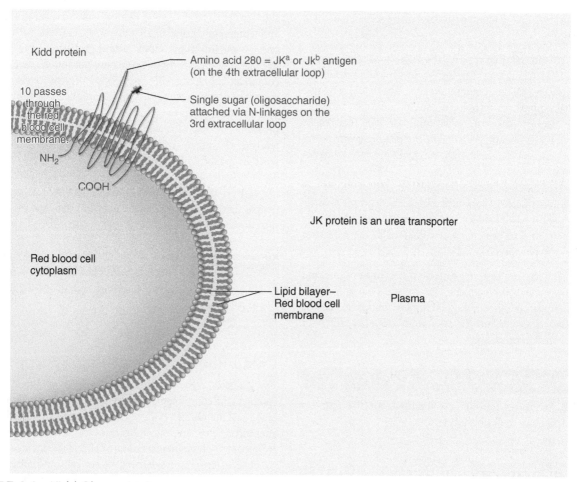

Kidd protein

Amino acid 280 = JK^a or Jk^b antigen
(on the 4th extracellular loop)

10 passes through the red blood cell membrane.

Single sugar (oligosaccharide) attached via N-linkages on the 3rd extracellular loop

NH₂

COOH

JK protein is an urea transporter

Red blood cell cytoplasm

Lipid bilayer–
Red blood cell
membrane

Plasma

 FIGURE 6-6 Kidd Glycoprotein

CASE IN POINT *(continued)*

You just received the properly labeled blood bank specimen on patient FH. You decide to collect some background information about her known historical antibodies before beginning the work-up knowing that she has a history of anti-E, anti-K, anti-Jk^a, anti-Fy^a, anti-M, and anti-Le^a.

1. Which of these antibodies normally react at room temperature and which react at 98.7° F (37° C)?
2. Which of these antibodies have been known to cause hemolytic transfusion reaction?
3. Which of these antibodies are the most immunogenic?
4. Which of the antibodies that are typically IgG in nature are destroyed by enzymes? Which are enhanced by enzymes?
5. Which antibody reactivity is enhanced by acidification?
6. Which antibody is destroyed with 0.2M DTT treatment?
7. Which antibody can be neutralized?

When you actually complete the work-up, you note that the Jk^a antibody is no longer detectable.

8. Can the patient receive red blood cells that contain the Jk^a antigen? Why or why not?

present with a negative antibody screen. If there is no historical record of the antibody, the patient may be transfused with Jk^a-positive cells. When this happens, the anti-Jk^a titer rises rapidly in an anamnestic response; complement is bound to the red blood cells, resulting in often severe hemolysis and a rapid drop in hemoglobin to pretransfusion levels. The level of antibody present may be too low to be detected by monospecific anti-IgG AHG reagent; the use of polyspecific AHG reagent, containing anti-C3d antibody, can detect the bound complement.

Lutheran and Xg Blood Group Systems

Antibody detection and identification antigen profiles usually also contain the typings for Lu^a, Lu^b, and Xg^a, although the antibodies are not often encountered.

Lutheran antigens are not fully developed at birth. There are 19 antigens in the Lutheran system, although Lu^a and Lu^b are usually the only phenotypes included on reagent antigen profiles. Lu^b is of high incidence and Lu^a occurs on 5–8% of red blood cells. Anti-Lu^a may be IgM or IgG whereas anti-Lu^b is usually IgG. Except for Au^a and Au^b, the other antigens in the Lutheran system are all high incidence, with only a handful of examples of the corresponding antibody in each case. Anti-Au^a and anti-Au^b are rarely encountered and are usually clinically insignificant, despite being IgG.

The Lu(a–b–) null phenotype is known to arise from three genetic situations:

1. Most red blood cells that appear to be Lu(a–b–) actually have a very low level of Lutheran antigens as a result of suppression due to the presence of a dominant *In(Lu)* gene. The *In(Lu)* gene also somewhat suppresses expression of P_1, i, In, and AnWj antigens.

2. There is also a recessive X-linked inhibitor gene that results in the Lu(a–b–) phenotype. None of the people having either inhibitor gene but the usual Lutheran genes produce Lutheran antibodies.

3. Lu(a–b–) red blood cells also may result from the recessive *LuLu* genotype, inheritance of two silent alleles. These people lack the Lu^a, Lu^b, and high-incidence Lu3 antigens and therefore may produce an anti-Lu3, which reacts with all cells except those of the Lu(a–b–) phenotype.

The Xg^a antigen results from a gene on the X chromosome, and it can be destroyed by ficin treatment. The antigen is not fully developed at birth. Apparently it is not especially immunogenic because anti-Xg^a is rarely detected. Anti-Xg^a does not cause either HDFN or hemolytic transfusion reactions.

> **☑ CHECKPOINT 6-6**
>
> What are the three genetic explanations for the existence of the Lu(a–b–) phenotype

OTHER BLOOD GROUP SYSTEMS WITH LIMITED CLINICAL SIGNIFICANCE[7]

There are a number of other blood group systems that appear on standard antigen profiles that have limited clinical significance but due to their presence are worth describing in the paragraphs that follow.

I and i Blood Group System

"I" is often referred to as standing for "individuality." There are two antigens involved in this system, as the name implies: I (pronounced as "big I") and i (pronounced as "little i"). The genetic basis for i expression has not been determined. At birth i antigen is expressed on red blood cells, usually most is converted to I antigen within the first 18 months of life. Thus, typical newborn red blood cells possess significant amounts of i antigen and no I antigen; adult RBCs contain significant amounts of the I antigen and undetectable, if any, i antigen. The i antigen lacks the more complex branching present on the I antigen. Figure 6-7 ■ illustrates the linear and branching structures that are responsible for the i and I antigens, respectively. The strength of I antigen expression varies among adults. Rarely, this conversion (from i to I antigen) does not occur and an adult may have primarily i expressed on the red blood cells.

Antibodies in this system are usually IgM *autoantibodies* (defined as antibodies against "self"). Autoanti-I (in this case an individual makes antibody against the I antigen that is located on his or her own cells) is commonly encountered when testing is performed at lower than 71.6° F (22° C). Dramatic increase in reactivity strength and temperature range of an autoanti-I can occur with *Mycoplasma pneumoniae* infections. **Cold autoagglutinins** (antibodies against self that react best at room temperature or lower) that react when a combination of I and ABH antigens are present are also not uncommon. The plasma of group A_1 and B producers of anti-IH will react with all adult group O cells such as screen and panel cells, but will probably be compatible with A and B donor cells, which have lower levels of H antigen. Table 6-9 ✴ presents the relative strength and reactivity patterns of these antibodies.

Clinically significant anti-I may be detected in adults who have not converted i antigen; provision of donor units from other I−i+ people may be necessary. Detection of anti-i has been associated with infectious mononucleosis.

> **☑ CHECKPOINT 6-7**
>
> Why does anti-I react negatively when tested with cord blood cells?

Chido/Rodgers Blood Group System

The antigens of the Chido/Rodgers system are located on the C4 complement component. The antigens are not intrinsic to the red blood cell membrane, but rather are adsorbed onto red blood cells after birth. There are nine antigens in the system; Ch1-6 and Rg1-2 are antigens of high incidence and WH is of low incidence.

Use of enzyme-treated red blood cells and antibody plasma neutralization are very helpful in identifying these antibodies. Enzymes destroy these antigens. Because the antigens are of high incidence, **crossmatch-compatible** (i.e., donor red blood cells that when tested with patient/recipient plasma or serum suggest that no reaction will take place *in vivo* if the cells are transfused to this patient) units may not be located. Although the antibodies are IgG, they have *low affinity*, which means that they do not bind well to their corresponding antigen. Consequently, transfused cells that are **crossmatch incompatible** (i.e., donor red blood cells that when tested with patient/recipient plasma or serum suggest that a reaction will take place *in vivo* if the cells are transfused to this patient) due to antibodies in the Chido/Rodgers system usually do not have a shortened survival.

Knops Blood Group System

Within the Knops blood group system, the Kn^a, McC^a, Sl^a, and Yk^a are high-incidence antigens, although Sl^a may be present on red blood cells of only 60% of people with African ethnicity. Kn^b, which is antithetical to Kn^a, is of low incidence. McC^b, which is antithetical to McC^a, has an incidence of 45% in populations of African ethnicity but has not been found in European populations. The antigens are weak at birth and later are expressed on complement receptor 1 (CR1). Ficin treatment of red blood cells does not affect these antigens, but 0.2M DTT may weaken or destroy them.

Antibodies within the Knops system are IgG, of low affinity, and are not known to cause shortened red blood cell survival after

I and i antigens are on the same molecules that carry ABH and Lewis antigens, but the Ii antigens are found on the interior of the 3 dimensional structure while the ABH and Lewis antigens are the terminal sugars and are on the exterior of the molecule.

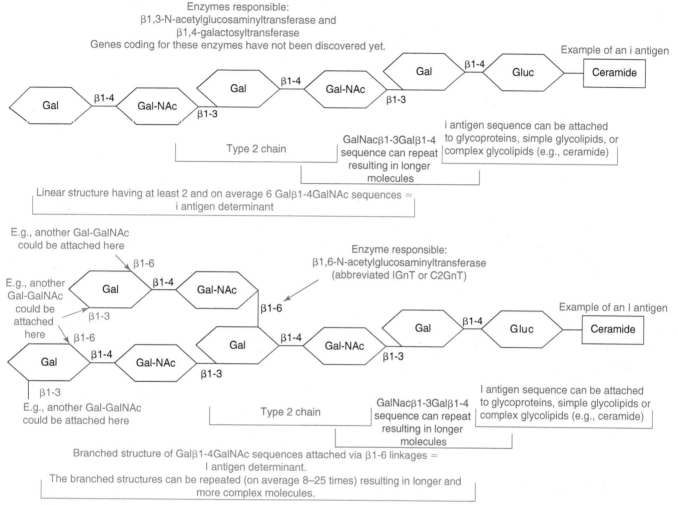

FIGURE 6-7   Schematic of I and i Antigens

transfusion of crossmatch-incompatible units. Antibodies with this set of characteristics but occurring at high titers were previously grouped together under the term *high titer, low avidity (HTLA)*

★ TABLE 6-9 Reactivity Patterns of Cold Autoantibodies

	Commonly Available Test Red Blood Cells						Rare Test Red Blood Cells	
	Adult				Cord		Adult	
Antibody	O	A₁	A₂	B	O	A	Bombay (H–)	I negative
Anti-I	4	4	4	4	0	0	4	0
Anti-i	0	0	0	0	4	4	0	4
Anti-H	4	0	2	1	4	2	0	4
Anti-IH	4	0	2	1	0	0	0	0

The numbers 0, 1, 2, 4 refer to reaction strengths that occur when the corresponding antibody is tested against the available test red blood cells (Chapter 3). Using a nonadditive tube technique incubated at 39.2° F (4° C).

antibodies. Many of the antibodies in the Knops system and also in several other systems were considered HTLA antibodies. HTLA is not used within the ISBT naming conventions as the corresponding antigens are not genetically related and therefore do not belong to the same blood group system.

JMH Blood Group System

The JMH antigen is a high-incidence antigen present on a glyco-sylphosphatidylinositol (GPI)-linked glycoprotein. People suffering from a rare blood cell membrane protein defect that results in an acquired hemolytic anemia known as **paroxysmal nocturnal hemoglobinuria (PNH)**, which should not be confused with paroxysmal cold hemoglobinuria (PCH), lack all GPI linked glycoproteins. Consequently, their red blood cells do not express any antigens that occur on GPI-linked glycoprotiens such as JMH, Yt, MER2, Emm, and those in the Cromer and Dombrock systems. Enzymes and 0.2M DTT destroy the JMH antigen.

Anti-JMH has most often been found in elderly patients, either as obvious autoantibody or probable autoantibody with antigen weakening with aging. Often the antibody is primarily of IgG4 subclass.

Bg Antigens

Human leukocyte antigens (HLA) are present on cells including white blood cells, platelets, and many tissue cells that are genetically determined by genes of the major histocompatibility complex (Chapter 18). Red blood cells, being non-nucleated, do not express HLA antigens in many people. However, expression of HLA antigens on red blood cells varies from person to person and even during the course of one person's life. Strong HLA expression on red blood cells is called *Bg* antigens. The most common Bg expression on red blood cells is Bg^a. Manufacturers of reagent red blood cells will try to avoid including Bg^a-positive cells in antibody screening sets as the inclusion can result in many "nuisance" positive reactions because antibodies to HLA antigens are not uncommon. When a known strongly positive Bg^a cell is included on a panel, the manufacturer will often identify it. Bg^a corresponds to HLA-B7; Bg^b and Bg^c show possible cross-reactivity with several HLA antigens. Bg is not considered a blood group system.

HLA antibodies are usually IgG and react weakly in serologic tests. They are clinically insignificant, problematic antibodies in the immunohematology (blood bank) laboratory but are vitally important in transplantation testing. If an HLA antibody is interfering with the detection of clinically significant antibodies, the plasma can be tested against red blood cells treated with chloroquin diphosphate or EDTA/glycine acid, both of which destroy Bg antigens. Of course, one must always be aware of what other red blood cell antigens are altered or destroyed by these reagents.

> ## ☑ CHECKPOINT 6-8
> Name two substances that can be used to diminish Bg reactivity.

Sd^a or Sid Antigen

The Sd^a (Sid) antigen has not been assigned to a specific blood group system; it is one of the antigens in the ISBT classification called *Series 901*, which encompasses antigens of high incidence where a genetic linkage to a blood group system has not yet been proven. This antigen is variable in red blood cell expression from person to person, weakens during pregnancy, and is not detected at birth. Ficin treatment of red blood cells enhances detection. A soluble form of the antigen is found in human urine on Tamm Horsfall glycoprotein. It is also present in high concentrations in guinea pig urine, resulting in both human and guinea pig urine being used in antibody-neutralization procedures. Antibody neutralizations help confirm the identity of an antibody to a high-incidence antigen, as well as help to uncover if other clinically significant antibodies are present.

The antibody is usually IgM. When observed microscopically, agglutinates exhibit a mixed-field, shiny, and refractile appearance, not characteristic of any other antibody specificity.

> ## ☑ CHECKPOINT 6-9
> Is anti-Sd^a a clinically significant antibody? Why or why not?

OTHER BLOOD GROUP SYSTEMS WITH CLINICAL SIGNIFICANCE[7]

The antibodies within the following blood group systems are clinically significant but are rarely encountered. Usually, the corresponding antigen is either of high or low incidence, resulting in a low occurrence of an antigen-negative recipient being transfused with an antigen-positive donor (Table 6-10 ✷).

Diego Blood Group System

The antigens in the Diego blood group system reside on a red blood cell transmembrane protein called Band 3 or AE1-transporter, which has several functions including a vital role in anion exchange. The more commonly encountered antibodies are to the low-incidence antigens, Wr^a and Di^a, which are more common in some Asian populations. Their antithetical high-incidence antigens are Wr^b and Di^b. The rest of the antigens in this blood group system are also of low incidence. Anti-Wr^a and anti-Di^a vary in their clinical significance from person to person, with some antibodies causing no or mild symptoms and other antibodies causing severe transfusion reactions or HDFN.

Yt Blood Group System

The Yt or Cartwright blood group system has two antigens. Yt^a is an antigen of high incidence; the incidence of Yt^b varies among different ethnicities. The antigens exist on a GPI-linked glycoprotein and therefore are absent from the red blood cells of people suffering from PNH. Anti-Yt^b is not clinically significant, but anti-Yt^a has been implicated in delayed hemolytic transfusion reactions.

Scianna Blood Group System

The Scianna blood group system has four more commonly encountered antigens; SC1 and SC3 are of high incidence and SC2 and SC4 are of low incidence. The null phenotype is SC−1,−2,−3. SC4 is also called Rd. SC1 and SC2 are antithetical. Neither anti-SC1 or anti-SC2 is clinically significant, but anti-SC4 can cause mild to severe HDFN and anti-SC3 can cause mild transfusion reactions or HDFN.

Dombrock Blood Group System

The antigens in the Dombrock blood group system are carried on a GPI-linked glycoprotein. Do^a and Do^b are antithetical. There are three antigens of high incidence: Gy^a, Hy, and Jo^a. The null phenotype is Gy^a(−). Antibodies in this blood group system do not cause HDFN but have been implicated in hemolytic transfusion reactions.

This is the first blood group system where genetic testing has in large part replaced serologic phenotyping.[8,9] In the Dombrock blood group system, two factors have contributed to the emergence of genetic testing as the primary methodology. First, there is no source of consistently reliable antisera. Second, the genetic polymorphisms are simple and have been well defined. In contrast, these two

★ TABLE 6-10 Information Related to Antigens with Less Commonly Encountered Antibodies

Blood Group Systems				
System	Antigens*	Incidence#	Location	Effect of Antigen-Altering Reagents
Diego	Di^b, Wr^b	High	AE-1 transporter	
	Di^a, Wr^a, Wd^a, Rb^a, WARR, ELO, Wu, Bp^a, Mo^a, Hg^a, Vg^a, Sw^a, BOW, NFLD, Jn^a, KREP, Fr^a, SW1	Low		
Yt	Yt^a	High	Acetylcholinesterase or AchE	Ficin varies DTT destroys
	Yt^b	Low, 30%; varies with ethnicity		
Scianna	Sc1, Sc3, STAR, SCER, SCAN	High	RBC adhesion protein: ERMAP	DTT varies
	Sc2, Rd	Low		
Dombrock	Do^a, Do^b	67%/82%	GPI-linked glycoprotein	DTT weakens
	Gy^a, Hy, Jo^a	High		
Colton	Co^a, Co3	High	Aquaporin-1 (AQP1)	
	Co^b	10%		
Gerbich	Ge2, Ge3, Ge4	High	Glycophorin C or D	Ficin destroys Ge2 and Ge4
	Wb, Ls^a, An^a, Dh^a, GEIS	Low		
Cromer	Cr^a, Tc^a, Dr^a, Es^a, IFC, UMC, WES^b, GUTI, SERF, ZENA, CROV, CRAM	High	Decay-accelerating factor (DAF)	DTT weakens
	Tc^b, Tc^c, WES^a	Low		
Indian	In^a, INFI, INJA	High	CD44 glycoprotein	Ficin and DTT destroy
	In^b	Low		
Ok	Ok^a	High		
Raph	MER2	High		
Gill	GIL	High	Aquaglyceroporin	
Rh-associated glycoprotein	Duclos	High		
	Ol^a	Low		
Blood Group Collections				
Ii	i	Low in adults		
Globoside	P^k, LKE	High		
Cost	Cs^a	High		
	Cs^b	34%		
Er	Er^a, Er3	High		Acid destroys
	Er^b	Low		
Vel	Vel, ABTI	High		
Antigens in the 901 series of high-incidence antigens				Antigens in the 700 series of low-incidence antigens
Lan, At^a, Jr^a, Emm, AnWj, Sd^a, PEL, MAM				By, Chr^a, Bi, Bx^a, To^a, Pt^a, Re^a, Je^a, Li^a, Milne, RASM, JFV, Kg, JONES, HJK, HOFM, SARA, REIT

*As of August 2008 update.

#High incidence: >90%; low incidence: <1%

conditions do not apply to most of the common blood group systems. Therefore, it is unlikely that genetic screening will supplant (replace) routine serologic phenotyping; rather, the two methodologies are increasingly used as complementary tests.

Colton Blood Group System

The three antigens in the Colton blood group system reside on aquaporin-1, a protein that is involved in the transport of water across the red blood cell membrane. Co^a, which is a high-incidence antigen, is antithetical to Co^b, which is a low-incidence antigen. Co3 is a common antigen that is absent on some very rare Co (a–b–) cells. The antibodies to these antigens are usually found in combination with other antibodies. The clinical significance varies from person to person, with some antibodies appearing to not shorten red blood cell lifespan and others causing mild to severe HDFN or hemolytic transfusion reactions.

Gerbich Blood Group System

Like the antigens of the MNS system, the Gerbich antigens are found on glycophorins; however, Gerbich antigens are found on glycophorin C and glycophorin D. The common phenotype present in almost 100% of people is Ge2,3,4. The rare null phenotype, also called Leach type, is Ge–2,–3,–4. There are also two rare deletion phenotypes: Ge–2,–3,4, which is also called Gerbich type, and Ge–2,3,4, which is also called Yus type. The Gerbich blood group system also includes a number of low-incidence antigens. Anti-Ge2 may cause hemolytic transfusion reactions and anti-Ge3 has been identified as the cause of both HDFN and transfusion reactions. The antibodies to the other Gerbich system antigens are not clinically significant or the significance is unknown due to the low number of cases studied.

Cromer Blood Group System

The antigens in the Cromer blood group system are expressed on the decay-accelerating factor (DAF), which is involved in regulation of the complement cascade (Chapter 1). DAF is a GPI-linked protein; therefore, the red blood cells in people suffering from PNH (proxysmal nocturinal hemoglobinuria) lack DAF and therefore lack all Cromer antigens. The antigens in the Cromer blood group system are either of high incidence or low incidence, although Cr^a, Tc^a, and Wes^a show variation in frequency between European and African ethnicities. Tc^a, Tc^b, and Tc^c are antithetical. The null phenotype is IFC(–), which is also called INAB. Antibodies in this system have not been implicated in HDFN, but some have caused hemolytic transfusion reactions. Most of the transfusion reactions reported have been mild, except for some case reports of anti-Tc^a, which has caused more severe reactions.

Indian Blood Group System

The Indian blood group system antigens are expressed on the CD44 protein. CD44 exists on a wide variety of tissue cells in addition to red blood cells. The In^a antigen is a low-incidence antigen, except in certain populations genetically originating around the Indian subcontinent such as Iranians, Arabs, and Indians. The In^b antigen is of high incidence. Both corresponding antibodies can cause a positive

DAT on cord cells as the antigens are expressed at birth, but there is no symptomatic HDFN. Anti-In^b has caused transfusion reactions of varying severities.

GIL Antigen

The GIL antigen is the only antigen in this blood group system. There have been only five case reports of GIL(–) people. The high-incidence antigen resides on the aquaglyceroporin protein, which is another protein involved in water transport. Anti-GIL has been reported to cause hemolytic transfusion reaction but no HDFN.

BLOOD GROUP SYSTEMS WITH UNKNOWN CLINICAL SIGNIFICANCE

In addition to blood group systems with known clinical significance, there is also a number of known blood group systems of which their clinical significance is not known. That being said, some of these blood group systems are not on antigen profiles, most likely due to their rarity of occurrence and the fact that they have no proven clinical significance.

OK Blood Group System

The OK blood group system consists of one antigen, Ok^a. It is a high-incidence antigen and so far all the people identified as Ok^a(–) have been of Japanese ethnicity. The clinical significance of anti-Ok^a has not been well defined, as only eight people have been identified as Ok^a(–).

RAPH Blood Group System

The RAPH blood group system also only has one antigen, called MER2. Originally, the antigen was identified by a reaction with a monoclonal antibody called MER2, hence the antigen's name. This was the first blood group antigen to be discovered through a reaction with a monoclonal antibody rather than an alloantibody. There have since been case reports of patients producing anti-MER2. As there have only been four examples of the antibody studied, the clinical significance has not been defined.

Rh-Associated Glycoprotein

Rh-associated glycoprotein (RHAG) is the latest blood group system identified in the ISBT classification. The genetics and biochemistry of this glycoprotein were discussed in Chapter 5. Two antigens are currently grouped in this system, the high-incidence Duclos antigen and the low-incidence Ol^a antigen. A third antigen has provisionally been assigned to this system, which illustrates that the number of antigens in any given blood group system changes over time as genetic studies provide clarity around each antigen's origin.

Review of the Main Points

- Many antigens have been determined to be on human red blood cells besides those in the ABO and Rh blood group systems.
- The International Society of Blood Transfusion (ISBT) has organized the human red blood cell antigens using uniform classification and terminology.[1] Related antigens are placed in a blood group system once the genetic basis is confirmed.
- Genetic terms of importance are dosage, homozygous, heterozygous, phenotype, genotype, and null phenotype.
- Antigen-altering reagents such as ficin and DTT are useful when dealing with patients with multiple antibodies.
- Antigen profiles, created by commercial manufacturers, consist of grids that indicate antigen make up of commercial red blood cells used for antibody detection or antibody identification.

- Antigen profiles are the primary component of antigrams (also known as panel sheets or profile sheets). Along with antigen profile grids, antigrams provide laboratorians with pertinent information about the commercial red blood cells that comprise a given panel or kit.
- Antigens can be divided according to biochemical characteristics. Protein antigens include Rh, Duffy, Kell, Kidd, and so on. Carbohydrate antigens include Ii, MN, Lewis, and so on.
- Protein antigens' corresponding antibodies are typically clinically significant (IgG) whereas carbohydrate antigens' corresponding antibodies are typically not clinically significant (IgM).
- Clinically significant antibodies are defined as those that result in shortened red blood cell survival in such situations as immune-mediated transfusion reactions and hemolytic disease of the fetus and newborn.

Review Questions

1. Select the antibodies that react optimally at room temperature: (Objective #7)

   A. Anti-M

   B. Anti-Le^a

   C. Anti-I

   D. Anti-S

2. Which of the following blood group system antibodies is known to bind complement? (Objective #7)

   A. Duffy

   B. Kidd

   C. Rh

   D. Lutheran

3. Choose the Kell blood group system phenotype that is associated with a homozygous expression of the Kell antigen: (Objective #3)

   A. (K+k−)

   B. (K+k+)

   C. (K−k+)

   D. (K−k−)

4. Which of the following blood group antigens has the highest frequency in the population? (Objective #4)

   A. Fy^a

   B. M

   C. K

   D. E

5. The Fy(a−b−) phenotype is most often found in which of the following blood donor populations? (Objective #4)

   A. European

   B. Asian

   C. African

   D. Hispanic

6. A technologist performed ficin treatment on a suspension of red blood cells. Select the expected change in antigen expression: (Objective #14)

   _____ C   A. Diminished

   _____ Fy^b B. Enhanced

   _____ Jk^a C. Unaffected

   _____ M

   _____ K

7. Treatment of red blood cells with _____ can destroy Kell system antigens. (Objective #15)

   A. 0.2M DTT

   B. Papain

   C. Acid pH 6.5

   D. LISS

8. Select the substance that is NOT able to inhibit or neutralize antibody reactivity: (Objective #15)

   A. Human saliva

   B. Pooled human plasma

   C. PEG

   D. Guinea pig urine

9. Characteristics of clinically significant antibodies include: (Objective #9)

    A. Ability to cross the placenta

    B. *In vivo* hemolysis of red blood cells

    C. Resulting anemia in newborns

    D. React optimally at room temperature

10. Chronic granulomatous disease (CGD) is associated with which of the following phenotypes? (Objective #9)

    A. En(a-)

    B. McLeod

    C. Rh null

    D. Kell null

11. Three days after transfusion of packed red blood cells, a patient experienced a decrease in hemoglobin and hematocrit to pretransfusion levels. An antibody screen and DAT were performed on a post-transfusion specimen and the results were positive. Repeat testing of the pretransfusion specimen confirmed that the antibody screen and DAT were both negative prior to the transfusion. What is the most likely explanation for these results? (Objective #10)

    A. The antibody screening reagents were expired and inert.

    B. The post-transfusion specimen was mislabeled.

    C. A low-titer antibody was present in the pretransfusion specimen.

    D. The technologist made a clerical error.

12. When an individual inherits both the Lewis (Le) gene and the secretor gene (Se), which of the following red blood cell phenotypes will be observed? (Objective #13)

    A. Le(a+b−)

    B. Le(a+b+)

    C. Le(a−b+)

    D. Le(a−b−)

13. Select the situations when the Le(a−b−) red blood cell phenotype can be identified. (Objective #13)

    A. Newborns

    B. Elderly

    C. Pregnancy

    D. Inheritance of Le gene

14. The characteristics of the I antigen include: (Objective #16)

    A. Straight chain structure

    B. Present at birth

    C. Reacts best at room temperature

    D. Varied expression among adults

15. Which of the following characteristics describe the Sid blood group antigen? (Objective #18)

    A. Mainly room temperature reactive

    B. Exhibit a mixed-field, shiny, and refractile appearance

    C. Variable expression in the population

    D. Highest quantity in urine

References

1. Daniels GL, Fletcher A, Garratty G, et al. Blood group terminology 2004: from the International Society of Blood Transfusion committee on terminology for red cell surface antigens. *Vox Sang* 2004; 87: 304–16.

2. International Society for Blood Transfusion. Working Party on Red Cell Immunogenics and Blood Group Terminology. Table of blood group systems [Internet]. Bristol; England: The Bristol Institute for Transfusion Services and the International Blood Group Reference Laboratory. Updated August 2010 [cited 18 July 2011]. Available from http://ibgrl.blood.co.uk/ISBTPages/ISBTTerminologyPages/Table%20of%20blood%20group%20systems.htm.

3. Code of Federal Regulations, Title 21, FDA. US government Printing Office, Washington, DC. 2005; 660(33); 121.

4. Hughes-Jones NC, Gardner B. The Kell system: Studies with radioactively labeled anti-K. *Vox Sang* 1979; 36: 31.

5. Vaughan JI, Manning M, Warwick RM, et al. Inhibition of erythroid progenitor cells by anti-Kell antibodies in fetal alloimmune anemia. *N Engl J Med* 1998; 338: 798–803.

6. Marsh WL, et al. Naturally occurring anti-Kell stimulated by E. coli enterocolitis in a 20-day-old child. *Transfusion* 1978; 18: 149–54.

7. Reid MD and Lomas-Francis C. *The Blood Group Antigen Facts Book*. New York: Academic Press.

8. Storry JR, Westhoff CM, Charles-Pierre D, Rios M, Hue-Roye K, Vege S, Nance S, Reid ME. DNA analysis for donor screening of Dombrock blood group antigens. *Immunohematology* 2003; 19(3): 73–6.

9. Reid ME. Complexities of the Dombrock blood group system revealed. *Transfusion*. 2005; 45: 92–9S.

Additional Resources

1. Roback, JD (ed). *Technical Manual*, 16th ed. Bethesda (MD): AABB; 2008.

2. Daniels GL. *The Human Blood Groups*, 2nd ed. Oxford (UK): Blackwell Science; 2002.

3. Harmening, DM. *Modern Blood Banking and Transfusion Practices*. 6th ed. Philadelphia (PA): F.A. Davis; 2012.

4. Mollison PL, Engelfriet CP, Contreras, M. *Blood Transfusion in Clinical Medicine*. 11th ed. Oxford (UK): Blackwell Scientific; 2005.

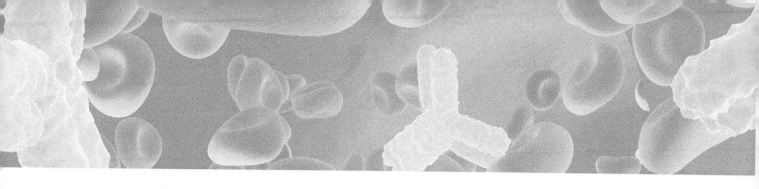

7

Pretransfusion and Compatibility Testing

COLLEEN YOUNG AND LISA DENESIUK

Chapter Objectives

Upon completion of this chapter, the student will be able to:

1. List the elements that should be discussed with a patient in order to obtain informed consent for transfusion.
2. Identify and describe the information that is included in a request for blood components.
3. Describe the timing and process of specimen collection for pretransfusion testing.
4. Discuss the uses for patient information including history in the transfusion service.
5. List the requirements and mandatory tests included in the receipt of blood products and pretransfusion testing for red blood cell transfusion.
6. Determine ABO compatibility for transfusion of red blood cell and plasma products.
7. Determine instances with justification when reflex testing should occur, select the tests that should be performed, and predict the results when appropriate.
8. Compare pretransfusion testing in adults to pretransfusion testing in neonates.
9. Describe pretransfusion testing for platelet, plasma, and fractionation products.
10. Describe the three methodologies used in transfusion medicine testing.
11. Describe the purpose of the crossmatch.
12. Compare and contrast antiglobulin, immediate spin, and electronic crossmatch procedures.
13. Describe the parameters that allow for electronic crossmatch.
14. Discuss ways to improve inventory control of blood products.
15. List the advantages and disadvantages of using the type and screen procedure.
16. Identify and describe the steps and procedures required in tagging and issuing blood products.
17. Describe the steps required at administration and postadministration of blood products.
18. Define uncrossmatched issue of packed red blood cell units.
19. List cases where incompatible red blood cells may be transfused.

Key Terms

ABO incompatibility
 (incompatibilities)
Allocating
Antiglobulin crossmatch
Autologous control
 (autocontrol; AC)
C:T ratio (crossmatched to
 transfused ratio)
Compatibility test (testing)
Compatible
Crossmatch (crossmatches)
Crossmatching
Donor cell antigen typing(s)
Electronic crossmatch
Fractionated product(s)
IAT crossmatch
Immediate spin crossmatch

Incompatible
Informed consent(s)
Issue
Major ABO incompatible/
 incompatibility
Minor ABO incompatible/
 incompatibility
Patient cell antigen typing(s)
Reflex test (s)|testing
Refractory
Regulation(s)
Rh-immune globulin (RhIg)
Serologic crossmatch
Standard(s)
Tagging
Type and screen (T & S)

What's Ahead?

The ideal pretransfusion test protocol would identify all clinically significant antibodies and incompatibilities between the recipient and donor, while ignoring all clinically insignificant antibodies and incompatibilities. Unfortunately, the ideal test does not exist and instead requirements try to find a balance that provides the greatest level of safety for the recipient. This chapter explores the requirements and the methods for pretransfusion and compatibility testing by addressing the following questions:

- What significant historical events contributed to the concepts of pretransfusion and compatibility testing?
- What regulations, standards, and protocols are associated with pretransfusion and compatibility testing?
- What administration and postadministration issues must be considered when blood is transfused?
- What special considerations must be taken into account if administering uncrossmatched or incompatible red blood cells?

CASE IN POINT

TK is a 62-year-old male with a history of cancer who is admitted to the hospital to undergo a cholecystectomy secondary to carcinoma. TK agrees that his surgeon can perform either a laproscopic or open surgery depending on the surgeon's assessment of TK's condition at the time of the operation. His surgeon orders preoperative laboratory tests that include a complete blood count (CBC), prothrombin time (PT)/international normalized ratio (INR), and type & screen (T & S). The physician places the order in the hospital information system and the patient is sent to the outpatient area to have the specimens collected.

HISTORICAL BACKGROUND

The requirements for pretransfusion testing have changed over time as the testing methods have developed. Requirements continue to change as knowledge in the field of transfusion medicine grows.

When the field of transfusion medicine was in its adolescence, much research was done on finding new methodologies or enhancing the current methods to detect more antibodies. Generally speaking, these testing phases and methods were added onto the existing testing protocols, resulting in more and more tests being performed. However, many of the antibodies detected by using a variety of test phases and methods were clinically insignificant. The profusion of testing in routine pretransfusion protocols peaked in the early to mid 1980s.

During the last two decades of the 20th century, researchers turned their attention to analyzing what constitutes the best mix of testing phases and methods. They searched for answers to questions such as: Does this test make the transfusion safer? Does this test add value for the recipient? Is the increased testing time and the resultant delay in transfusion a larger safety risk than the safety benefits, if any,

delivered by the test result? Based on this research, most pretransfusion testing protocols were pared down and new testing formats, such as the *electronic crossmatch*, were developed.

REGULATIONS AND STANDARDS

Regulations are rules made by governments that support implementation of laws (Chapters 20 and 21). **Standards** are issued by accreditation organizations and are guidelines that outline an expected level of quality. Regulations are mandatory, whereas standards may be mandatory or voluntary. For example, in the United States, the Code of Federal Regulations (CFR) 21 outlines many of the requirements around blood donation and a commonly used voluntary standard is the AABB (an organization formerly known as the American Association of Blood Banks but due to the expansion of the organization's scope now goes only by the acronym AABB) Standards for Blood Banks and Transfusion Services.

Regulations and standards outline the minimum requirements for both donor and recipient (a term used interchangeably with patient) testing. These minimum standards are developed to ensure that transfusion is as safe as possible. Blood banks and transfusion services must meet the minimum requirements, but facilities may choose to perform additional tests. The decision to perform or not perform additional tests may be driven by the availability of resources: human, financial, and technological. However, equally important in the decision-making process is the particular situation of the transfusion service; for example, the medical services provided in the facility or facilities that the transfusion services supports, the patient population supported, and the distance between the transfusion service and their blood supplier.

RECEIPT OF BLOOD PRODUCTS

When blood products are received from a blood collection facility not affiliated with the transfusing institution, certain standards must be followed to verify that the products are correctly labeled. For red blood cell units or granulocytes, which may have 20–50 ml of red blood cells (RBCs), ABO retyping is required, as is **crossmatching** (that is, the act of testing donor red blood cells with patient/recipient plasma) with the recipient's sample. In the United States, Rh(D) retyping must be performed on all units labeled as Rh(D) negative. The blood for testing is obtained from a sterilely sealed segment attached to the unit of RBCs (Figure 7-1 ■). Confirmatory testing for weak D does not need to be repeated at the receiving institution; weak D testing is performed at the original collection facility. Blood products (discussed in more detail in Chapter 11) with few RBCs (plasma, cryoprecipitate, or platelet products) do no generally get retested for ABO or Rh type at the receiving institution. Visual inspection of the products and clerical checks are performed on all products.

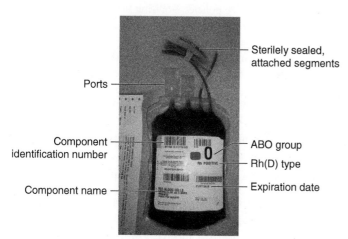

Ports
Sterilely sealed, attached segments
Component identification number
ABO group
Rh(D) type
Component name
Expiration date

■ **FIGURE 7-1** Unit of Red Blood Cells
Source: Gretchen James.

Transfusion centers that also collect blood donors do not need to reconfirm the blood typing performed at their own institution.

PRETRANSFUSION REQUIREMENTS

Pretransfusion requirements encompass all aspects of preparing to provide patients with blood components. Requirements include obtaining *informed consent* (a concept described in detail in the next section), formally requesting products, collecting and testing patient specimens, and selecting appropriate blood components for transfusion. Pretransfusion testing increases the safety of blood transfusion and improves patient care.

Informed Consent

Informed consent is one of the cornerstones of transfusion safety. In order for patients to give informed consent, they must first be educated about the risks and benefits of transfusion, as well as any alternatives that may be available to them. This education is the responsibility of the physician ordering the transfusion, with the aid of the nursing or laboratory staff.[1]

Consent is considered informed when a description of the risks, benefits, and viable treatment alternatives are provided in language the patient or the legal representative can comprehend. The description should be specific to the patient's condition and the blood product he or she would receive. The patient or the legal representative must have the opportunity to ask questions and the right to refuse the transfusion without suffering punitive reactions or a decrease in the quality of care received.

Patients are often most concerned about the risk of exposure to infectious diseases, but other transfusion risks occur much more frequently, such as transfusion-related circulatory overload or febrile nonhemolytic transfusion reactions (Chapters 12 and 13). Some of the noninfectious complications can be fatal, so transfusion is never undertaken lightly and it is important that the patient be aware of complications that could be associated with transfusion.

Facilities are required to have policies in place to govern the informed consent process. Consent for transfusion may be done at the time of admission in conjunction with consent for other medical treatment or it may be obtained separately when the need to transfuse is identified. Regardless of when consent is obtained, patients must have the opportunity to ask questions and must be given the right to accept or refuse transfusion.[1] If the patient is unable to give consent due to incapacitation or inability to comprehend, the legal medical next of kin must be educated before giving consent (or denying it for religious or other beliefs).

Requests for Blood Components

Physicians or other authorized health professionals are responsible for ordering blood components for transfusion.[1] The request for blood components is a critical control point that impacts the entire pretransfusion testing process. Consideration must be given to the following when blood components are ordered:

- The name of the physician placing the order must be indicated.
- Orders should be placed to ensure sufficient time to perform complete testing.

- Requests should include enough clinical information and patient history to ensure that appropriate products will be provided.

- Requests must include the number and type(s) of component(s) required.

- There should be sufficient information on the request form to allow adequate identification of the patient.

- Requests may be verbal but they should be followed up with a written request form.[2, 3]

Requests for blood components should be documented in the patient's health record as well as transmitted to the transfusion service. The documentation may be hard copy or electronic. The hard copy form sent to the transfusion service is often called a *requisition*.

At minimum, there must be two independent patient identifiers on the request for transfusion. These usually include the patient's first and last name and a unique identification number, usually a hospital or blood bank identification number. Other acceptable types of identification may include the patient's date of birth, driver's license number, or other forms of photographic identification.[3] Facilities should have policies outlining the acceptance criteria for requests and should not accept those that do not meet the minimum requirements.[1, 2] Policies should also state what actions may be taken to manage requests that do not meet minimum requirements. Specific requirements associated with select blood products are detailed in the following sections.

☑ **CHECKPOINT 7-2**

What is the minimum number of patient identifiers that must be included on a request for transfusion?

A. One
B. Two
C. Three
D. Four

Red Blood Cells

Most pretransfusion sample collection and testing requirements are intended to reduce the risks associated with transfusing incompatible red blood cells.[3] Transfusion of incompatible red blood cells can result in a hemolytic transfusion reaction (Chapter 12) that may be life-threatening. The majority of hemolytic transfusion reactions that occur are due to errors in sample or patient identification.[4, 5]

Specimen Collection

Specimen collection is the first critical step in ensuring positive patient and sample identification. The individual collecting the specimen is responsible for ensuring that it is collected from the patient for whom the transfusion is requested and that the sample is labeled correctly with key information.

Patient identification may be done using eye-readable or machine-readable information or a combination of both. Machine-

readable information may be encoded into one- or two-dimensional barcodes or into a radio frequency identification (RFID) chip. Machine-readable information tends to be the most reliable as it is less prone to human error; however, machine-readable systems require an investment in infrastructure such as computer systems and readers in order to create and translate the encoded information.[6] One-dimensional barcodes are used to encode small pieces of information such as an identification number. Two-dimensional barcodes and RFID chips have a much larger data capacity and can encode more information, such as all key patient identifiers, in a single scan.[7]

Key patient identifiers on the request for transfusion must be checked against the information presented by the patient prior to specimen collection. For inpatients, this information is usually presented in the form of a hospital wristband. Some facilities may also require wristbands for outpatient sample collection or there may be other mechanisms in place to ensure that traceability is maintained for these patients. Regardless of the system in place, an effective link must be created between the patient and the specimen and, ultimately, with the blood component that will be transfused.[2]

At minimum, two points of identification should be checked. These may include given name and family name, date of birth, and identifying patient number.[3] When it is not possible to access the minimum patient identifiers—for example, an unknown patient presenting in a trauma situation—there should be at least one identifier that links the patient, the specimen, and the components to be transfused. Many facilities use sets of stickers with unique number sequences that can be affixed to requests for transfusion, hospital wristbands, specimens, and component tags. These numbers create a positive identification link and are often referred to as blood bank numbers.[2, 3]

Once collected, specimens must be labeled before leaving the patient bedside. Labeling must include two independent patient identifiers, the date of collection, and a means to identify the individual who drew the specimen.[1] Specimens may be labeled by hand or by using preprinted labels. Although each labeling method has advantages and disadvantages, at least one published study has demonstrated that, in the absence of a machine-readable identification system, hand-labeled tubes impart the lowest risk of labeling errors.[8] Facilities may also have policies requiring that a second individual verify the patient identification and specimen labeling prior to leaving the patient bedside.

Upon receipt in the blood bank, specimens must be checked carefully against the request for transfusion to ensure the following:

- Key identifying information is identical on the specimen and on the request for transfusion.

- The date of specimen collection and a means to identify the individual drawing the specimen are present.

- All information is presented legibly and accurately.[1, 2]

Specimens that do not meet the above criteria should be rejected and a request should be made to recollect the specimen. Numerous studies have shown that strict adherence to specimen collection and identification guidelines significantly reduces the risk of hemolytic transfusion reactions.[4, 5]

CASE IN POINT (continued)

TK arrives in the outpatient laboratory collection area. The phlebotomist pulls up the T & S order and prints computer-generated stickers that contain the patient's information. The phlebotomist asks TK to state his full name then compares the information given by the patient to the specimen labels and the patient's hospital wristband, which was applied to the patient's wrist upon admission. This process is performed to ensure proper identification of the patient before collection of the blood specimens. The specimens are collected and labeled in front of the patient.

1. At a minimum, what information *must* be on the T & S specimen?

Patient History

Patient history is of particular importance when transfusing red blood cells. With the exception of antibodies to ABO antigens, virtually all antibodies capable of causing a hemolytic transfusion reaction are produced in response to exposure to foreign red blood cell antigens, usually through previous transfusion or pregnancy. Over time, in the absence of a stimulus, these antibodies may fall below detectable levels. They can then cause a delayed hemolytic reaction when a new exposure in the form of an antigen-positive red blood cell transfusion occurs. Likewise, recent pregnancy or transfusion may stimulate antibodies that are not detectable at the time of specimen collection but may be detectable at a later time. For this reason, specimens beyond 3 days after collection should not be used for pretransfusion testing for patients who have been recently transfused or are pregnant.[2]

Patient history is an important source of information for previous pretransfusion testing results. Testing history is used to confirm ABO and Rh(D) typings as a means of verifying correct patient identification or, conversely, for identifying potential errors in patient identification or specimen collection. Historical test results may also include previously identified red blood cell antibodies that are not detectable in the current specimen; this information can be used to select appropriate red blood cell components, thereby preventing a possible delayed hemolytic transfusion reaction (Chapter 12).

Reviewing patient history is also essential when selecting components for transfusion. Many patients needing transfusion have special requirements, such as irradiated products for immunocompromised patients or washed red blood cells for patients with anti-IgA antibodies. A review of patient history helps to ensure that patients receive the safest products for their particular circumstances[1] (Chapters 10 and 17).

☑ CHECKPOINT 7-3

List two ways that exposure to foreign red blood cell antigens can occur.

Mandatory Tests

At minimum, pretransfusion testing for red blood cell transfusion must include the following three tests that comprise the minimum required components of the immunohematology test known as **type and screen (T & S)**. In the event that discrepancies or a positive antibody screen test occur, additional tests may need to be performed to complete a type and screen. The three tests that comprise a type and screen are:

- ABO group
- Rh(D) type
- Antibody screen test (looking for red blood cell antibodies)

Transfusion of even a small volume of ABO-incompatible red blood cells can cause an immediate and potentially life-threatening hemolytic transfusion reaction. For this reason, correct ABO typing (Chapter 4) of the patient prior to transfusion is a critical step. ABO typing must include patient red blood cell testing with anti-A and anti-B reagent antisera (forward grouping) and patient plasma testing with A_1 and B reagent red blood cells (reverse grouping).[1] Typing must be performed on a current sample; red blood cells cannot be released for transfusion based on historical test results.

Facilities may have policies that require that ABO typing be performed at least twice prior to releasing red blood cells for transfusion. Depending on the facility's policies, the second typing may be obtained by one or more of the following methods: historical records, two tests on the same specimen, tests of two specimens drawn at the same time, or tests on two specimens drawn independently. Some facilities that accept two tests on the same specimen specify that different people must perform the testing. Some facilities that require tests on independently drawn specimens will issue group O red blood cells until a second specimen is drawn and tested. These policies are intended to reduce the risk of errors in patient identification and specimen collection.[9]

When selecting red blood cells for transfusion based on patient ABO type, the components may be ABO identical or ABO compatible (Table 7-1 ✱). ABO-compatible red blood cells lack the corresponding ABO antigen to the naturally occurring ABO antibodies in the patient's plasma (Chapter 4). In the event that a patient's ABO type cannot be determined in accordance with facility policies, group O red blood cells may be issued for transfusion until the patient's ABO type has been resolved.

Rh(D) typing is the second most significant red blood cell antigen typing for most patient populations (Chapter 5). The Rh(D) antigen is highly immunogenic and Rh(D)-negative patients who

✱ **TABLE 7-1** ABO Compatibility of Red Blood Cells

		Patient (Recipient) ABO Group			
		O	A	B	AB
Donor (Component)	First Choice ABO Identical	O	A	B	AB
	Alternatives ABO Compatible	None	O	O	O, A, B

are exposed to the antigen have a relatively high likelihood of developing the corresponding antibody. Studies done in the 1960s using healthy volunteers demonstrated that 80–90% of Rh(D)-negative people receiving repeat exposures to Rh(D)-positive blood formed an anti-D antibody. Hospitalized Rh(D)-negative patients were found to be much less likely to make anti-D than healthy volunteers, with only around 30% forming antibodies when given Rh(D)-positive blood (Chapter 5).[27] Preventing the formation of anti-D is especially important for female patients who may become pregnant in the future because this antibody can cause severe hemolytic disease of the fetus and newborn (HDFN) if the fetus is Rh(D) positive (Chapter 14).

In most situations patients who type as Rh(D) negative should receive Rh(D)-negative red blood cells. However, in cases of shortage or extremely high utilization, male patients and females who are beyond childbearing years may be switched to Rh(D)-positive red blood cells as long as their plasma does not contain anti-D. Most facilities will have policies in place with regard to transfusion of Rh(D)-positive red blood cells to Rh(D)-negative patients. Rh(D)-positive patients can safely receive either Rh(D)-positive or Rh(D)-negative red blood cells, although Rh(D)-negative red blood cells are normally reserved for Rh(D)-negative patients.

In some institutions, testing for weak Rh(D) is not performed when Rh-typing recipients for transfusion. Patients who type as Rh(D) negative with routine Rh typing receive Rh(D)-negative blood without performing extended Rh testing to look for weak Rh(D). This is not the case when testing donors for Rh type. Donors who appear Rh(D) negative from the initial Rh testing get additional Rh(D) testing through the antiglobulin phase to identify any donors with weak Rh(D) antigens. The units of blood from weak Rh(D)-antigen donors are labeled as Rh(D) positive. Giving weak Rh(D)-antigen-positive donor blood to Rh(D)-negative patients could result in the formation of an anti-D antibody. On the other hand, giving Rh(D)-negative units to a patient with weak Rh(D) antigen themselves will not result in the formation of an antibody (Chapter 5).

The final critical stage of pretransfusion testing is screening to detect unexpected red blood cell antibodies. These are antibodies to red blood cell antigens that are not part of the ABO system. Ideally, the screening method should detect only clinically significant red blood cell antibodies that are known to potentially cause hemolytic transfusion reactions.

To maximize the sensitivity of the screening test and to ensure that low levels of red blood cell antibody can be detected, screening cells must not be pooled and should be selected to provide at least one expression of all significant antigens in the panel.[1] Where possible, at least one homozygous expression of each significant antigen should be present. This is especially important for Jk^a, Jk^b, Fy^a, Fy^b, S, and s, as these antigens tend to show dosage (Chapter 8).[3]

The method must include an IAT phase to detect IgG antibodies that react at 98.6° F (37° C).[1] Optional testing may include incubation at room temperature, quick spin after incubation at 98.6° F and/or complement detection in the IAT phase through the use of polyspecific antihuman globulin. These optional tests are designed to detect IgM antibodies and complement, which may aid in identifying unexpected antibodies. However, antibodies detected in these optional phases are not generally considered to be clinically significant unless they also react with anti-IgG in the IAT phase.[2] An **autologous**

control (**autocontrol; AC**) (a test in which patient cells are tested with the patient's own plasma) or direct antiglobulin test (DAT) is not recommended as part of routine pretransfusion antibody screen testing.[2] For patients who do not have a high likelihood of needing blood, pretransfusion testing may not proceed beyond these three mandatory tests as long as no unexpected antibodies are present.

☑ **CHECKPOINT 7-4**

Identify the mandatory tests that are part of a pretransfusion testing work-up.

Reflex Tests

Reflex tests are automatically performed as a result of inconclusive or unexpected results found during mandatory testing. These tests include methods to resolve ABO blood group discrepancies and positive antibody screen tests.

Resolution of ABO grouping discrepancies may involve additional patient red blood cell testing with anti-A,B and anti-A_1 and patient plasma testing with A_2 and O reagent red blood cells. More complex testing may be required to resolve some discrepancies (Chapter 4). If an ABO grouping cannot be resolved before the patient requires blood, group O red blood cells may be provided for transfusion.[2]

Positive antibody screen results will normally require additional testing of patient plasma against a panel of red blood cells with known antigen determinants, a test referred to as antibody identification. To perform this test, commercial cells with known antigenic determinants are tested against patient/recipient plasma or serum to confirm or exclude antibodies to various red blood cell antigens (Chapter 8). Once the antibody or antibodies present in the patient plasma are identified, the patient is usually typed for the corresponding antigen(s). This test, referred to as **patient cell antigen typing**, consists of combining patient red blood cells with commercial antisera that contain the identified antibodies and examining for agglutination. If the patient's red blood cells type as negative for the corresponding antigen, this provides additional confirmation that the antibody has been correctly identified.[2] Antigen typing may be difficult to perform on patients who have been transfused in the past 3 months, as circulating donor red blood cells may cause false-positive or false-negative test results. Therefore, whenever possible, patient antigen typing should be performed on a pretransfusion specimen.[2]

Once the identity of any clinically significant antibodies has been confirmed, either through testing or through review of historical records, donor red blood cell components that are negative for the corresponding antigen(s) must be selected. This test, which may be referred to as **donor cell antigen typing**, consists of testing donor RBCs against known commercial antiserum. Depending on the frequency of antigens in the donor population, large numbers of donor units may have to be screened to identify **compatible** red blood cell units. The term compatible refers to the interpretation of the *crossmatch* test in which there is no reaction between donor red blood cells and patient plasma. This desired result suggests that no *in vivo* reaction will occur if these donor cells are given to the patient. All donor units that will be issued for transfusion to patients with clinically significant antibodies must have the corresponding antigen typings confirmed prior to release[1] (Chapter 8).

CASE IN POINT (continued)

The T & S specimen for patient TK is sent to the laboratory for testing. When it arrives, the laboratorian reviews both the request form and specimen to ensure all information is complete and accurate. The laboratorian centrifuges the specimen and reviews the patient history. She notes that patient TK has been transfused in the past. TK's historical record indicates that he is A Rh(D) positive and no other information is noted.

2. Why is it important to review a patient's blood bank history prior to transfusion?

3. At a minimum, what tests need to be performed when a T & S is ordered?

Compatibility Testing

Compatibility testing, also known as a **crossmatch**, is performed prior to release of red blood cells for transfusion. The compatibility test uses *in vitro* testing of patient/recipient plasma and donor red blood cells to to predict if patient/recipient plasma will react *in vivo* with donor RBCs if transfused.

Immediate spin phase testing (room temperature) is conducted to detect any **ABO incompatibilities** (that is, an antigen-antibody reaction that takes place as a result of two different blood types being mixed together that cannot co-exist). Donor red blood cell reactions with unexpected recipient/patient red blood cell antibodies may also be detected.

Historically, crossmatching was often performed at three standard test phases: (1) immediate spin at room temperature, which will detect ABO incompatibilities; (2) after addition of an enhancement and incubation at 98.6° F (37° C); and (3) after an IAT procedure using polyspecific antihuman globulin reagent, often referred to as an **antiglobulin crossmatch** or **IAT crossmatch**. Testing conducted in phases 2 and 3 above is designed to detect unexpected patient antibodies directed against corresponding antigens on the donor cells.

If agglutination occurred in any of these test phases, the unit was considered **incompatible** (the interpretation of a crossmatch test in which a reaction occurs between donor red blood cells and patient plasma; this indicates that if given, these donor red blood cells will cause the undesired result of an *in vivo* reaction) and thus was not released for transfusion. Today, laboratories may choose to use less test phases or may use other crossmatch methods for routine testing. For example, some laboratories may choose to perform testing designed to only detect ABO incompatibilities (known as an **immediate spin crossmatch**) or an *electronic crossmatch* (a concept described in detail later in this chapter) if the current and historical results indicate that the patient/recipient has not developed any unexpected antibodies to red blood cell antigens. An IAT crossmatch is required when the patient is known to have a clinically significant antibody.

☑ CHECKPOINT 7-5

What phases of testing are used in the immediate spin (IS) and antiglobulin (IAT) crossmatching procedures?

Considerations for Neonates

Special consideration must be given to pretransfusion testing of specimens from neonates (Chapter 14). Because infants under the age of 4 months rarely produce red blood cell antibodies, certain tests are affected.[3] The ABO group of the neonate is determined only by the forward typing of patient red blood cells with commercial anti-A and anti-B antisera. Plasma from neonates when tested against A_1 and B cells (that is, a reverse typing) may demonstrate no reactivity or results may show passive maternal anti-A or anti-B. Some facilities include anti-A,B and a DAT in routine neonatal pretransfusion testing. With antibody screening, the major concern is detecting and identifying possible passive maternal red blood cell antibodies. For this reason, either neonatal or maternal plasma may be used for testing.[1] In order to reduce the risk of a transfusion reaction due to passive maternal anti-A or anti-B, many facilities have policies in place to transfuse only group O red blood cells to neonates.[3]

Specimen Retention

Once pretransfusion testing is complete, patient specimens and *segments* (small portions of donor blood that extend from the donor bag in the form of a tube; the tube is systematically divided into small sealed sections called segments for the purpose of testing without introducing outside contaminants into the donor bag; see Chapter 10 for details) from each RBC unit tested must be retained by the laboratory for a minimum of 7 days after transfusion.[1] In the event of a patient transfusion reaction, these samples are required, along with a post-transfusion patient specimen, for investigation into the cause of the reaction (Chapter 12).

Platelets

The critical pretransfusion test for platelet transfusion is ABO typing. The reason for this is that anti-A and anti-B present in the plasma portion of the platelet component can potentially react with A and B antigens on a patient's red blood cells, referred to as a **minor ABO incompatibility** because the causative ABO antibody is in the blood component and is therefore in a limited quantity. Also, platelets express ABH antigens, so recipient anti-A and anti-B may bind to these antigens and cause the platelets to be cleared from the patient's circulation, referred to as a **major ABO incompatibility** because the causative ABO antibody is in the recipient's plasma and will continue to be produced. However, because platelets have a very short shelf life and it is not always possible to provide ABO-identical platelets, patients may be given ABO major–incompatible platelets as a second choice or may even receive ABO minor–incompatible or both major and minor–incompatible platelets in some situations.[2] Most facilities will have policies in place for selecting the ABO group of platelets for transfusion (Table 7-2 ✳).

Numerous studies have been published with regard to the effects of ABO-incompatible platelet transfusion. The greatest concern is

✳ **TABLE 7-2** ABO Compatibility of Platelets

		Patient (Recipient) ABO Group			
		O	A	B	AB
Donor (Component)	First Choice	O	A	B	AB
	Second Choice	A*, B*, AB*	AB*	AB*	A#, B#
	Third Choice	N/A	B*, O	A*, O	O

First choice, ABO identical; Second choice, donor plasma is ABO compatible with recipient red blood cells, except for recipient group AB; Third choice, donor plasma is ABO compatible with recipient red blood cells; #, Group A or B donors have antibodies in the plasma that are incompatible with the recipient red blood cells, but group A and B people tend to have lower ABO antibody titers compared to group O people; *, Recipient plasma has ABO antibodies that are incompatible with the donor platelets.

✳ **TABLE 7-3** ABO Compatibility of Plasma

		Patient (Recipient) Blood Group			
		O	A	B	AB
Donor (component)	ABO compatible	O, A, B, AB	A, AB	B, AB	AB

HLA or HPA typing, identification of patient antibodies, and identification of platelet components with HLA or HPA types that will likely result in an acceptable platelet increment when tranfused[2, 13] (Chapters 16 and 18).

☑ **CHECKPOINT 7-6**

How could the transfusion of an apheresis platelet unit trigger a hemolytic transfusion reaction in a recipient?

with minor ABO incompatibility and generally relates to transfusion of apheresis or buffy coat pooled platelets. This is because of the large volume of plasma present from a single donor in these components (Chapter 10). If the donor plasma contains very high titer anti-A or anti-B, it is possible for the patient to experience a hemolytic transfusion reaction if their red blood cells express the corresponding A or B antigen. Although reactions are rare, the consequences for patients can be serious.[10, 11] Because group O blood donors have been shown to be more likely to have high titers of anti-A and anti-B, some facilities restrict the transfusion of group O apheresis or pooled buffy coat platelets to group O patients. Other facilities may have policies and procedures in place to reduce the plasma volume of ABO minor–incompatible platelets prior to transfusion (Chapter 10).

Concerns have also been identified with the transfusion of ABO major–incompatible platelets because platelets with antibodies attached will be cleared from the patient's circulation, potentially reducing the effectiveness of the platelet transfusion.[2] A meta-analysis of studies investigating the impact of ABO compatibility on platelet transfusion outcomes concluded that ABO-identical platelet transfusions resulted in a higher post-transfusion platelet increment in recipients; however, as yet there has been no correlation of these results to actual patient morbidity and mortality outcomes.[12]

Rh(D) typing is an important secondary test when selecting platelets for transfusion. Platelet components can contain small amounts of donor red blood cells that may cause the recipient to mount an immune response. For this reason, it is recommended that Rh(D)-negative patients receive platelets prepared from Rh(D)-negative donors.[2] When this is not possible, Rh(D)-negative patients may be given a post-transfusion dose of **Rh-immune globulin (RhIg)** (Chapter 14) to prevent the formation of anti-D due to any Rh(D)-positive red blood cells that may have been transfused in the platelet component.[2]

Some patients who receive multiple transfusions of platelet components will become **refractory** (Chapter 16). This means that they fail to demonstrate an incremental increase in platelet count post transfusion. This phenomenon can sometimes be seen in an ABO major mismatch platelet transfusion or it may be due to the development of antibodies to human leukocyte antigens (HLA) or human platelet antigens (HPA).[13] In the case of antibodies to HLA or HPA, additional pretransfusion testing may include patient

Plasma Products

As with platelet components, the most critical pretransfusion test for plasma products is patient ABO group. In the case of plasma products, only minor ABO compatibility is of concern because these products contain no cells and therefore no ABH antigens (Table 7-3 ✳). Rh(D) type may be performed in conjunction with the ABO group, but patient Rh(D) type is not used when selecting plasma for transfusion.

Fractionation Products

Generally, administration of **fractionated products**, comprised of plasma proteins, does not necessitate pretransfusion testing. The one exception is the administration of Rh-immunoglobulin (RhIg). Rh(D) typing is critical for this product when used for either of its major indications.

When used to prevent the formation of anti-D, RhIg is given only to Rh(D)-negative patients. Also, assessment of the need for postnatal administration of RhIg normally includes Rh(D) typing of the neonate, as the product is usually administered to the mother only if the infant is Rh(D) positive (Chapter 14).

When RhIg is used in the treatment of idiopathic thrombocytopenic purpura (ITP), it is only effective in Rh(D)-positive patients, so Rh(D) typing is necessary for these patients prior to administration of the product (Chapter 16).[14]

PRETRANSFUSION TEST METHODS

Currently, there are three methodologies used for transfusion medicine testing: tube/microplate testing, gel testing, and solid-phase testing. All three methodologies can be performed manually and some methodologies have automated or semi-automated options.

There are also three methods for achieving the required crossmatch requirements: immediate spin, antiglobulin/IAT, and electronic. Laboratories must define policies that outline what type of crossmatch will be performed under which circumstances.

Tube/Microplate Testing

Tube testing was historically used for all transfusion medicine testing and is still a common procedure. Tube testing can be used to complete:

- ABO typing/grouping (Chapter 4)
- Rh(D) typing (Chapter 5)
- Antibody screening (Chapter 3) and identification (Chapter 8)
- Crossmatching (as discussed in this chapter)
- Antigen typing (Chapter 8)
- DAT/direct antiglobulin testing (Chapter 3)

Additives are often used if antibody screening and identification is performed by tube testing (Chapter 3). The additives enhance the antigen–antibody interaction, which reduces the incubation time and increases the sensitivity of the test. Common additives include albumin, low ionic strength saline (LISS), and polyethylene glycol (PEG).

Agglutination testing in microplates is a smaller-scale version of tube testing. Microplate testing was historically used more often in donor centers where the number of specimens tested was high. Although automation is relatively new to transfusion service laboratories, automation in donor centers has been around for a long time. The earliest automated or semi-automated procedures used microplate for routine testing of donor specimens, such as ABO group, Rh(D) type, antibody screen, and certain transmissible disease tests (Chapter 9).

Gel Testing

Gel testing uses a different method to visualize the agglutination of red blood cells, which is the basis of most immunohematology (transfusion medicine) tests. In tube testing, the agglutination is visualized as clumps of cells in the tube or microplate well. In gel testing, the agglutination is visualized by the capture of red blood cells within the gel column (Chapter 3) (Figure 7-2 ■). If the correct gel cards are available, gel testing can be used for all the same routine tests as tube testing, namely, ABO grouping, Rh(D) typing, antibody screening and identification, crossmatching, antigen typing, and direct antiglobulin test. Gel testing can be performed manually or on an automated machine (Figure 7-3 ■).

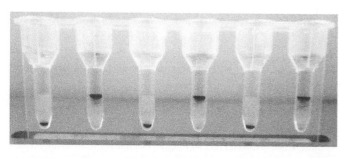

Negative	Positive	Negative	Positive	Negative	Positive
			Result		

■ **FIGURE 7-2** Negative and Positive Results in Gel Test
Source: Lisa Denesiuk.

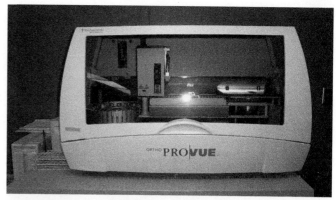

■ **FIGURE 7-3** Ortho Clinical Diagnostics ProVue®
Source: Lisa Denesiuk.

Solid-Phase Testing

Solid-phase testing is used primarily for antibody screening and identification. The testing relies on antigen coated wells on a microplate (Chapter 3). For antibody screening and identification, plates that have wells precoated with red blood cell antigens are usually used. Positive results are visualized as a smooth coating of indicator cells and negative results are visualized as a solid dot of indicator cells (Figure 7-4 ■). Solid-phase testing can be performed manually or on an automated machine (Figures 7-5 ■ and 7-6 ■). Automated machines that use solid-phase testing for antibody screening and identification usually use microplate hemagglutination for ABO and Rh(D) testing.

Crossmatches may be performed by solid-phase testing, but would require the testing laboratory to coat a microplate well with the donor red blood cell stroma. This step adds time and complexity to the procedure; therefore, most laboratories that perform manual solid-phase testing choose a faster method such as tube for performing crossmatch testing.

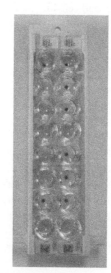

Result	
Negative	Negative
Positive	Negative
Positive	Negative
Positive	Positive
Positive	Negative
Positive	Negative
Negative	Negative
Positive	Positive

■ **FIGURE 7-4** Negative and Positive Results in Solid-Phase Test
Source: Lisa Denesiuk.

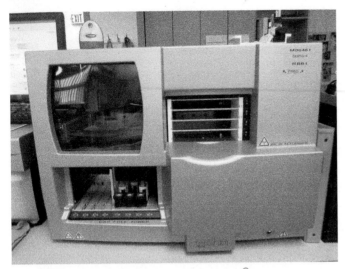

FIGURE 7-5 Immucor Galileo Echo®
Source: Lisa Denesiuk.

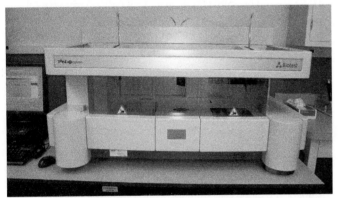

FIGURE 7-6 Biotest Tango Optimo®
Source: Janet Young.

Immediate Spin Crossmatch

Testing that occurs when donor red blood cells are physically tested against the recipient/patient plasma is called a **serologic crossmatch**. As previously mentioned this testing may occur at several test phases. An immediate spin crossmatch, which occurs at room temperature, is designed to detect ABO incompatibilities. A suggested procedure to perform this test is to add one drop of a 3–5% saline-washed donor red blood cell suspension to two drops of recipient/patient plasma in a test tube.[15] The tube is then gently mixed, centrifuged for approximately 30 seconds, and then read immediately for agglutination. ABO incompatibilities should result in hemolysis and/or gross agglutination of the donor cells.

As there is no incubation or IAT phase in the immediate spin crossmatch, most non-ABO antibodies will not be detected. Therefore, the immediate spin crossmatch should only be used if the recipient appears not to have a clinically significant antibody. Checks of previous testing results on the recipient, which may identify a clinically significant antibody that is no longer reactive, are a critically important step in preventing hemolytic transfusion reactions.

Cold-reactive (room temperature) antibodies other than ABO may cause a positive reaction in the immediate spin crossmatch. If an immediate spin crossmatch is positive, laboratories may repeat the immediate spin crossmatch but using either a prewarm technique (Chapter 8) or an incubation phase. Other laboratories will repeat the crossmatch but using their antiglobulin crossmatch technique (Table 7-4 ✱).

Laboratories that use an electronic crossmatch (discussed later in this chapter) will often perform an immediate spin crossmatch if their laboratory information system (LIS) is not working.

Antiglobulin (IAT) Crossmatch

Like immediate spin crossmatches, antiglobulin crossmatches are serologic in nature. Both immediate spin and antiglobulin (using the IAT technique, hence the name of this section) crossmatches are serologic. Historically, laboratories performed antiglobulin crossmatches as part of their regular pretransfusion work-ups. The current protocols followed in immunohematology/blood bank laboratories vary. It is thus important that each laboratory generate and follow policies that meet their regulatory and accreditation requirements for determining when an antiglobulin crossmatch is required and when other methodologies, as noted in the following paragraph, may be performed.

As previously eluded to, laboratories usually use the same IAT technique for the antiglobulin crossmatch that they use for their antibody screens. For example, a laboratory that performs their routine antibody screens using a tube technique and PEG as an additive will perform their antiglobulin crossmatch by tube technique using PEG as an additive. The exception is laboratories that use solid-phase testing for their routine antibody screens. Crossmatching can be done by solid-phase testing but it is labor intensive. Therefore, many laboratories that use solid-phase testing for their antibody screens will choose an alternate method for their antiglobulin crossmatches. Often, this is a tube technique using either LISS or PEG as an additive because tube procedures require minimal specialized equipment and materials when compared to the gel technique.

Some laboratories choose to routinely perform an antiglobulin crossmatch for all recipients; others use the antiglobulin crossmatch only for certain recipients. The antiglobulin crossmatch should detect incompatibilities between donor and recipient due to both ABO and non-ABO antibodies. Therefore, an antiglobulin crossmatch should always be performed if the recipient is known to have a clinically significant antibody. Often the donor red blood cells will have been antigen-typed so that only donors negative for the corresponding antigen(s) will be crossmatched.

There may be slight variations between laboratories when defining a clinically significant antibody. Therefore, corresponding policies must clearly define this definition. An example of such a policy would be one that states that an antiglobulin crossmatch will be performed if the following situations are encountered:

- If the current antibody screen is positive, regardless of the results of the antibody investigation.

- If there is a historical record or current identification of a clinically significant antibody.

There is usually a list of common clinically significant antibodies that are known to be capable of causing hemolytic transfusion reactions, either in the same policy or in a related policy. Common

✳ **TABLE 7-4** Example Algorithms for Follow-Up to a Positive Immediate Spin Crossmatch

Example 1

Initial Results: Negative antibody screen; no ABO or Rh discrepancies; no history of a clinically significant antibody; positive immediate spin crossmatch with one donor unit

Step 1	Check that ABO group recorded on blood supplier label on donor unit is compatible with ABO group of recipient.	Most common cause of this discrepancy is accidentally choosing a unit of the wrong ABO group.
Step 2	If ABO groups appear compatible, then remove a new segment from unit. Retest the new segment for ABO group and in the immediate spin crossmatch. May also want to regroup the patient sample for ABO.	Rules out a mix-up of segments, especially if dealing with more than one unit at one time. Also confirms ABO group of unit. Rules out transcription or technical errors that might have caused an incorrect ABO group to be recorded for the patient.
Step 3	If ABO retesting results confirm original results and immediate spin crossmatch repeat is still positive, perform an IAT crossmatch.	If IAT crossmatch is negative, unit is probably safe to transfuse. Positive reaction may be due to a clinically insignificant cold antibody. A room temperature or cold incubated panel may identify the cold antibody, if identification is required.
Step 4	If the IAT crossmatch is positive, crossmatch a different donor unit. The positive result can be further investigated: • Perform a DAT on a segment of the donor unit. If positive, discard the unit or return to the blood supplier as per procedure. • Test patient's plasma against red blood cells that are known to be positive for low-incidence antigens, if available.	A positive IAT crossmatch may be due to one of the following: • Donor unit has a positive DAT. • Recipient has an antibody to a low-incidence antigen and donor is positive for the corresponding antigen.

Example 2

Initial Results: Negative antibody screen; no ABO or Rh discrepancies; no history of a clinically significant antibody; positive immediate spin crossmatch with all donor units

Step 1	Check that ABO group of recipient and donors are compatible.	ABO incompatibility could cause this discrepancy.
Step 2	If ABO groups are compatible, repeat the immediate spin crossmatch using a saline replacement technique.	Saline replacement technique should dissipate rouleaux, if present. Suspect rouleaux if the recipient has a diagnosis where unusual plasma proteins may be present and/or microscopically the agglutination appears like a stack of coins and/or the hematology laboratory has reported rouleaux when performing white cell differential. *Note:* Rouleaux may sometimes cause an apparent ABO incompatibility.
Step 3	If the crossmatch is still positive using saline replacement, repeat the crossmatch using an IAT technique or, less preferred, using a prewarm technique.	A cold agglutinin may be responsible for the positive results. Most cold agglutinins will not react in the IAT technique. A room temperature or cold incubated panel may identify the cold antibody, if identification is required. Prewarm technique may also be used to negate the cold agglutinins, and may be required if the IAT technique is still positive. However, prewarm should be used with caution as the technique has been shown to sometimes give false-negative results with clinically significant warm antibodies.

clinically significant antibodies include those of the Rh, Kell, Duffy, and Kidd blood group systems as well as anti-S and anti-s in the MNS blood group system.[2] The policy may include other antibodies that occur with relative frequency in a particular laboratory because of the ethnic mix of its patient population.

☑ **CHECKPOINT 7-7**

When should the antiglobulin crossmatch technique be selected to determine the compatibility between donor blood and recipient plasma?

Electronic Crossmatch

An **electronic crossmatch** uses logic tables located in a laboratory information system (LIS) to detect ABO incompatibilities between a patient and a donor.[16] The recipient's plasma is not physically tested against the donor cells. The electronic crossmatch, also called the computer crossmatch or computer-assisted crossmatch, has been used in Canada and many European countries since the late 1980s. Implementation of the electronic crossmatch in the United States has been slower due to various regulatory and financial issues, but is gaining popularity.

The elements usually required for an electronic crossmatch include:

• A method for the LIS to determine the ABO group of the donor

• A method for the LIS to determine the ABO group of the recipient

• Software that allows the LIS to compare the ABO groups of the donor and recipient

• Logic tables that will not allow ABO-incompatible red blood cell units to be allocated or issued

• Quality checks in the LIS that ensure that policies around when an electronic crossmatch is acceptable are followed

Donor units are retyped for ABO group alone or both ABO group and Rh(D) type upon receipt in the transfusion service laboratory. Many LIS that allow for electronic crossmatching will require that each ABO/Rh individual tube, gel microtube, or microplate well result be recorded in the LIS; for example, the graded result for the donor cells tested against anti-A, anti-B, and anti-D. The results can be entered into the LIS by a laboratorian or may be transferred from an automated instrument via an interface. The LIS often will then require a laboratorian to interpret the ABO or ABO/Rh group. The LIS compares the interpretation to the results using logic tables. If the interpretation and results do not correlate, an error message occurs and the unit is not available for crossmatching.

Similarly, the results for the ABO group, Rh(D) type, and antibody screen performed on the recipient's sample are recorded in the LIS. Interpretations are compared to the results and all discrepancies must be resolved or an electronic crossmatch cannot be performed.

Electronic crossmatching systems require two ABO tests on the recipient.[1] Each laboratory must define in its policies what is acceptable as two ABO test results. Some laboratories will only issue group O red blood cell units until an ABO test has been performed on two specimens drawn at different times from the same recipient.[1] Other laboratories will accept two ABO test results performed on the same recipient specimen or on two specimens drawn at the same time.

The LIS should not allow an electronic crossmatch to be performed if the antibody screen result for the current specimen is interpreted as positive. Similarly, the LIS should check antibody identification results from all testing on the recipient, both current and historical. Some systems will not allow an electronic crossmatch if there is any result in the antibody identification field. Other systems may be able to assess the results and determine if the antibody(ies) identified are clinically insignificant or clinically significant. Some LIS will also check other result fields, such as special transfusion requirements, either for any comment or for certain comments and will block the electronic crossmatch function according to the parameters set up in its logic tables.

If all the parameters that allow for an electronic crossmatch are met, an ABO-compatible red blood cell unit will be assigned to the recipient's file and a tag or label will be printed (Table 7-5 ✱).

All LIS systems should be validated upon implementation and after updates are installed.[1] Some facilities will also revalidate their information systems on a periodic basis. If using an electronic crossmatch, it is important for the validation to challenge the logic tables.

✱ **TABLE 7-5** Parameters for Electronic Crossmatch

Laboratory information system (LIS) supports an electronic crossmatch, has been validated, and is currently functional.
Current patient sample has a negative antibody screen by an IAT methodology and results are in the LIS.
Patient history has been checked and there is no history of a clinically significant antibody.
Current patient sample has been typed for ABO/Rh and results are interpreted in the LIS.
Two ABO/Rh typings have been performed on the patient and the results are in the LIS.
Donor cells have been retyped and results are in the LIS.

Common and uncommon scenarios, which include both instances where an electronic crossmatch should be allowed and an electronic crossmatch should not be allowed, should be presented to the LIS during the validation (Table 7-6 ✱).

Downtime procedures are vital in a laboratory that performs electronic crossmatches because the crossmatch function depends on a functioning LIS. Commonly, immediate spin crossmatches will be performed instead of electronic crossmatches during downtime. ABO retyping of the recipient sample may be required, depending on what test results, if any, are available from backup systems. There must also be some way to identify the recipients that require an antiglobulin crossmatch. If this is not possible, then an antiglobulin crossmatch should be performed on all specimens during downtime. Downtime procedures also encompass back-entry of results once the LIS is functioning again.

☑ CHECKPOINT 7-8

When computer selection of ABO-compatible red blood cells is utilized in transfusion services, this is also called

_____.

CASE IN POINT *(continued)*

The testing on patient TK is completed and he is type A Rh(D) positive with a negative antibody screen. His specimen is placed in the refrigerator for storage.

TK's surgery turned out to be more extensive then the surgeon had initially anticipated. The team decided to perform an open cholecystectomy and requested 4 units of red blood cells and 2 units of plasma. The laboratorian begins the crossmatch prior to issuing the red blood cells. Two A Rh(D)-positive red blood cell units are selected from inventory for this patient.

4. What is the minimum testing that must be performed to ensure compatible red blood cell products for TK?
5. You currently have 4 units of plasma thawed and available for issue in the blood bank. Two units are group O and 2 units are group AB. Which type of units should be issued to this recipient and why?
6. Do you need to consider the patient's Rh(D) type when issuing plasma?

INVENTORY CONTROL

Managing inventory to reduce discards to the lowest amount was and sometimes still is a complicated process. Historically, the crossmatch was the most common request made of the transfusion service. Red blood cell units would be tagged for a particular recipient and would remain set aside for that recipient until the crossmatch specimen expired. Units could expire while sitting tagged or, more often, would miss an opportunity to be used for a recipient that was being

✳ **TABLE 7-6** Examples of Validation Scenarios for Electronic Crossmatch

Test Result	Sample Validation Scenarios
ABO/Rh	• Enter results and interpretations for each ABO/Rh group to validate that the LIS will accept the interpretations. • Transpose ABO-forward groupings and/or transpose ABO-reverse groupings to validate that the LIS will reject the interpretation. • Leave a required result field blank to validate that the LIS will reject the interpretation. • Enter results that require investigation, such as mixed-field agglutination, and validate that the LIS performs in the manner that you expect. • Enter results for donor retyping where the interpretation and results match and where they do not match to validate that the LIS will accept or reject interpretations appropriately.
Antibody screen	• Enter negative antibody screen results and a negative interpretation to validate that the LIS will accept the interpretation. • Enter positive antibody screen results and a positive interpretation to validate that the LIS will accept the interpretation. • Enter negative antibody screen results and a positive interpretation or vice versa to validate that the LIS will reject the interpretation.
Electronic crossmatch	• Allocate and issue a unit of the same ABO group to a patient whose results meet all the criteria for an electronic crossmatch to validate that the LIS will allow issue. • Allocate and issue a unit of a compatible, but not identical ABO group to a patient whose results meet all the criteria for an electronic crossmatch to validate that the LIS performs in the manner that you expect. • Allocate or issue* a unit to a patient who has a history of a clinically significant antibody to validate that the LIS will not allow an electronic crossmatch. • Allocate or issue a unit to a patient who has a positive antibody screen result to validate that the LIS will not allow an electronic crossmatch. • Allocate or issue a unit to a patient who has a history of a clinically insignificant antibody to validate that the LIS performs in the manner that you expect. • Allocate or issue a unit to a patient who has only one ABO result to validate that the LIS will not allow an electronic crossmatch. • If the LIS uses other fields, such as transfusion requirements, challenge the LIS with results in these fields where an electronic crossmatch should be rejected and, if any exist, where an electronic crossmatch should be allowed to validate that the LIS performs in the manner that you expect.

LIS, laboratory information system; *, Some LIS block the electronic crossmatch at the allocation step. Others may allow allocation in some scenarios but will not allow issue.

transfused because they were set aside for a recipient that ended up not requiring a transfusion. Units would be set aside for surgical patients just in case they were needed and often the units were not needed. Practices such as double **tagging**, where an older unit would be tagged with the information for two or more recipients and would be issued to the first recipient requiring a transfusion, were common. Knowing that blood components have a finite supply, laboratory and clinical professionals continue to explore ways to maximize usage and minimize wastage. Three concepts associated with inventory control are detailed in the next sections: surgical blood order schedule, type and screen process, and redistribution systems.

Surgical Blood Order Schedule

One of the earliest innovations in inventory control was the surgical blood order schedule.[17] This is a list of recommended number of units for each surgery type. It is based on what is usually transfused in the majority of patients undergoing that particular surgery in that particular facility.

Surgical blood order schedules have been published by various institutions to act as guidelines for others.[2, 18] These are good starting points, but each institution should also consider their individual circumstances. For example, how far away is the hospital from their blood supplier? A rural hospital that receives blood once per day from their supplier may crossmatch units for a Cesarean section, whereas an urban hospital located 15 minutes away from their blood supplier may not crossmatch any units for this surgery, which has a low risk

of transfusion. Which blood-saving techniques, if any, are available to their surgeons? A hospital that has a cell-salvaging device may be able to transfuse fewer units during the majority of hip replacement surgeries than a hospital that does not have this equipment. Generally, over time, the number of units recommended for most surgeries has decreased as medical and surgical improvements have been implemented as well as research into appropriate blood usage has progressed.[2]

The surgical blood order schedule is used as a guideline by physicians in one institution or region. The majority of patients scheduled for the same surgery would have the same number of units ordered on their presurgical crossmatch. However, physicians still have the discretion to order more units based on their knowledge of the circumstances of a particular patient. For example, more units may be ordered for a patient with an underlying medical condition that would result in a more complex surgery or a patient with a bleeding disorder.

Type and Screen

When surgical blood use was studied in order to create surgical blood order schedules, it became apparent that some surgeries were performed with the majority of patients not requiring a transfusion. This led to the adoption of a *type and screen*, as detailed below, being recommended as routine presurgical bloodwork for these patients.

A type and screen (T & S), as previously defined and also called a *group and screen*, consists of an ABO group, Rh(D) type, and antibody screen. Historically, the theory behind the type and screen was to identify patients with positive antibody screens or testing discrepancies in advance of these individuals potentially needing transfusions.[19] A full investigation and crossmatch, usually of two red blood cell units, would be performed in these cases and the blood would be available for surgery. In the majority of patients, the antibody screen is negative and units could be crossmatched quickly if the patient required a transfusion either during or after surgery. No units would be set aside at the time of the pretransfusion testing. The type and screen meant that units that in the past would have been set aside for patients who would not usually use them were now left in the available stock.

One risk associated with performing a type and screen is the fact that an antibody to a low-incidence antigen may be missed by the antibody screen test but found during the crossmatch because one of the donor units is positive for the corresponding antigen. This is obviously a rare occurrence. Another problem that can arise is clinically insignificant reactions occurring in the crossmatch, usually related to the fact that the recipient's plasma was refrigerated between the time the initial antibody screen was performed and the subsequent crossmatch was performed. In either case, the availability of crossmatched red blood cell units is delayed while an investigation into the unexpected positive result is completed.

During the 1990s, many countries, for example Canada and France, experienced blood scandals related to the presence of human immunodeficiency virus (HIV) and hepatitis C virus in the blood supply.[20, 21] The subsequent disillusionment of donors with the blood establishment, coupled with the fears associated with the emergence of HIV, resulted in some of the most severe blood shortages the medical community had experienced to that point. Further efforts to maximize the usage of the available stock were investigated.

Research showed that widespread use of the type and screen resulted in virtually no increase in transfusion reactions compared to the full antiglobulin crossmatch used in the past.[22, 23] The obvious next step was questioning whether a full antiglobulin crossmatch added any safety for recipients in whom no clinically significant antibody had ever been detected.

Laboratories began performing type and screen procedures on all patients regardless of whether a crossmatch was ordered or not. If the antibody screen is negative and the patient has no history of a clinically significant antibody, red blood cell units are not to be crossmatched until an order to transfuse is received. Once the order to transfuse is received, ABO-compatible units are tagged based on the results of either an immediate spin or electronic crossmatch. Either technique requires very little time (Table 7-7 ✱).

Now, except for those recipients with a positive antibody screen or a history of a clinically significant antibody, all the red blood cell units remain in the available inventory until an order for transfusion, rather than an order for crossmatch, is placed. At the time that surgical blood order schedules were first being proposed, common metrics used to assess inventory management included the discard rate and the crossmatched to transfused ratio, commonly called the **C:T ratio**.[24] In facilities that use the electronic crossmatch, the C:T ratio should approach 1, making this metric obsolete (meaning that the units crossmatched are almost always transfused). Additionally, discard rates are usually lowered as the oldest red blood cell unit is available for issue to the next recipient requiring transfusion. Turnover of stock improves and average age of the unit at transfusion may decrease, especially in the common A and O blood groups.

Redistribution Systems

Improvements in materials and methods used in blood transportation as well as increased regionalization and cooperation among health care facilities have led to redistribution systems, especially for platelet and red blood cell units. Redistribution systems allow a donor unit that is nearing its expiry date to be transported from a low-usage site to a high-usage site. Sometimes this is accomplished via a blood supplier and other times it occurs directly between two transfusion services.

All of these advancements combined have led to ever decreasing discard rates in many facilities. Discard rates are also affected by the nature of the blood component. Platelet units, which have the shortest lifespan, generally have the highest discard rates. Conversely, frozen plasma products, with typical expiry dates of at least a year from the date of donation, have the lowest discard due to outdate rate. With red blood cell units, the blood groups in highest demand—for example, group O Rh(D) negative—generally have the lowest discard rate but also the highest incidence of stock shortages. Conversely, despite all efforts, the discard rate for group AB red blood cell units is often much higher than other groups, simply because there are fewer group AB recipients requiring transfusion.

✱ **TABLE 7-7** Example Algorithm for Routine Pretransfusion Testing

Step 1	Order for crossmatch or type and screen is made by physician.
Step 2	Pretransfusion sample is drawn and labeled using proper identification procedures.
Step 3	Transfusion service records are checked for previous results on the patient.
Step 4	ABO group, Rh type, and IAT antibody screen are performed on the current sample.
	Depending on policy, the ABO/Rh type may be performed twice if no previous results are available.

If the current antibody screen is negative, there are no discrepancies in the ABO/Rh type and no history of clinically significant antibodies:	If the current antibody screen is positive and/or the patient has a history of clinically significant antibodies:
• The sample is stored according to procedure.	• Perform antibody investigation, including antigen typing of donor units, as required.
• When units are required, perform either an electronic crossmatch or an immediate spin crossmatch according to procedure.	• Perform an IAT crossmatch to obtain the requested number of compatible donor units or to obtain two compatible donor units if a type and screen was ordered.

PRODUCT RELEASE PROTOCOLS

Issue is defined in transfusion medicine as the release of a product for clinical use.[1] It is usually the last step for a laboratory to catch a mistake before the unit moves outside their realm of influence. For example, the blood center issues blood components to a transfusion service or the transfusion service issues a red blood cell unit to a clinical unit such as an operating room or nursing unit.

Each time that a blood component is moved from one facility to another, such as being issued from a blood supplier to a transfusion service, it should be inspected twice: (1) upon being packed for transport and (2) upon being received (Chapter 10). The physical appearance of the unit is assessed for abnormalities and often the label on the unit is checked (Table 7-8 ✱). Similar visual inspection checks are often performed as part of *each* process that moves the blood component closer to being transfused.

Allocating

Allocating, sometimes also called *tagging*, is the process of applying a label or tag that contains the recipient information and usually also the donor unit information, to the selected donor unit (Figure 7-7 ■). Allocating can be considered a separate process or it can be considered the last step in the crossmatch process or the first step in the issuing process. The label or tag should be reviewed for legibility,

✱ **TABLE 7-8** Visual Inspection Steps

Check physical appearance of product and condition of storage container:	
Red blood cells	• Before bag is disturbed and if supernatant layer is visible, check for turbidity, hemolysis, white particulate matter, gross lipemia, and purple or brown color. Green-colored plasma due to use of birth control pills is acceptable, but RBCs with green coloration of the plasma due to bacterial infection by *Pseudomonas* species or liver disease must be quarantined. • Check that red blood cell mass is usual dark red color, not black or purple. • Check for visible clots. • Check for visible blood in the ports. • Check that the color of the segments is similar to color of red blood cell mass in the primary bag (not darker or lighter). • Mix bag by inversion and check for leakage. • Apply gentle pressure to the bag and check that seams are intact. • Check that at least one port is covered and that all ports are intact. • Check expiration date and time.
Plasma/platelets	• Check for unusual debris or particulate matter. • Check for visible clots. • Check for visible plasma in the ports. • Mix bag by inversion and check for leakage. • Apply gentle pressure to the bag and check that seams are intact. • Check that at least one port is covered and that all ports are intact. • Check expiration date and time. • Depending on the policies of your facility concerning acceptable limits for red blood cell contamination and/or lipemia, check that unit meets acceptable limits.
Fractionation products	• Check for debris. • Check for broken or cracked vials. Insufficient volume may also signal previous leakage. • Check that seals are intact. • Check for turbidity or cloudiness in products that are normally clear. • Check the expiration date and time.
If the unit is allocated to a specific patient, check the tag or label:	
All products	• Compare the unit/lot number of the bag/vial to the tag/label. • Check all the patient information on the tag/label for correctness, completeness, and legibility and be sure that it matches the information provided by the clinical staff. The patient information must include at least two identifiers and may include the patient's name, date of birth, an identification number used by the facility, and/or an identification number used specifically by the transfusion service. Some computerized systems may require electronic input of data via bar code or RFID scan. • Compare all information on the tag/label and bag/vial to what is in the laboratory information system or manual documentation system.
Red blood cells	• Check that ABO group of recipient and donor are compatible. • Compare blood center's ABO/Rh type on donor bag to ABO/Rh type on the tag/label. • Check interpretation of crossmatch test.
Platelets	• Check that ABO/Rh type of recipient and donor meet your facility's policies. • Compare blood center's ABO/Rh type on donor bag to ABO/Rh type on the tag/label.
Plasma products	• For large-volume plasma products, check that ABO group of recipient and donor are compatible. Some facilities will allow issue of ABO-incompatible cryoprecipitate AHF. • Compare blood center's ABO type on donor bag to ABO type on the tag/label. Rh type may or may not be reported for plasma products.

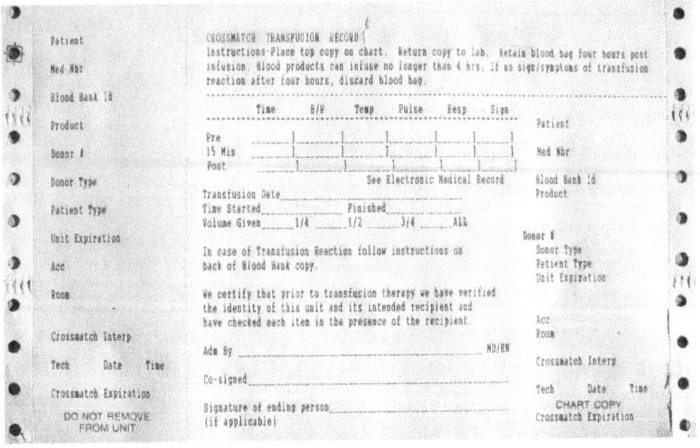

Patient
Med Nbr
Blood Bank Id
Product
Donor #
Donor Type
Patient Type
Unit Expiration
Acc
Room
Crossmatch Interp
Tech Date Time
Crossmatch Expiration
DO NOT REMOVE FROM UNIT

CROSSMATCH TRANSFUSION RECORD
Instructions-Place top copy on chart. Return copy to lab. Retain blood bag four hours post infusion. Blood products can infuse no longer than 4 hrs. If no sign/symptoms of transfusion reaction after four hours, discard blood bag.

	Time	B/P	Temp	Pulse	Resp	Sign
Pre						
15 Min						
Post						

See Electronic Medical Record

Transfusion Date______
Time Started______ Finished______
Volume Given___ 1/4 ___ 1/2 ___ 3/4 ___ ALL

In case of Transfusion Reaction follow instructions on back of Blood Bank copy.

We certify that prior to transfusion therapy we have verified the identity of this unit and its intended recipient and have checked each item in the presence of the recipient.

Adm By ______ MD/RN
Co-signed______
Signature of ending person______
(if applicable)

Patient
Med Nbr
Blood Bank Id
Product
Donor #
Donor Type
Patient Type
Unit Expiration
Acc
Room
Crossmatch Interp
Tech Date Time
CHART COPY
Crossmatch Expiration

FIGURE 7-7 Example of a Blood Product Allocation Label

Source: Janet Young.

correctness, and completeness. It is also very important to ensure that the donor unit number on the transfusion service's label or tag corresponds with the unit number on the label that was attached by the blood supplier to the donor unit. Close attention must be paid, especially if more than one donor unit is being tagged at the same time. Transfusion services may have donor units with similar numbers in their inventory at the same time. Some laboratories have policies that state that only one donor unit or only units for one recipient can be tagged at the same time. The use of barcodes and barcode scanners can reduce, but will not eliminate, errors.

☑ CHECKPOINT 7-10

The process of affixing a label with recipient information to a blood unit is called:

A. Labeling
B. Scanning
C. Tagging
D. Crossmatching

Issuing Procedures

In a transfusion service, issuing refers to transferring the donor unit from the laboratory to the clinical staff. Both the recipient information and the donor information are checked carefully during this step (Table 7-8). A visual inspection should also be performed. The issue date and time must be documented.[1] Many laboratories will also document the identity of the person or people performing the verifications.

Historically, the issue step involved a member of the nursing staff coming to the laboratory to retrieve the unit. The nursing staff member, a laboratory staff member, or, more commonly, both would check the information on the tag or label and the donor unit. Laboratories have adapted their policies to achieve similar safety checks when hospitals have implemented other transport options, for example, pneumatic tube systems. These systems can improve patient care by increasing the speed that a donor unit arrives at the patient bedside.

CASE IN POINT *(continued)*

The requested blood products are tagged for patient TK. A visual inspection of the blood products is performed by the laboratorian at the time of issue.

7. Name some abnormalities that should be looked for when performing a visual inspection of blood products.

Remote Storage

Blood components, usually red blood cell units, can be issued from the laboratory to a remote refrigerator, which is a blood bank refrigerator located away from the transfusion service. Remote refrigerators are more common in large facilities or hospital systems that have more than one building. Nursing and operating room staff must have clear policies that ensure that the blood components are stored appropriately when not under the control of the transfusion service.

Despite these policies, there is always a concern that a blood component may be removed and returned to the refrigerator without the knowledge of transfusion services. Manufacturers have developed refrigerators that remain locked unless a valid code is entered. Staff members scan the barcode of the blood components that they are putting into or taking out of the refrigerator. Some systems also produce barcodes that contain the recipient information. The software attached to these refrigerators monitors who unlocked the refrigerator, at what time, and what unit was removed or returned. Some refrigerators act like a vending machine, dispensing only the unit requested rather than unlocking the door. The request is usually made by scanning a barcode that contains the patient information or by entering a code that equates to a request for uncrossmatched red blood cell units. The stored data can be downloaded by the transfusion service and analyzed to determine if a blood component can be returned to inventory. The data download also acts as documentation of the storage conditions for the blood components.

Another popular alternative to remote refrigerators is to use a validated cooler style transport system to temporarily store a number of units assigned to a particular patient. This allows the units to be right at the bedside and therefore is particularly popular in operating room theaters or for patients undergoing procedures that require multiple blood components, such as plasma exchange or extracorporeal membrane oxygenation.

Return to Inventory

Based on the validation of the temporary storage system, policies should be developed that define if and when unused units will be returned to inventory. For example, some laboratories will only return blood components to inventory if the cooler has not been opened, as evidenced by an intact tamper-evident seal, and if the cooler has been out of the transfusion service for less than the maximum time that the validation has shown the cooler can maintain an adequate temperature. Other laboratories include a temperature-monitoring device, such as a data logger, in the cooler and base their decision on the temperature recording.

Similarly, laboratories should have policies that outline when a single unit issued to a patient care unit can be returned to inventory or when it should be discarded. In the past, this was often based on a particular timeframe that would ensure that the majority of blood components would still be at an acceptable temperature. For example, less than 30 minutes was and is a popular time frame for policies around blood components that need to be refrigerated. Time-based policies usually apply to full-size blood components, not smaller units or aliquots, which would change temperature faster. Conversely, the same time frame is usually applied to larger units such as apheresis plasma or double-volume red blood cells, which may take longer to change temperature. Time-based policies assume that the unit is kept at room temperature during the time that it is outside of the transfusion service.

Time-based policies are acceptable and are still popular, but some laboratories have implemented tools that try to provide better monitoring of the conditions that the blood component encountered. For example, laboratories may monitor the temperature of the blood component upon return using either a conventional thermometer or an infrared thermometer. This addresses the issue of the volume of the blood component affecting the length of time that it takes to reach an unacceptable temperature. However, it does not identify if the temperature of the blood component reached an unacceptable limit but then returned to acceptable. In an effort to address this concern, manufacturers have developed temperature monitors that are applied directly to the blood component. Any glue used to adhere the monitor to the unit must be approved for use on blood bags. Most of these monitors are one-time use. There are more options to monitor high temperatures, most commonly >50° F (>10° C), as this is usually the biggest concern around refrigerated components that are at room temperature while on the patient care unit. However, there are also monitors that identify <33.8° F (1° C) or that combine both ends of the acceptable temperature limit. No matter what policies are used to determine that components remain at acceptable temperatures, all units that are being returned to inventory after issue must be visually inspected.[1]

ADMINISTRATION

Safety checks continue once the blood component leaves the transfusion service. Before the blood is administered, the nursing staff should double-check that all documentation is correct (Table 7-9 ✳). A bedside check of the patient identification and donor unit identification should be performed. Some hospitals have policies that require two nursing staff members to perform the identification checks. The checks are documented; for example, the staff members may do one or more of the following: sign the tag attached to the blood component, enter their codes in an information system that produces electronic health records, and/or record their actions in a hardcopy health record. Other institutions allow one staff member to perform the bedside checks.

Manufacturers have developed information systems that try to decrease the number of incidents of transfusion to the wrong recipients. These usually use either a barcode or a RFID to capture patient information. The system links information in pharmacy, transfusion service, surgical, and other health care services. At the bedside, when the patient is to receive a transfusion or a medication, for example, the nursing staff member uses a device to scan the identification band on the patient. The patient's identification information is retrieved from the RFID embedded in the armband or the barcode on the armband. The nursing staff member is then prompted to scan the label that is attached to the blood component or the medication. This label will have the patient information generated by the transfusion service or the pharmacy as well as the blood component or medication information. The patient information from the two sources is compared and the nursing staff member is alerted if they do not match. Some systems will continue on to prompt the staff member to the next step in the process, for example, taking and entering the recipient's vital signs. Some systems will also erect physical barricades, for example, locking the recipient's intravenous pump, if the patient information does not match. All of the systems must have some way to accommodate emergency transfusion of uncrossmatched red blood cell units.

Another policy designed to decrease errors at the bedside requires the nursing staff member to perform a bedside ABO grouping on the recipient before administering the blood component.[25]

Transfusion services should ensure that clinical staff members have clear policies that guide their actions throughout the transfusion. Such policies likely include ones that address:

- How to handle various blood components
- What administration systems and administration fluids are acceptable and not acceptable
- How often vital signs should be checked
- How to identify if a transfusion reaction is occurring
- What to do if a transfusion reaction is suspected

Often, the best policies and procedures are created by cooperative efforts between the laboratory and clinical staff.

✳ **TABLE 7-9** Safety Checks Performed Before Administration

Clinical staff members should check the following before beginning administration of a blood product.	
Documentation in chart	• Order to transfuse has been documented, including identification of the ordering physician, component type, number of units or volume/dose of product, infusion rate, and any special transfusion requirements. • Informed consent for transfusion has been obtained and documented.
Physical condition of recipient	• Vital signs should be taken before administration, after administration, and at intervals during administration as defined in policy. • IV access has been established.
Identification of recipient	• Check identity of the recipient at the bedside. • Confirm identity against tag/label on product. • Bedside ABO check if required by policy.
Identification of donor	• Check donor unit number or product lot number on bag/vial against tag/label. • Confirm ABO and/or Rh-type compatibilities between donor and recipient if required for product being transfused.

POST ADMINISTRATION

When documentation occurs on the label or tag on the blood component, this tag or the bag with the label is often returned to transfusion services. A duplicate record is kept on the patient's health record or chart. Any signs or symptoms of a transfusion reaction should be documented. If the hospital's various information systems are linked, data may be stored electronically.

Transfusion services may use the information on returned tags or bag labels to review the documentation of all transfusions or to perform audits of selected transfusions. Alternately or additionally, audits of patient health records may be performed. Adherence to procedures and policies designed to protect patient safety is checked. For example, the transfusion service may verify that informed consent was documented, that vital signs were taken at the beginning and end of the transfusion, and that the blood component was transfused in less than the maximum time allowed.

UNCROSSMATCHED RED BLOOD CELLS

Any time that a red blood cell unit is issued for a patient before all testing is completed the unit is considered "uncrossmatched" (Table 7-10 ✳). The physician determines that the patient is at a greater risk if the transfusion is delayed than if uncrossmatched blood is used.

The most common scenario is a patient who needs blood urgently to stabilize his or her condition, often before blood specimens have even been drawn. In these cases, group O red blood cells are issued. Most transfusion services will try to issue group O Rh(D)-negative units whenever possible but local conditions and stock levels sometimes force the use of group O Rh(D)-positive units. An individual's historical blood group should never be used to issue nongroup O red blood cell units; testing on a current sample is required. A crossmatch specimen should be drawn and tested as soon as possible. If the antibody screen and/or crossmatch test is positive, the physician should be notified immediately. There should be documentation of the physician's order for uncrossmatched blood. Hospitals must also have some way to identify patients who arrive unresponsive and without identification.

INCOMPATIBLE RED BLOOD CELLS

Sometimes compatible blood cannot be found for a recipient (Table 7-11 ✳). The physician must weigh the risks to the patient of having no transfusion versus transfusing red blood cells that test incompatible. If the recipient is *hemodynamically* (i.e., relating to the forces involved in the circulation of blood) unstable, most experts agree that red blood cells should not be withheld, even if incompatible.[26] Ideally, red blood cell units should always be ABO compatible because ABO-incompatible red blood cell transfusion will cause an immediate hemolytic transfusion reaction, which may be fatal.

Often when incompatible blood is given, the recipient is monitored more closely for signs or symptoms of a transfusion reaction. Sometimes the physician will order a slower than usual rate of transfusion, although the transfusion must still be completed within the allowable maximum of 4 hours.

Some institutions will try what is known as a *biologic* or *in vivo crossmatch* if incompatible red blood cells are to be transfused.[?] A small amount of the red blood cell unit (e.g., 50 mL) is transfused slowly. After a short interval such as 30 minutes, a blood sample is drawn and tested for signs of hemolysis (e.g., an increase in free plasma hemoglobin). If no signs of hemolysis are present, the transfusion proceeds slowly and cautiously.

In many instances what is seen in the test tube does not perfectly correlate with what happens in the body. For example, many recipients who have a warm autoantibody tolerate transfusion the same as recipients with a negative antibody screen, although all red blood cell units appear incompatible during testing (Chapter 15).

✳ TABLE 7-10 Examples of Uncrossmatched Red Blood Cell Issue

Red blood cell units are considered uncrossmatched if
- No current pretransfusion sample has been collected.
- Current pretransfusion sample has been collected, but has not been tested.
- ABO-compatible units are being issued but antibody screen or identification is not yet complete.

Red blood cell units may be considered uncrossmatched if the investigation of an ABO or Rh discrepancy is not complete, depending on the facility's protocols.

✳ TABLE 7-11 Common Reasons for Incompatible Red Blood Cell Issue

- Patient has a warm autoantibody.
- Patient has multiple antibodies including one or more clinically insignificant antibodies; the red blood cells are antigen negative for all clinically significant antibodies that have been identified in the patient but are still positive in the IAT crossmatch due to the clinically insignificant antibodies; it is unlikely that units negative for all the corresponding antigens will be found or the patient requires transfusion before units negative for all the corresponding antigens can be found.
- Patient has an antibody to a high-incidence antigen that is known to be clinically insignificant.
- Patient has an antibody to a high-incidence antigen where the clinical significance of the antibody is unknown and no antigen-negative units are available.
- Patient has an antibody to a high-incidence antigen that is known to be clinically significant, but no antigen-negative units are available and transfusion is urgently required.
- Depending on the facility's policies, some transfusion services will consider units that are incompatible by their primary antibody screen/IAT crossmatch method to be incompatible even if the units are compatible when tested using a less sensitive technique, for example, nonadditive tube or prewarm techniques.

Review of the Main Points

- Regulations and standards outline the minimum requirements related to blood donors and blood recipients.
- Requirements are intended to reduce the risks associated with transfusion.
- Informed consent consists of the following elements: informing the patient of the risks and benefits of the transfusion, informing the patient of any alternatives that are available, giving the patient the opportunity to refuse or accept the transfusion, and documenting that the informed consent process has occurred.
- A request for transfusion should contain the following elements: name of the physician or authorized health professional who is requesting the transfusion, adequate identification of the patient, number and type of components requested, and clinical information and patient history to ensure that any need for specialized products is identified.
- At least two identifiers must link the patient: the pretransfusion specimen and the blood components chosen for transfusion.
- Patient identification may be eye-readable, machine-readable, or both. Machine-readable identification tools include one-dimensional barcodes, two-dimensional barcodes, and radio frequency identification chips.
- Patient history can help identify collection errors, can help prevent delayed hemolytic transfusion reactions, can help ensure that patients who require specialized products receive the correct product, and can aid antibody identification.
- Mandatory pretransfusion patient testing consists of ABO group, Rh(D) type, and red blood cell antibody screen.
- Red blood cells selected for transfusion must be ABO compatible with the recipient's plasma.
- Red blood cells are issued based on ABO test results from a current specimen, not on historical ABO results.
- Plasma products selected for transfusion should be ABO compatible with the recipient's red blood cells.
- Policies must define what is acceptable for platelet and cryoprecipitate AHF transfusions.
- Pretransfusion testing is not usually required prior to fractionation product infusion, except for Rh(D) typing when Rh immune globulin is requested.
- Reflex tests are used to resolve ABO or Rh typing discrepancies, to identify red blood cell antibodies, and to choose compatible red blood cell components.

- Three methods used to perform pretransfusion tests are tube, gel, and solid phase.
- Crossmatch is used to prevent issue of an ABO-incompatible red blood cell component.
- Crossmatch options include antiglobulin, immediate spin, and electronic. Policies must define when each crossmatch option is acceptable.
- Visual inspections check the physical condition of the blood product and are performed prior to transport, upon receipt, prior to issue, and prior to administration.
- Allocating and issuing procedures maintain the identification link with the patient.
- Inventory management processes reduce blood component discards due to outdating. Practices may include surgical blood order schedule, use of type and screen, and redistribution systems.
- Temperature of the blood products must be kept within acceptable limits during transport and storage.
- Patients undergoing a transfusion should be monitored throughout the procedure for signs and symptoms of a transfusion reaction.
- Uncrossmatched blood is red blood cell components that are issued before the completion of all pretransfusion testing.
- Group O red blood cell components can be issued as uncrossmatched when a specimen or current ABO test results are not available. A pretransfusion specimen should be drawn and tested as soon as possible.
- Some patients may be transfused with red blood cells that appear incompatible, but the red blood cells must still be ABO compatible.
- Some instances where incompatible red blood cell components may be transfused include patients with a warm autoantibody, patients with an antibody to a high-incidence antigen, or patients with multiple antibodies.
- It is the responsibility of the physician to determine if the risk of transfusing uncrossmatched or incompatible red blood cells is greater than the risk of not receiving a transfusion at that point in time.

Review Questions

1. Which of the following tests are mandatory to perform on red blood cell units that have just been received from a blood supplier? (Objective #5)

   A. ABO typing

   B. Rh(D) typing

   C. Weak D test

   D. Extended antigen phenotype

2. The process of obtaining informed consent for a blood transfusion: (Objective #1)

   A. Provides the patient with a description of risks, benefits, and viable treatment alternatives

   B. Is specific to the patient's condition and type of blood product that will be transfused

   C. Requires the opportunity for questions to be asked

   D. Requires the right to refuse the transfusion

3. What information is needed when a blood component is requested for transfusion to a patient? (Objective #2)

   A. Name of the ordering physician

   B. Clinical information and patient history

   C. Number and type of component to be transfused

   D. Donor name and contact information

4. A hemolytic transfusion reaction can be caused by: (Objective #3)

   A. Patient identification error at the time of transfusion

   B. Product viability

   C. Specimen labeling error at the time of collection

   D. Reagent QC failure

5. Select the appropriate patient identifiers for specimen labeling that should be checked for accuracy against the request for transfusion. (Objective #4)

   A. Full name of patient

   B. Date of birth

   C. Medical/hospital record number

   D. Number sequence/blood bank numbers

6. Why should specimens be used no more than 3 days after collection in patients who have been recently transfused or who are pregnant? (Objective #3)

   A. Delayed hemolytic transfusion reactions may not be detected.

   B. Recent pregnancy or transfusion may stimulate antibodies that are not detectable at the time of collection.

   C. Clinically significant antibodies may fall below detectable levels after the transfusion.

   D. Patient identification errors may not be identified.

7. Steps to reduce ABO blood typing errors in the laboratory include: (Objective #5)

   A. Compare current ABO typing results to a historical record.

   B. Perform two separate ABO typing tests on the same specimen.

   C. Perform ABO typing tests on two specimens drawn independently.

   D. Perform ABO typing tests on two specimens drawn at the same time.

8. What type of red blood cells should be issued when an ABO blood type cannot be determined prior to the request for transfusion? (Objective #6)

   A. Group O

   B. Group O or Group A

   C. Group A or Group AB

   D. Group O, Group A, Group B, or Group AB

9. Select the requirements for the manufacture of screening cells that are used in the antibody screening test for pretransfusion testing. (Objective #5)

   A. Must be blood group O

   B. Must be from a single donor (not pooled)

   C. Should contain at least one expression of all significant antigens

   D. Must contain a homozygous form of all antigens

10. Why is patient cell antigen typing, as part of the reflex testing process, performed only on pretransfusion specimen? (Objective #7)

    A. Circulating patient cells may cause false-negative results

    B. Circulating patient cells may stimulate antibody production

    C. Circulating donor cells may cause false-positive results

    D. Circulating donor cells may be below detectable levels

11. ABO incompatibility of red blood cells for transfusion is detected at the _____ phase of the major crossmatch test. (Objective #12)

    A. Immediate spin (I.S.)

    B. 98.6° F (37° C)

    C. IAT

    D. Coombs control cells

12. Which of the following blood products does *not* require any pretransfusion testing? (Objective #9)

    A. Red blood cells

    B. Fresh frozen plasma

    C. Single-donor platelets

    D. Plasma protein fraction

13. Which pretransfusion test method uses antigen coated wells on a microplate for the identification of clinically significant antibodies? (Objective #10)

    A. Gel

    B. Solid phase

    C. Tube

    D. PEG

14. A patient is scheduled for hip replacement surgery and a pretransfusion work-up, including crossmatch for 2 units of red blood cells, is requested. Although the patient has a history of anti-Fy^a, the antibody screen in the current sample is negative by gel method. What type of crossmatch test should be performed? (Objective #12)

    A. Immediate spin major crossmatch

    B. Antiglobulin major crossmatch

    C. Electronic crossmatch

    D. Minor crossmatch

15. Disadvantages of using the type and screen (T & S) procedure in pretransfusion testing include: (Objective #15)

    A. Antibody to rare antigens may not be detected.

    B. High-incidence antigens may not be identified.

    C. Clinically significant antibodies are always detected.

    D. More false-positive transfusion reactions are reported.

16. Which of the following procedures is important for the safe administration of blood products? (Objective #17)

    A. Document checks

    B. Vital sign checks

    C. Transfusion reaction reporting

    D. Emergency transfusion

17. A red blood cell unit is considered "uncrossmatched" when it is issued: (Objective #18)

    A. Prior to a surgical procedure

    B. Prior to laboratory test completion

    C. Without a physician's order

    D. Without informed consent

References

1. AABB. *Standards for blood banks and transfusion services*, 27th ed. Bethesda (MD): AABB Press; 2011.

2. Roback JD, Grossman BJ, Harris T, Hillyer CD, editors. *Technical manual*, 17th ed. Bethesda (MD): AABB Press; 2011.

3. White J. Pre-Transfusion testing. *ISBT Science Series* 2009; 4:37–44.

4. Murphy MF, Stearn BE, Dxik WH. Current performance of patient sample collection in the UK. *Transfus Med.* 2004; 14: 113–21.

5. Stainsby D, Russell J, Cohen H, Lilleyman J. Reducing adverse events in blood transfusion. *Br J Haematol.* 2005; 131: 8–12.

6. Davis R, Geiger B, Gutierrez A, Heaser J, Veeramani D. Tracking blood products in blood centres using radio frequency identification: a comprehensive assessment. *Vox Sang.* 2009; 97: 50–60.

7. Pavlidis T, Swartz J, Wang YP. Information encoding with two-dimensional bar codes. *Computer* 1992; 25: 18–28.

8. Gonzalez-Porras JR, Graciani IF, Alvarez M, Pinto J, Conde MP, Nieto MJ, Corral M. Tubes for pretransfusion testing should be collected by blood bank staff and hand labelled until the implementation of new technology for improved sample labeling. Results of a prospective study. *Vox Sang* 2008; 95: 52–6.

9. Goodnough, LT, Viele M, Fontaine MJ, Jurado C, Stone N, Quach P, Chua L, Chin ML, Scott R, Tokareva I, Tabb K, Sharek PJ. Implementation of a two-specimen requirement for verification of ABO/Rh for blood transfusion. *Transfusion* 2009; 49: 1321–8.

10. Pierce RN, Reich LM, Mayer K. Hemolysis following platelet transfusion from ABO-incompatible donors. *Transfusion* 1985; 25: 60–2.

11. Mair B, Benson K. Evaluation of changes in hemoglobin levels associated with ABO-incompatible plasma in apheresis platelets. *Transfusion* 1998; 38: 51–5.

12. Shehata N, et al. ABO-identical versus nonidentical platelet transfusion: a systematic review. *Transfusion* 2009; 49: 2442–53.

13. Slichter SJ. Algorithm for managing the platelet refractory patient. *J Clin Apher* 1997; 12: 4–9.

14. Bussel JB, Granziano JN, Kimberly RP, Pahwa S, Aledort IM. Intravenous anti-D treatment of immune thrombocytopenic purpura: analysis of efficacy, toxicity, and mechanism of effect. *Blood* 1991; 77: 1884–93.

15. Butch SH, Judd WJ, Steiner EA, Stoe M, Oberman HA. Electronic verification of donor-recipient compatibility: the computer crossmatch. *Transfusion* 1994; 34: 105–9.

16. Judd WJ. Requirements for the electronic crossmatch. *Vox Sang* 1998; 2: 409–17.

17. Friedman BA, Oberman HA, Chadwick AR, Kingdon KI. The maximum surgical blood order schedule and surgical blood use in the Untied States. *Transfusion* 1976; 16: 380–7.

18. Petride M, Stack G. *Practical guide to transfusion medicine.* Bethesda (MD): AABB Press; 2001.

19. Peterson DM, Roxby DJ, Seshadri R. Is the indirect antiglobulin crossmatch justified? *Pathology* 1987; 19: 121–3.

20. Weinberg PD, Hounshell J, Sherman LA, Godwin J, Ali S, Tomori C, Bennett CL. Legal, financial, and public health consequences of HIV contamination of blood and blood products in the 1980s and 1990s. *Ann Intern Med* 2002; 136: 312–9.

21. Krever H. *Final report: Commission of Inquiry on the Blood System in Canada.* Ottawa: The Commission; 1997.

22. Pinkerton PH, Coovadia AS, Goldstein J. Frequency of delayed hemolytic transfusion reactions following antibody screening and immediate-spin crossmatching. *Transfusion* 1994; 34: 87–8.

23. Heddle NM, O'Hoski P, Singer J, McBride JA, Ali MA, Kelton JG. A prospective study to determine the safety of omitting the antiglobulin crossmatch from pretransfusion testing. *Br J Haematol* 1992; 4: 579–84.

24. Davis SP, Barrasso C, Ness PM. Maximizing the benefits of type and screen by continued surveillance of transfusion practice. *Am J Med Technol* 1983; 49: 579–82.

25. Migeot V, Tellier S, Ingrand P. Diversity of bedside pretransfusion ABO compatibility devices in metropolitan France. (English abstract). *Transfus Clin Biol* 2003; 10: 26–36.

26. Ness PM. How do I encourage clinicians to transfuse mismatched blood to patients with autoimmune hemolytic anemia in urgent situations? *Transfusion* 2006; 11: 1859–62.

27. Frohn C, Dümbgen L, Brand JM, Görg S, Luhm J, Kirchner H. Probability of anti-D development in D− patients receiving D+ RBCs. *Transfusion* 2003; 43: 893–98.

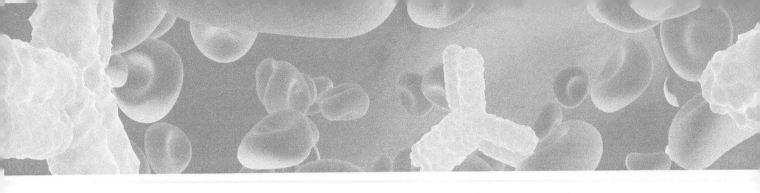

8 Identification of Unexpected Antibodies

STEPHANIE CODINA AND ELAINE J. SCOTT

Chapter Objectives

Upon completion of this chapter, the student will be able to:

1. Determine when antibody identification is necessary.
2. Correctly interpret panel results by ruling out or ruling in significant antibodies.
3. Differentiate alloantibodies and autoantibodies based on test results.
4. Determine when additional testing is necessary to complete antibody identification.
5. Identify additional tests that may need to be done in given scenarios and predict the desired results.
6. Calculate the number of donor units that should be screened to obtain a given number of antigen-negative donor red blood cell units.
7. Identify the appropriate pieces of historical information that should be obtained when performing antibody identification.
8. List the common antigens that are enhanced by enzymes and destroyed by enzymes.
9. Describe how statistical validity is achieved in antibody identification.
10. Cite examples of situations in which mixed-field agglutination reactions can be observed.
11. Identify and describe the antibodies that can be neutralized, including the appropriate medium necessary for success.
12. Describe the different methods that are used for elution of red blood cell antibodies.
13. Describe the typical pretransfusion testing results seen when a warm autoantibody is present.
14. Choose and explain the procedures that are routinely used to identify alloantibodies in the presence of either a warm or cold agglutinin.
15. Describe the procedure for antibody titration.
16. Discuss the clinical usefulness of antibody titration.
17. Define the concept of polyagglutination.
18. Explain how the different types of polyagglutination are differentiated.

Chapter Outline

Key Terms

Adsorption
Antigen typing
Antigram
Autocontrol (AC)
Avidity
Cold agglutinin(s)
Cryptic autoantigen(s)
Dosage
Elution
Enzyme(s)
Exclusion
Neutralization

Panagglutination
Panagglutinin
Polyagglutinable
Polyagglutination
Potentiator(s)
Rouleaux
Titration
Titration score
Unexpected antibody
   (antibodies)
Warm autoantibody
   (antibodies)

What's Ahead?

Red blood cell antibodies must be detected and identified to avoid serious transfusion complications. Studies estimate 0.5% of transfusions will induce the formation of an alloantibody. This number can increase up to 60% in chronically transfused patients, making antibody identification a common task in the transfusion medicine laboratory.[1] Even though antibody identification is a routine laboratory procedure, it can be one of the most challenging tasks performed by laboratory personnel.

This chapter addresses the following questions:

- How are antibodies to red blood cell antigens identified in the laboratory?
- What laboratory techniques are used in antibody investigations?
- How does the laboratory choose the safest donor units for transfusion when the recipient has an antibody or antibodies?

CASE IN POINT

MG is a 57-year-old male transferred from a nearby community hospital. The patient has been diagnosed with a malignant neoplasm and was transferred due to a suspected intraparenchymal bleed. Upon arrival, the patient's hemoglobin and hematocrit were 6.2 g/dL (62 g/L) and 18.6% (0.19), respectively. A crossmatch for 4 units of packed red blood cells was ordered and 4 units of fresh frozen plasma were placed on hold.

ANTIBODY DETECTION REVIEW

The provision of compatible blood for transfusion begins with determining whether the patient has any unexpected red blood cell antibodies. An antibody screen is used to detect these antibodies (Chapter 7). The antibody screen must include an indirect antiglobulin test (IAT) phase using unpooled group O red blood cells (Chapter 3). Commercial sets of antibody screen cells include red blood cells that are antigen positive for the most commonly encountered corresponding antibodies. Currently three methods are routinely used to detect antibodies: tube, gel, and solid-phase testing (Chapter 3). Regardless of the method used to perform the antibody screen, a positive result must be investigated to identify the antibody or antibodies present.

☑ CHECKPOINT 8-1

What test is routinely used to determine if a patient has developed an unexpected antibody?

RESOLUTION OF A POSITIVE ANTIBODY SCREEN

Antibody identification begins with testing of patient plasma against a panel of red blood cells with known phenotypes. Laboratories generally use commercially prepared reagent red blood cells, but panel cells can also be prepared in-house. Each panel should

have an **antigram**. The antigram is a chart that shows the antigenic makeup of each cell in the panel. The results that are obtained when the panel cells are tested against the patient's plasma are compared to the antigram to determine the identity of antibody(ies) in the specimen.

Selection of an Antibody Panel

Both screening and identification panel cells are prepared from group O donors. Group O donors are used because these cells do not contain A or B antigens. Because the blood type of a patient requiring an antibody identification can vary, group O panel cells eliminate the chance of an ABO antibody in the patient's serum or plasma. It is important to keep in mind here that ABO antibodies (Chapter 4) are expected based on the ABO type of the patient. The antibody identification process seeks to identify **unexpected antibodies** (antibodies other than those in the ABO system found in plasma directed against corresponding red blood cell antigens).

Reagent red blood cells should have a negative direct antiglobulin test (DAT) to prevent false-positive reactions in the IAT phase used for antibody screening and identification.[2] Each vial of reagent red blood cells comes from an individual donor, who has been typed for the common red blood cell antigens. The United States Food and Drug Administration (FDA) requires that each lot of screening and identification cells has at least one cell that demonstrates each of the following antigens: D, C, E, c, e, K, k, Fy^a, M, N, S, and s.[3] These, however, are the minimum requirements. Most reagent screen sets or panels also have known positives for the P$_1$, Le^a, Le^b, Fy^b, Jk^a, and Jk^b

antigens.[4] For screening and panel identification purposes, cells with the greatest number of homozygous expressions are ideal.

The primary difference between antibody screening and antibody identification is the number of cells used for testing. Antibody screening is generally performed using two to four different donor cells, while antibody identification uses cells from a larger number of donors. Manufacturers choose panel cells so that they produce a distinctive pattern of positive and negative reactions for the most commonly encountered antibodies.[5] The number of cells that should be tested varies by laboratory, method, and antibody. However, additional cells must be tested and/or other antibody identification methods must be employed if the initial testing does not yield a clear reactivity pattern.

A good rule of thumb is to begin antibody identification by testing a panel of 8–12 cells using the same method that was employed in the antibody screen. Usually any commercial or in-house prepared panel is used. However, the choice of cells for testing can be altered based on known results. For example, if a patient has a history of an anti-D, testing Rh(D+) cells will not be helpful to the identification process because the anti-D will react with these cells and may mask other reactions. Figure 8-1 ▇ provides an example of a reaction pattern caused by an anti-D.

> ### ☑ CHECKPOINT 8-2
>
> What antigens does the FDA mandate must be demonstrated in each reagent screen cell set?

Patient History

An accurate patient history can be very helpful during antibody identification testing.[5] Key questions for consideration consist of:

- Has the patient ever been transfused or pregnant?
- If the patient has been transfused, did any transfusions occur in the last 3 months?
- What medications is the patient currently taking?
- Are there other medications that the patient has taken in the last 3 months?

If the patient has a history of transfusion or pregnancy, the potential for immune-mediated antibodies exists. If the patient has never been pregnant or transfused, the positive antibody screen is likely due to naturally occurring antibodies such as a nonspecific cold antibody, anti-Le^a or anti-Le^b.

If the patient has been transfused within the previous 3 months, donor cells may still be circulating in the patient's bloodstream. Antigen typing results may not be valid and a positive DAT may be evidence of a delayed serological transfusion reaction.

Lastly, an accurate medication history is helpful. Some drugs such as cephalosporins, procainamide, intravenous penicillin, or α–methyldopa (aldomet) will coat red blood cells and cause a positive DAT (Chapter 15). Therapeutic regimens that include antilymphocyte or antithymocyte globulin can mimic alloantibodies in a patient's plasma. Treatment with intravenous immune globulin (IVIG), which may contain various red blood cell antibodies, or with Rh-immune globulin (RhIg), which contains anti-D and occasionally anti-C, can

Donor	D	C	c	E	e	K	k	Fy^a	Fy^b	Jk^a	Jk^b	Le^a	Le^b	P$_1$	M	N	S	s	Patient Results Gel IAT
I	+	+	0	0	+	+	+	0	+	+	0	+	0	0	+	0	+	+	3+
II	+	0	+	+	0	0	+	0	+	0	+	0	+	0	0	+	0	+	3+
III	0	0	+	0	+	0	+	+	0	+	+	0	+	+	+	0	+	0	0

Donor	D	C	c	E	e	K	k	Fy^a	Fy^b	Jk^a	Jk^b	Le^b	Le^b	P$_1$	M	N	S	s	Patient Results Gel IAT
1	+	+	0	0	+	+	+	0	+	+	+	0	0	0	0	+	0	+	3+
2	+	+	0	0	+	0	+	0	+	0	+	+	0	0	+	0	+	0	3+
3	+	+	0	0	+	0	+	+	0	+	0	0	0	+	0	+	0	+	3+
4	+	0	+	+	0	0	+	+	0	+	0	0	0	+	+	0	+	+	3+
5	+	0	+	+	0	0	+	0	+	+	0	+	0	+	+	0	0	+	3+
6	0	+	+	0	+	0	+	0	+	+	+	+	0	+	+	+	0	+	0
7	0	0	+	0	+	+	+	+	+	+	0	0	+	+	+	+	0	+	0
8	0	0	+	0	+	+	+	+	0	+	+	+	0	+	+	0	+	0	0
9	0	0	+	0	+	0	+	0	+	0	+	0	+	0	+	+	0	+	0
10	0	0	+	0	+	0	+	+	+	+	+	0	0	+	0	+	0	0	0
Autocontrol																			0

0 = no agglutination

+ = agglutination (with or without strength of reaction noted in front)

▇ **FIGURE 8-1** Screen Cell and Panel Cell Antigram Results for an Anti-D

cause a positive antibody screen, DAT, and/or eluate due to passive antibodies.

Autocontrol and Direct Antiglobulin Test (DAT)

An autocontrol or DAT should be tested whenever an antibody panel is run.[6] An **autocontrol** consists of testing patient plasma against patient cells by the same method used to test the panel cells. A positive DAT result indicates *in vivo* coating of red blood cells with IgG or complement (Chapter 3). A positive autocontrol result will not differentiate *in vivo* or *in vitro* coating of red blood cells because the test is incubated, often with an enhancement reagent. Therefore, a DAT should be performed on a patient's red blood cells when the autocontrol is positive.

Both the autocontrol and DAT can help to distinguish autoantibodies from alloantibodies.[7] Generally speaking, an autoantibody may be present if the autocontrol or DAT is positive. However, a serological transfusion reaction (Chapter 12) should also be considered if the patient has been transfused within 90 days of the test because donor red blood cells may still be circulating in the patient's bloodstream.

Test Phases and Enhancement Reagents

Gel and solid-phase testing provide IAT results and are very sensitive techniques. Tube testing allows for more variation in technique, which can sometimes be helpful in identifying antibodies.

A variety of phases can be used with tube testing, such as immediate spin and incubation at different temperatures as well as the required IAT phase (Chapter 3). Knowledge of antibody characteristics (Chapter 6) can aid in choosing appropriate additional incubation temperatures, test phases, and/or test methods that might be beneficial in resolving difficult antibody problems. Figure 8-2 ■ illustrates a reaction pattern of two antibodies where each reacts at a different test phase.

Tube testing can be performed without enhancement or using one of a variety of enhancement reagents, such as albumin, low ionic strength saline (LISS), or polyethylene glycol (PEG) (Chapter 3). Enhancement reagents are also called **potentiators**. In general, the more sensitive the test methodology, the less specific the testing becomes because more nonspecific reactions or clinically insignificant antibodies will be detected. PEG is the most sensitive enhancement reagent, but also has the highest false-positive rate of up to 2.9%.[8]

Testing by a variety of methodologies, if available, including different enhancement reagents in tube testing and nontube methods, can sometimes help to resolve difficult antibody problems, such as multiple antibodies, nonspecific patterns, or weakly reactive results.

CASE IN POINT (continued)

A type and crossmatch specimen was collected from MG in an EDTA tube, labeled properly and sent to the transfusion service. A check of the patient's history recorded in the laboratory information system (LIS) showed that in 1988 while in the hospital for a coronary artery bypass graft procedure he tested as B Rh(D) positive with a negative antibody screen, but that by 1998 the patient had developed an anti-C.

MG's current results are as follows: B Rh (D) positive, positive antibody screen using PEG, positive DAT using polyspecific antihuman globulin (anti-IgG, C3d), and monospecific anti-IgG. The antibody screen results were as follows:

Donor	D	C	c	E	e	K	k	Fy^a	Fy^b	Jk^a	Jk^b	Le^a	Le^b	P$_1$	M	N	S	s	IS	IAT	CC
I	+	+	0	0	+	+	+	0	+	+	0	+	0	0	+	0	+	+	0	3+	
II	+	0	+	+	0	0	+	0	+	0	+	0	+	0	0	+	0	+	0	0	+
III	0	0	+	0	+	0	+	+	0	+	+	0	+	+	+	0	+	0	0	0	+

0, no agglutination; +, agglutination (with or without strength of reaction noted in front).

The positive reactions of the screening cells fit the anti-C pattern perfectly. However, the laboratorian called the referring hospital and learned that the community hospital laboratory had identified an anti-K in the patient's plasma. The anti-C was not detected in their laboratory and they did not know the patient had a history of anti-C. Two B Rh(D)-positive, K-negative units, with an unknown C phenotype, had been transfused to the patient the previous day at the community hospital.

1. What are the possible causes of the positive reaction with screen cell I?
2. What should the laboratorian do next?

Donor	D	C	c	E	e	K	k	Fyᵃ	Fyᵇ	Jkᵃ	Jkᵇ	Leᵃ	Leᵇ	P₁	M	N	S	s	IS	IAT	CC
																			Patient Results		
1	+	+	0	0	+	+	+	0	+	+	+	0	0	0	0	+	0	+	0	0	+
2	+	+	0	0	+	0	+	0	+	0	+	+	0	0	+	0	+	0	1+	0	+
3	+	+	0	0	+	0	+	+	0	+	0	0	0	+	0	+	0	+	0	0	+
4	+	0	+	+	0	0	+	+	0	+	0	0	0	+	+	0	+	+	0	2+	
5	+	0	+	+	0	0	+	0	+	+	0	+	0	+	0	0	0	+	1+	2+	
6	0	+	+	0	+	0	+	0	+	+	+	+	0	+	+	+	0	+	1+	0	+
7	0	0	+	+	+	0	+	+	+	+	0	0	0	+	+	+	0	+	0	2+	
8	0	0	+	0	+	+	+	+	0	+	+	+	0	+	+	0	+	0	1+	0	+
9	0	0	+	0	+	0	+	0	+	0	+	0	+	0	+	+	0	+	0	0	+
10	0	0	+	0	+	0	+	+	+	+	0	0	+	0	+	0	+	0	0	0	+
																	Autocontrol		0	0	+

0 = no agglutination

+ = agglutination (with or without strength of reaction noted in front)

This specimen contains two distinct antibodies. The anti-Leᵃ represented in pink, reacts best at room temperature as demonstrated by the results in the immediate spin phase. The anti-E, represented in green, reacts best at 37° C and shows positive results in the IAT phase because the IAT includes a 37° C incubation step.

FIGURE 8-2   Example Panel Results Caused by Two Antibodies

Exclusion (Rule Out)

Antibody identification *exclusion* (rule out) requires knowledge, understanding, and skill. The following sections describe the process and considerations related to exclusion (rule out).

Process

Exclusions should be performed once the initial antibody identification cells are tested and the corresponding reactions are recorded on a copy of the panel antigram. An exclusion or rule out consists of crossing off the antigens that did not react with the patient specimen; generally only antigens that are homozygous are used to exclude an antibody. For preliminary antibody identification we can tentatively assume that an antibody is not present if the patient's plasma result is negative when tested against the corresponding antigen.[5, 9] Figure 8-3 ■ illustrates the steps taken in the rule-out process.

☑ **CHECKPOINT 8-4**

Describe the rule out or exclusion process.

Dosage

If a person inherits the same allele at a particular locus, they are called homozygous for the red blood cell antigen and their red blood cell antigen is called a *double dose* (Chapter 6), for example, someone with a *CC* genotype whose red blood cell phenotype is C+c−. If an individual inherits two antithetical alleles, the person is heterozygous and their cells carry a single dose of antigen, for example,

someone with a *Cc* genotype whose red blood cell phenotype is C+c+.

Dosage occurs when an antibody reacts differently with cells that have homozygous versus heterozygous antigen expression.[5] An antibody demonstrating the dosage effect will react weaker with cells that are heterozygous for the corresponding antigen and stronger with homozygous cells. Thus, homozygous cells are used in exclusions to prevent ruling out an antibody that is showing dosage. Some antibodies showing dosage may react only with homozygous cells.

Common Exceptions to Homozygous Exclusion

There are exceptions to the rule advocating the use of only homozygous cells for exclusion of an antibody.

- D and P1 antigens do not have antithetical alleles; cells are either positive or negative for these antigens and dosage effect is not seen. Antibodies to D and P1 can be ruled out based on negative reactions with one or more antigen-positive cells.
- Cellano (k) is a high-frequency antigen present in >99% of all individuals. This makes finding a cell that demonstrates homozygosity for the K antigen difficult. Therefore, an anti-K may have to be ruled out using one or more heterozygous cells.
- The chance of finding a dCe/dCe or dcE/dcE antibody screening cell is very small, 0.01% and 0.03%, respectively.[10] Therefore, the presence of anti-C and anti-E in a patient who has produced anti-D will likely have to be decided based on the reactions of heterozygous cells.

Figure 8-4 ■ illustrates some common exceptions to homozygous rule out.

CASE IN POINT (continued)

An initial antibody panel was run on MG's sample using tube technique with PEG enhancement and the results are as follows:

Donor	D	C	c	E	e	K	k	Fy^a	Fy^b	Jk^a	Jk^b	Le^a	Le^b	P$_1$	M	N	S	s	IS	IAT	CC
1	+	+	0	+	+	+	+	+	0	+	0	0	+	+	0	+	0	+	0	3+	
2	+	+	0	0	+	0	+	+	0	0	+	+	0	+	+	0	+	+	0	2+	
3	+	0	+	+	0	0	+	0	+	+	0	0	+	0	+	+	+	0	0	0	I
4	+	0	+	0	+	0	+	+	0	+	+	0	+	+	+	+	0	0	0	0	+
5	0	+	+	0	+	0	+	+	0	+	0	+	0	+	+	+	+	+	0	3+	
6	0	0	+	+	+	0	+	+	+	+	0	0	+	+	+	+	+	+	0	0	+
7	0	0	+	0	+	+	+	0	+	0	+	0	+	+	+	+	+	+	0	3+	
8	0	0	+	0	+	0	+	+	0	0	+	0	+	+	+	+	+	+	0	0	+
9	0	0	+	0	+	0	+	+	0	0	+	+	0	0	+	0	0	+	0	1+	

0, no agglutination; +, agglutination (with or without strength of reaction noted in front).

3. What antibodies are ruled out?
4. What previously identified antibody or antibodies is/are reacting?
5. What antibodies are not ruled out?
6. Is the reaction pattern explained by the patient's history?

Donor	D	C	c	E	e	K	k	Fy^a	Fy^b	Jk^a	Jk^b	Le^a	Le^b	P$_1$	M	N	S	s	IS	IAT	CC
1	+	+	0	0	+	+	+	0	+	+	+	0	0	0	0	+	0	+	0	0	+
2	+	+	0	0	+	0	+	0	+	0	+	+	0	0	+	0	+	0	0	0	+
3	+	+	0	0	+	0	+	0	+	+	0	0	0	+	0	+	0	+	0	0	+
4	+	0	+	+	0	0	+	+	0	+	0	0	0	+	+	0	+	+	0	+	
5	+	0	+	+	0	0	+	0	+	+	0	+	0	+	+	0	0	+	0	0	+
6	0	+	+	0	+	0	+	0	+	+	+	+	0	+	+	+	0	+	0	0	+
7	0	0	+	+	+	0	+	+	+	+	0	0	+	+	+	+	0	+	0	+	
8	0	0	+	0	+	+	+	+	0	+	+	+	0	+	+	0	+	0	0	+	
9	0	0	+	0	+	+	0	0	+	0	+	0	+	0	+	+	0	+	0	0	+
10	0	0	+	0	+	0	+	+	+	+	0	0	+	0	0	+	0	+	0	+	
															Autocontrol				0	0	+

0 = no agglutination

+ = agglutination

The antibodies that we are ruling out are highlighted in yellow and the cells with antigens on which we ruled them out are highlighted in pink.

FIGURE 8-3   Example of Rule Out Process

Step 1: Find the first cell that is reacting negatively in all phases. In this example, cell #1 has negative reactions in both IS and IAT phases.

Step 2: Cross out all the antigens demonstrating a homozygous expression on this cell. In this example, for cell #1 cross out D, C, e, Fy^b, N, and s. Do not cross out Jk^a or Jk^b because cell #1 is demonstrating a heterozygous expression of these antigens.

Step 3: Repeat the process for each cell on the panel that is reacting negatively in all phases. For example, the next cell with all negative reactions is cell #2 and it is homozygous for k, Jk^b, Le^a, M, and S.

Donor	D	C	c	E	e	K	k	Fyª	Fyᵇ	Jkª	Jkᵇ	Leª	Leᵇ	P₁	M	N	S	s	IS	IAT	CC
1	+	+	0	0	+	+	+	0	+	+	+	0	0	0	0	+	0	+	0	2+	
2	+	+	0	0	+	0	+	0	+	0	+	+	0	0	+	0	+	0	0	2+	
3	+	+	0	0	+	0	+	0	+	+	0	0	0	+	0	+	0	+	0	2+	
4	+	0	+	+	0	0	+	+	0	+	0	0	0	+	+	0	+	+	0	2+	
5	+	0	+	+	0	0	+	0	+	+	0	+	0	+	+	0	0	+	0	2+	
6	0	+	+	0	+	0	+	0	+	+	+	+	0	+	+	+	0	+	0	0	+
7	0	0	+	+	+	0	+	+	+	+	0	0	+	+	+	+	0	+	0	0	+
8	0	0	+	0	+	+	+	+	0	+	+	+	0	+	+	0	+	0	0	0	+
9	0	0	+	0	+	0	+	0	+	0	+	0	+	0	+	+	0	+	0	0	+
10	0	0	+	0	+	0	+	+	+	+	0	0	+	0	+	0	+	+	0	0	+
																		Autocontrol	0	0	+

0 = no agglutination

+ = agglutination (with or without strength of reaction noted in front)

The sample contains an anti-D, highlighted in green. Antibodies ruled out by homozygous cells are highlighted in yellow. Antibodies ruled out using heterozygous cells are highlighted in pink. P1, which does not have an antithetical antigen, is ruled out using the cell highlighted in turquoise.

FIGURE 8-4 Example Showing Common Exceptions to Homozygous Rule Out

CONFIRMATION OF ANTIBODY IDENTIFICATION

Confirmation of antibody identification requires utilizing statistical measures and performing a testing technique known as *antigen typing*. These two important concepts are described in the following sections.

Statistical Measures

The probability, or *p* value, is a statistical measure that predicts the likelihood of an outcome. The *p* value is calculated by considering the fixed distribution of a known antigen on the panel cells and the pattern of agglutination that is obtained when tested against a patient's plasma.[9] Care must be taken in applying *p* values from published tables in complex antibody patterns to ensure that the underlying statistical principles apply in each particular case.[11]

However, a general rule exists that is based on *p* value as calculated from Fisher's exact test; an antibody must react with three antigen-positive cells and must not react with three antigen-negative cells to be statistically proven.[5] If a specimen contains multiple antibodies, the rule must be applied to each antibody independently in order to be valid.

For example, if a patient's plasma contains anti-K, anti-C, and anti-E, one must prove each antibody is present by testing the following combinations of red blood cells and obtaining the appropriate reactions:

- Three *positive* reactions on three cells that are phenotype K+, C−, E−
- Three *positive* reactions on three cells that are phenotype K−, C+, E−
- Three *positive* reactions on three cells that are phenotype K−, C−, E+
- Three *negative* reactions on three cells that are phenotype K−, C−, E−

Red blood cells that are homozygous for an antigen should be used whenever possible for the positive cells. Since homozygous positive cells possess more antigen sites than heterozygous positive cells, they are more likely to react with weak antibodies that might otherwise be missed. Some important considerations must be made when using this method to prove the presence or absence of an antibody. First, a consistent pattern of reactivity cannot be the only factor used to identify an antibody.[11] All other common clinically significant antibodies must be ruled out before identification can be made. Conversely, antibody identification does not rely solely on the exclusion process; the pattern of reactivity should also be considered in case an antibody that is present has been ruled out based on an aberrant reaction with one cell. Lastly, accurate identification should be made only after considering all characteristics of an antibody such as reaction temperature, dosage, and other available information.

Antigen Typing

Antigen typing, which determines the phenotype of the tested red blood cells, can be used to help prove an antibody is present and to rule out antibodies that are not present. In theory, a person cannot make antibodies corresponding to the antigens that he or she possesses. Therefore, once the antigens present on a person's red blood cells are known, one can determine which antibodies that person has the ability to make.

Antigen typing is performed by testing a specific known antiserum with patient or donor red blood cells. If the antiserum reacts positively, the red blood cells have the corresponding antigen. The red blood cells lack the corresponding antigen if they do not react with the antiserum. Several different brands of commercially prepared antisera are available in a variety of different specificities. Antigen typing cannot be performed on patients who have been transfused within the previous 3 months because donor red blood cells are still circulating and will interfere with testing results.

CASE IN POINT (continued)

After the initial panel was run, selected red blood cells were chosen to help rule in or rule out the suspected antibodies. The results of the selected red blood cell panel by traditional tube technique using PEG enhancement are as follows:

Donor	D	C	c	E	e	K	k	Fyᵃ	Fyᵇ	Jkᵃ	Jkᵇ	Leᵃ	Leᵇ	P₁	M	N	S	s	IS	IAT	CC
10	+	+	0	0	+	0	+	0	+	+	+	0	+	+	+	0	0	+	0	1+	
11	+	0	+	+	0	0	+	0	0	+	0	+	0	+	+	0	0	+	0	1	
12	0	0	+	+	+	0	+	0	+	+	0	+	0	0	+	0	+	+	0	1+	
13	0	0	+	0	+	+	+	0	+	0	+	0	+	+	0	+	0	+	0	3+	
14	0	0	+	0	+	0	+	+	0	+	+	+	0	0	0	+	0	+	0	W+	
15	0	0	+	0	+	+	0	+	+	0	+	0	+	+	+	+	0		0	3+	

0, no agglutination; +, agglutination (with or without strength of reaction noted in front).

7. What additional antibody has been identified?
8. Which red blood cells have been used to confirm the identity of each antibody?

FINDING COMPATIBLE BLOOD

Once antibody identification is complete, compatible blood must be found. IAT crossmatch-compatible red blood cell units should be negative for the antigens that correspond to a patient's antibodies when the antibody is clinically significant (Chapter 7). When a clinically insignificant antibody (Chapter 6) is identified, the red blood cell units for transfusion do not need to be antigen-typed but should still be crossmatch compatible in the IAT if the antibody is currently reacting.

The Hardy-Weinberg equation is used to calculate the frequency of alleles and genotypes within a population. The frequency of one of the alleles must be known and certain assumptions are made. A simple formula is used to calculate how many donor units to type for a particular antigen in order to find the number of donor units needed[12]. For example, if a patient with anti-C needs 2 units of blood, the formula is:

$$\frac{\text{Number of units needed}}{\text{Incidence of phenotype}} = \text{Number of units to screen}$$

The frequency of the C allele in the general population is 70%, which means that approximately 30% of donor units are *negative* for C. The antigen frequencies for the most commonly antigens tested on a typical antibody identification panel is located in the Case-In-Point entry at the end of this section.

In this example, the incidence of C-negative donor units is 0.30. A step-by-step calculation of this value follows:

Step 1: Determine the percentage of antigen-*negative* individuals. In this case we are given that 70% of the population is positive for the C antigen. Thus, 100% − 70% = 30% are C antigen negative.

Step 2: Convert the value obtained in step 1 to a decimal number. In this example, 30% = .30.

Step 3: Fill in the appropriate values into the formula and determine the resulting value. In this case,

2 units needed/0.30 (decimal version of antigen-negative individuals = 6.66 = screen 7 donor units

When more than one antibody is present, the same formula is used but the incidence of both antibodies is considered.

For example, if both anti-c and anti-E are present, the formula is calculated as:

Step 1: Determine the percentage of antigen-*negative* individuals. In this case, the frequency of the c allele in the general population is 80%, which means that approximately 20% of donor units are *negative* for c.

The frequency of the E allele in the general population is 30%, which means that approximately 70% of donor units are *negative* for E.

Step 2: Convert each value obtained in step 1 to a decimal number. In this example, 20% = .20 (c antigen negative) and 70% = .70 (E antigen negative).

Step 3: Multiply the values (i.e., the incidences of the desired phenotypes) obtained in step 2:

0.2 × 0.7 = 0.14

Step 4: Fill in the appropriate values into the formula and determine the resulting value. In this case, if 4 units of donor blood are needed, the formula is:

4 units needed/0.14 (the value obtained in step 3 above; i.e., the product of the decimal version of antigen-negative individuals)

4/0.14 = 28.6 = Screen 29 donor units

CASE IN POINT *(continued)*

Antigen typing could not be performed on MG because he had been transfused recently at the community hospital. The following antigen frequency chart is used in this laboratory to determine the number of donor units that should be screened:

Antigen Frequency Chart (% values)

D	C	c	E	e	K	k	Fy^a	Fy^b	Jk^a	Jk^b	Le^a	Le^b	P$_1$	M	N	S	s
85	70	80	30	98	10	99	65	80	77	73	22	72	79	78	72	55	89

9. What phenotype is required in the donor units for transfusion to MG?
10. How many donor units should be screened?

While this method works well much of the time for choosing the number of donor units to screen, the formula is based on probabilities and is not exact. Many factors will affect the number of antigen-positive or -negative donor units that are found, such as ethnicities in the donor population and prescreening of donor units.

☑ CHECKPOINT 8-5

What equation can be used to estimate the number of donors that need to be phenotyped to find compatible blood for a patient with an antibody?

OTHER TECHNIQUES USED IN ANTIBODY IDENTIFICATION

Sometimes specialized techniques must be used in the antibody identification process. Five of these important techniques are described in the sectons that follow.

Enzymes

Enzymes are proteins that increase the rate of a chemical reaction. In transfusion medicine, enzymes are used to alter red blood cell antigens. The most commonly used enzymes are ficin and papain. Less commonly used enzymes are bromelin, pronase, trypsin, and chemotrypsin. Some red blood cell antigens are destroyed by enzymes, whereas the reactivity of other antigens is enhanced.[13] Table 8-1 ✳ lists the effect of enzymes on common red blood cell antigen sites.

Antigens that are destroyed by enzymes are likely to reside on the part of the molecule that the enzyme removed from the red blood cell membrane. Theories that explain the enhancement of certain antigens include removal of sialic acid from the red blood cell membrane; this reduces the net negative charge of the red blood cell enhancing agglutination. Removal of part of the molecule on which the red blood cell antigen resides may make the antigen more physically accessible to its corresponding antibody; this is called a reduction in *steric hindrance*. Different enzymes may affect the same antigen in different ways. Table 8-2 ✳ lists the effects of both common and less commonly used enzymes on some red blood cell antigen sites.

✳ **TABLE 8-1** Effect of Ficin or Papain on Red Blood Cell Antigen Sites

Enhanced	Destroyed
D	Fy^a
C	Fy^b
E	M
c	N
e	
C^w	
Jk^a	
Jk^b	
Le^a	
Le^b	
P1	

☑ CHECKPOINT 8-6

What common antigens are destroyed by ficin?

Enzyme-treated red blood cells are generally used in two circumstances. If a weakly reactive antibody is present, enzyme-treated red blood cells may be tested in an effort to enhance the reactivity and possibly clarify the reaction pattern or confirm the presence of the antibody. Second, use of enzyme-treated red blood cells can often help differentiate antibodies when multiple antibodies are present in a sample. If one or more of the identified antibodies is to an antigen that is destroyed by enzyme treatment, testing the plasma against a panel of enzyme-treated red blood cells may reveal additional antibodies that were masked in the testing with untreated red blood cells. Comparing the reaction strength of the same red blood cells when untreated and when enzyme-treated can help differentiate which antibodies are present. Some antibody reactions may disappear, some may get stronger, and others will be unaffected.

Enzyme treatment can be performed in two ways: the one-step technique and the two-step technique.[5] In the one-step technique, enzyme is added as an enhancement medium to the tube containing

✳ **TABLE 8-2** Effect of Various Enzymes on Select Red Blood Cell Antigen Sites

Antigen Site	Enzyme					
	Papain	Bromelin	Ficin	Pronase	Trypsin	Chymotrypsin
S	Weakened	Variable	Weakened	Destroyed		Destroyed
Fy	Destroyed	Destroyed	Destroyed	Destroyed		Destroyed
M/N	Destroyed	Destroyed	Destroyed	Destroyed	Destroyed	
k					Destroyed[1]	
Lu		Unknown[2]		Destroyed	Destroyed	Destroyed

[1] The k antigen is only destroyed when a combination of trypsin and chymotrypsin is used.

[2] No definitive information is available for the effect of bromelin on the Lu antigens.

test plasma and red blood cells. The enzyme is incubated with the test samples and carried through the IAT phase of testing. The two-step technique requires treatment of the red blood cells with enzyme and washing prior to the addition of patient plasma. The two-step method is often preferred because the enzymes in the one-step technique are added directly to the patient's plasma and any antibodies present may be damaged. Also, the pH at which the enzyme reacts is different from the pH at which optimal antigen antibody uptake occurs. Both of these problems are resolved in the two-step method. Commercially prepared enzyme-treated red blood cells are also available and allow the laboratory to proceed directly to the second step of the two-step technique.

Untreated red blood cells must be used in tandem with the enzyme-treated red blood cells to identify all antibodies present in a test sample. Otherwise, antibodies to enzyme-labile antigens will not be detected. Figure 8-5 ■ illustrates how use of enzyme-treated red blood cells can be beneficial when multiple antibodies are present in the same patient specimen.

Neutralization

Neutralization is the inactivation of an antibody by combining it with a soluble form of the corresponding antigen. Some blood group antigens can be found in soluble forms in body fluids such as plasma, urine, and saliva. Table 8-3 ✳ lists sources of soluble blood group antigens. The fluids containing these antigens can be used to neutralize their corresponding antibody in patients' plasma.

Inactivation of the antibody can aid in identification of a suspected antibody that does not react with an ideal pattern. Also, antibodies that react with the majority of panel cells—for example, an anti-P1, an anti-Sd^a, or a combination of anti-Le^a and anti-Le^b—can be neutralized to discover if they were masking the presence of other underlying antibodies.

In a neutralization technique, the appropriate neutralizing fluid is added to an aliquot of the patient's plasma. As a control, another aliquot of patient's plasma is diluted to the same degree with an inert fluid such

Donor	D	C	c	E	e	K	k	Fy^a	Fy^b	Jk^a	Jk^b	Le^a	Le^b	P$_1$	M	N	S	s	Untreated IAT	Enzyme IAT	CC
1	+	+	0	0	+	+	+	0	+	+	+	0	0	0	0	+	0	+	1+	2+	
2	+	+	0	0	+	0	+	0	+	0	+	+	0	0	+	0	+	0	1+	2+	
3	+	+	0	0	+	+	0	0	0	+	0	+	0	+	0	+	0	+	0	0	+/+
4	+	0	+	+	0	+	+	0	+	0	0	0	+	+	0	+	0	0	0	+/+
5	+	0	+	+	0	0	+	0	+	+	0	+	0	+	+	0	0	+	1+	0	/+
6	0	+	+	0	+	0	+	0	+	+	+	+	0	+	+	+	0	+	1+	2+	
7	0	0	+	+	+	0	+	0	+	+	0	0	+	+	+	+	0	+	1+	0	/+
8	0	0	+	0	+	+	+	+	0	+	+	+	0	+	+	0	+	0	1+	2+	
9	0	0	+	0	+	0	+	0	+	+	0	+	0	+	+	0	0	+	1+	2+	
10	0	0	+	0	+	0	+	0	+	+	0	0	+	0	0	+	0	+	1+	0	/+
																Autocontrol			0	0	+/+

0 = no agglutination

\+ = agglutination (with or without strength of reaction noted in front)

■ **FIGURE 8-5** Example Reaction Pattern Using Enzyme Treated Red Blood Cells

Initial exclusion performed on the untreated panel is shown in pink and demonstrates that all clinically significant antibodies are ruled out except anti-Fy^b, anti-Jk^b, and anti-Le^b. Using enzyme treated red blood cells, a clear pattern with increased strength of reaction emerges for anti-Jk^b shown in blue. Fy^b and Le^b are both present on the panel cells that decreased in reactivity after enzyme treatment, shown in green. The Fy^b antigen is enzyme labile and the Le^a antigen is enzyme stable, therefore, we can assume that anti-Fy^b is present in this plasma specimen. Further testing is needed to confirm the anti-Fy^b. In addition, this example demonstrates the necessity of comparing an untreated panel to an enzyme treated panel. The anti-Fy^b would have been missed if only an enzyme treated panel had been tested.

✳ **TABLE 8-3** Sources of Neutralizing Substances

Substance	Corresponding Antibody(ies)	Source
Lewis substance (available commercially)	Anti-Le^a, anti-Le^b	Saliva: Le^a found in a Le^a+ person Le^a and Le^b found in Le^b+ person
P$_1$ substance (available commercially)	Anti-P$_1$	Hydatid cyst fluid, or can be prepared from pigeon egg whites
Sd^a substance	Anti-Sd^a	Urine from an Sd^a+ person
Chido and Rodgers substances	Anti-Ch, anti-Rg	Plasma from a Ch+ or Rg+ person
I substance	Anti-I	Breast milk, amniotic fluid

as saline. Both mixtures are incubated at the temperature where binding of the antibody and its corresponding soluble antigen is optimal. Then each mixture is tested against a panel of red blood cells using an IAT technique. If the suspected antibody was present in the plasma, the neutralized plasma should be negative with the red blood cells that are positive for the corresponding antigen, while the diluted plasma should remain positive. Sometimes an antibody will be only partially neutralized and the strength of reaction will decrease but not become negative. If the diluted plasma shows no reactivity with the antigen-positive red blood cells, then the neutralization is invalid because the negative reactions of the neutralized plasma may be due to dilution rather than neutralization. Figure 8-6 ■ illustrates an example of P$_1$ neutralization.

> ☑ **CHECKPOINT 8-7**
>
> Name at least one antibody that can be neutralized by soluble antigen.

Elution

Samples with a positive DAT may need to be evaluated by using an **elution**. Elution frees antibody that is bound to a red blood cell and can be used for several purposes. The following sections describe the uses, methods, and technical factors associated with an elution.

Uses

There are numerous uses for the elution technique. Identification and brief descriptions of these uses are introduced below.

- An elution can be used to identify one or more antibodies attached to the red blood cell membrane. This is useful in cases of suspected hemolytic disease of the fetus and newborn (HDFN) or hemolytic transfusion reactions. The antibody recovered in a usable form for testing is called an *eluate*. The eluate can be tested against screening cells and panel cells to identify the antibody.

- An elution may concentrate antibody and therefore can be used to prepare antisera or to detect and identify weakly reactive antibodies.

Donor	D	C	c	E	e	K	k	Fy^a	Fy^b	Jk^a	Jk^b	Le^a	Le^b	P$_1$	M	N	S	s	Untreated IAT	Neut IAT	Diluted IAT	CC
1	+	+	0	0	+	+	+	0	+	+	+	0	0	0	0	+	0	+	0	0	0	+/+/+
2	+	+	0	0	+	0	+	0	+	0	+	+	0	0	+	0	+	0	0	0	0	+/+/+
3	+	+	0	0	+	+	0	0	0	+	0	+	0	+	0	+	0	+	2+	0	2+	/+/
4	+	0	+	+	0	0	+	+	0	+	0	0	0	+	+	0	+	0	1+	0	1+	/+/
5	+	0	+	+	0	+	0	+	+	0	+	0	0	+	+	0	0	+	0	0	0	+/+/+
6	0	+	+	0	+	0	+	0	+	+	+	+	0	+	+	+	0	+	0	0	0	+/+/+
7	0	0	+	+	+	0	+	0	+	+	0	0	+	+	+	+	0	+	2+	0	1+	/+/
8	0	0	+	0	+	+	+	+	0	+	+	0	+	+	+	0	+	0	2+	0	2+	/+/
9	0	0	+	0	+	0	+	0	+	0	+	0	+	+	+	+	0	+	1+	0	Wk	/+/
10	0	0	+	0	+	0	+	0	+	+	0	0	+	0	0	+	0	+	0	0	0	+/+/+
																		Autocontrol	0	0	0	+/+/+

0 = agglutination

Wk = weak agglutination (in tube tests agglutination is seen only microscopically)

+ = (with or without strength of reaction noted in front)

■ **FIGURE 8-6** Example of P1 Neutralization

An anti-P1 is suspected in the initial panel because 5 out of 7 P1 positive red blood cells are reacting. All the clinically significant antibodies are ruled out except for anti-Fy^a as shown by the red blood cells highlighted in yellow. The reaction pattern is not clear cut because 2 P1 positive red blood cells are not reacting. In addition, the homozygous K cell is reacting, which raises the possibility of a weaker than usual anti-K that is only reacting with homozygous cells. The plasma that has been incubated with P1 substance shows no reactivity, while the plasma diluted with saline is still reacting with all of the same red blood cells as untreated plasma. This indicates that likely all of the reactions are due to an anti-P1.

- Elution can be used to prepare DAT-negative red blood cells for further testing. If the patient has not been recently transfused, intact red blood cells can be used for antigen typing or the cells can be used in **adsorption** techniques such as a warm autoadsorption. Adsorption methods are used to selectively remove an antibody from plasma by adding red blood cells with the corresponding antigen under conditions that will enhance the antibody–antigen binding. Both phenotyping and autoadsorption are often used in the investigation of autoimmune hemolytic anemias (Chapter 15).
- An elution can be combined with adsorption techniques to remove specific antibody or antibodies. This can help identify antibodies when multiple antibodies are present.
- Adsorption and elution techniques can also be used to detect a weakly reactive antigen, such as a weak ABO subgroup.

☑ CHECKPOINT 8-8

List at least two reasons for performing each of the following: (1) an elution or (2) a combination of adsorption and elution.

Methods

Elution releases bound antibody from the red blood cell antigens by disrupting the structure of the binding site, reversing the forces of attraction that keep the antigen–antibody complexes together or changing the thermodynamics of the antigen–antibody reaction. Many elution methods exist, but no single method is optimal in all situations. The selection of an elution method is based on ease of performance, preparation time, reagent availability, thermal characteristics of the antibody to be removed (if known), and personal preference.

Methods that are best at releasing cold-reactive antibodies or antibodies that have a broad temperature range of reactivity include Lansteiner and Miller heat elution, Weiner's freeze–thaw method, Lui's freeze–thaw method, and sonication. These techniques are useful for removing antibodies from the red blood cells in HDFN due to ABO antibodies. In the heat elution method, the increased temperature results in increased molecular motion, which in turn disrupts the antigen–antibody bond. Similarly, sonication uses ultrasound waves to physically disrupt the antigen–antibody bond. The freeze–thaw methods cause ice crystals to form, resulting in hemolysis of the red blood cells and therefore, release of the antibody.

Elution methods that are better suited for recovering warm-reactive alloantibodies or autoantibodies include use of organic solvents such as ether, xylene, methylene chloride, and chloroform; or acids such as digitonin, citric, or glycine. Organic solvents are not widely used due to their hazardous properties and the regulations imposed on the use of these reagents by federal authorities. Some organic solvents are highly flammable, toxic, or carcinogenic. Organic solvents alter the structure of the antibody molecule or disrupt the red blood cell membrane in order to dissociate the antibody. Acid-based methods are used in some commercial kits. Acid lowers the pH, which reverses the attraction of the antigen–antibody complex. Buffer must be added to the resulting eluate to reestablish a neutral pH. All of these methods result in destruction of red blood cells.

Elution procedures that remove antibody but leave the red blood cells intact include gentle heat, chloroquine, and acid glycine–EDTA methods. The resulting red blood cells can then be used for phenotyping or autoadsorption. Chloroquine may denature antigens in the Rh blood group system; glycine–EDTA denatures Bg, Er[a], and antigens in the Kell blood group system.

Technical Factors

Preparation of a successful eluate can be influenced by several factors[5]:

- Improper technique such as incomplete removal of organic solvents or the wrong pH of the eluate can cause the test red blood cells to hemolyze or stick together.
- Inadequate stroma removal can interfere with the reading of the test.
- Insufficient washing of the sensitized red blood cells before eluting the antibody can cause contamination of the eluate with plasma antibody. To determine whether the washing process was sufficient, the supernatant from the last wash should be tested for antibody activity and show a negative reaction.
- Washed red blood cells should be transferred to a clean test tube before eluting the antibody to avoid detecting any free antibody binding to the glass surface during the wash phase or from the original plasma.
- Bound IgM antibody may dissociate from red blood cells during the wash phase if cells are allowed to sit in the wash solution for prolonged periods of time. An uninterrupted washing process and saline at 39.2° F (4° C) may be used to minimize the loss of bound antibody.
- Eluates prepared in saline can be unstable. Eluates should be tested as soon as possible after preparation. Alternately, eluates may be stored frozen after the addition of albumin. The eluate can also be prepared with media other than saline, such as albumin or antibody-free plasma.

Adsorption

As previously introduced, adsorption is a technique used to remove an antibody or antibodies from plasma. Adsorption is done most often to remove autoantibodies from a patient's specimen in order to see if other antibodies are present in the plasma. Two types of adsorption, described in the following sections, are typically used depending on the situation: autologous adsorption and allogenic adsorption.

Autologous Adsorption

Autologous adsorption is the preferred method to remove autoantibodies. However, patient history is vital when determining which method to employ. Autologous adsorption cannot be used if the patient has been transfused within the previous 3 months because the patient's specimen will also contain donor red blood cells. Even a small amount of donor red blood cells can result in the unintentional removal of significant alloantibodies. In addition, if the patient is severely anemic, the sample may not contain enough red blood cells to perform the autoadsorption.

CASE IN POINT (continued)

Patient MG had a positive DAT that was not yet resolved. The laboratorian performed an acid elution on the patient's red blood cells using a commercial kit. The resulting eluate was initially tested against a three-cell antibody screen, A₁ cells and B cells. The results are as follows:

Donor	D	C	c	E	e	K	k	Fyᵃ	Fyᵇ	Jkᵃ	Jkᵇ	Leᵃ	Leᵇ	P₁	M	N	S	s	IS	IAT	CC
I	+	+	0	0	+	+	+	0	+	+	0	+	0	0	+	0	+	+	0	3+	
II	+	0	+	+	0	0	+	0	+	0	+	0	+	0	0	+	0	+	0	0	+
III	0	0	+	0	+	0	+	+	0	+	+	0	+	+	+	0	+	0	0	0	+
A₁																			0	0	+
B																			0	0	+

0, no agglutination; +, agglutination (with or without strength of reaction noted in front).

The laboratorian subsequently tested the eluate against a panel of cells:

Donor	D	C	c	E	e	K	k	Fyᵃ	Fyᵇ	Jkᵃ	Jkᵇ	Leᵃ	Leᵇ	P₁	M	N	S	s	IS	IAT	CC
1	+	+	0	+	+	+	+	+	0	+	0	0	+	+	0	+	0	+	0	3+	
2	+	+	0	0	+	0	+	+	0	0	+	+	0	+	+	0	+	+	0	3+	
3	+	0	+	+	0	0	+	0	+	+	0	0	+	0	+	+	+	0	0	0	+
4	+	0	+	0	+	0	+	+	0	+	+	0	+	+	+	+	0	0	0	0	+
5	0	+	+	0	+	0	+	+	0	+	0	+	0	+	+	+	+	+	0	3+	
6	0	0	+	+	+	0	+	+	+	+	0	0	+	+	+	+	+	+	0	0	+
7	0	0	+	0	+	+	+	0	+	0	+	0	+	+	+	+	+	+	0	0	+
8	0	0	+	0	+	0	+	+	0	0	+	0	+	+	+	+	+	+	0	0	+
9	0	0	+	0	+	0	+	+	0	0	+	+	0	0	+	0	0	+	0	0	+

11. What is the probable cause of the reactions obtained in the eluate?

Autologous adsorption consists of treating the patient's own red blood cells with proteolytic enzymes or ZZAP, which is a mixture of thiol and protease, to elute the bound autoantibodies off of the red blood cells. Next, the washed, treated red blood cells are incubated with the patient's plasma at the temperature that appears optimal for the autoantibody. The free autoantibodies in the plasma will bind to the antigen sites on the red blood cells, leaving any alloantibodies in the plasma. Several adsorptions may be necessary to remove all the autoantibodies. Once all autoantibodies are adsorbed, as demonstrated by a negative autocontrol using the adsorbed plasma, the adsorbed plasma can then be tested by routine antibody detection and identification methods.

Allogenic Adsorption

Allogenic adsorption may be used when a patient with an autoantibody has been transfused. If the patient's phenotype is known, red blood cells with a similar phenotype may be used for the allogenic adsorption. More commonly the patient's phenotype is not known; separate aliquots of plasma are adsorbed with several group O red blood cells that have different phenotypes. Allogenic adsorption is also used either alone or paired with elution techniques to separate mixtures of antibodies to allow for identification.

When choosing red blood cells for adsorption, the antigens that stimulate the most clinically significant antibodies are considered, for example, C, E, c, e, K, Fyᵃ, Fyᵇ, Jkᵃ, Jkᵇ, S, and s. Donor red blood cells are treated with ZZAP or enzymes prior to testing or a potentiator, such as polyethylene glycol, is used to increase antibody uptake. If treated red blood cells are used, some of the antigens will be destroyed and the phenotype of the cells for these antigens does not need to be considered. After adsorption, each aliquot of adsorbed plasma is tested against antibody screen and if necessary, panel red blood cells.

This procedure requires a great deal of technical expertise because donor red blood cells adsorb both autoantibodies and alloantibodies. Result interpretation must take into account the phenotype of the adsorbing cells, the reaction of each aliquot of adsorbed plasma to the screen or panel cell, and the phenotype of the screen or panel red blood cell. Figure 8-7 ▇ illustrates an example of an allogenic adsorption.

As well as requiring a high degree of technical expertise to interpret the results, allogenic adsorptions run the risk of not detecting a clinically significant antibody if a weakly reactive alloantibody is diluted or an antibody to a high-frequency antigen is adsorbed. Autoantibodies that are only partially absorbed may mimic the reaction pattern of alloantibodies.

plasma being incubated at a lower temperature. Sometimes when dealing with cold-reactive autoantibodies, the autoantibodies may be stripped off the red blood cells simply by washing with warm saline.

Alternately, *rabbit erythrocyte stroma* can be used to adsorb certain antibodies. The rabbit erythrocytes contain antigen sites similar to those of I, H, and IH and therefore remove cold autoantibodies, which often have these specificities.[14] Furthermore, rabbit erythrocyte stroma removes anti-B and antibodies in the P blood group system (anti-P_1). Plasma adsorbed by this method should not be used for ABO typing. Rabbit erythrocyte stroma will also decrease the strength of or completely remove other IgM antibodies from plasma, including clinically significant antibodies.[15] However, rabbit erythrocyte stroma remains the adsorption medium of choice when an autoadsorption cannot be performed because a patient with a cold autoantibody has been recently transfused.

Rabbit erythrocyte stroma is available in commercial kits. Patient plasma and stroma are incubated together at 39.2° F (4° C). The absorbed plasma is then tested using a routine IAT technique to detect any alloantibodies that are still present in the plasma.

☑ CHECKPOINT 8-9

What chemicals may be used to treat cells used in adsorptions?

☑ CHECKPOINT 8-10

What common antibodies are removed by adsorption with rabbit erythrocyte stroma?

Rabbit Erythrocyte Stroma

Cold autoantibodies often have to be removed to ensure they are not masking the reactions of more clinically significant antibodies. If the patient has not been recently transfused, an autoadsorption can be performed with enzyme- or ZZAP-treated patient cells and

Titration

Titration is a technique used to measure the strength (concentration) of an antibody. Serial dilutions are made of the antibody containing plasma and tested against selected red blood cells to determine

Phenotype of adsorbing cells	Antibodies potentially removed from the plasma	Antibodies, if present, left in the plasma
R1R1 Jk(a-b+)	Autoantibody + alloanti- D, C, e, Jk^b	Anti-c, E, Jk^a, K, S, s, Fy^a, Fy^b
R2R2 Jk(ab)	Autoantibody alloanti- D, E, c, Jk^a	Anti-e, C, Jk^b, K, S, s, Fy^a, Fy^b
rr Jk(a-b+)	Autoantibody + alloanti- c, e, Jk^b	Anti-D, C, E, Jk^a, K, S, s, Fy^a, Fy^b

Each aliquot of plasma was tested against screening cells using a gel technique. Cells used to rule out antibodies using the plasma adsorbed with the R1R1 Jk^a negative cells are highlighted in yellow. Cells used to rule out antibodies using the plasma adsorbed with the R2R2 Jk^b negative cells are highlighted in pink. The anti-D is ruled out using the plasma adsorbed with the rr Jk^a negative cell, highlighted in green. The most likely antibody present in addition to the autoantibody is anti-Jk^a. This would need to be confirmed by testing the adsorbed plasmas with more red blood cells.

Donor	D	C	c	E	e	K	k	Fy^a	Fy^b	Jka	Jk^b	Le^a	Le^b	P$_1$	M	N	S	s	R1R1	R2R2	rr
I	+	+	0	0	+	+	+	0	+	+	0	+	0	0	+	0	+	+	2+	0	2+
II	+	0	+	+	0	0	+	0	+	0	+	0	+	0	0	+	0	+	0	0	0
III	0	0	+	0	+	0	+	+	0	+	+	0	+	+	+	0	+	0	2+	0	2+

(IAT results using plasma adsorbed with: R1R1, R2R2, rr)

0 = no agglutination

+ = agglutination (with or without strength of reaction noted in front)

▇ **FIGURE 8-7** Example of Allogenic Adsorption

ZZAP treated group O donor red blood cells were used for allogenic adsorption. ZZAP destroys K, Fy^a, Fy^b, S, and s antigens. Therefore only C, E, c, e, Jk^a, and Jk^b antigens were considered when choosing the adsorbing cells.

Antibody Sample	Dilution:	1:1	1:2	1:4	1:8	1:16	1:32	1:64	1:128	1:256	1:512	1:1024	Titer	Score
1	Strength	4+	4+	4+	3+	2+	1+	1+	+/−	+/−w	0	0	64	
	Score	12	12	12	10	8	5	5	3	2	0	0		69
2	Strength	3+	2+	2+	1+	1+	1+	1+	+/−	+/−w	0	0	64	
	Score	10	8	8	5	5	5	5	3	2	0	0		51
3	Strength	1+	1+	1+	1+	1+	1+	1+	1+	1+	+/−	0	256	
	Score	5	5	5	5	5	5	5	5	5	3	0		48

0 = no agglutination

+/− = weak macroscopic reaction

+/−w = no agglutination seen macroscopically, agglutination visible microscopically

+ = agglutination (with or without strength of reaction noted in front)

Sample 1 and 2 both have a titer of 64 but sample 1 has a stronger avidity than sample 2.

Sample 3 has a higher titer than sample 1 and 2 but a lower avidity.

FIGURE 8-8   Titration Results of Antibodies with Different Titers and Avidities

the highest dilution causing a positive reaction. The result or titer is expressed as the reciprocal of the highest plasma dilution reacting at 1+. For example, if the highest dilution showing a 1+ reaction is 1:64, the titer is 64.

Titers can also be resulted as a score, where a number is assigned to each positive reaction in the titration based on the strength of the reaction. A 4+ reaction is assigned a score of 12, 3+ a score of 10, 2+ a score of 8, 1+ a score of 5, +/− a score of 3, and a weak +/− a score of 2. The sum of these scores reflect the total binding strength of antigen and antibody molecules, a concept known as the **titration score** or **avidity**. This can be useful for comparing how an antibody reacts to different red blood cells or comparing how different antibodies react to the same red blood cell. Two antibodies can have the same titer but different titration scores, demonstrating the same strength but differing avidity, as determined after performing the calculations described earlier. Figure 8-8 ▪ illustrates titration results.

Titration is most commonly used for determining antibody activity and the potential severity of HDFN in alloimmunized pregnant women (Chapter 14).

Titration can also be a useful aid in identifying antibodies to certain high-incidence antigens, such as Kn[a], McC[a], Ch, Rg, Cs[a], Yk[a], and JMH. These antibodies typically show a weak, variable reaction pattern but the antibody has a high titer. These antibodies were formerly called high-titer, low-avidity antibodies (HTLA). A titration can distinguish between a characteristic high-titer, low-avidity antibody and a weakly reactive antibody with a low titer.

Reliable results from titration are technique dependant and care must be taken to perform the titration with consistency. Uniform pipetting for each dilution is important. Pipette tips should be changed with each dilution. If possible, fresh red blood cells should be used for testing and the cell suspension should be the same for each tube and each titration if comparing titers. Incubation time and temperature and centrifugation time and speed should be consistent.

☑ **CHECKPOINT 8-11**

How is a titration performed?

SPECIAL PROBLEMS IN ANTIBODY IDENTIFICATION

Unfortunately, there are times when special problems are encountered during antibody identification testing. The next sections identify and describe a plethora of such problems that may be encountered. Suggested resolution steps are included as appropriate.

All or Most Cells Reacting

Samples where all or most screen and panel red blood cells are reacting positive present a difficult challenge. If all cells are reacting, no antibodies can be excluded.

If the autocontrol or DAT is negative and the patient has been transfused or is pregnant, then the reactions are likely due to alloantibodies. Both combinations of multiple antibodies and a single antibody to a high-incidence antigen may cause this pattern of reactivity. If the autocontrol or DAT is positive and the patient has not been transfused recently, then the results are likely due to an autoantibody, either warm-reactive, cold-reactive, or both. If the autocontrol or DAT is positive and the patient has been transfused recently, the results may indicate either an autoantibody or a delayed serological transfusion reaction. False-positive panreactivity may occur with rouleaux or antibodies to reagents.

Multiple Antibodies

Many combinations of antibodies are easily identified based on the exclusion process. However, certain combinations of antibodies may cause all or most cells tested to react positively, making antibody exclusion and subsequent identification very difficult.

A combination of techniques is usually required to identify the specificity of each antibody present within a complex mixture of them. The technique(s) that should be used in such cases depend(s) on which antibodies are suspected. Tasks that assist in identifying appropriate additional techniques include:

- Assess the patient history for previous testing results, previous transfusions, and previous pregnancies.
- Assess any variation in strengths of reaction.

- Test the plasma using different methods. If using a tube method, utilize different enhancement medium and/or incubation temperature.

- If possible, phenotype the patient to identify which alloantibodies the patient could develop. Phenotype results can also be used to exclude alloantibodies.

- Test the plasma using enzyme-treated cells. Less commonly, cells may be treated with other reagents such as chloroquine, acids, or sulfhydryl agents. Each reagent will affect different antigens. The most common sulfhydryl reagent used in transfusion medicine is dithiothreitol (DTT).

- Test the plasma with cord cells, as completion of this task may provide clues to an antibody's identity because some antigens are well developed at birth and others are not.

- Allogenic adsorption followed by elution can sometimes separate antibodies between the plasma and the eluate. Adsorption/elution studies can also help identify antibodies that mimic antibody combinations, such as anti-G (Chapter 8).

- Dilution or titration may help separate specificities that have different titers. Some antibodies show a characteristic pattern upon dilution. For example, a strong autoanti-I may react with adult and cord cells equally when undiluted, but when diluted may show the characteristic weaker reactions with cord cells.

- DTT can be used to treat plasma as well as cells. DTT will weaken or destroy IgM antibodies in plasma, but not IgG antibodies.

Antibodies to High-Incidence Antigens

The typical reaction pattern when a patient has developed an antibody to a high-incidence antigen is a negative autocontrol or DAT, but all (or nearly all) screen, panel, and donor red blood cells reacting positive. Testing with rare selected cells that lack the antigen is the best way to confirm the specificity of the antibody. If rare cells are not available, testing the patient's plasma against treated cells may provide clues to the antibody's identity. As well, knowing the patient's ethnicity can be helpful.

Warm Autoantibodies

Warm autoantibodies may cause a condition known as *autoimmune hemolytic anemia* (Chapter 15). A **warm autoantibody** reacts with the patient's own red blood cells at body temperature. The typical pattern of reactivity is a positive autocontrol and DAT and all screen, panel, and donor red blood cells reacting positive. When an antibody causes all cells tested to agglutinate, this is called **panagglutination**. Therefore, a warm autoantibody is sometimes called a **panagglutinin**. Often the patient has not been recently transfused. If an eluate is prepared, it generally reacts with all cells tested. Occasionally, an autoantibody will show specificity to one antigen.

The most important issue when identifying an autoantibody is determining whether underlying alloantibodies are present. Patients with warm autoantibodies appear to have an increased sensitivity to alloimmunization as compared to other patient populations. Studies show that 12–40% of patients with warm autoantibodies also have underlying alloantibodies.[5, 16, 17]

If the patient has not been transfused in the last 3 months, an autoadsorption can be performed and the adsorbed plasma tested for alloantibodies. Any red blood cell donor units chosen for transfusion must be antigen negative for any corresponding, clinically significant alloantibody that is present. As well, the patient's cells can be phenotyped for antigens of clinical significance. The cells may have to be treated to remove antibody prior to phenotyping if the antiserum requires an IAT phase. If transfusion is required, many laboratories will provide phenotypically matched red blood cell donor units.

If the patient has been transfused, allogenic adsorptions may be used to identify any underlying alloantibodies. However, if phenotypically matched red blood cell donor units are available, allogenic adsorption may not be necessary.

☑ CHECKPOINT 8-12

What is panagglutination?

Cold Agglutinins

Cold agglutinins are those antibodies that optimally react at temperatures between 39.2° F (4° C) and 77° F (25° C) and can be autoantibodies or alloantibodies. They are differentiated by running an autocontrol or DAT. Since body temperature is closer to 98.6° F (37° C), these antibodies rarely cause destruction of transfused red blood cells. These antibodies do create problems in the laboratory because they interfere with ABO typing and can mask the reactions of more clinically significant antibodies.[18] The next sections describe cold autoantibodies, cold alloantibodies, a technique designed to detect clinically significant antibodies in the presence of cold agglutinins, and concerns and possible resolutions of cold agglutinins appearing during cardiac surgery.

Cold Autoantibodies

Cold agglutinin syndrome, which is also called *cold hemagglutinin disease* or *cold autoimmune hemolytic anemia*, can occur when cold autoantibodies react at body temperature (Chapter 15). Cold autoantibodies include the specificities to I, i, I^T, IH, and Pr antigens; autoanti-I is the most common. Although the autoantibodies can be distinguished using cord and adult red blood cells, identification is generally not necessary. Antibody titer and thermal amplitude are considered good indicators of clinical significance for cold-reacting autoantibodies. Thermal amplitude and titer are performed by serially diluting the patient's serum or plasma and testing the titers at different temperatures, such as 39.2° F (4° C), room temperature, 86° F (30° C), and 98.6° F (37° C). If cold autoantibodies may be masking alloantibodies, the autoantibodies can be removed from plasma by autoadsorption using a low temperature or by adsorption with rabbit erythrocyte stroma.

Cold Alloantibodies

Cold alloantibodies include specificities such as anti-M, anti-N, anti-P1, anti-P, anti-P^k, anti-Le^a, anti-Le^b, and anti-Lu^a. These antibodies rarely cause *in vivo* hemolysis, especially when reactions occur below body temperature.[18] Three simple techniques for avoiding detection of cold alloantibody when using a tube method are eliminating the immediate spin reading, eliminating microscopic readings, and testing with anti-IgG instead of polyspecific antihuman globulin.

Prewarm Technique

Prewarming is another technique that has been used to detect the presence of clinically significant antibodies in the presence of cold reacting antibodies. Plasma and cells are warmed separately at 98.6° F (37° C) prior to testing in an attempt to avoid binding of cold antibodies. As well, if performing a tube technique, warm saline may be used for the wash step in the IAT. The prewarm technique is controversial in antibody detection because research shows warming the plasma causes a decrease in the reactivity of 40–47% of clinically significant antibodies.[19] Therefore, the prewarm technique should ideally not be used until antibody specificity has been identified. Prewarm is also used to resolve ABO discrepancies due to cold antibodies (Chapter 4).

Cold Agglutinin Concerns and Resolutions During Cardiac Surgery

Cold agglutinins have been a concern during cardiac surgery because patients are routinely placed into a systemic hypothermia.[20] A few reports exist of cold antibodies causing problems during surgery and, for those that did, the problems resolved when the patient was warmed. If cold agglutinins are a concern for surgery, thermal amplitude and titer are good predictors of potential complications. If problems are expected or encountered, the blood or the patient's body temperature may be kept above the temperature at which the cold antibody reacts or a plasma exchange to remove the cold agglutinins may be performed prior to surgery.

Delayed Hemolytic or Serologic Transfusion Reaction

A delayed hemolytic or serologic transfusion reaction (Chapter 12) caused by multiple alloantibodies may show the same pattern of reactivity as a warm autoantibody. With a delayed hemolytic reaction the patient exhibits symptoms of hemolysis, whereas in a delayed serologic reaction the DAT becomes positive but the patient does not exhibit symptoms of hemolysis.

Several studies suggest that blood transfusion induces the formation of autoantibodies without the development of *autoimmune hemolytic anemia*. One study showed nearly 5% of patients studied formed a warm or cold autoantibody following transfusion and 34% of patients studied formed a positive DAT with subsequent formation of alloantibodies.[21] Patients with an autoantibody developed a positive DAT and panagglutinin in the eluate following transfusion of compatible blood. The DAT can remain positive for up to 300 days, which is well after the donor red blood cells have been cleared from the system. The cause of this phenomenon has been associated with an isoimmune reaction stimulated by transfusion that causes a temporary, false autoimmunity. However, further research is necessary to definitively state the cause and effect.

Rouleaux

Rouleaux is caused by unusual properties in a patient's plasma that can aggregate red blood cells and mimic agglutination. This pseudo-agglutination is not due to antibodies but to a change in the surface charge on the red blood cell. This can occur as a result of various intravenous injections or an abnormal concentration of serum proteins due to the patient's clinical condition. The intravenous solutions include high-molecular-weight dextran, polyvinylpyrrolidone (PVP), hydroxyethylstarch (HES), or fibrinogen. Abnormal protein concentrations in the plasma may be seen in disease states such as multiple myeloma, Waldenstrom's macroglobulinemia, cirrhosis, or hyperviscosity syndrome.

Rouleaux formation most commonly interferes with any test combining red blood cells with patient plasma. The IAT is not usually affected because the plasma is washed away, if using a tube methodology. ABO typing and the immediate spin phase of the antibody screen and/or crossmatch are places where rouleaux may cause interference.

Microscopically, rouleaux formation characteristically appears as refractile, shiny clumps that resemble a "stack of coins." Figure 8-9 illustrates the difference between rouleaux and agglutination. Occasionally, in strong rouleaux formation, the characteristic stacks are not as obvious and can be confused with true agglutination. It is necessary to differentiate rouleaux from true agglutination in the antibody screen and crossmatch to determine the presence of any underlying antibodies of clinical significance. This can be done by performing a saline replacement procedure (Chapter 4).

☑ CHECKPOINT 8-13

How is rouleaux commonly described?

Antibodies to Reagents

Just as patients make antibodies to blood group antigens, they can make antibodies to drugs or chemicals. Occasionally laboratories will run across antibodies directed toward a drug or chemical present in the reagents used to test the specimen.[22] Table 8-4 ✳ lists examples of substances commonly found in reagents. Initially, the reaction pattern mimics that of an antibody directed toward a high-frequency antigen. However, the crossmatch with donor red blood cells will be negative. Differences in reactivity may appear if cells from different manufacturers are tested.

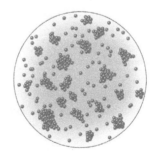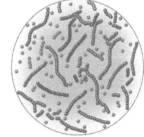

Agglutination:
• Irregularly shaped clumps
• Difficult to detect red cell borders

Rouleaux:
• Orderly rows
• Distinct borders
• Resembles a fallen stack of coins

■ **FIGURE 8-9**   Agglutination versus Rouleaux
Source: Lisa Denesuik.

★ **TABLE 8-4** Common Reagent Chemicals that Have Induced an Antibody Response

Type of Chemical	Name of Chemical	Resolution
Antibiotics	Neomycin Chloramphenicol Gentamycin	Wash reagent red blood cells prior to testing
Sugars	Glucose	Inhibit by adding glucose to test medium
Dyes	Acriflavine Yellow #5 tartrazine	Wash patient red blood cells to remove patient plasma prior to testing
Bacteriostatic/ antifungal reagents	Paraben® Thimerosal Sodium azide	Wash patient red blood cells to remove patient plasma prior to testing
Miscellaneous	EDTA Citrate Inosine	Wash reagent red blood cells prior to testing

Neomycin, chloramphenicol, and gentamycin are used in reagent red blood cell suspensions. EDTA and citrate are used by some manufacturers in reagent A and B red blood cell suspensions. EDTA can interfere with blood typing if the patient has antibodies that react with polycarboxyl groups. Conversely, citrate inhibits some reactions when present. Inosine is also used in reagent red blood cell suspensions. Interference by any of these chemicals can be remedied if the reagent red blood cells are washed prior to testing.

Sugars such as glucose are used in red blood cell suspending mediums. Antibodies to sugars appear to bind to the red blood cell membrane in a fashion similar to penicillin. Washing the reagent cells will not eliminate the reaction. However, the reaction will be inhibited if the sugar in question is added to the patient's plasma.

Dyes and bacteriostatic/antifungal reagents are used in antisera. Reactions encountered when a patient has antibodies to the reagents used in antisera can be eliminated if the patient cells are washed prior to testing. This removes the patient plasma that contains the antibodies.

Antibodies to Human Leukocyte Antigens

Antibodies directed toward human lymphocyte antigens (HLA) are generally considered clinically insignificant with regard to red blood cell transfusion (Chapter 18). They have been associated with febrile, nonhemolytic transfusion reactions and can cause platelet refractoriness[23] (Chapter 16). However, there have been reports that indicate antibodies to HLA may be responsible for a decreased survival rate of some transfused red blood cells.[24, 25] Antibodies to HLA can interfere with detection and identification of clinically significant antibodies.

HLA molecules are expressed on immature red blood cells that contain nuclei but often disappear as the erythrocytes mature. Occasionally, HLA persist on mature red blood cells. Three specificities have been termed Bennet-Goodspeed (Bg) antigens. Bg^a, Bg^b, and Bg^c correspond to HLA-B7, HLA-B17, and HLA-A28/A2 respectively.

Antibodies to HLA are not easy to identify in pretransfusion testing for a number of reasons. First, the corresponding antigens show variable expression on red blood cells. This results in varying reaction strengths during testing. Second, antigen sites decrease in expression during storage. As a result, antibody reactivity appears inconsistent over time. Third, antibodies to HLA are often multispecific and are not directed toward a single HLA site. Fourth, few commercially prepared panel cells are tested for specific HLA epitopes.

Antibodies to HLA can be adsorbed using pooled human platelets. Adsorption can confirm that the nonspecific reactions were due to a HLA antibody and can allow identification of clinically significant antibodies, which may have been masked by the HLA antibody reactivity. Crossmatch-compatible blood should be given when antibodies to HLA are reactive in pretransfusion testing.

Antibodies to Low-Incidence Antigens

An antibody to a low-incidence antigen may occur alone or in combination with other alloantibodies. Specificities include Wr^a, Kp^a, Js^a, C^w, Di^a, Go^a, SC2, Mi^a, Lu^a, Co^b, and Yt^b. Typical patterns of reactivity include the following:

- The antibody screen is negative but one donor unit is incompatible if an IAT crossmatch is performed.
- There is a cell reacting on the panel that is not explained by the antibody or antibodies identified.
- The patient appears to have experienced a delayed hemolytic or serologic transfusion reaction but the antibody screen is negative.

An antibody to a low-incidence antigen may not be detected in the antibody screen because the screening red blood cells are all negative for the corresponding antigen. If a patient has a history of an antibody to a low-incidence antigen, donor units should be tested by an IAT crossmatch, even if the antibody screen is negative. If available, a panel cell that is positive for the corresponding antigen can be run to determine if the antibody is reacting or to confirm the identity of the antibody.

Incompatible Crossmatch with Undetermined Cause

Occasionally, a crossmatch is positive or incompatible when donor units are negative for the antigens that correspond to the antibodies identified in the patient plasma. Crossmatch incompatibility may also be seen when the patient's antibody screen is negative. The primary causes for this include:

- The antibody may be A or B in origin. Screening cells are group O, so anti-A and anti-B antibodies will not react in the screen.
- The donor red blood cells may contain a low-frequency antigen that was not present on antibody screening or identification cells.
- Antibody detection red blood cells may lack antigens such as f(ce) that the red blood cells used in the crossmatch possess. Often, f antigen positivity is presumed based on the Rh phenotype of the cells (Chapter 5).
- Donor red blood cells may be fresher than reagent red blood cells. Therefore, labile antigens on the donor cells may be stronger than those on the stored, reagent red blood cells. This occurrence should be rare if using manufactured reagent red blood cells because manufacturers must meet specific regulations.
- Rarely, donor cells may have a positive DAT or may react with all sera, a concept known as **polyagglutinable**.

- The donor red blood cells may have homozygous expression of antigens that are heterozygous on the antibody screen cells. Antibodies can be missed if screening cells exhibit heterozygous expressions of antigens or if heterozygous cells are used for exclusion and the antibody is showing dosage.

Mixed-Field Agglutination

Samples that contain two separate populations of red blood cells may demonstrate mixed-field agglutination in testing. When using a tube methodology, mixed-field agglutination characteristically appears as a few tight clumps of red blood cells in a field of unagglutinated cells microscopically or macroscopically as large clumps (2–4+) of red blood cells in a cloudy background. Figures 8-10 ▦

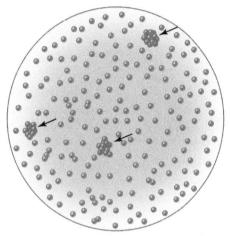

Rare clump of red blood cells (arrows) against a background of free cells.

▦ **FIGURE 8-10**   Weak Mixed-Field Agglutination Viewed Microscopically
Source: Lisa Denesuik.

and 8-11 ▦ illustrate mixed-field agglutination in tube tests. When the tube is initially rocked, a stream of unagglutinated cells or "tail" can be seen coming off the cell button if there is mixed-field agglutination. If using the gel testing system, mixed-field agglutination is seen as agglutinated cells on top of the gel and unagglutinated cells at the bottom of the tube. Figure 8-12 ▦ illustrates mixed-field agglutination in a gel test.

Mixed-field agglutination is usually seen in the ABO or Rh(D) typing (Chapters 4 and 5). During antibody identification, it may be seen in the DAT if the positive DAT is due to a delayed hemolytic or serologic transfusion reaction (Chapter 12). If antigen phenotyping is performed on a specimen where the patient has been recently transfused, mixed-field agglutination can be seen in the tests where the patient and donor are phenotypically different. And lastly, mixed-field agglutination can occasionally be seen in the antibody screen. Anti-Sd^a and anti-Lu^a characteristically produce a mixed-field agglutination reaction.

Polyagglutination

Polyagglutination refers to a state in which the surface membrane of a person's red blood cells is altered in a way that exposes carbohydrates that are not normally seen.[26] The result is that affected patient red blood cells react with all adult plasma except that of self.

Figure 8-13 ▦ illustrates the chemical structure of **cryptic autoantigens** (a concept also known as and in many cases formerly known as *cryptantigens*). Antibodies to these cryptic autoantigens are naturally formed in adult plasma in response to environmental exposures similar to the formation of ABO antibodies (Chapter 4).

Cell buttons in bottom of test tubes

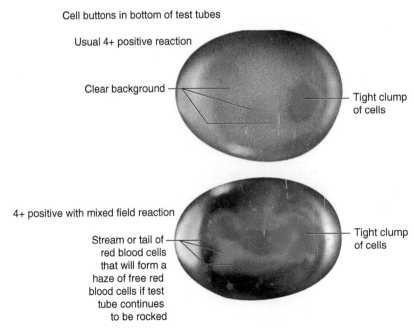

Usual 4+ positive reaction

Clear background

Tight clump of cells

4+ positive with mixed field reaction

Stream or tail of red blood cells that will form a haze of free red blood cells if test tube continues to be rocked

Tight clump of cells

▦ **FIGURE 8-11**   Macroscopic Mixed-Field Agglutination
Source: Stephanie Codina.

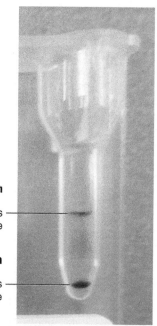

After centrifugation

Agglutinated red blood cells
remain at the top of the microtube

After centrifugation

Unagglutinated red blood cells
are at the bottom of the microtube

■ **FIGURE 8-12**   Mixed-Field Agglutination in Gel

© Ortho Clinical Diagnostics Inc. 2010

Source: Lisa Denesuik.

☑ CHECKPOINT 8-14

What is polyagglutination?

Polyagglutinable red blood cells react or agglutinate when tested against normal adult plasma or serum. Conversely, agglutination is not seen when the cells are tested against cord sera from infants less than 2 months of age or the person's own plasma or serum. Consequently, polyagglutinable cells have a negative reaction in an autocontrol, but polyagglutinable donor red blood cells have a positive reaction if used in a serologic crossmatch and polyagglutinable donor or recipient cells have a positive reaction if antigen-typed with a human source antiserum. As most antisera in use today are clonal rather than human source, polyagglutinable cells are often undetected in routine testing.

Polyagglutinable red blood cells may be the cause of an unexplained hemolytic transfusion reaction (Chapter 12). If the recipient's cells are polyagglutinable, hemolysis may occur when blood products that contain plasma are transfused. Even in the patient population where this causes the most concern, which is infants with necrotizing entercolitis, hemolysis attributed to the polyagglutination is an unusual event.[27] A minor crossmatch, which consists of the donor plasma tested against the recipient's red blood cells, can help identify this rare transfusion reaction. Even more uncommon would be a reaction caused by polyagglutinating donor cells issued via electronic crossmatch (Chapter 7).

Plant lectins can be used to differentiate the types of polyagglutination.[28] Lectins are prepared from extracts of seeds that have been found to react with specific carbohydrates on red blood cell membranes. These extracts can be made from the seeds by the blood bank or transfusion service laboratory or can be purchased commercially ready to use from a manufacturer. In the proper dilutions, the extracts have highly specific reaction patterns and may be used to delineate the identity of the antigen on a patient's polyagglutinating red blood cells. Polyagglutination results from an acquired or inherited abnormality of the RBC membrane, resulting in the exposure of "cryptic autoantigens." These autoantigens are normally hidden and all adult human sera contain antibodies to the cryptic antigens. Some of the cryptic autoantigens include T, Tn, Tk, Th, and Tx and therefore polyagglutination is sometimes referred to as "T activation." Lectins are used for other purposes in transfusion medicine; for example, Dolichos biflorus extract can also be used to differentiate A_1 cells from A_2 cells. Table 8-5 ✳ lists the reaction patterns of polyagglutinable red blood cells with lectins.

The following sections describe three categories of polyagglutination worthy of discussion in this chapter: those acquired passively via cryptic autoantigen activation, a category known as VA (which refers to Virginia, the state where the first known case occurred), and polyagglutination of the inherited variety.

Passively Acquired Cryptic Autoantigen Activation

Polyagglutination can be passively acquired or inherited.[28] The acquired form occurs when a carbohydrate that is usually hidden is exposed. Acquired polyagglutination has been associated with microbial infection, myeloproliferative disorders, and myelodysplasia. Acquired polyagglutination is a transient condition that resolves within weeks or months. Known instances of polyagglutination associated with microbial infection include:

- T activation occurs when a patient is exposed to bacteria that produce neuraminidase.[29] Neuraminidase removes sialic acid (neuraminic acid) from the red blood cell membrane and exposes the normally hidden T antigens. The two most common organisms associated with T activation are *Clostridium perfringens* and *Streptococcus pneumoniae*. However, species of *Bacteroides*, species of *Actinomyces*, influenza viruses, and several other microorganisms have been associated with T activation. T activation is most commonly seen in infants with necrotizing enterocolitis and children with serious pneumococcal infections. The clinical significance of T activation has been debated, but no clear relationship between anti-T and hemolysis has been determined.

- Th activation is likely a mild form of T activation in which bacterial neuraminidase cleaves off a lesser amount of the sialic acid exposing Th receptors instead of T receptors. Th activation has been associated with *Corynebacterium aquaticum*.

- Tk activation occurs when bacterial endo-β-galactosidases cleave galactose from the red blood cell membrane, exposing the Tk receptor. The bacterial strains *Bacteroides fragilis*, *Escherichia freundii*, and *Flavobacterium keratolyticus* have been associated with Tk activation.

- Tx activation occurs when pneumococcal enzymes expose the Tx sites on red blood cells.

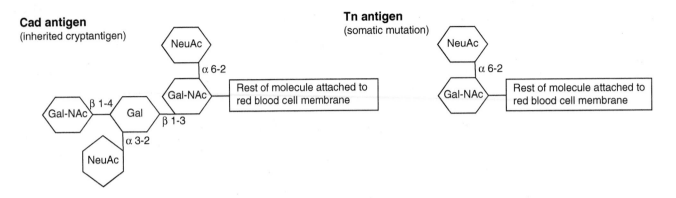

Cad antigen
(inherited cryptantigen)

Tn antigen
(somatic mutation)

T antigen
(acquired)

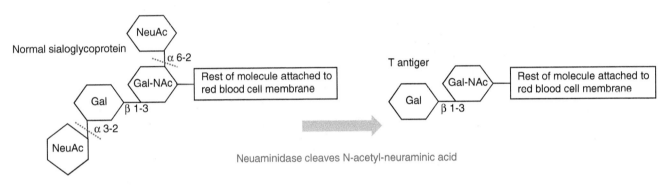

Neuaminidase cleaves N-acetyl-neuraminic acid

Tk antigen
(acquired)

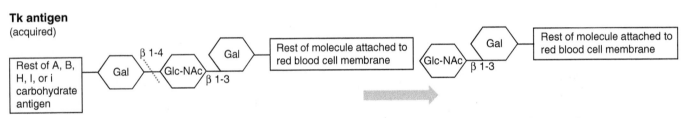

Endo and/or exo β-galactosidases produced by bacteria cleave the antigens exposing the crypantigen

Legend:
Gal = galactose
NeuAc = N-acetyl-neuraminic acid (sialic acid)
Glc-NAC = N-acetylglucosamine
Gal-NAc = N-acetylgalactosamine

FIGURE 8-13   Structure of Cryptic Autoantigens

✱ TABLE 8-5 Reaction Patterns of Polyagglutinable Red Blood Cells Tested with Lectins

Lectin Name	Cryptic Autoantigens Resulting in Polyagglutinable Red Blood Cells										
	T	Tn	Tk	Th	Tx	Cad	NOR	MHP	VA	HEMPAS	Tr
Gl. Max	+	+	0	0	0	+	0	+	0	+	+
Gr. simplicifolia I	0	+	0	0	0	0	0	0	0	0	+
Gr. Simplicifolia II	0	0	+	0	0	0	0	+w	0	0	+
A. hypogea	+	0	+	+	+	0	0	+w	0	0	+
S. sclarea	0	+	0	0	0	0	0	0	0	0	+w
S. horminum	0	+	0	0	0	+	0	+w	0	0	+w
H. pomatia	+	+	0	+	NT	+	0	+	+mf	+	+
D. biflorus	0	+	0	0	0	+	0	0	0	0	0
P. lunatus	0	0	0	0	0	0	0	0	0	0	0

0, no agglutination; +, agglutination; +w, weak agglutination; +mf, mixed-field agglutination; NT, not tested.

In addition to the above listed mechanisms, T, Tn, and Tk activation can occur in malignancies. The T antigen is present on approximately 90% of carcinomas and T cell lymphomas. T cell lymphomas also express the Tn antigen and Tk is associated with colorectal carcinoma.

VA Polyagglutination

VA polyagglutination is characterized by polyagglutination and persistent hemolytic anemia.[26] The condition presents with a decreased number of H receptors. VA appears to be a form of acquired polyagglutination, but no bacteria have been identified as the cause of the change to the H receptor and the condition appears persistent rather than transient.

Inherited Polyagglutination

The inherited forms of polyagglutination arise from somatic mutations. The mutation may cause the cells to express an antigen that is not present on normal adult red blood cells and to which most adults have the corresponding antibody. Or the mutation may cause a deficiency in an enzyme that is required for normal red blood cell membrane or red blood cell antigen development; the defect may expose a cryptantigen that is normally hidden. Unlike the acquired forms of polyagglutination, the inherited forms do not resolve. Descriptions of cryptantigens associated with inherited forms of polyagglutination are as follows:

- Cad is a very low-frequency antigen that is expressed on red blood cells.[26] Cad-positive cells are considered polyagglutinable because anti-Cad is found in nearly all human plasma. All Cad-positive red blood cells have strongly expressed Sd^a antigens in addition to the Cad pentasaccharide. For this reason, the Cad antigen reacts very strongly with anti-Sd^a.

- NOR is an inherited form of polyagglutination that produces two neutral glycolipids on the red blood cell membrane.[30] The genetic background of the NOR phenotype is not known, but the condition appears to be inherited in a dominant manner. The agglutination of NOR red blood cells is inhibited by hydatid cyst fluid and avian P1 glycoproteins, suggesting NOR may be related to the P1 glycolipid.

- Hemoglobin M-Hyde Park is associated with a form of polyagglutination caused by two defective cell membrane sites.[31] The first is associated with a reduction in the sialylation of O-linked oligosaccharides on sialoglycoproteins. The second is caused by an exposed N-acetylglucosaminyl residue on the red blood cell membrane.

- The acronym HEMPAS stands for hereditary erythroblastic multinuclearity with a positive acidified serum test.[32] HEMPAS is an autosomal recessive form of congenital dyserythropoietic anemia type 2 in which there are increased amounts of i antigen on the red blood cells that hemolyze when exposed to anti-i. Most patients with HEMPAS have a normocytic anemia.

- Tr polyagglutination is a recently identified form of polyagglutination.[28] Research suggests that Tr polyagglutination is caused by inheriting a defective transferase that results in decreased glycosylation. Multiple cell lineages, including red blood cells, are affected.

Review of the Main Points

- Panels of cells with known phenotypes are used to determine antibody specificity.
- Exclusion is the ruling out of an antibody when the patient's plasma does not react with a red blood cell that is known to be homozygous positive for the corresponding antigen.
- A general rule of thumb for antibody confirmation is negative reactions with at least three cells known to be negative for the corresponding antigen and positive reactions with at least three cells known to be positive for the corresponding antigen.
- Antibody confirmation includes phenotyping the patient for the corresponding antigen, unless the patient has been transfused in the last 3 months.
- Donor cells chosen for transfusion should be antigen negative for any corresponding clinically significant antibody identified in the patient's plasma.

- A crossmatch using an indirect antiglobulin test (IAT) should be performed whenever a patient is known to have clinically significant antibodies or when the antibody screen is positive.
- Enzyme treatment of red blood cells enhances some antigens and destroys others.
- Neutralization uses soluble antigen to inactivate an antibody.
- Elution frees antibody that is bound to the red blood cell membrane.
- Elution may be used to identify the antibody that was bound to the red blood cells or may be used to obtain red blood cells that are free of the previously bound antibody.
- Autoadsorptions use the patient's own red blood cells to remove a warm or cold autoantibody from the plasma.
- Alloadsorption use red blood cells of known phenotypes to remove antibodies from plasma.

- Titration measures the strength of an antibody.
- Plasma with multiple antibodies may show variation in strength of reaction, or may react differently if tested using different methods, at different phases, or at different temperatures.
- Complicated mixtures of antibodies may require use of a variety of identification techniques including testing against enzyme-treated red blood cells, testing against red blood cells treated with other chemicals, testing against cord red blood cells, adsorption combined with elution studies, dilution of the plasma, and/or treatment of the plasma with DTT.
- Patients with warm autoantibodies typically have the following reaction pattern: positive DAT, positive autocontrol, positive with all screen, panel, and donor red blood cells.
- When an autoantibody is present, underlying alloantibodies may be detected by testing autoadsorbed plasma.
- Patients with warm autoimmune hemolytic anemia are often given phenotypically matched red blood cells if transfusion is required.
- Autoadsorptions and phenotyping should not be performed on patients who have been transfused in the last 3 months.
- Polyagglutination describes red blood cells that agglutinate with normal adult plasma but not when tested with plasma from infants or in an autocontrol.
- Polyagglutination can be inherited or passively acquired.
- Passively acquired polyagglutination is usually associated with a bacterial infection.
- Reaction patterns with lectins can differentiate the different types of polyagglutination.

Review Questions

1. The autocontrol tube in an antibody identification study consists of: (Objective #5)

   A. Panel cells and patient plasma

   B. Screening cells and patient plasma

   C. Patient cells and patient plasma

   D. Check cells and patient plasma

2. Anti-K is identified in an antibody identification rule-out procedure. The autocontrol tube on the panel study shows negative results. What is the patient's expected red blood cell phenotype? (Objective #3)

   A. (K+k−)

   B. (K+k+)

   C. (K−k+)

   D. Both A and C

3. Enzyme treatment of red blood cells assists with the identification of which of the following sets of antibodies? (Objective #5)

   A. Anti-M and anti-Fy^b

   B. Anti-C and anti-Jk^a

   C. Anti-K and anti-S

   D. Anti-Fy^a and anti-c

4. A blood bank technologist receives a request for 3 units of packed red blood cells for a patient who has both Anti-Jk^b and Anti-K in the plasma. The antigen frequency of Jk^b is 73% and that of K is 10%. How many units of blood will need to be tested to find 3 compatible units? (Objective #6)

   A. 3

   B. 7

   C. 10

   D. 12

5. Select the antibody whose corresponding antigen is destroyed by enzyme treatment: (Objective #8)

   A. Anti-Fy^a

   B. Anti-D

   C. Anti-Jk^a

   D. Anti-K

6. Statistical validity for the identification of anti-C on a panel study is achieved through: (Objective #9)

   A. One C+ cell with positive results and one C− cell with negative results

   B. One C+ cell with negative results and one C− cell with positive results

   C. Three C+ cells with positive results and three C− cells with negative results

   D. Three C+ cells with negative results and three C− cells with positive results

7. Choose the antigen that is an exception to homozygous exclusion of an antibody: (Objective #2)

   A. Fy^b

   B. D

   C. C

   D. S

8. Mixed-field agglutination is commonly observed when: (Objective #10)

   A. Group O packed red blood cells are transfused to an Group A patient

   B. Anti-Sd^a is identified in the plasma

   C. Patient has a delayed hemolytic transfusion reaction

   D. All of the above

9. Match the neutralization substances with the source of origin: (Objective #11)

    1. _____1. I substance

    2. _____2. Lewis substance

    3. _____3. P₁ substance

    4. _____4. Sdᵃ substance

    A. Saliva

    B. Hydatid cyst fluid

    C. Urine

    D. Breast milk

10. Polyagglutinable red blood cells will react with which of the following sera? (Objective #17)

    A. Cord blood sera

    B. Autologous sera

    C. Human source reagent antisera

    D. All of the above

11. Which elution method is recommended for removal of antibodies from the red blood cell membrane in suspected cases of hemolytic disease of the fetus and newborn (HDFN) due to ABO incompatibility? (Objective #12)

    A. Glycine pH 3.0

    B. Freeze–thaw

    C. Ether

    D. Methylene chloride

12. A warm autoantibody is identified in a specimen from a 32-year-old male patient. The patient was transfused with 2 units of packed red blood cells 2 months ago. Which type of procedure should be performed to rule out the presence of alloantibodies? (Objective # 14)

    A. Autoadsorption

    B. Elution

    C. Allogeneic adsorption

    D. Plasma dilution

13. Select the substance that can be used to destroy IgM class antibodies in plasma: (Objective #14)

    A. Dithiothreitol

    B. Chloroquine

    C. Ficin

    D. Sdᵃ + urine

14. A plasma specimen demonstrates 2+ agglutination strength with 10 out of 10 panel cells in an antibody identification study. The autocontrol tube is negative. The antibody specificity is most likely: (Objective #2)

    A. Anti-C

    B. Anti-D

    C. Anti-k (cellano)

    D. Anti-Fyᵇ

15. Warm autoantibodies are characterized by all of the following *except*: (Objective #13)

    A. Strong positive DAT

    B. Positive plasma reactions with all panel cells

    C. Optimal reactivity at 98.6° F (37° C)

    D. Compatible crossmatch with all donor cells tested

References

1. Young PP, Uzieblo A, Trulock E, Lublin DM, Goodnough LT. Autoantibody formation after alloimmunization: are blood transfusions a risk factor for autoimmune hemolytic anemia? *Transfusion* 2004; 44: 67–72.
2. Salamat N, Bhatti FA, Yaqub M, Hafeez M, Hussain A, Ziaullah. Indigenous development of antibody screening cell panels at Armed Forces Institute of Transfusion (AFIT). *Journal of the Pakistan Medical Association* 2005; 55(10): 439–43.
3. Food and Drug Administration. (2005). Code of Federal Regulations, Title 21, volume 7, (21CFR660). Washington DC: US Government Printing Office.
4. Garratty G. Screening for RBC antibodies—what should we expect from antibody detection RBCs. *Immunohematology* 2002; 18: 71–7.
5. Roback JD, et al. *Technical Manual*, 17th ed. Bethesda (MD): AABB; 2011.
6. Judd WJ, Barnes BA, Steiner EA, Oberman HA, Averill DB, Butch SH. The evaluation of a positive direct antiglobulin test (autocontrol) in pretransfusion testing revisited. *Transfusion* 1986; 26: 220–4.
7. College of American Pathologists. *Autoimmune Hemolytic Anemia*. J-A 2006. Northfield, IL: College of American Pathologists; 2006.
8. Shirey RS, Boyd JS, Ness PM. Polyethylene glycol versus low-ionic-strength solution in pretransfusion testing: a blinded comparison study. *Transfusion* 1994; 34: 368–70.
9. Harris RE, Hochman HG. Revised p values in testing blood group antibodies. Fisher's exact test revisited. *Transfusion* 1986; 26: 494–9.
10. Harmening DM. *Modern blood banking and transfusion practices*, 5th ed. Philadelphia (PA): F.A. Davis Company; 2005.
11. Kanter MH, Poole G, Garratty G. Misinterpretation and misapplication of p values in antibody identification: the lack of value of a p value. *Transfusion* 1997; 37: 816–22.
12. Casina TS. Estimating the ability to find compatible blood when alloantibodies are encountered. *AABB News* 2002; Jul/Aug: 36.
13. Strobel E. Use of the enzyme method for antibody identification. *Clin Lab* 2004; 50: 575–80.
14. Rabbit Erythrocyte Stroma for Adsorption of Cold Agglutinins Anti-I, Anti-H, or Anti-IH package insert, version 368-4. Norcross (GA): *Immucor-Gamma*; 2005.
15. Waligora SK, Edwards JM. Use of rabbit red cells for adsorption of cold auto-agglutinins. *Transfusion* 1983; 23: 328–30.
16. Ahrens N, Pruss A, Kähne A, Kiesewetter H, Salama A. Coexistence of autoantibodies and alloantibodies to red blood cells due to blood transfusion. *Transfusion* 2007; 47: 813–6.

17. Maley M, Bruce DG, Babb RG, Wells AW, Williams M. The incidence of red cell alloantibodies underlying panreactive warm autoantibodies. *Immunohematology* 2005; 21: 122–5.

18. Judd WJ. How I manage cold agglutinins. *Transfusion* 2006; 46: 324–6.

19. Leger RM, Garratty G. Weakening or loss of antibody reactivity after pre-warm technique. *Transfusion* 2003; 43: 1611–4.

20. Heltze GA. Should we worry about cold-reactive antibodies in cardiac surgery? [Internet]. Sacramento: California Blood Bank Society e-Newwork Forum; 1999 [cited 2006 Sept 10]. Available from http://www.cbbsweb.org/enf/1999_2000/coldabsurg.html.

21. Pampee PY, Uzieblo A, Trulock E, Lublin DM, Goodnough LT. Autoantibody formation after allommunization: are blood transfusion a risk factor for autoimmune hemolytic anemia. *Transfusion* 2004; 44: 67–72.

22. Garratty G. In vitro reactions with red blood cells that are not due to blood group antibodies: a review. *Immunohematology* 1998; 14: 3–13.

23. Buetens O, Shirey RS, Goble-Lee M, Houp J, Zachary A, King KE, Ness PM. Prevalence of HLA antibodies in transfused patients with and without red cell antibodies. *Transfusion* 2006; 46: 754–6.

24. Chikako T, Ohto H, Miura S, Yasuda H, Ono S, Ogata T. Delayed and acute hemolytic transfusion reactions resulting from red cell antibodies and red cell-reactive HLA antibodies. *Transfusion* 2005; 45: 1925–9.

25. Nance ST. Do HLA antibodies cause hemolytic transfusion reactions or decreased RBC survival? *Transfusion* 2003; 43: 687–90.

26. Klein HG, Anstee DJ. *Mollison's Blood Transfusion in Clinical Medicine*, 11th ed. Malden (MA): Wiley-Blackwell; 2005.

27. Boralessa H, Modi N, Cockburn H, Maide R, Edwards M, Roberts I, Letsky E. RBC T activation and hemolysis in a neonatal intensive care population: implications for transfusion practice. *Transfusion* 2002; 42: 1428–34.

28. Halverson GR, Lee AH, Øyen R, Reiss RF, Hurlet-Jensen A, Reid ME. Altered glycosylation leads to Tr polyagglutination. *Transfusion* 2004; 44: 1588–92.

29. Crookston KP, Reiner AP, Cooper LJN, Sacher RA, Blajchman MA, Heddle NM. RBC T activation and hemolysis: implications for pediatric transfusion management. *Transfusion* 2000; 40: 801–12.

30. Duk M, Lisowska E, Moulds J. Polyagglutinable NOR red blood cells found in an American family and a Polish family have the same unique glycosphingolipids. *Transfusion* 2006; 46: 1264–5.

31. King MJ, Liew YW, Moores PP, Bird GW. Enhanced reaction with Vicia graminea lectin and exposed terminal N-acetyl-D-glucosaminyl residues on a sample of human red cells with Hb M- Hyde Park. *Transfusion* 1988; 28: 549–55.

32. McKenzie SB. *Clinical Laboratory Hematology*, 2nd ed. Upper Saddle River (NJ): Prentice Hall; 2009.

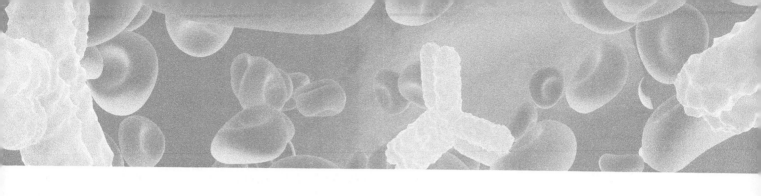

9

Donor Selection, Phlebotomy, and Required Testing

HANNAH ACEVEDO

Chapter Objectives

Upon completion of this chapter, the student will be able to:

1. Identify the regulatory agencies that oversee blood donations and describe the function of each.
2. Identify the procedures that are performed as part of the blood donation process.
3. Discuss the regulatory requirements for the development, modification, and completion of the Donor History Questionnaire (DHQ).
4. Evaluate educational materials that must be provided to prospective donors.
5. Expound on the rationale for each question present on the health history questionnaire.
6. Articulate the reasons for deferral of blood donors and whether the deferral is designed to prevent harm to the donor or the recipient.
7. Discuss the difference between permanent, temporary, and indefinite deferrals and provide an example of each.
8. Identify the acceptable criteria for the physical examination of a blood donor that is in accordance with AABB standards.
9. State the shelf life of the common anticoagulants and additive solutions that are used in whole blood collection procedures.
10. Discuss the criteria for a low-volume whole blood unit collection.
11. Describe the different types of adverse donor reactions to blood donation, including the reasons why they occur.
12. Diagram the basic schema for collection of platelets by the automated process of plateletpheresis.
13. Compare and contrast the automated red blood cell collection process with the automated platelet collection process.
14. Differentiate between the donor requirements for autologous versus allogeneic donations.
15. Assess the risks and benefits of designated or directed donations.
16. Identify the infectious disease tests that are performed on donated blood.
17. Describe confidential unit exclusion and why it is such an important part of the blood donation process.
18. Discuss the rationale for leukoreduction and irradiation of donor blood.
19. Identify the circumstances that require a donor lookback.

Key Terms

Allogeneic donation(s)
Apheresis
Autologous donation(s)
Community donation(s)
Confidential unit exclusion
    (CUE)
Deferred Donor Directory
    (DDD)
Designated donation(s)
Directed donation(s)
Donor Deferral Registry
    (DDR)
Donor History Questionnaire
    (DHQ)

Donor lookback
Hematoma(s)
Indefinite deferral
Infiltration(s)
Permanent deferral
Plasmapheresis
Plateletpheresis
Preoperative autologous
    donation (PAD)
Quantity not sufficient
    (QNS)
Satellite bag(s)
Temporary deferral
Therapeutic phlebotomy

CASE IN POINT

A local blood center is experiencing critical shortages of donor red blood cells. The blood center works with local television and radio stations to begin a campaign plea asking people to donate blood. A group of coworkers heard a radio announcement and decided they would donate blood at the local blood center after work.

What's Ahead?

Donating blood is by far one of the most important acts individuals can do to help patients in need, be it for their own future needs or for others. This chapter details the selection, phlebotomy, and required testing associated with blood donation by addressing the following questions:

- What is the difference between autologous, allogenic, and directed/designated donations?
- What agencies regulate blood donation practices?
- What are the components of the blood donation process?
- What is the purpose of providing potential blood donors with education materials to review prior to donation?
- What is the purpose of the Donor History Questionnaire (DHQ)?
- What are the three categories of blood donor deferrals?
- What are the minimum acceptable vital signs and hemoglobin/hematocrit values required for individuals to donate blood?
- What is the purpose of a Confidential Unit Exclusion (CUE)?
- Why are blood donors required to remain in the area after giving blood?
- What is apheresis?
- What is the most common type of reaction that donors may experience?
- What is the purpose of these three special donations: autologous, directed, and therapeutic?
- What blood bank tests are run on blood donation samples after collection?
- What are some examples of infectious disease tests that are currently required by the FDA on donated blood?

INTRODUCTION

Blood centers are responsible for supplying a safe and adequate blood supply to the community. Because blood can only be provided by people, recruiting them to donate is a crucial step in ensuring that blood is available for the patients who need to be transfused. Only a very small percentage of people who are eligible actually donate blood. Blood centers are constantly working to increase the number of people who donate. In addition, manufacturers of automated blood collection equipment work to develop instruments that can be used to optimize each donation for particular blood components.

Blood is most often donated voluntarily; however paid donor programs are permitted in some countries, while payment is forbidden in others. A unit of blood must be labeled to identify it as being from a person who donated blood as a volunteer or was paid for their blood. There is concern that if a person is paid that they may not reveal information during the health history that would disqualify them from giving blood.

There are many different types of donations that can be made, including whole blood, automated double red blood cells (RBC), automated red blood cells with two units of plasma (RBCP), plasmapheresis, and plateletpheresis. Donations may be made by donors for their own use, which is called **autologous donation**. **Allogeneic donations** are given for use by someone other than the donor. This

may be for a specific recipient, which is called a **directed or designated donation** or for use by any recipient, which is called a **community donation**.

REGULATORY AGENCIES

Blood centers in the United States are regulated by several agencies. The Food and Drug Administration (FDA) licenses blood centers. Only blood centers licensed by the FDA can routinely ship blood across state lines. Blood centers must follow the regulations in the Code of Federal Regulations (CFR) parts 211 and 600-799. In the early 1990s, the FDA started to regulate blood centers as manufacturers and required them to follow "Good Manufacturing Practices," which are found in part 211 of the CFR.

Each country establishes its own regulations for blood centers and sometimes for transfusion services. The regulations cover similar broad topics such as donor and recipient safety. However, the details in the regulations and manner of enforcement will differ due to political, geographical, economical, and population diversity among the various countries.

The AABB, formerly called the American Association of Blood Banks, publishes *Standards for Blood Banks and Transfusion Services* (hereafter referred to as AABB Standards), which are voluntarily

✱ **TABLE 9-1** Areas of Regulation for Blood Centers

- Donor selection
- Blood collection
- Blood testing
- Component production
- Blood and component shipment
- Blood and component storage
- Premises (fixed, temporary, and mobile) where blood is collected
- Premises where blood is processed
- Premises where blood and components are stored

followed by transfusion services and blood centers that choose to be accredited by the AABB. The AABB Standards are updated every 2 years. Although AABB accreditation is not required, following the AABB Standards are considered the standard of care for blood centers and are followed by most facilities even if they choose not to be accredited by the AABB.

Many plasma fractionation companies are located in Europe and are regulated by the European Union (EU) Standards. Blood centers that supply plasma or other blood components for further manufacturing to these facilities must also comply with the EU Standards, which are published as the Directive of the European Parliament and of the Council. Areas of regulation are listed in Table 9-1 ✱.

☑ **CHECKPOINT 9-1**

Which regulatory agency publishes standards of practice that are followed by most transfusion services and blood centers?

DONOR HEALTH HISTORY SCREENING

The blood donation process includes registering the donor, obtaining the donor's health history, performing a "mini" physical exam, and collecting blood. These procedures are performed using manual methods, automated methods, or a combination of both. The process is designed to minimize the risks for both donor and recipient (Table 9-2 ✱).

Registration

Donors must present some form of identification at the time of registration. It is extremely important to ensure the correct identification of the person attempting to donate. Most blood centers require the identification to contain the donor's full name and some other identifying information such as a date of birth or a photograph. The EU requires positive identification of the donor, which is defined as the use of the donor's name and picture identification.[1] Another form of positive identification is fingerprint scans. Some computer-assisted donor interviews take the donor's picture at the time of registration and save this in the donor's permanent electronic file.

During the registration process demographic information is obtained from the donor. The donor's name, address, and date of birth are basic identifying information obtained. A Social Security number may also be obtained, but donors may prefer not to give their Social Security number due to fear of identity theft. Therefore, the use of the Social Security number has been eliminated by many blood centers. If a computer system is used to register the donor, an identifying number is often assigned by the computer that can be used for identification at future blood donations. Additional information such as race and ethnicity may be asked to identify donors for specific antigen testing or for research studies.

The donor's date of birth is not only an identifying statistic but is also used to verify the age of the donor. In most states, donors who are at least 17 years of age can donate without parental consent. In many states, 16-year-olds may donate if they have parental consent. Age requirements are defined by state regulations.

The donor's name must be checked against a list of donors who have been deferred from donating blood on a previous donation or donation attempt.[2] This list is referred to as a **donor deferral registry (DDR)** or **deferred donor directory (DDD)**. This is often done using a computer with a database of deferred donors, but if a computer is not available, a printed report must be used. The FDA recommends that the DDR be checked prior to donating blood to prevent the collection of blood from a donor who is still deferred. The DDR check is often done at the time of registration but must be completed prior to releasing the unit of blood for distribution to prevent the release of blood from a donor who was previously deferred and does not reveal the information that resulted in the deferral on a later donation attempt.

☑ **CHECKPOINT 9-2**

State an acceptable form of positive identification for a potential blood donor.

Education

Blood donors must be given educational material to read prior to donating blood. This material must include information about infectious diseases that may be transmitted by blood transfusions, the signs and symptoms of acquired immune deficiency syndrome (AIDS), and the importance of providing accurate answers on the donor questionnaire and of not donating if they think their blood should not be used for transfusion for any reason. Donors must be told which laboratory tests will be performed on their blood and that certain agencies will be notified of abnormal or positive results as required by state law. During the health history interview process the donor must acknowledge that he or she has read the educational materials presented. The educational materials available from the FDA and AABB website are not to be changed with regard to order, content, and wording. The use of different fonts or colors is permitted, as well as making the educational materials into a brochure, handout, or poster presentation.

★ TABLE 9-2 Processes for Minimizing Risk to Donor and Recipient

Minimizing Risk to the Donor	
Step or Process	**Rationale**
Date of birth/age General health questions Questions about previous health conditions Questions about medications Question about pregnancy Taking the donor's vital signs	Helps to determine that the donor is healthy enough to donate and would be at low risk for any health problem related to donation.
Questions about previous donation intervals Maximum donation volumes	Maximum donation frequencies and maximum volume/donation are chosen to allow the donor's body time to replace the elements donated (e.g., blood volume, red blood cells, platelets, clotting factors, and other proteins in plasma)
Informed consent	Ensures that the donor is aware of the risks of donation and has voluntarily chosen to participate.
Hemoglobin or hematocrit check	Minimizes the risk that the donor will become anemic by donating whole blood or red blood cells.
Other laboratory tests if required as part of pheresis program (e.g., platelet count, plasma protein level)	Ensures that the donor is capable of returning or maintaining normal levels after or between donations.
Venipuncture site cleaning	Minimizes risk of infection at venipuncture site.
Donors are usually lying down or reclining during donation	To prevent injury due to a fall if the donor faints or has a seizure during the donation.
Postdonation care such as pressure on the venipuncture site, remaining at the blood center/mobile clinic for a period of time, drinking fluids, and eating a snack.	Minimizes the risk of postdonation injuries. Ensures that the donor will be close to qualified medical help during the time period when a serious reaction is likely to occur.
Minimizing the Risk to the Recipient	
Step or Process	**Rationale**
Identification of the donor	Ensures that the donor has not been previously deferred.
Questions about previous health conditions Questions about medications	Minimizes the risk that the blood or blood component from the donor will have elements such as cancer cells, medications, or abnormal proteins that could harm the recipient.
Educational materials Questions about infectious disease exposure Questions about sexual activities and sexually transmitted diseases Questions about travel Questions about blood exposure Infectious disease tests Confidential unit exclusion	Minimizes the risk that the blood or blood component will transmit a blood-borne pathogen.
Laboratory tests on the donor such as the hematocrit and on the donor blood such as infectious disease testing	Ensures that the blood component meets minimum requirements and therefore will produce the desired effect in the donor.
Checking the venipuncture site for lesions Venipuncture site cleaning Diversion pouch	Minimizes the risk of bacterial contamination of the blood and blood components.
Requirements for shipping, storage, and preparation of blood and blood components	Ensures that the blood component meets minimum requirements and therefore will produce the desired effect in the donor.

Donor History Questionnaire

Once the donor has been registered and found to be eligible to donate from the deferral registry check, the health history screening of the donor must be performed. The donor health history screening process is a very important step in protecting the safety of the blood supply. A qualified physician must determine the eligibility of the donor. This responsibility may be delegated to another trained individual under the physician's direction. This is done by the physician approving written standard operating procedures (SOP) to be

followed in determining the donor's eligibility. Any questions about the donor's eligibility must be directed to the facility's medical director. It is the medical director's decision as to whether a donor may be accepted or not.

The AABB has developed a full-length (sometimes called uniform) **Donor History Questionnaire (DHQ)**, which has been approved by the FDA.[3] The DHQ was developed to ensure that the donor gets a consistent message and that the questions asked are thorough and meet the AABB Standards as well as the FDA

CASE IN POINT (continued)

The group of donors is immediately greeted by blood center staff when they arrive at the donation location. Each donor provides identification and is asked to read a pamphlet about the infectious diseases that can be transmitted via blood transfusion. A blood center employee checks the donor deferral list to ensure that none of the potential donors have been previously deferred.

1. Why is it important to know if a donor has been previously deferred?

One of the donors asks how much donors get paid for donating blood. The blood center employee informs him that donation is strictly voluntary and no one is paid for blood donation.

2. Why is payment for blood donation a discouraged practice?

regulations. In the United States, the FDA-approved DHQ cannot be modified or edited with regard to order, content, or wording, with the exception of making the screening criteria more restrictive (e.g., increasing the time for deferral after aspirin ingestion from 48 hours to 72 hours) or to add local additions of questions, which must be placed at the end of the DHQ. The order of the standard questions was developed with design experts who tested the cognitive recall of donors answering the questions. Whereas previous versions of donor questionnaires had questions grouped around specific donor or recipient risk factors, the latest versions put many questions in reverse chronological order. The chronological order helps donors remember travel and illness history better. Formatting changes are permitted, such as changes in shading, columns or rows, spacing, size, or color. An example of a donor history questionnaire is shown in Figure 9-1 ■.

Questions are added as new diseases or viruses emerge that may be transmitted through a blood transfusion. Questions are removed or modified as new blood screening tests are developed and approved by the FDA or if the risk of the disease diminishes. An example of this is the risk of severe acute respiratory syndrome (SARS). This disease was identified as a risk in several countries in 2003 by the Centers for Disease Control (CDC). By 2006, the number of cases of SARS declined and the CDC did not consider any country as a risk for SARS. The questions related to identifying donors who may have had contact with people with SARS were no longer required.[4] The AABB notifies institutions of the changes in donor documents and the timeline for implementation. The DHQ must be periodically updated by the blood center, within the AABB's specified timeframe.

Another example is having lived in or traveled to Africa. Certain African countries have an increased risk of exposure to a rare strain of the human immunodeficiency virus (HIV) called HIV group O (outlier group), which could not always be detected by early HIV tests. Questions were added to the DHQ related to African travel and sexual contact with someone who was born in or lived in certain parts of Africa. These questions were designed to identify donors who may be at risk for contracting HIV group O infections. In 2007, a test for HIV that also detected the group O strain was licensed by the FDA. Any blood center testing their blood donors with this test, could stop asking the questions related specifically to Africa.[3]

Health history questions are asked to protect the donor as well as the recipient of the donated blood. The questions may be asked by a donor historian (interviewer) or may be self-administered by the donor. Self-administered health history questionnaires may be presented in several ways such as on printed forms where the donor reads the questions and records an answer on the form or by audio and/or video presentation of the questions where the donor listens to a recording or watches a video and records the answers on a form. A computer-assisted interactive interview where the donor reviews the questions on a computer screen and enters the answers electronically is also acceptable. Whatever method is used for the self-administered questionnaire, a donor historian must review the donor's answers.

When the questions are asked by a donor historian, good interview techniques must be followed. The donor historian should speak slowly enough to ensure the questions are clear and are understood by the donor. The donor must be given enough time to thoroughly respond to each question.

Some questions on the DHQ are considered to be capture questions and cover a broad topic. If a capture question is answered yes, additional follow-up questions need to be asked to obtain adequate information to qualify the donor. There are also some questions called attention questions that apply only to either males or females to ensure the donors are carefully understanding and answering each question.

Other countries in the developed world use similar questionnaires and methods to administer the questionnaire, although there are differences in the details. Some are obvious, such as the fact that European countries will not have questions about time spent in Europe on their questionnaires. Some blood centers in other countries voluntarily choose to be accredited by the AABB. They use the questionnaire mandated by their regulatory agencies rather than the DHQ and ask for a variance if there are differences that do not meet the AABB Standards.

Deferrals fall within three categories (Table 9-3 ✱). A **temporary deferral** occurs when a donor has had an exposure that results in a risk to the potential recipient for a limited period of time. An example would be a donor who is vaccinated for yellow fever, which results in a 2-week deferral for the prospective donor. A **permanent deferral** occurs when a donor has a condition or exposure that causes them to never be eligible to donate blood for someone else again. An example would be having a positive laboratory test result for certain viruses, such as HIV or hepatitis C, or having had a previous exposure to certain treatments or medications, such as human growth hormone or etretinate (Tegison). An **indefinite deferral** means the prospective donor is unable to give blood to someone else for an unspecified period of time due to current regulatory requirements. However, this requirement could change in the future, allowing the donor to give blood. An example of an indefinite deferral in the United States is having spent 3 months or more in England during the years of 1980–1996.

Are you		Yes	No
1	Feeling healthy and well today?	☐	☐
2	Currently taking an antibiotic?	☐	☐
3	Currently taking any other medication for an infection?	☐	☐
Please read the Medication Deferral List.		**Yes**	**No**
4	Are you now taking or have you ever taken any medications on the Medication Deferral List?	☐	☐
5	Have you read the educational materials?	☐	☐
In the past 48 hours		**Yes**	**No**
6	Have you taken aspirin or anything that has aspirin in it?	☐	☐
In the past 6 weeks		**Yes**	**No**
7	Have you been pregnant or are you pregnant now? (Males: check "I am male.") ☐ I am male	☐	☐
In the past 8 weeks have you		**Yes**	**No**
8	Donated blood, platelets or plasma?	☐	☐
9	Had any vaccinations or other shots?	☐	☐
10	Had contact with someone who had a smallpox vaccination?	☐	☐
In the past 16 weeks		**Yes**	**No**
11	Have you donated a double unit of red cells using an apheresis machine?	☐	☐
In the past 12 months have you		**Yes**	**No**
12	Had a blood transfusion?	☐	☐
13	Had a transplant such as organ, tissue, or bone marrow?	☐	☐
14	Had a graft such as bone or skin?	☐	☐
15	Come into contact with someone else's blood?	☐	☐
16	Had an accidental needlestick?	☐	☐
17	Had sexual contact with anyone who has HIV/AIDS or has had a positive test for the HIV/AIDS virus?	☐	☐
18	Had sexual contact with a prostitute or anyone else who takes money or drugs or other payment for sex?	☐	☐
19	Had sexual contact with anyone who has ever used needles to take drugs or steroids, or anything not prescribed by their doctor?	☐	☐
20	Had sexual contact with anyone who has hemophilia or has used clotting factor concentrates?	☐	☐
21	Had sexual contact with a male who has ever had sexual contact with another male? (Males: check "I am male.") ☐ I am male	☐	☐
22	Had sexual contact with a person who has hepatitis?	☐	☐
23	Lived with a person who has hepatitis?	☐	☐
24	Had a tattoo?	☐	☐
25	Had ear or body piercing?	☐	☐
26	Had or been treated for syphilis or gonorrhea?	☐	☐
27	Been in juvenile detention, lockup, jail, or prison for more than 72 hours?	☐	☐
In the past three years have you		**Yes**	**No**
28	Been outside the United States or Canada?	☐	☐
From 1980 through 1996,		**Yes**	**No**
29	Did you spend time that adds up to three (3) months or more in the United Kingdom? (Review list of countries in the UK)	☐	☐
30	Were you a member of the U.S. military, a civilian military employee, or a dependent of a member of the U.S. military?	☐	☐
From 1980 to the present, did you		**Yes**	**No**
31	Spend time that adds up to five (5) years or more in Europe? (Review list of countries in Europe.)	☐	☐
32	Receive a blood transfusion in the United Kingdom? (Review list of countries in the UK.)	☐	☐

■ **FIGURE 9-1** Example Donor History Questionnaire

Are you		Yes	No
From **1977 to the present**, have you		Yes	No
33	Received money, drugs, or other payment for sex?	☐	☐
34	Male donors: had sexual contact with another male, even once? (Females: check "I am female.") ☐ I am female	☐	☐
Have you **EVER**		Yes	No
35	Had a positive test for the HIV/AIDS virus?	☐	☐
36	Used needles to take drugs, steroids, or anything **not** prescribed by your doctor?	☐	☐
37	Used clotting factor concentrates?	☐	☐
38	Had hepatitis?	☐	☐
39	Had malaria?	☐	☐
40	Had Chagas' disease?	☐	☐
41	Had babesiosis?	☐	☐
42	Received a dura mater (or brain covering) graft?	☐	☐
43	Had any type of cancer, including leukemia?	☐	☐
44	Had any problems with your heart or lungs?	☐	☐
45	Had a bleeding condition or a blood disease?	☐	☐
46	Have any of your relatives had Creutzfeldt-Jakob disease?	☐	☐

FIGURE 9-1 *continued*

The following questions are taken from the DHQ.[5]

Are you feeling well and healthy? This question is designed to establish that the donor is in general good health and free from infectious disease, colds, or other illnesses. Donors who do not feel well should not donate blood until the underlying cause is determined, the illness has run its course, and the donor feels well.

Are you currently taking an antibiotic? Donors should be free of any disease or infection that may be transmitted through their blood. The reason for taking antibiotics should be clarified and an evaluation performed to determine if the donor is eligible to donate. If the donor has an infection, they should not donate until the course of antibiotics is completed and the infection has resolved. Antibiotics, if given only for acne treatment and not for infection (such as tetracycline), do not result in a deferral at most centers. Antibiotics are used for acne treatment less commonly than in the past.

★ TABLE 9-3 Definitions and Examples of the Different Types of Deferrals Adapted from the AABB/FDA Donor History Questionnaire User Brochure

DEFINITIONS	
Term	**Definition**
Attention Question	Strategically developed and placed questions design to determine if a potential blood donor is paying attention
Capture Question	A global question designed to determine if further specific information is required to assess the potential donor or not
Self-Administered Questionnaire	A term that refers to a potential donor completing the donor questionnaire without assistance; such forms are still reviewed upon completion to determine donor eligibility
TYPES OF DEFERRAL	
Indefinite Deferral	Based on current regulatory donor requirements, potential donors grouped into this category are referred from blood donation as long as these requirements are in force.
Permanent Deferral	When select criteria are met, such as when a donor indicates that he/she has hepatitis C, which is known to be transmitted in blood, donation is deferred forever.
Temporary Deferral	There are some instances, such as an individual who was transfused within the previous 12 months, when potential donors are not currently eligible but after a designated wait period, may donate blood.

Source: http://www.fda.gov/downloads/BiologicsBloodVaccines/BloodBloodProducts/ApprovedProducts/LicensedProductsBLAs/BloodDonorScreening/UCM213473.pdf%20

Are you currently taking any other medications for an infection?   Viral, fungal, or parasitic infections are treated with medications other than antibiotics. The reason for taking any medication for an infection must be investigated to determine if the donor has a fungal, viral, parasitic, or other infection that may be transmitted through blood.

Are you now taking or have you ever taken any medications on the medication deferral list?   A medication deferral list should be provided to the donor to read (Table 9-4 ✳). The medication list contains names of medications and length of time the donor should be deferred after discontinuation of the medication. It also includes information in plain language about why a medication causes a deferral. Some medications on the list result in permanent deferral from donating blood whereas others result in deferral for a certain period of time after the medication is stopped. The medication deferral list given to donors to read contains only the most common medications that cause donor deferral; the complete list of medications contains hundreds of medications. Other medications that the donor may be taking would be identified through follow-up questions based on answers to the Donor History Questionnaire.

Some medications have side effects that could be harmful to the blood transfusion recipient or to a fetus if the recipient is pregnant. Etretinate (Tegison) is a medication that results in a permanent donor deferral, even if the donor is no longer taking the medication. The permanent deferral is designed to prevent possible teratogenicity to the fetus in a pregnant recipient.

Other medications were previously produced from materials that may have had the potential to transmit a communicable disease to the person taking it. Examples of these medications are growth hormone from human pituitary glands and insulin obtained from cows, which have been associated with the transmission of prion diseases.

Hepatitis B immune globulin (HBIG) is given to a person who had been exposed to hepatitis and the donor should be deferred for 1 year from the time the HBIG was received. An exposure to the hepatitis B virus would require a 12-month deferral as well. Experimental or unlicensed products have unknown or untested potential for harm and the deferral period is often for 1 year from the last time the product was given.

In the United States, the medication deferral list, like the educational materials, may be reformatted, but the order, content, and wording must not be changed in accordance with the AABB and FDA.

Have you read the educational materials?   The donor must be given the opportunity to read the educational materials prior to answering the health history questions. If the donor answers no to this question, they must be given time to read the materials prior to continuing with the questions. If the donor refuses to read the information, they must be deferred from donating.

In the past 48 hours have you taken aspirin or anything that has aspirin in it?   Donors who are taking or have taken aspirin or an aspirin-containing medication should not be the only source of platelets as in plateletpheresis. Platelet function is irreversibly inactivated by aspirin. The donor may, however, donate other types of blood products if they have taken aspirin within 48 hours of the donation. The medication sheet contains the names of drugs that inhibit platelet function, such as clopidogrel (Plavix), and require a 2-week deferral if the collection is to be a plateletpheresis product.

✳ **TABLE 9-4** Example Medication Deferral List

Medication Name(s)	Common Condition(s) Treated	Deferral Period
Proscar© (finasteride)	Prostate gland enlargement	1 month
Avodart© (dutasteride)	Prostate gland enlargement	6 months
Propecia© (finasteride)	Baldness	1 month
Accutane© (Amnesteem, Claravis, Sotret, isotretinoin)	Severe acne	1 month
Soriatane© (acitretin)	Severe psoriasis	3 years
Tegison© (etretinate)	Severe psoriasis	Permanent
Growth hormone from human pituitary glands	Delayed or impaired growth	Permanent
Insulin from cows (bovine or beef insulin)	Diabetes	Indefinite
Hepatitis B immune globulin (different from the hepatitis B vaccine)	After exposure to hepatitis B	12 months
Plavix (clopidogrel)	Reduce the chance for heart attack and stroke in people at increased risk	• 14 days—platelet donation • No deferral—whole blood with no platelet component production
Ticlid (ticlopidine)	Reduce the chance for heart attack and stroke in people at increased risk	• 14 days—platelet donation • No deferral—whole blood with no platelet component production
Feldene (piroxicam)	Mild to moderate arthritis pain	• 2 days—platelet donation • No deferral—whole blood with no platelet component production
Experimental medication or unlicensed (experimental) vaccine	Associated with a research protocol	1 year or as determined by donor center medical director

In the past 6 weeks, female donors: Have you been pregnant or are you pregnant now? Males check "I am male." A female who is pregnant or who has been pregnant in the past 6 weeks should not donate blood. The "I am male" choice should be chosen by male donors. This question is considered to be an attention question. It indicates that donors who self-administer the questionnaire are paying attention to the questions they answer. If a male answers yes or no to this question, it would be an inappropriate answer and further action must be taken by the donor interviewer reviewing the responses. The blood center develops a policy on what that action should be and generally involves questioning the potential donor for possible error or further explanation. If a computer-assisted interview is utilized, it may be configured so this question is not asked of male donors. If the questions are asked in person by a donor interviewer, the question again does not have to be asked of male donors.

In the past 8 weeks have you donated blood, platelets, or plasma? This question is one that is asked to protect the donor and ensure they do not donate more frequently than the regulations allow. The whole blood donation interval is a minimum of every 8 weeks. Serial plasmapheresis, plateletpheresis, or leukapheresis donors may not donate more often than once every 2 days, with a maximum of two times a week and 24 times per year. For infrequent plasma donors, the minimum time between donations should be at least 4 weeks. Source plasma donors donate more frequently than once every 4 weeks; they follow additional regulations and are not usually collected at blood centers.

In the past 8 weeks have you had any shots or vaccinations? Some vaccinations contain live attenuated viruses and bacteria. Examples of these vaccines are German measles (rubella) and chicken pox or shingles (varicella-zoster); also, measles (rubeola), mumps, oral polio (Sabin), oral typhoid, and yellow fever. Donors who have received these vaccinations should not donate blood for 4 weeks (rubella and varicella-zoster) and 2 weeks (the others), respectively (Table 9-5 ✳). In general, no deferral is required for toxoids, synthetic or killed viral, bacterial, or rickettsial vaccines, if the prospective donor is symptom-free and afebrile. The deferral period should be defined by the blood center medical director and be included in the procedure for donor qualification.

After smallpox (variola) vaccination, donors are deferred for a minimum of 21 days, but several variables affect the length of deferral. If the scab at the vaccination site has not come off when the donor comes in to donate, the donor is deferred until the scab falls off spontaneously. If the scab is gone but did not come off by itself, the donor is deferred until 56 days after the vaccination date. If the scab came off on its own, it is more than 21 days since the day of vaccination, and the potential donor had no illness or complications related to the vaccine, the donor may donate. If the donor had complications from the vaccination (see the next question for examples of complications), the donor must be deferred for 14 days after the symptoms resolved.

In the past 8 weeks have you had contact with someone who had a smallpox vaccination? The smallpox vaccination contains a live weak strain of vaccinia virus, which is another orthopox virus closely related to smallpox but which causes a much

✳ **TABLE 9-5** Vaccination Deferrals

Immunization Deferrals				
See FDA Guidance	**One Year**	**Four Weeks** Live Attenuated	**Two Weeks** Live Attenuated	**No Deferral** Toxoids, Synthetic, or Killed
Variola (smallpox)	Unlicensed vaccines	Rubella (German measles)	Rubeola (measles)	Anthrax
		Varicella-Zoster (chicken pox and shingles)	Mumps	Cholera
			Polio (Sabin)—oral	Diptheria, pertussis, and tetanus (DPT)
			Yellow fever	Hepatitis A
			Typhoid—oral	Hepatitis B
				Human papilloma (HPV)—recombinant
				Influenza
				Influenza—intranasal live attenuated
				Lyme disease
				Paratyphoid
				Pneumococcus polysaccharide
				Polio (Salk)—injection
				Rabies
				Rocky Mountain Spotted Fever
				Typhoid—injection

milder illness called vaccinia. The antibodies made in response to exposure to the vaccinia virus will protect against smallpox either completely or result in a much milder course of illness. Around 30% of unvaccinated people die from smallpox, lacking the protective antibodies to vaccinia. A donor who has had contact with the vaccination site, bandages covering the vaccination site, or any other material, such as clothing, that may have come in contact with an unbandaged site may have been exposed to the live virus and should not serve as a donor. If a potential donor has had such contact, they should be further questioned about having a new skin rash, skin sore, or severe complication since the contact was made. Severe complications include a rash resembling blisters on a small or large area of the body, necrosis or dead tissue in the area of exposure, encephalitis (brain inflammation), infection of the cornea of the eye, and localized or systemic reaction in someone with a chronic skin condition such as eczema.

If the donor had a rash, then the blood center must evaluate whether the scab separated spontaneously or was removed. The donor may be accepted if it has been 14 days or more since the symptoms went away and there was spontaneous scab separation. If the scab did not separate spontaneously, then the donor should be deferred for 3 months from the date of the contact's vaccination. If the date of the contact's vaccination is unknown, the potential donor is deferred for 2 months from the current date.

In the past 16 weeks have you donated a double unit of red blood cells using an apheresis machine? Donors who donate 2 units of red blood cells using an *apheresis* (this concept is described in the automated collections section later in the chapter) instrument should not donate more frequently than once every 16 weeks.

In the past 12 months have you had a blood transfusion? Due to the possibility of a blood component transmitting an infectious disease, a donor who has received an allogeneic transfusion of red blood cells, plasma, platelets, or other blood component should not donate for 12 months. Donors who have received only an autologous blood transfusion do not have to be deferred, although inquiry into the reason for the autologous transfusion should be made as it could be a cause for deferral (e.g., in preparation for major surgery).

In the past 12 months have you had a transplant such as organ, tissue, or bone marrow? Due to the possibility of the transplant transmitting an infectious disease, a donor who has received an allogeneic transplant should not donate blood for 12 months after transplant. An autologous transplant is not reason for a deferral, although the reason for the transplant may be cause for deferral.

In the past 12 months have you had a graft such as bone or skin? Again, due to the possibility of the allogeneic bone or skin graft transmitting an infectious disease, a donor should not donate for 12 months after such a graft. Autologous bone or tissue graft is not reason for deferral, but the surgery to implant the bone or skin might result in deferral.

In the past 12 months have you come in contact with someone else's blood? If human blood comes in contact with a donor's open wound, mucous membrane, or nonintact skin, an infectious disease could be transmitted to the donor. The donor must be deferred for 12 months from the date of the contact.

In the past 12 months have you had an accidental needle-stick? A 12-month deferral is also indicated for a person who has had a needlestick with a needle used on another person. Any other sharp injury from an instrument used on another person would also defer the donor for 12 months.

In the past 12 months have you had sexual contact with anyone who has HIV/AIDS or has had a positive test for the HIV/AIDS virus? Anyone who has had sexual contact with a person with clinical or laboratory evidence of HIV infection must be deferred for 12 months from the date of the last sexual contact. HIV may be transmitted through sexual contact with an infected person.

The following four questions ask about sexual contact with persons who are at risk for having HIV or other diseases that may be transmitted through sexual contact. The donors should be deferred for 12 months from the date of the last sexual contact.

In the past 12 months have you had sexual contact with a prostitute or anyone else who takes money, drugs, or other payment for sex? Due to the risk of exposure to infectious diseases, anyone who has had sexual contact with a prostitute must be deferred for 12 months from the date of the last sexual contact.

In the past 12 months have you had sexual contact with anyone who has ever used needles to take drugs or steroids, or anything *not* prescribed by their doctor? Use of needles includes intravenous use or risk of contact with blood and blood vessels; skin popping, which is injection under the skin; mainlining, which is arterial injection; and any other use of a needle to administer drugs.

In the past 12 months have you had sexual contact with anyone who has hemophilia or has used clotting factor concentrates? Clotting factor concentrates manufactured from human plasma have a risk of transmitting HIV or hepatitis. Therefore, anyone who has had sexual contact with someone who has received any of these concentrates should be deferred for 12 months.

Female donors: In the past 12 months have you had sexual contact with a male who has ever had sexual contact with another male? Males check: "I am male." Due to the possible risk of exposure to HIV, female donors with such sexual contact should not donate for 12 months from the date of the last sexual contact with a man who has ever had sex with another man.

In the past 12 months have you had sexual contact with a person who has hepatitis? Hepatitis may be transmitted through sexual contact, especially hepatitis B. The donor must be deferred for 12 months from the date of the last sexual contact.

In the past 12 months have you lived with a person who has hepatitis?   There is a risk of acquiring hepatitis when living with a person who has hepatitis. Sharing of bathrooms, eating utensils, razors, toothbrushes, or other personal hygiene items have the potential for transmitting hepatitis from the infected person to the another person.

In the past 12 months have you had a tattoo?   People who have a new tattoo are deferred for 12 months from the date of the tattoo due to the risk of transmission of infectious disease. An exception is made for tattoos applied with sterile needles and nonreusable ink in a state-regulated tattoo parlor. The term *tattoo* includes tattoo touchups, tattoos applied by oneself, and those applied by others, as well as cosmetic tattoos, such as permanent makeup.

In the past 12 months have you had ear or body piercing?   If the ear or body piercing is performed using single-use equipment, there is no deferral. Otherwise, the deferral is for 12 months from the date of the piercing due to the risk of infectious disease transmission.

In the past 12 months have you had or been treated for syphilis or gonorrhea?   People who have had syphilis or gonorrhea, been treated for either disease, or have had a confirmed positive screening test for syphilis are deferred for 12 months from the date the treatment is completed.

In the past 12 months have you been in juvenile detention, lock-up, or prison for more than 72 hours?   People who have been detained or incarcerated in a facility for more than 72 hours are at a higher risk for exposure to infectious diseases. It doesn't matter why the person was incarcerated. The person is deferred for 12 months after their release from the facility.

In the past 3 years have you been outside the United States or Canada?   Immigrants, refugees, or citizens coming from a country endemic for malaria, the parasitic disease caused by infection with parasites in the genera *Plasmodium*, should be deferred for 3 years after they leave the endemic area and must not have had symptoms for malaria for at least 3 years. If a person has traveled to an area considered to be endemic for malaria, they are deferred for 12 months. The person is deferred for 12 months whether or not they have taken malaria prophylaxis. If they contracted malaria, they are deferred for 3 years after treatment or the last time that they had symptoms, whichever is last. Malaria risk areas are identified by the CDC and are updated as necessary. Donors who have traveled to Iraq must be deferred for 12 months after leaving Iraq because they may have been exposed to the parasitic diseases caused by *Leishmania* species known as leishmaniasis.

The following four questions are asked due to the small risk of developing variant Creutzfeldt-Jakob disease (vCJD) after eating beef from England. If a person did acquire vCJD, there is a possibility of transmitting the disease through a blood transfusion.

From 1980 through 1996, did you spend time that adds up to 3 months or more in the United Kingdom? Review a list of countries in the UK.   Donors must be given a list of countries that are part of the United Kingdom (UK) to ensure they understand which countries are included. These countries include the Channel Islands, England, Falkland Islands, Gibraltar, Isle of Man, Northern Ireland, Scotland, and Wales. People who spent a cumulative 3 months or more in the UK from 1980 to 1996 are indefinitely deferred from donating blood.

From 1980 through 1996, were you a member of the U.S. military, a civilian military employee, or a dependent of a member of the U.S. military?   Anyone who spent a cumulative 6 months or more associated on a military base in Belgium, the Netherlands, or Germany from 1980 through 1996 is indefinitely deferred. Those who were on a military base in Spain, Turkey, Italy, or Greece for 6 months or more from 1980 through 1996 are also indefinitely deferred.

From 1980 to the present, did you spend time that adds up to 5 years or more in Europe? Review list of countries in Europe.   People who have spent a cumulative 5 years or more in Europe are indefinitely deferred. The countries on the list for deferral of donors includes Albania, Austria, Belgium, Bosnia-Herzegovina, Bulgaria, Croatia, Czech Republic, Denmark, Finland, France, Germany, Greece, Hungary, Republic of Ireland, Italy, Liechtentein, Luxembourg, Macedonia, Netherlands, Norway, Poland, Portugal, Romania, Slovak Republic, Slovenia, Spain, Sweden, Switzerland, United Kingdom, and the Federal Republic of Yugoslavia.

From 1980 to the present, did you receive a blood transfusion in the United Kingdom or France?   People who were transfused in the UK or France since 1980 are indefinitely deferred.

The following three questions are asked to determine if the donor is at risk for HIV or other infectious diseases that may be transmitted through sexual contact. Donors must have read the educational materials provided. Not all donors define sex or sexual contact the same way.

From 1977 to the present, have you received money, drugs, or other payment for sex?   People who have used sex for trade are at a higher risk of sexually transmitted diseases, including HIV and some forms of hepatitis.

Male donors: From 1977 to the present, have you had sexual contact with another male, even once? Females: Check "I am female."

Have you ever had a positive test for the HIV/AIDS virus?

Have you ever used needles to take drugs, steroids, or anything *not* prescribed by your doctor?   People who have in the past or present used a needle to take nonprescribed drugs are indefinitely deferred due to the potential of transmission of infectious diseases. Needles that are shared may transmit disease.

Have you ever used clotting factor concentrates?   People who have been exposed to clotting factor concentrates are deferred indefinitely due to the possibility of the concentrates transmitting disease. While diseases such as hepatitis C were more likely to have been transmitted prior to the advent of current laboratory testing, this deferral still applies. An exception is made for donors who had a one-time use of factor concentrates for a medical condition, which will trigger a 12-month deferral.

Have you ever had hepatitis?   People who have had any type of viral hepatitis after age 11 are deferred indefinitely. If the donor had an "unknown" type of hepatitis before their 11th birthday, they are eligible to donate. This is because most hepatitis in children 10 years old and younger is hepatitis A. If the donor knows that they have had a positive test for or been diagnosed with hepatitis B or hepatitis C at any age, they are indefinitely deferred.

Have you ever had malaria?   People who have had malaria and have been treated appropriately for the disease are deferred for 3 years after they became asymptomatic. Malaria is transmitted by blood so it is important that the donor not have malaria or any risk of having malaria at the time of donation.

Have you ever had Chagas' disease?   People who have had Chagas' disease are indefinitely deferred. Chagas' disease is caused by the parasite *Trypanosoma cruzi* and it may be transmitted through blood. Currently there is no cure for this disease.

Have you ever had babesiosis?   People who have ever had babesiosis are indefinitely deferred since it can be transmitted through a blood transfusion and life-long parasitemia can follow recovery from illness. *Babesia* species are tick borne and can survive in RBCs and platelets.

Have you ever received a dura mater (or brain-covering) graft?   People who have received a dura mater graft from a human may be at risk for Creutzfeldt-Jakob disease (CJD) and are indefinitely deferred.

The next three questions are asked to determine if a person should donate blood if they have had certain medical conditions. Their eligibility to donate blood must be determined after further investigation and questioning of the donor. Each blood center must determine acceptable criteria and develop procedures to protect both the donor and potential recipients.

Have you ever had any type of cancer, including leukemia?

Have you ever had any problems with your heart or lungs?

Have you ever had a bleeding condition or a blood disease?

Have any of your relatives had Creutzfeldt-Jakob disease?   Donors who have a first-degree blood relative with CJD are indefinitely deferred. If the donor has had a laboratory test, such as gene sequencing, that shows the donor does not have a mutation associated with familial CJD, then the donor is eligible. If a donor does not know if any of their blood relatives have had CJD, they are eligible to donate. Only donors who know they have a relative who has or had CJD are deferred.

☑ CHECKPOINT 9-3

List three categories of blood donor deferrals.

CASE IN POINT *(continued)*

Each donor is given a Donor History Questionnaire to complete.

3. Donor #2 received a tattoo approximately 3 months ago. Can she still donate blood or should she be deferred? Why?

4. Donor #3 visited an area of Mexico that is endemic for malaria 13 months ago. Should he be deferred?

Physical Examination

In addition to the health history questions, the donor's vital signs must be taken and a hemoglobin or hematocrit check must be performed (Table 9-6 ✶). The AABB Standards require a donor's temperature to be less than or equal to 99. 5° F (37.5° C).[6] The blood pressure must have a systolic pressure less than or equal to 180 mm Hg and a diastolic pressure no higher than 100 mm Hg. The donor's pulse should be taken for at least 15 seconds and be 50–100 beats per minute. If the donor is athletic, a pulse less than 50 beats per minute may be acceptable. The pulse should also be regular. If the pulse is irregular, further questioning of the donor must be done to attempt to determine the reason for the irregular pulse.

For whole blood donations, a hemoglobin check can be performed using copper sulfate solution with a specific gravity of 1.053. A drop of blood from a fingerstick is put into a vial of the copper sulfate solution and if it falls to the bottom of the solution within 15 seconds, the blood has a hemoglobin level of at least 12.5 g/dL (125 g/L). The minimum hemoglobin level for an allogeneic whole blood donation is 12.5 g/dL (125 g/L). For automated double-RBC donations, the hemoglobin must be at least 13.3 g/dL (133 g/L). There are also instruments that may be used to determine the donor's hemoglobin or hematocrit from a capillary blood specimen obtained by fingerstick (Figure 9-2 ■).

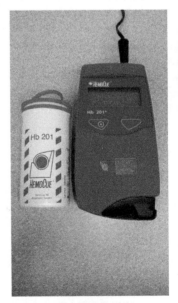
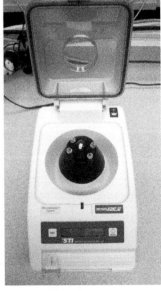

| Point of collection hemoglobin analyzer | Micro hematocrit analyzer |

■ **FIGURE 9-2**   Hemoglobin and Hematocrit Instruments
Source: Janet Young.

✳ **TABLE 9-6** Physical Examination Requirements and Restrictions

Physical Exam Criteria	Allogeneic Donation	Autologous Donation
Age	State law or ≥16 years of age	
Weight	110 lb (50 kg)	
Maximum Volume	10.5 mL/kg donor weight, including blood for laboratory testing	
Blood Donation Interval	8 weeks after whole blood donation 16 weeks after 2 unit RBC collection 4 weeks after infrequent plasmapheresis ≥2 days after plasma-, platelet-, or leukapheresis	
Temperature	≤99.5° F (37.5° C)	
Hemoglobin/hematocrit	≥12.5 g/dL (≥125 g/L)/ ≥ 38% (≥0.38) (not earlobe puncture)	≥11.0 g/dL (≥110 g/L)/ ≥ 33% (≥0.33)
Blood pressure	Systolic ≤180 mmHg Diastolic ≤100 mmHg	
Pulse (taken for at least 15 secs)	50–100 beats per minute and regular <50 bpm if an athlete	
Additional requirements		An order from patient's physician is required to donate All collections must be completed >72 hours prior to anticipated time of surgery

If the copper sulfate hemoglobin screening test fails, a hematocrit may be performed on a capillary blood specimen. Except for automated double-RBC donations, the hematocrit must be at least 38% (0.38) for allogeneic donations. For automated double-RBC collections, the hematocrit must be at least 40% (0.40). For automated single RBC collections, the requirement varies with the instrument used for the collection. For autologous donations, the requirements are lower; the hemoglobin must be at least 11.0 g/dL (110 g/L) or the hematocrit must be at least 33% (0.33).

Finally, the skin on both forearms, which is where the phlebotomy will occur, should be checked for any lesions, evidence of intravenous (IV) drug use, and ease of access.

☑ CHECKPOINT 9-4

What is the minimum required hemoglobin level for an allogeneic whole blood donation? What is the minimum required hematocrit level?

CASE IN POINT (continued)

Next, each donor was given a mini physical exam in which their vital signs were taken and hemoglobin levels checked. This blood center uses copper sulfate to determine whether the hemoglobin level is greater than or less than 12.5 g/dL (125 g/L).

5. The blood from donor #2 floated on the copper sulfate solution. What does this mean?

6. Should this donor be allowed to donate? Why or why not?

Consent

The donor's consent must be obtained prior to the actual donation. The consent form is often incorporated into one document with the Donor History Questionnaire. The consent form generally includes an attestation by the donor that he or she has truthfully answered the history questionnaire and understands the potential harm to others that could arise from untruthful answers; consent for transmissible disease testing, and any required notifications arising from the test results; consent for the blood donation procedure including agreement that the risks of the procedure are understood by the donor; consent for the blood to be used by the blood collecting facility; and agreement to contact the blood collecting facility if the donor decides after the donation that the blood should not be used.

The donor must sign and date the consent. The donor interviewer or reviewer of the donor questionnaire must also sign and date the health history record. When an automated procedure will be performed, the informed consent must contain a description of the procedure, the maximum donation frequency or minimal interval, a description of foreseeable risks, an opportunity to refuse the procedure, a right to ask questions, and an indicator that the donor has reviewed the information about AIDS and understands he or she should not donate if at risk of HIV infection.

Confidential Unit Exclusion

Donors must be given a confidential way to indicate that their blood should not be used for transfusion. This is referred to as **confidential unit exclusion (CUE)** and can be accomplished by a variety of methods.[6] A barcode label system can be used where the donor is given a card with two barcode labels. One label is identified as a "yes" label and indicates that the donor feels it is safe to use his or her blood. The other label is identified as a "no" label that indicates the donor believes he or she may not be a suitable donor. The donor selects one label and places it on the health history record. The barcode is scanned after the donation process and the donations from donors who selected the "no" barcode are discarded. A problem with this method is that the donor can accidentally select the wrong barcode label.

Another method is to give the donor instructions to call the blood center after the donation and ask that the blood collected not be used. A card with the donation number and a telephone number to call is given to the donor. The donor should be informed that even if they want to exclude their blood from being used after it has been donated, it will be tested and they will be notified of any positive results.

The donor must also be informed of circumstances when testing will not be performed. For instance, if a full unit of blood is not collected, testing may not be performed. Usually this information is included in the educational materials given to the donor prior to starting the health history interview. The CUE is one of the most important ways to ensure donated blood is safe for the recipient. Pressure from family, friends, or coworkers may cause someone to donate when he or she realizes they should not. The CUE provides a confidential way to indicate this when more open ways may not be acceptable to the donor.

> ### ☑ CHECKPOINT 9-5
>
> Why is the confidential unit exclusion (CUE) an important part of the blood donation process?

PHLEBOTOMY

Once the health history is complete, the donor is ready for the phlebotomy. For whole blood donations there are collection sets available in a variety of configurations. The type of collection set used is determined by the type of components to be produced (Chapter 10). Collection sets are available for collecting 450 mL (+/−45 mL) and 500 mL (+/−50 mL) of whole blood. The decision of which one to use is made by the blood facility, based on the blood products needed at the time. Donor requirements are the same for either volume of blood collected. It is important not to collect more than the maximum amount of blood allowed, which should be considered before using the 500 mL blood bag for a smaller donor. The maximum volume of blood that may be collected is 10.5 mL/kg of body weight. Therefore, for a donor who is the minimum weight of 110 pounds or 50 kg, the maximum whole blood that should be collected is 525 mL including the lab samples.

The whole blood collection set consists of one main bag used to collect the blood and other smaller bags attached to the main bag with plastic tubing. These bags are referred to as **satellite bags** and are used when the whole blood is made into various components such as platelets, plasma, cryoprecipitate, and red blood cells. Most often used are double- or triple-collection bag sets (Figure 9-3 ■). The blood collection sets must be approved by the FDA. They must be sterile and free from any extraneous material. The main blood bag used for the collection of the whole blood contains an anticoagulant. The two anticoagulants used for whole blood collection in the United States are citrate phosphate dextrose (CPD) and citrate phosphate double dextrose (CP2D). When red blood cells are stored using only these anticoagulants, they have a shelf life of 21 days.

Whole blood is not frequently utilized as such in the United States. Therefore, one of the satellite bags of most collection sets contains an additive solution (AS) to extend the shelf life of the red blood cell component to 42 days, twice the length of units without the additive solution. The additive solutions used in the United States include AS-1, AS-3, and AS-5. These solutions are different formulations of saline, adenine, glucose, and mannitol (SAGM). The additive solution is added to the red blood cells in the component preparation

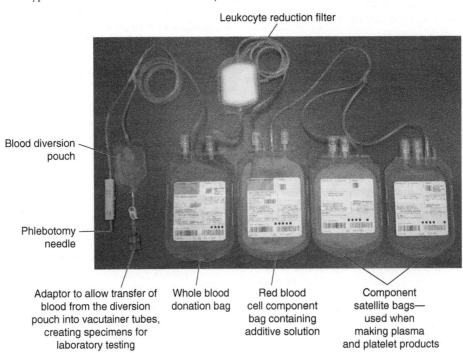

Leukocyte reduction filter

Blood diversion pouch

Phlebotomy needle

Adaptor to allow transfer of blood from the diversion pouch into vacutainer tubes, creating specimens for laboratory testing

Whole blood donation bag

Red blood cell component bag containing additive solution

Component satellite bags— used when making plasma and platelet products

■ **FIGURE 9-3** Blood Collection Set

Source: Janet Young.

laboratory after the plasma has been removed from the whole blood (Chapter 10).

Another anticoagulant/preservative in the main collection bag of some blood collection sets is citrate phosphate dextrose adenine (CPDA-1). The adenine (used for making ATP) is a nutrient in this solution that has been FDA approved for storing whole blood or RBC for 35 days.

Whole blood collection sets may also have a filter in the configuration that is used to remove white blood cells from the blood collected. In this type of configuration, the main collection bag is above the filter with another whole blood bag and the attached satellite bags below the filter (Figure 9-3) to receive the leukoreduced blood. The blood is filtered and collected into the bags below the filter and then components are prepared from the filtered whole blood. In other configurations, the cellular components (rather than the whole blood) are filtered to achieve prestorage leukoreduction.

Several whole blood collection sets are usually packaged together inside a foil pouch. Once that pouch is opened, the expiration date of the bags inside is shortened. The manufacturer's instructions determine the length of time the blood bags may be used. A large-bore needle, often a 16-gauge needle, is attached to the collection set. The needle size must be large enough to prevent hemolysis of the RBC and to allow the blood to flow fast enough to prevent the clotting process to start before the blood reaches the anticoagulant in the collection bag.

Prior to performing the phlebotomy, the donor's identity must be confirmed and compared with the DHQ. A unique identification number must be placed on the DHQ, the blood collection bag, and the tubes used for donor testing. This number is a confidential way of tracking the donated blood from collection through the actual transfusion to the recipient. Blood centers accredited by the AABB use an international donor identification numbering system called ISBT 128 (Chapter 10).

Selecting the vein to be used for the venipuncture is important. For whole blood the needle should be inserted into a vein large enough to accommodate the needle size. It should also be one that is anchored so that it doesn't roll when the needle is inserted. Usually a vein in the antecubital area of the arm is used. A tourniquet or slightly inflated blood pressure cuff applied to the upper part of the arm can be used to help distend the vein. This often makes it easier to find an appropriate vein.

Once the venipuncture site is selected, the area of the arm must be cleaned by using an antiseptic arm scrub. There are several products commercially available. Some consist of an alcohol scrub followed by application of an iodine solution in concentric circles, moving outward from the selected site for the needle entry. Other products only require the use of one agent. Because some people are sensitive to iodine, it is useful to have a product on hand that does not contain iodine as part of the arm-cleansing regimen. Whichever product is selected, the manufacturer's instructions must be followed for the arm scrub to ensure the area is effectively cleaned. Once the arm is prepared, the clean area must not be touched again until after the needle is inserted. The needle is inserted with the bevel side up to penetrate through the skin more smoothly and to allow the blood to easily flow into the needle.

Most blood collection sets have a sample diversion pouch on one side of a Y connector, which allows the first 20–40 mLs of blood collected to be diverted into the pouch (Figure 9-3). Once a sufficient amount of blood is collected in the diversion pouch, the pouch is sealed off and the blood is allowed to flow into the tubing on the other side of the Y connector and into the blood bag. It is extremely important that the blood collected is sterile; there are several ways to potentially contaminate it. Scrubbing the arm prior to the venipuncture may not completely remove all bacteria. A plug of skin may be removed when inserting the needle and this skin may harbor bacteria. In addition, bacteria may be found in subcutaneous hair follicles and glands or in areas with irregular skin or scarring at sites of repeated needle entries as in frequent donors. These areas may not be disinfected thoroughly using the normal scrub process. It has been shown that the first few milliliters of blood have the highest potential for bacterial contamination. Diverting this blood to the diversion pouch prior to allowing blood to flow into the blood collection bag has been shown to decrease the risk of bacterial contamination of the collected blood.[7] The blood collected in the diversion or sample pouch is transferred to tubes and used as the donation specimens for testing. The specimen tubes must be labeled with the same unique donor identification number that was placed on the blood bag. The FDA requires that the number must be placed on the tubes prior to filling them.

Most whole blood donations are completed within 5–10 minutes. If the donation takes too long, there is a risk that coagulation may begin. This can affect the quality of blood components used for clotting factors and platelets or result in the destruction of the entire unit if clots form in the whole blood. Blood collections requiring extended phlebotomy time should be identified so the component laboratory can carefully check for clots and determine the best components to be produced from the whole blood. If the flow of blood is very slow, a clot may form in the needle and block the flow of the blood. The collection process is discontinued when this happens and the donation may not have enough blood to be used by the blood center. These units are referred to as **quantity not sufficient (QNS)**, or *shorts*, and cannot be used for transfusion. When a phlebotomy is discontinued before the entire amount of blood is collected (300–400 mL of whole blood for the 450 +/− 45 mL collection set or 333–449 mL of whole blood for the 500 +/− 50 mL bag) and no clot is present, the red blood cells prepared from this unit are labeled "Red Blood Cells Low Volume." No other components may be made from a low-volume collection. An example of when a low-volume red blood cell unit might be collected is if the donor should have a vasovagal reaction and the collection is discontinued.

To ensure that an acceptable amount of blood is collected in the blood bag, a scale is utilized during the collection process. There are many different types of scales available. Some are a simple trip scale, which has an indicator that shows when the proper amount of blood fills the collection bag. Other commonly used instruments are a combination of an automatic mixer and scale (Figure 9-4 ■).

During the collection process, frequent mixing of the blood is necessary to ensure proper anticoagulation of the unit. When a trip scale is used, the blood must be manually mixed thoroughly and at regular intervals during the collection to prevent the blood from clotting. When electronic mixers are used, the blood is constantly mixed as well as weighed during the collection. Whichever method is used, the scales must undergo routine quality control checks to ensure that

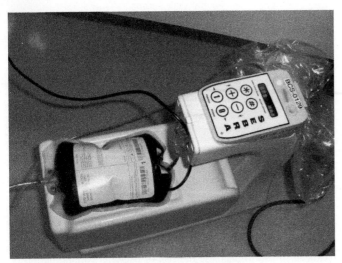

■ **FIGURE 9-4** Blood Collection Scale

Source: Janet Young.

they are accurate. The amount of blood collected at each whole blood donation cannot exceed 10.5 mL per kilogram of donor weight.[6] A donor must therefore weigh at least 110 lbs to be able to collect 450–500 mL of whole blood. Exceptions for weight may be made in certain circumstances, but a smaller blood volume needs to be collected and the volume of anticoagulant decreased appropriately.

Once an acceptable amount of blood is collected, the tourniquet is released and the tubing below the needle is clamped to stop the blood flow. When the needle is removed from the donor's vein, it is pulled into a protection device that covers the sharp end to protect from needlestick accidents. The donor is asked to hold a piece of gauze, applying pressure over the venipuncture site. The arm should be held straight (not bent) to help prevent a hematoma from forming. Once the bleeding stops, a pressure bandage is placed on the arm and the donor is instructed to leave the bandage on for several hours.

☑ CHECKPOINT 9-6

What are satellite bags, and why are they used in a whole blood collection?

 ### CASE IN POINT *(continued)*

The phlebotomy was started on all donors after consent was obtained.

7. Donor #1 asks why the needle has to be so large. How would you answer this question?
8. The blood center collects the whole blood in bags containing either CPD or CPDA-1 anticoagulant. What is the shelf life of the blood if left in the CPD? CPDA-1?
9. Would the shelf life change if an additive solution (AS-1, AS-3, or AS-5) were added to the CPD units after processing?

POST DONATION

The donor must be given post donation information concerning possible complications such as bruising, bleeding, or faintness and what to do if a complication should occur. The donor is sent to a refreshment area and asked to remain in the area for several minutes while consuming a beverage and a snack. This is because most donor reactions that occur happen within the first few minutes after the donation process. The time the donor is asked to wait in the refreshment area varies according to state or blood center regulation. California, for example, has a state regulation that the donor must wait in the collection area for 15 minutes or more.

After collection, the unit of whole blood is placed in a container that will cool the blood down to between 33.8 and 50° F (1 and 10° C), unless platelets are to be produced from the blood. If platelets are to be manufactured, the blood should be placed in a container that will cool the blood down to 68–75.2° F (20–24° C). The blood sample tubes collected for testing must also be placed into a monitored environment.

 ### CASE IN POINT *(continued)*

One day after donating a unit of whole blood, donor #4 wakes up with a fever of 102° F (38.9° C), sore throat, and general malaise. She calls the blood center to report her symptoms. The blood center feels that her symptoms are not a result of donating blood.

10. Should any other action be taken?

AUTOMATED COLLECTIONS

Apheresis is a procedure in which whole blood is removed from the body and a specific component is retained, while the remainder of the blood is returned to the donor. It can be used as a treatment modality for the removal of RBCs, WBCs, platelets, or plasma depending on the particular disease entity. Apheresis is the primary treatment or a common adjunct treatment for patients suffering from several diseases. For example, RBCs are sometimes removed in patients with certain serious complication of sickle cell disease or severe intracellular erythrocyte parasitemias such as malaria. Likewise, the removal of plasma from a patient can decrease the amount of an undesirable antibody present while excess number of platelets or immature WBCs (blasts especially) may be removed in myeloproliferative syndromes or leukemia. Another use of apheresis is to collect donor hematopoietic progenitor cells (stem cells) for marrow replacement in patients with leukemia or lymphoma or autologous stem cells for myeloma patients and others. Apheresis can also be used to collect specific blood products or any combination of blood products from blood donors.

The number of blood components collected by automation is growing rapidly as technology progresses. Figure 9-5 ■ shows one example of the numerous apheresis instruments available. There are instruments available that can collect two units of RBCs and return the plasma to the donor. The AABB Standards say to follow the instrument operator's manual when collecting these donors; however,

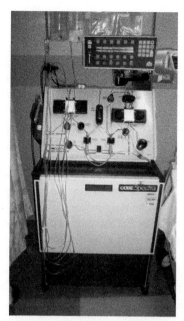

FIGURE 9-5 Apheresis Instrument

Source: Janet Young.

the collection shall not exceed a volume predicted to result in a donor hematocrit of less than 30% (0.30) or a hemoglobin value of less than 10.0 g/dL (100 g/L) after volume replacement. Donor requirements for a double-RBC collection are more stringent than for whole blood. Requirements are also different for males and females. For example, one manufacturer requires that male donors be at least 5'1" (155 cm) and weigh 130 pounds (59 kg), whereas female donors must be 5'5" (165 cm) and weigh at least 150 pounds (68 kg). Both genders must have a hematocrit of at least 40% (0.40) or a hemoglobin level of 13.3 g/dL (133 g/L) prior to collection. During the donation, saline is given to the donor to replace some of the blood volume removed. Donors must wait 16 weeks to donate again after donating a double RBC.

Sometimes 1 unit of RBCs and the equivalent of 2 units of fresh frozen plasma are collected. The donor criteria for this type of donation are the same as for whole blood donations. Again, saline is given to the donor to replace some of the additional blood volume removed as compared to a whole blood donation. Donors are deferred from donating for 8 weeks because only 1 unit of RBC is collected during this type of donation. A single unit or approximately 200 mLs of RBC can be donated once every 8 weeks.

Plasma collected by automation (**plasmapheresis**) may be donated once every 4 weeks. A maximum volume of 500 mL of plasma, excluding the amount of anticoagulant, can be collected from donors weighing 175 pounds (79 kg) or less at each donation. The total volume collected from a donor must not exceed 12.0 liters within a rolling 12-month timeframe. For donors weighing more than 175 pounds (79 kg), a maximum volume of 600 mL of plasma can be collected at each donation, not to exceed 14.4 liters within a rolling 12 months.

Plateletpheresis is the removal of platelets from the whole blood, with the plasma and RBCs being returned to the donor. Enough platelets can be removed from a single donor to produce a therapeutic dose for a patient, thereby avoiding exposure to multiple donors to achieve one therapeutic dose. Several companies produce instruments

that perform plateletpheresis. With technological advances, two or more therapeutic doses of platelets can sometimes be collected from one donor with a single procedure. The platelet count on the apheresis product must be sufficiently high to be able to split the product into a double dose or sometimes a triple dose of platelets. The donor requirements for donating platelets by automation are the same as for whole blood, with an additional requirement of a platelet count of at least $150 \times 10^3/\mu L$ ($150 \times 10^9/L$). Aspirin and piroxicam (Feldane) must be stopped for 48 hours prior to collection and the donor must be off of antiplatelet drugs such as clopidogrel (Plavix) for 2 weeks. It is important for the donor's safety to ascertain why he or she is on the antiplatelet medication and check with their doctor first to be sure they can safely stop the drug. A platelet count is not required prior to the first donation or if there have been more than 4 weeks since the last donation. However, having an accurate platelet count at the time of the donation increases the accuracy of the predicted amount of platelets collected by the instrument. Donors are eligible to donate a single plateletpheresis unit every 48 hours, not to exceed two donations in 7 days. The interval between a double or triple plateletpheresis donation should be at least 7 days. A maximum of 24 platelet donations can be made in a rolling 12-month period.[8]

The FDA requires that the amount of plasma and RBCs lost during each plateletpheresis procedure be recorded and the cumulative loss tracked over time. The requirements for plasma loss include the amount of plasma collected during platelet collections. The RBC loss includes the residual whole blood remaining in the collection set at the end of the procedure, whole blood in the sample tubes collected for laboratory testing, and any concurrent RBC collected in addition to the platelets. The accumulated laboratory data for plateletpheresis donors must be monitored by qualified staff and donor platelet counts less than $100 \times 10^3/\mu L$ ($100 \times 10^9/L$) must be reported to the medical director.

Plasma should be evaluated for hemolysis during and after the collection. If hemolysis is noted, the procedure should be stopped and the reason for the hemolysis thoroughly investigated. If there are visibly apparent RBCs in the platelet component, a hematocrit is then performed on the component. If more than 2 mL of RBCs are present in the platelet component, a blood sample from the donor must be attached for compatibility testing with the potential recipient.

When 1 unit of RBCs is collected, the donor is deferred for 8 weeks. If only 1 unit of RBCs is collected, the donor may donate platelets or plasma by apheresis within 8 weeks if the extracorporeal RBC loss during the apheresis collection is less than 100 mL. Most instruments used for automated platelet collections meet this requirement.

☑ CHECKPOINT 9-7

A donor is eligible to donate a double-RBC collection by apheresis every _____ weeks.

DONOR REACTIONS

Although most blood donations are completed without any difficulties, occasional donors experience an adverse reaction. The most common type of donor reaction is a vasovagal reaction which can cause the donor to faint. When a unit of whole blood is removed from the body, a portion of the person's blood volume is removed rapidly. If the donor stands up quickly from the donor chair, a certain percentage of blood gravitates to their feet. When the blood flow decreases, the normal response of the body is to try to restore the blood flow. The heart rate increases and blood vessels constrict to keep the blood pressure up, while the heart pumps more blood with each heartbeat. Normally, the blood flow is restored with no symptoms noticed. However, in a vasovagal reaction the body's response is abnormal. The heart rate does not increase and the blood vessels do not constrict, but instead may dilate. This results in a decrease of blood flow to the brain and sometimes a drop in blood pressure as well. The donor may lose consciousness. Symptoms of a vasovagal reaction include weakness, sweating, dizziness, pallor, and nausea. Donors may vomit, have convulsions, or have incontinence of urine or feces.

Other occurrences that are not uncommon are **hematomas** or **infiltrations**. A hematoma results from blood leaking from the vein and can be caused in several ways. The needle may be inserted too far initially and puncture both the proximal and distal sides of the vein, causing blood to leak into the surrounding tissue during the phlebotomy process. Removing the needle from the donor's arm prior to releasing the tourniquet increases the chance of hematoma because increased pressure is still on the vein. Not putting enough pressure on the venipuncture site after the needle is removed is the third cause of a hematoma.

Infiltrations are caused by fluid going into the interstitial tissue instead of the vein. This happens if a needle is not inserted into the vein far enough and the return pressure causes the needle to come further out of the vein. If any part of the bevel of the needle is outside the vein, fluid will go into the surrounding tissue. Infiltration can happen during automated blood collections when blood or saline is returned to the donor. Donor collection staff must be trained in handling various types of donor incidents or reactions. They should be certified in cardiopulmonary resuscitation (CPR).

> **☑ CHECKPOINT 9-8**
>
> What is the most common type of adverse reaction to a blood donation?

SPECIAL DONATIONS

There are three instances in which donations are made for a reason other than an allogenic donation: autologous, directed, and therapeutic. A description of each special donation type follows.

Autologous

An autologous donation is donating blood for one's own use; if this is done in preparation for surgery, it is referred to as **preoperative autologous donation (PAD)**. Autologous donation is not permitted if the donor has a clinical condition for which there is a risk of bacteremia. The time between autologous donations can be less than the interval required for allogeneic donations. The minimum hematocrit requirement is 33% (0.33) or if hemoglobin level is used minimum of 11.0 g/dL (110 g/L) for autologous whole blood and 35% (0.35) for autologous automated double RBCs (Table 9-6). These

donations are reserved for the patient's use only and cannot be placed into the regular inventory if not used by the donor. All donations by the patient-donor must be completed more than 72 hours before the time of planned surgery or transfusion. The units are labeled "For Autologous Use Only" and are stored in a separate location in the refrigerator from the allogeneic units. A method to ensure that the autologous units are given to a patient before any allogeneic units is strongly advised. Two other methods of decreasing the use of allogeneic blood for surgery patients are intraoperative blood recovery or normovolemic hemodilution, which are discussed in Chapter 11.

A shorter health history questionnaire can be used for autologous donors. The patient's physician must evaluate the patient first to determine if the patient's health is robust enough to permit blood donation. The surgeon or physician ordering the transfusion determines the number of units of blood that the patient will need for his or her surgery and the patient's physician and the transfusion medicine director will decide if the patient can donate this number of units in the time before surgery.

The patient may have a history that would normally exclude him or her from donating allogeneic blood for other patients, but would allow donation for him- or herself. For example, weight and age requirements do not apply to autologous donors unless their health might be endangered. The donor's blood, however, might be a risk to the phlebotomy and blood center staff, who should take precautions when collecting or processing blood from these donors. The patient's/donor's blood may also test positive for infectious diseases, if such testing is done. Testing of autologous donors beyond ABO and Rh is only required if the blood is shipped to another facility and only for the first donation collected during each 30-day period.[6] Some infectious diseases may disqualify further donations either as result of a blood center policy or because some hospital transfusion service medical directors may not accept units of blood with certain positive test results. These policies are specific to each transfusion center and are communicated to the blood collection center.

> **☑ CHECKPOINT 9-9**
>
> True or False: If an autologous blood unit is not transfused, it may be placed into regular inventory to be transfused to another patient.

Directed

Directed (designated) donations are blood donations made and identified to be used specially by a particular patient. In some countries, where a volunteer blood donation program is not well established, directed donations make up the bulk of the blood donations. In other countries, including those in North America, directed donations are uncommon.

In the mid-1980s when AIDS was determined to be transmitted through blood transfusions, even those patients living in countries with long established blood systems wanted acquaintances or family members to donate blood for them, a concept that was termed designated or directed donations. With the improvements in testing for HIV and other infectious agents, patient requests for directed donations have again tapered off. In some collection centers, the patient signs a request form and lists the names of people the patient would accept as a blood donor. The request contains the patient's blood type as well as the number of units required for the patient's operation or transfusion. Most blood centers also require a physician to sign the request. In other centers, donors arrive and identify the person they wish to donate for after the patient or family contacted them with a request to donate. Infectious disease testing is performed on all directed donation units. Directed donor units have special labeling and are stored in a separate refrigerator or separate location in the refrigerator from the allogeneic units intended for use for any patient who needs them.

This type of donation may lead to increased risks for the patients. For example, it is not advisable for a man to donate blood for his wife if she is of childbearing age, as this exposes her to antigens that may be present in future offspring, putting the fetus or baby at risk for hemolytic disease of the fetus and newborn (Chapter 14). First-degree relatives may increase the risk of transfusion-associated graft versus host disease, which can be fatal unless the units are irradiated to prevent this (Chapter 12). Numerous studies determined that directed donations are no safer than blood from the general public. There is concern that people asked to donate may not be completely honest when revealing their health history information. A donor may fear that he or she might be asked sensitive questions, which is information the donor may not want to reveal to the patient, friends, or family members. Often friends and family members go together to the blood center to donate and would be aware if someone was deferred, perhaps adding to the pressure. Furthermore, if a donor tests positive for any of the viral marker tests, their blood would be quarantined and the patient would be notified that they needed another donor, which could again lead to questions as to why the blood was not available for the patient.

The units of blood are identified as having been donated for a specific patient. Blood centers have different policies as to whether these units of blood may be placed in the general blood inventory if they were not used by the patient for whom they were designated or if they were incompatible with the patient. Some blood centers do not allow the crossover to the general blood inventory. Health history questionnaires, donor requirements, and laboratory testing (including infectious disease testing) must be the same as for any other allogeneic donation.

Allogeneic donations from unrelated volunteer donors may be set aside or collected for a specific patient because of antigen matching. Two common situations are plateletpheresis donors who are HLA-matched for a patient who is platelet refractory (Chapters 16 and 18) and donors who are RBC antigen–matched for a sickle cell patient on a transfusion protocol for stroke prevention (Chapter 17). Antigen typing is also done on RBC units to be given to patients with one or more RBC antibodies (there is a Rare Donor Registry for units with rare phenotypes). These units may cross over to the general inventory if the specified patient does not use them because the donors have met the same criteria as other allogeneic donors and the components have undergone the same testing as other allogeneic components. The labels on these units are the same as on other allogeneic units.

Therapeutic

Therapeutic phlebotomy is a procedure to remove blood from a patient, generally with a myeloproliferative disorder or neoplasm causing a high hematocrit. This category of phlebotomy is only performed with a physician's order and may be done every few weeks as needed. Patients with iron storage disorder (hereditary hemochromatosis) may also have phlebotomy performed. Generally, these units are not utilized for patients, but are discarded. The units could be used with a variance from the FDA if they met all the allogeneic criteria and are labeled with the condition for which the donor is being phlebotomized.

DONOR BLOOD TESTING

Blood donations must be tested for ABO group, Rh type, weak D when needed, and red blood cell antibody screening. Infectious disease testing *currently* required by the FDA on units intended for allogeneic use includes tests for syphilis, hepatitis B, hepatitis C, human T-cell lymphotrophic virus (HTLV), HIV, and West Nile virus (WNV). The required infectious disease testing must use FDA-licensed tests for antibodies to HIV (anti-HIV 1/2), hepatitis C virus (anti-HCV), human T-cell lymphotrophic virus (anti-HTLV I/II), and hepatitis B core antigen (anti-HBc). Also required are FDA-licensed tests for the surface antigen for hepatitis B (HBsAg) and nucleic acid testing (NAT) for HCV ribonucleic acid (RNA), HIV-1 RNA, and WNV RNA. The last required test is a serologic test for syphilis (Table 9-7 ✶). It is important to note here that the list of required tests is adjusted as necessary to ensure the safest blood supply possible.

Other tests, like antibodies to *Trypanosoma cruzi* (*T. cruzi*), the causative agent of Chagas' disease, is licensed by the FDA for screening blood donors and recommended for use. In January 2007, many blood centers started screening donated blood for anti–*T. cruzi* as the standard of care. Hepatitis B virus nucleic acid testing for DNA (HBV NAT) is FDA-licensed and also performed at most blood centers.

Blood samples with a positive antibody screen are tested further for antibody identification. Units of RBC prepared from donations with a positive antibody screen should have minimal amounts of plasma. Blood components, other than the RBCs, should not be used for the transfusion. The identification of the antibody must be recorded on the final label of the blood component unless the final RBC component is one that has had all of the plasma removed, such as washed RBC or frozen/deglycerolized RBC. This unit of RBCs may be given to a patient negative for the antigen to the donor's antibody. Many blood centers do not use RBCs from donors with antibodies and defer them from donation.

For most infectious disease tests, a positive screening test is repeated in duplicate. If two out of three results are positive, it is considered as repeat reactive or positive. A confirmatory test, if available, is performed. Positive confirmatory test results in the deferral of the donor from being an allogeneic blood donor. The donor must be notified of any confirmed positive test results. Blood components that test repeatedly reactive for any of the infectious disease tests must not be used for transfusion, except if they are for autologous donations. In addition, some positive test results must be provided to state health agencies as required by various state regulations. A **donor lookback** is performed whenever a repeat donor tests positive for an infectious disease when the donor was previously negative. In the donor lookback, the blood center checks which patient(s) received the blood products from this donor's previous donation and whether

---

☑ CHECKPOINT 9-10

How is a directed donation defined?

★ **TABLE 9-7** Table of Required Infectious Disease Testing using FDA-Licensed Tests

Testing For	Infectious Agent
Antibodies to:	Human immunodeficiency virus (anti-HIV1/2)
	Hepatitis C virus (anti-HCV)
	Human T-cell lymphotrophic virus (anti-HTLV-I/II)
	Hepatitis B core antigen (anti-HBc)
Antigens	Hepatitis B surface antigen (HBsAg)
Nucleic acid (NAT)	Hepatitis C ribonucleic acid (RNA)
	Human immunodeficiency virus—1 RNA
	West Nile virus (WNV) RNA
Serologic test (antibodies to nontreponemal antigens for screening and/or specific treponemal [syphilis] antigens for confirmatory testing)	Rapid plasma reagin (RPR)—nontreponemal
	Venereal disease research lab (VDRL)—nontreponemal
	Fluorescent treponemal antibody with absorption (FTA-ABS)—treponemal
	Treponema pallidum hemagglutination (TPHA)
Not currently required, usually tested	Antibody to *Trypanosoma cruzi*
	NAT for Hepatitis B virus (HBV) deoxyribonucleic acid (DNA)

the patient(s) contracted the disease for which the donor now tests positive. Generally, the transfusion medicine director sends a letter notifying the recipient's physician of the possible exposure to the disease with instructions on how to proceed with testing.

Physicians may request cytomegalovirus (CMV)–negative blood components for patients who are immunocompromised and known to be CMV negative. Some donations may be tested for CMV antibodies (total IgG and IgM) and the blood components labeled as CMV seronegative. Leukoreduction reduces exposure to CMV also because the virus is found within the WBCs. Seronegative, leukoreduced blood

products carry the least risk for infection with CMV. In other circumstances, such as RBC replacement for sickle cell patients, the RBC units can be tested for the presence of hemoglobin S.

As the causative agent for infectious diseases that are transmitted by blood are identified, new tests are developed. Donor blood testing may be performed under a research protocol to obtain information for submission to the FDA for licensure. The donor must give consent to participate in these research studies. The regulatory and accreditation agencies evaluate the research results to determine the need or benefit of using the test in routine blood donor screening.

Review of the Main Points

- The process defined as individuals who donate blood for their own future use is known as autologous donation.
- Allogenic donations occur when individuals donate blood for use by individuals other than themselves.
- Blood donated for a specific individual is considered as a directed or designated donation.
- The regulatory agencies in the United States that oversee blood donations vary by blood donation center location and may include the Food and Drug Administration (FDA), the Code of Federal Regulations (CFR), the organization formerly known as the American Association of Blood Banks, known as the AABB, and the European Union (EU) Standards.
- There are four components of the blood donation process: (1) registering the donor; (2) obtaining the donor's health history; (3) performing a "mini" physical exam; and (4) collection of the blood.
- Donors are given education material to read prior to donating blood to inform them about potential infectious diseases transmitted in blood, the signs and symptoms of acquired immune deficiency syndrome (AIDS), and the importance of providing accurate answers on the Donor

History Questionnaire (DHQ) and of not donating if they believe their blood should not be used for transfusion.

- Potential donors are required to complete a DHQ because this serves as an important step in protecting the safety of the blood supply.
- A temporary deferral occurs when it is determined that the donor may not donate for a limited amount of time due to potential exposure or vaccination.
- When it is determined that the donor has a condition or exposure that causes them to never be eligible to donate blood, the donor is put on permanent deferral.
- In instances when potential donors have a risk factor that under current regulatory requirements has an unknown deferral timeframe, the donor is placed on an indefinite deferral until such time that the regulations are changed resulting in the donor being acceptable for donating blood.
- AABB Standards require that potential donors have the following minimum vital signs and hemoglobin/hematocrit values upon physical examination prior to blood donation: (1) body temperature—less than or equal to 99.5° F (37.5° C); (2) systolic pressure of less than or equal to 180 mm Hg and

a diastolic pressure of no higher than 100 mm Hg; (3) pulse of 50–100 beats per minute tested over at least 15 seconds (less than 50 beats per minute is acceptable for athletes); (4) a value of at least 12.5–13.3 g/dL (125-133 g/L) hemoglobin, depending on the method used; (5) 38–40% (0.38-0.40) hematocrit value, depending on the donation method to be done; (6) a minimum of 11.0 g/dL (110 g/L) hemoglobin or hematocrit of at least 33% (0.33) for autologous donations.

- The purpose of a confidential unit exclusion (CUE) is to provide a confidential way for donors to indicate that their blood should not be used for transfusion.
- Blood donors are required to remain in the area after donation because most donor reactions occur within the first few minutes after completion of the process.
- Apheresis is defined as a procedure in which whole blood is removed from the body and a specific component is retained, while the remainder is returned to the donor.

- The most common post–blood donation reaction experienced by donors is a vasovagal reaction, which can cause the donor to faint.
- Autologous donations are done when individuals wish to donate blood for their own future use.
- Donations made for a specific individual are referred to as directed donations.
- Therapeutic donations are defined as instances in which individuals undergo phlebotomy to remove blood due to a medical condition.
- Blood donations must be tested for ABO group, Rh type, and weak D when deemed necessary and red blood cell antibody screening. In instances when a positive antibody screen is obtained, antibody identification must be done.
- Examples of FDA-required infectious disease assessments include tests for syphilis, hepatitis B and C, West Nile virus, HIV, and HTLV.

Review Questions

1. The blood donation process includes: (Objective #2)
   A. Donor registration
   B. Health history
   C. Physical examination
   D. Blood collection

2. According to regulations, the Donor History Questionnaire (DHQ) form: (Objective #3)
   A. May not be modified with respect to formatting
   B. Is not modified when new diseases or viruses emerge
   C. May not be modified or edited with respect to content or wording
   D. May not be modified to make screening criteria more restrictive

3. Select the medications that are on the permanent deferral list: (Objective #7)
   A. Etretinate (tegison)
   B. Proscar
   C. Accutane
   D. Growth hormone of human origin

4. Match the donor history with the appropriate deferral period: (Objective #7)
   1. _____ Babesiosis 2 years ago
   2. _____ Treatment for malaria 1 year ago
   3. _____ Blood transfusion 5 months ago
   4. _____ Sibling has Creutzfeldt-Jakob disease
   5. _____ Lived in United Kingdom from 1991 until 1993

   A. Permanent deferral
   B. Temporary deferral

5. According to AABB standards, the physical examination of an acceptable blood donor must include: (Objective #8)
   A. Pulse between 50 and 100 bpm
   B. Hemoglobin at least 10.5 g/dl
   C. Systolic pressure less than or equal to 180 mmHg
   D. Temperature less than or equal to 99.8° F (37.5° C)

6. Select the shelf life for a blood product that is preserved with each type of anticoagulant: (Objective #9)
   1. _____ CP2D
   2. _____ CPD with AS-1
   3. _____ CPD
   4. _____ CPDA-1

   A. 21 days
   B. 35 days
   C. 42 days

7. Which of the following criteria describe a low-volume unit collection? (Objective #10)
   A. Amount of blood collected is 450 +/− 45 ml
   B. No clot must be present in the collection bag
   C. Plasma must be removed and labeled for use within 6 hours of collection
   D. Blood unit label states "quantity not sufficient"

8. Most donor reactions occur within a few _____ after the donation process. (Objective #11)
   A. Minutes
   B. Hours
   C. Days
   D. Weeks

9. What is the deferral period after the donation of a single plateletpheresis unit? (Objective #12)

A. 24 hours

B. 48 hours

C. 3 days

D. 7 days

10. Mr. C developed a hematoma immediately after donation of a unit of whole blood. Which of the following steps in the collection process may have caused this to occur? (Objective #11)

A. The needle penetrated the distal part of the vein.

B. The needle was removed from the donor's arm after release of the tourniquet.

C. Adequate pressure was placed on the venipuncture site after the needle was removed.

D. The needle insertion caused fluid to penetrate surrounding tissue.

11. Which donor requirement distinguishes an autologous donation from an allogeneic donation? (Objective #14)

A. Photo identification is not required

B. Time interval between donations may be shorter

C. All transmissible disease test results must be negative

D. Weight and age requirements may be waived

12. Choose the circumstances when a directed donation can present a greater risk to the recipient: (Objective #15)

A. A man donates for his mother

B. Husband donates for his wife who is pregnant

C. Directed unit tests positive for a transmissible disease

D. Directed unit is crossed over to general inventory

13. Select the transmissible disease test that is *not* required to be performed on allogeneic donor blood: (Objective #16)

A. WNV

B. HTLV

C. CMV

D. Syphilis

14. What procedure should be performed when a repeat donor tests positive for an infectious disease marker that was not present in the previous donation? (Objective #19)

A. Confidential unit exclusion

B. Donor recheck

C. Review of Donor History Questionnaire (DHQ)

D. Donor lookback

15. Which unit modification reduces the exposure to CMV? (Objective #18)

A. Irradiation

B. Leukoreduction

C. Fractionation

D. Centrifugation

References

1. Official Journal of the European Union. *Commission Directive 2004/33/EC*, August 2, 2003.
2. Food and Drug Administration, Code of Federal Regulations, Part 606.160(e), Washington, D.C., April 1, 2005.
3. Food and Drug Administration, Guidance for Industry: Implementation of Acceptable Full-Length Donor History Questionnaire and Accompanying Materials for Use in Screening Donors of Blood and Blood Components, October, 27, 2007.
4. Food and Drug Administration, Guidance for Industry: Revised Recommendations for the Assessment of Donor Suitability and Blood Product Safety in Cases of Suspected Severe Acute Respiratory Syndrome (SARS) or Exposure to SARS , September 16, 2003.
5. American Association of Blood Banks, Blood Donor History Questionnaire Version 1.3, May 2008.
6. *Standards for Blood Banks and Transfusion Services*, 27th ed. Bethesda (MD): AABB; 2011.
7. Bruneau C, Perez P, Chassaigne M, Allouch P, Audurier A, Gulian C, Janus G, Boulard G, De Micco P, Salmi LR, Noel L. Efficacy of a new collection procedure for preventing bacterial contamination of whole-blood donations. *Transfusion* 2001; 41: 74–81.
8. Food and Drug Administration, Guidance for Industry for the Collection of Platelets by Automated Methods, December 2007.

Additional Resources

1. www.aabb.org
2. www.fda.gov/cber/blood.htm

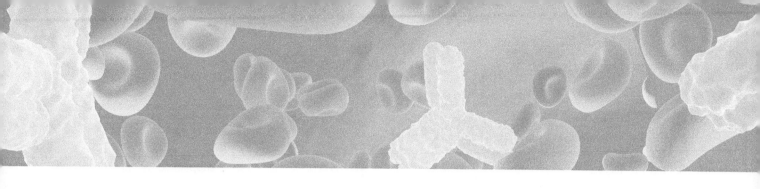

10

Blood Products
Preparation, Storage, and Shipment of Blood Components

COLLEEN YOUNG

Chapter Objectives

Upon completion of this chapter, the student will be able to:

1. Identify the major historical events that have contributed to the development of blood component production.
2. List the anticoagulants used in blood banking and explain the functions of the individual constituents of these anticoagulants.
3. Identify the components that can be prepared from whole blood.
4. Compare the types of transfusable plasma that can be prepared from whole blood with regard to processing and storage conditions and plasma protein levels.
5. Explain how cryoprecipitated antihemophilic factor (AHF) is prepared from plasma.
6. Identify the major plasma proteins present in AHF.
7. Compare the two methods used to prepare platelet components from whole blood and discuss the advantages and disadvantages of each method.
8. Discuss the principle for collecting blood components by apheresis.
9. Identify the types of blood components that can be collected by apheresis.
10. List the critical information that must be included on a blood component label.
11. Explain how ISBT 128 labeling of blood components enables an effective transfer of critical blood component information.
12. Define the term "red cell storage lesion."
13. Describe the adverse effects of storage on blood components.
14. Discuss ways that the adverse effects of storage can be moderated.
15. Describe the proper storage conditions for blood components that are prepared from whole blood.
16. Describe the conditions that must be met when transporting blood components.
17. Describe the principle of phase change materials that may be used in blood component transportation systems.
18. List the various types of modifications that may be made to blood components and explain the purpose of these modifications

(continued)

Chapter Objectives (continued)

19. Explain the difference between an open and a closed system for modifying blood components.
20. Discuss the impact of blood component modifications on storage conditions and component expiration.
21. Explain the principle for fractionating proteins from plasma.
22. Identify the three major categories of proteins that can be fractionated from plasma.
23. Describe the process for preparing proteins using recombinant technology.
24. Discuss the advantages of recombinant proteins over fractionated plasma proteins.

Key Terms

Apheresis
Apoptosis
Circular of information
Closed system(s)
ISBT 128
Labile plasma protein(s)
Open system(s)
Phase-change material(s)
Plasma press(es)
Red cell storage lesion(s)
Relative centrifugal force (RCF)
Satellite bag(s)
Satellite container(s)
Sterile docking
Tubing sealer(s)

CASE IN POINT

You work for a large hospital system that currently contracts with a local blood supplier for all blood products. Your contract is about to end and a new blood supplier has entered the market. The new supplier is physically much closer to your facility and its prices are very similar to the current supplier. However, there will be changes in the availability of some blood products. The senior administrative team at your facility has asked you to evaluate the differences based on your patient population to determine whether the new blood supplier can be considered.

What's Ahead?

The majority of blood component production is performed at blood centers that collect and process large numbers of blood donations. While some blood bankers may not have an opportunity to be directly involved in the processes discussed in this chapter, it is important to develop an understanding of the origin of blood products.

Separation of whole blood into components provides the best opportunity to maximize the value of each blood donation and is an integral part of transfusion medicine. It also ensures that patients receive only the portions of a donation that they require, thereby contributing to better patient care.

This chapter addresses the following questions:

- How are blood components prepared from a whole blood donation?
- Can individual blood components be collected from a blood donor?
- Why can some blood components be stored longer than others?
- How can blood components be modified to meet the specific needs of patients?
- Where do manufactured plasma protein products come from?

HISTORICAL BACKGROUND[1]

Until the discovery and development of anticoagulants in the early 1900s, human-to-human blood transfusions were restricted to collection and immediate transfusion or direct vein-to-vein connections between the donor and the recipient. This process created many challenges for physicians, particularly due to the tendency of the donor blood to clot, impeding the transfer of blood to the patient. The development of citrate as an anticoagulant in 1914 provided the first opportunity to remove this obstacle and pushed forward the development of transfusion.

The next challenge for transfusion medicine pioneers was to find a way to store donor blood prior to transfusion. Storage meant that blood could be collected before it was needed, allowing physicians to treat patients as soon as the requirement for transfusion was identified. In 1915, Richard Weil discovered that refrigerating donor blood prolonged the shelf life, allowing it to be stored for short periods of time. In 1916, Francis Rous and J.R. Turner discovered that, by adding glucose to citrate anticoagulant, they were able to extend storage by several days. These developments led to the establishment of

the first blood bank in Leningrad in 1932. The first American blood bank was opened by Bernard Fantus at the Cook County Hospital in Chicago in 1937. Fantus was the originator of the term *blood bank*.

A number of major advances occurred through the 1940s. Edward Cohn discovered that, by exposing plasma to cold ethanol at various temperatures and acidity levels, he could precipitate specific proteins, such as albumin, from donor plasma. John Elliot developed the first manufactured blood container in 1940, a glass bottle that was widely adopted by the Red Cross. In 1943, J.F. Loutit and Patrick L. Mollison developed a new anticoagulant preservative solution called acid citrate dextrose (ACD). ACD permitted the collection of larger volumes of blood with a higher ratio of blood to anticoagulant volume and also allowed for longer storage of collected blood. All of these developments made important contributions to the successful treatment of soldiers injured in World War II.

In 1950, the most significant advance in the preparation of blood components from whole blood occurred. Carl Walter and W.P. Murphy, Jr., developed the plastic blood bag, creating a collection system that allowed centrifugation and easy separation of individual blood components from whole blood. This innovation led to the development of component-specific patient therapies, allowing optimum utilization of every whole blood donation.

The 1960s and 1970s brought important developments resulting in a procedure in which whole blood is removed from the body and a specific component is retained while the remainder of the blood is returned to the donor, a process known as **apheresis**. Stated in another way, apheresis involves the collection and separation of whole blood into components at the time of donation. This automated process allows collection of specific blood components, such as platelets or plasma, rather than whole blood from a donor. In 1964, the process for obtaining apheresis plasma from donors was introduced and in 1972 the first successful cellular apheresis methods were developed. Apheresis technologies have provided a very efficient means of collecting the most appropriate components from each individual donor.

BLOOD BANK ANTICOAGULANT PRESERVATIVE SOLUTIONS

Anticoagulants are used primarily to prevent the activation of clotting factors and maintain blood in a liquid state for transfusion. Anticoagulants used in blood banking are citrate based, binding calcium and blocking the coagulation cascade. They also contain preservatives that extend the shelf life of blood components.

The anticoagulant preservative solutions that have been approved for blood bank use in the United States are citrate–phosphate–dextrose (CPD), citrate–phosphate–dextrose–dextrose (CP2D), acid–citrate–dextrose (ACD), and citrate–phosphate–dextrose–adenine solution (CPDA-1).[2] A list of the constituents found in these solutions and the purpose of each constituent is provided in Table 10-1 ✱.

☑ CHECKPOINT 10-1

Which of the constituents in anticoagulant preservative solutions prevents blood from clotting?

Table 10-2 ✱ shows the amounts of the constituents for each of the anticoagulant preservative solutions and their respective shelf lives.

PRODUCTION OF BLOOD COMPONENTS FROM WHOLE BLOOD

Whole blood is collected from a donor into a plastic collection bag containing anticoagulant. The volume of anticoagulant in the bag will vary based on the target amount for whole blood collection volume in order to maintain the appropriate ratio of anticoagulant to whole blood. Generally speaking, 63 mL of anticoagulant is used to collect a target volume of 450 mL whole blood, while 70 mL of anticoagulant will permit a target collection volume of 500 mL whole blood.[2]

The collection set also includes a number of **satellite containers** (also referred to as **satellite bags**) that are integrally attached to the main collection bag with hollow tubing. Satellite bags become the storage containers for the blood components prepared from the donation. The entire collection set is sterile on the inside and the satellite containers allow whole blood to be separated into individual blood components in a **closed system**. A closed system ensures that no foreign contaminants in the outside environment, such as bacteria, can enter the system. Figure 10-1 ■ shows a collection set with two attached empty satellite containers. A description of whole blood and components that can be made from it follows. It is important to note that although the purpose of generating blood components is to isolate specific blood components, small amounts of residual cells and/or plasma proteins that are not part of the targeted component may be contained in the product. For example, a unit of red blood cells typically contains residual white blood cells, platelets, and plasma proteins. Under most circumstances these small amounts of residual substances do not cause harm to a patient after transfusion. Modifications to blood products, as discussed later in this chapter, may be performed before or during transfusion to eliminate such potential problems when indicated.

✱ **TABLE 10-1** Constituents of Approved Blood Bank Anticoagulant Preservative Solutions

Constituent	Purpose	Associated Anticoagulants
Sodium citrate	Binds calcium and prevents initiation of coagulation	CPD CP2D ACD CPDA-1
Citric acid	Creates an acidic environment to slow down glycolysis that occurs through cell metabolism	CPD CP2D ACD CPDA-1
Dextrose	Provides a source of sugar for cell metabolism	CPD CP2D ACD CPDA-1
Monobasic sodium phosphate	Buffer to maintain pH	CPD CP2D CPDA-1
Adenine	Maintains ATP levels during cell metabolism	CPDA-1

★ **TABLE 10-2** Contents of Anticoagulant Preservative Solutions[4]

Anticoagulant-Preservative	Trisodium Citrate	Citric Acid	Monobasic Sodium Phosphate	Dextrose	Adenine	Shelf Life
Anticoagulant citrate–dextrose A (ACD-A)*	22.0 g/L	8.0 g/L	0	24.5 g/L	0	21 days
Citrate–phosphate–dextrose (CPD)	26.3 g/L	3.27 g/L	2.22 g/L	25.5 g/L	0	21 days
Citrate–phosphate–dextrose–dextrose (CP2D)	26.3 g/L	3.27 g/L	2.22 g/L	51.1 g/L	0	21 days
Citrate–phosphate–dextrose–adenine (CPDA-1)	26.3 g/L	3.27 g/L	2.22 g/L	31.9 g/L	0.275 g/L (27.5 mg/100mL)	35 days

*ACD is used for apheresis components.

Whole Blood

Whole blood contains all of the plasma and cellular components of blood. It is not typically used for transfusion anymore because most patients do not require all of the elements present in whole blood. Fresh, whole blood is sometimes used by the military in cases requiring massive transfusion support.[3] Separating whole blood into components allows multiple patients to benefit from a single blood donation. On average, whole blood has a volume of 450 or 500 mL and a minimum hematocrit of 0.38 (38%).[4] Figure 10-2 ■ shows a schematic of a whole blood donation.

Red Blood Cells

Red blood cells are the component that most people think of when they think about blood transfusion. Red blood cells are prepared by centrifuging whole blood in a very large centrifuge that can hold anywhere from 6 to 12 whole blood collection sets. Centrifugation causes the heaviest components of whole blood to settle at the bottom of the collection bag and the lighter components to stay on top. In general, red blood cells tend to concentrate at the bottom of the container, followed by white blood cells and platelets, which usually settle on top of the red blood cell layer. The top portion of a centrifuged collection bag contains the liquid plasma portion of whole blood.

After centrifugation, the blood unit is placed into a device known as a **plasma press**, also called an *expresser*, that is designed to apply firm, even pressure to the bag, forcing plasma out through the connection tubing into an empty satellite container. A plasma press may be a simple spring-driven manual device or it may be a more sophisticated semi-automated device. Semi-automated plasma presses are usually fluid- or pump-driven and may have optical sensors that cause the equipment to stop pressing at the appropriate time to optimize the quality of the components, for example, preventing red blood cells from entering the plasma component.

Once the plasma has been pressed, the resulting red blood cells and plasma bags can be separated by using a **tubing sealer** to close off the connection tubing and then detaching the components at the

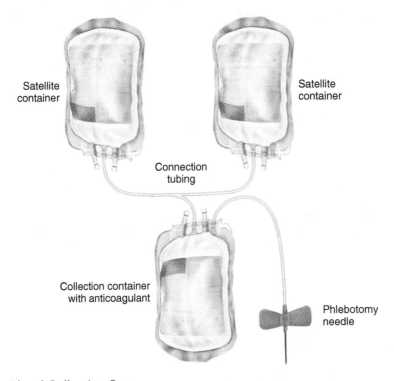

Satellite container

Satellite container

Connection tubing

Collection container with anticoagulant

Phlebotomy needle

■ **FIGURE 10-1**   Whole Blood Collection Set

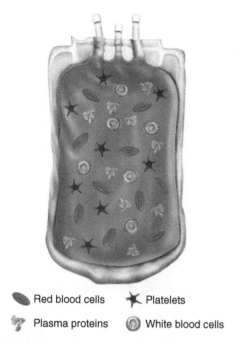

Red blood cells   ★ Platelets

🦠 Plasma proteins   ◉ White blood cells

■ **FIGURE 10-2**   Whole Blood

seals. Tubing sealers ensure that the system remains closed and that sterility is maintained. Electronic tubing sealers use high-frequency radio waves to generate heat that melts the plastic tubing and seals it closed. Figure 10-3 ■ shows how a whole blood unit is separated into a red blood cell and a plasma component.

A red blood cell component will generally have a volume of 225–350 mL and a hematocrit of 0.65 (65%) to 0.80 (80%). If an additive solution is used to prolong shelf life, the final volume of the component will vary from 300 to 400 mL and the hematocrit will be somewhat lower, at 0.55–0.65 (55–65%). The hemoglobin in a patient who is not actively bleeding is expected to increase 1 g/dL for each unit of blood transfused.[2] A typical red blood cell unit prepared from whole blood contains 50–80 grams of hemoglobin.[4]

☑ **CHECKPOINT 10-2**

How does a tubing sealer maintain the sterility of a blood component?

Plasma

Plasma separated from whole blood can be used for different purposes, depending on the collection, processing, and storage conditions. In most cases, plasma is stored frozen to preserve the activity of **labile plasma proteins**. Labile plasma proteins are proteins that break down easily during refrigerated storage or standing at room temperature. Examples of labile proteins include coagulation factors V and VIII.

Plasma for Transfusion

Plasma for transfusion is generally processed and frozen as soon as possible after separation from red blood cells. Frozen plasma must be thawed prior to transfusion and may be stored in a thawed state

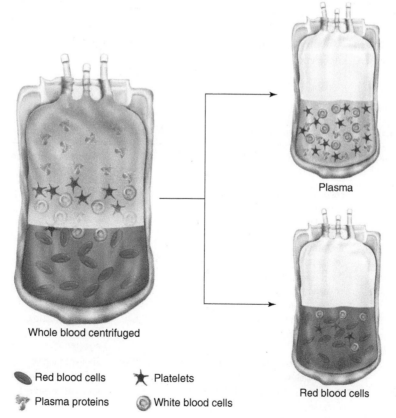

Whole blood centrifuged

Plasma

Red blood cells

🔴 Red blood cells   ★ Platelets

🦠 Plasma proteins   ◉ White blood cells

■ **FIGURE 10-3**   Whole Blood Separated into Red Blood Cells and Plasma for short periods of time with minimal impact on its effectiveness. Plasma is considered to have 1 unit of each coagulation factor in every 1 mL of fresh frozen plasma (FFP). Whole blood–derived plasma components vary in volume but normally range from 200 to 300 mL.[2] Table 10-3 ✳ identifies the types of transfusable plasma, processing and storage conditions, and differences in plasma protein levels.

Cryoprecipitated Antihemophilic Factor

Fresh frozen plasma can be further processed to produce cryoprecipitated antihemophilic factor (AHF) and plasma, cryoprecipitate reduced, as noted in Table 10-3. When frozen FFP is thawed slowly at 33.8–42.8° F (1–6° C) (instead of rapidly in a circulating 98.6° F [37° C] water bath), proteins that are insoluble in the cold will precipitate out. After centrifugation, the majority of the plasma is extracted from the precipitated protein sediments into a satellite container. Plasma extraction may be done by gravity or with a plasma press. Figure 10-4 ■ shows how cryoprecipitated AHF is prepared from FFP.

The cold-insoluble proteins that precipitate out of solution include Factor VIII, fibrinogen, von Willebrand factor (vWF), Factor XIII, and fibronectin. A small volume of residual plasma, 15 mL or less, is left with these factors in the component. Each cryoprecipitated AHF component prepared from whole blood must contain a minimum of 80 international units (IU) of Factor VIII and 150 mg of fibrinogen.[2]

The plasma that is extracted from the precipitate is called plasma, cryoprecipitate reduced. It is acceptable for use in transfusion but has some restrictions because it has been depleted of the coagulation proteins that are contained in cryoprecipitated AHF. As such, it cannot be used interchangeably with fresh frozen plasma; for example, it should not be given to a patient with Factor XIII deficiency.[4]

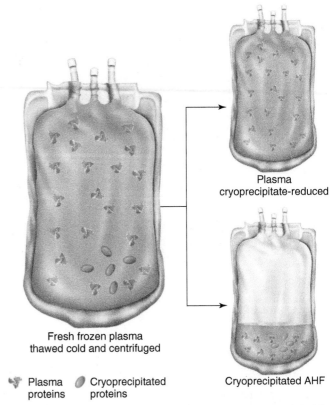

Plasma cryoprecipitate-reduced

Fresh frozen plasma thawed cold and centrifuged

Cryoprecipitated AHF

🦐 Plasma proteins   〇 Cryoprecipitated proteins

■ **FIGURE 10-4**   Production of Cryoprecipitated AHF

☑ **CHECKPOINT 10-3**

How many units of cryoprecipitated AHF should be given if 240 international units (IU) of Factor VIII is requested for transfusion?

✳ **TABLE 10-3** Transfusable Plasma Components from Whole Blood[2, 4]

Transfusable Plasma Component	Processing and Storage Conditions	Plasma Protein Levels
Fresh frozen plasma (FFP)	• Processed and placed in freezer within 8 hours of collection for CPD, CD2D, or CPDA-1 or within 6 hours for ACD. • Stored frozen (≤−64° F [≤−18° C] for 12 months or (≤−149° F [≤−65° C] for 7 years). • Once thawed, may be stored for 24 hours in the refrigerator.	Levels of stable and labile proteins are similar to that of freshly collected plasma.
Plasma frozen within 24 hours after phlebotomy (FP or FP24)	• Processed and placed in a freezer within 24 hours of collection. • Stored frozen.	Levels of stable proteins are similar to that of FFP. Factor V levels are similar to FFP; Factor VIII levels are somewhat reduced.
Thawed plasma	Prepared from FFP thawed at 86–98.6° F (30–37° C) and stored refrigerated for up to 5 days.	Levels of stable proteins are similar to that of FFP. Factor V and Factor VIII levels drop through the storage period.
Liquid plasma	Plasma extracted from whole blood up to 5 days after expiration, stored refrigerated or frozen.	Similar to thawed plasma with more significant reductions in Factor V and Factor VIII levels.
Plasma, cryoprecipitate reduced	FFP thawed at 33.8–42.8° F (1–6° C). Separated into cryoprecipitated AHF and plasma, cryoprecipitate reduced; stored frozen.	Reduced levels of FVIII, vWF, fibrinogen, FXIII, and fibronectin.

CASE IN POINT *(continued)*

The plasma products that each blood center provides are different. You purchase FFP from your current blood supplier. The new blood supplier makes only limited amounts of FFP and sells mostly FP24.

1. What is the primary difference between FFP and FP24?
2. Is there any difference in expiration date between FFP and FP24?

Plasma wastage in your hospital has been high. Your Laboratory Medical Director has asked the medical staff to consider transfusing thawed plasma with a 5-day expiration to all patients requiring plasma to help decrease plasma wastage.

3. What is the advantage of turning a frozen FFP or FP24 into thawed plasma versus thawed FFP or thawed FP24?
4. What is the disadvantage of using thawed plasma over thawed FFP or thawed FP24?
5. If the medical staff decides to switch to thawed plasma, will it matter whether the frozen product is FFP or FP24?

Solvent/Detergent-Treated Plasma

In a large-scale controlled manufacturing environment, plasma from up to 2,500 donors can be pooled and treated with a solvent/detergent solution. The solution inactivates lipid-enveloped viruses such as human immunodeficiency virus (HIV), hepatitis B virus (HBV), and cytomegalovirus (CMV) by breaking down the lipid envelope. Viruses without envelopes such as hepatitis A virus (HAV) and parvovirus are not inactivated by the solvent/detergent process and must be treated with a second process to inactivate them. The pooled plasma is then aliquoted into 200 mL bags and stored frozen. The process causes a slight reduction in all coagulation proteins, but its use is similar to FFP.[2] Solvent-/detergent-treated plasma is currently not licensed in the United States or Canada, but is in use in Europe.

Plasma for Further Manufacturing

Instead of preparing transfusable plasma components for direct transfusion to patients, plasma may be sent to manufacturers that can separate out individual proteins, such as albumin or specific coagulation factors, for patient use. Plasma that is intended to be used for this process is called recovered plasma or plasma for manufacture.

Platelets

Production of platelet components from whole blood donations requires special handling of a whole blood unit starting from the time of collection. Platelet function is impaired following storage at colder temperatures,[5] so donations must be maintained at room temperature during all stages of collection, storage, and production.[2] There are two approved methods for extracting platelet components from whole blood donations. The platelet-rich plasma (PRP) method produces a single platelet component from a single whole blood donation and is widely used in the United States. The buffy coat (B/C) method produces a pool of platelets from four to six whole blood donations and is the most common method in Europe and in Canada. Both processes are two-stage, requiring two separate centrifugation and extraction steps to produce the platelet component.

☑ CHECKPOINT 10-4

Which type of platelet component, single platelet or pooled platelet, has less risk for transmission of a blood-borne pathogen?

Platelet-Rich Plasma Production

The first stage of PRP production is the recovery of platelet-rich plasma from a whole blood donation. This is achieved by centrifuging the whole blood at a low **relative centrifugal force (RCF)**. Relative centrifugal force is a measure of how much gravitational force (*g*-force) is applied to the bag during centrifugation and is a function of the speed of rotation, the amount of time that the centrifugal force is applied, and the radius of centrifugation. Generally, the radius of centrifugation remains constant, so RCF can be manipulated by changing the time of centrifugation and/or the speed of rotation. Lowering the RCF, also referred to as a "soft spin," applies less gravitational force to the whole blood, causing the platelets to remain suspended in the plasma rather than being forced down onto the red blood cell layer.

The centrifuged whole blood is placed on a plasma press and the platelet-rich plasma is expressed into an empty satellite container. Figure 10-5 ■ shows the production of platelet-rich plasma and a red blood cell component from whole blood.

The second stage of PRP production is the preparation of a platelet concentrate. The platelet-rich plasma is centrifuged at a relatively high RCF, also called a "hard spin," causing the platelets to concentrate or aggregate into a pellet at the bottom of the bag. The bag is then placed on a plasma press that expresses the majority of the supernatant plasma into another empty satellite container. The platelet-rich plasma is then allowed to rest on the counter, letting the aggregated platelets resuspend into the supernatant plasma. Figure 10-6 ■ shows the production of a platelet component and a plasma component from the platelet-rich plasma.

A single component of PRP produced from whole blood will contain a minimum of 5.5×10^{10} platelets and a total volume of 40–70 mL.[4] There may be a small number of residual red blood cells present, but the total number cannot exceed 1.0×10^9 red blood cells per component.[2] Adult transfusion normally requires four to eight PRP platelet components, each prepared from one whole blood donation.[4]

☑ CHECKPOINT 10-5

Each unit of platelet-rich plasma (PRP) prepared from whole blood contains a minimum of _____ platelets per component.

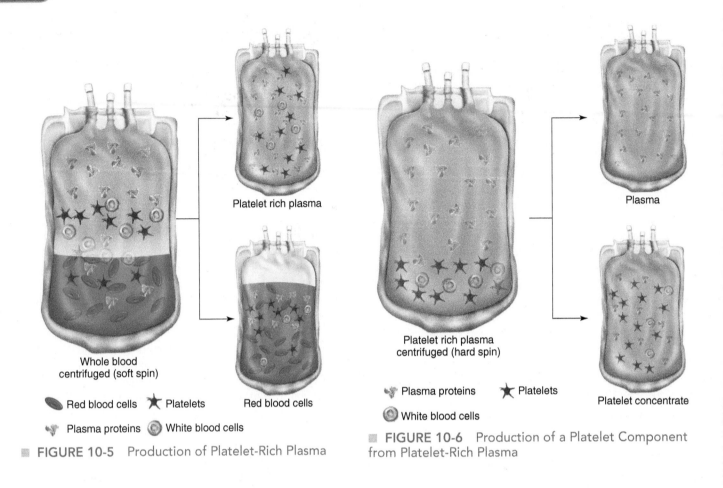

FIGURE 10-5 Production of Platelet-Rich Plasma

Whole blood centrifuged (soft spin)

Platelet rich plasma

Red blood cells

Red blood cells | Platelets

Plasma proteins | White blood cells

FIGURE 10-6 Production of a Platelet Component from Platelet-Rich Plasma

Plasma

Platelet rich plasma centrifuged (hard spin)

Platelet concentrate

Plasma proteins | Platelets

White blood cells

Buffy Coat Production

The buffy coat (B/C) platelet production method reverses the steps that are used in PRP production. In B/C production, the whole blood is first subjected to a hard spin. This causes the red blood cells to concentrate at the bottom of the unit, followed by the white blood cells and the platelets that sit on the red blood cell layer in a "buffy coat." The plasma remains at the top of the bag.

The centrifuged whole blood is placed on a semi-automated plasma press. Pressing depends on the type of collection bag and placement of the empty satellite containers. In a "top/top" configuration, the plasma is first expressed into an empty satellite container, followed by the buffy coat layer into a second empty satellite container. In a "top/bottom" configuration, the plasma is pressed up into an empty satellite and the red blood cells are simultaneously pressed down into another empty satellite; the B/C remains in the collection container. Figure 10-7 ■ shows how a whole blood donation is processed into a red blood cell component, a plasma component, and a buffy coat.

The second stage of B/C platelet production starts with pooling buffy coats prepared from four to six whole blood donations, along with either one plasma component or a bag of platelet additive solution. The plasma or additive solution is used to suspend the platelets and provide nutrients during storage. Pooling is achieved by **sterile docking** the connection tubing of the satellite containers together. Sterile docking is done using a small bench-top device that welds

connection tubing together while maintaining a closed system. The four to six buffy coats and the plasma or additive solution are all pooled together into one satellite container.

The B/C pool is centrifuged using a soft spin. This causes the red blood cells and white blood cells to move toward the bottom of the bag, but the platelets remain suspended in the plasma or additive solution. The centrifuged pool is placed on a semi-automated plasma press and the pooled platelet concentrate is expressed into a platelet storage container. Because buffy coats are very rich in white blood cells, the pooled platelet concentrate is usually pressed through a filter that traps the majority of white blood cells and prevents them from entering the platelet component. The red blood cells and white blood cells that remain in the pooling container are discarded. Figure 10-8 ■ shows the production of a pooled platelet component from a buffy coat pool.

A B/C pooled platelet component will contain a variable number of platelets per component depending on the number of buffy coats pooled. In Canada, a standard pool is prepared from four buffy coats and will have a minimum of 240×10^9 platelets per pooled component and a volume of approximately 300 mL.[6] One pooled B/C platelet is generally considered a normal adult dose for transfusion.

Comparing Platelet Production Methods

Table 10-4 ✶ shows the differences between the PRP and B/C methods for preparing platelet components.

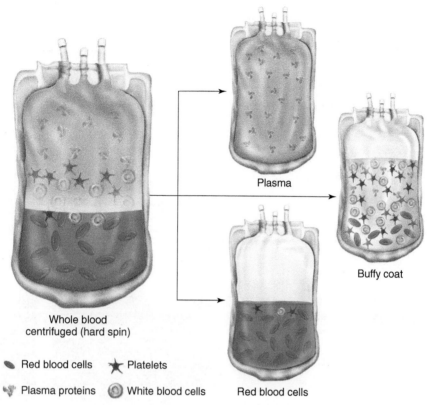

Plasma

Buffy coat

Whole blood
centrifuged (hard spin)

Red blood cells

🫘 Red blood cells   ⭐ Platelets

🦠 Plasma proteins   ⚪ White blood cells

FIGURE 10-7   Production of a Buffy Coat from Whole Blood

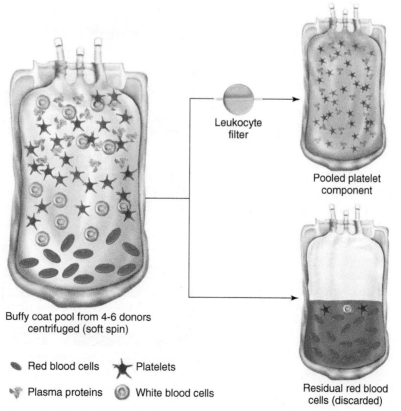

Leukocyte
filter

Pooled platelet
component

Buffy coat pool from 4-6 donors
centrifuged (soft spin)

Residual red blood
cells (discarded)

🫘 Red blood cells   ⭐ Platelets

🦠 Plasma proteins   ⚪ White blood cells

FIGURE 10-8   Production of a Pooled Platelet Component from a Buffy Coat Pool

✳ **TABLE 10-4** Comparison Chart for Platelet Components Produced from Whole Blood

Production Method	Processing	Key Advantages	Key Disadvantages
Platelet-rich plasma (PRP)	• Soft spin to produce platelet-rich plasma • Hard spin to concentrate platelets • Resuspension of aggregated platelets into supernatant plasma	• Individual components allow dosing based on patient needs (e.g., pediatric use) • Red blood cells from the whole blood donation are not lost during processing	• Concentrating platelets into a pellet causes platelet activation and platelet aggregation • Soft spin of whole blood traps a significant amount of plasma and platelets in the red blood cell layer
Buffy coat (B/C)	• Hard spin to concentrate platelets in the buffy coat layer • Pooling and soft spin to remove red blood cell contamination	• Concentrating platelets in the buffy coat layer reduces platelet activation and results in better platelet quality • Hard spin of whole blood minimizes the amount of plasma and platelets trapped in the red blood cell layer	• Pooled product is not ideal for pediatric use • Some red blood cells are lost in the buffy coat • Requires the use of specialized equipment, such as a semi-automated plasma press and sterile docking device

☑ **CHECKPOINT 10-6**

Which platelet component, single platelet or pooled, is preferred for the transfusion of a newborn infant?

Granulocytes

Granulocytes, sometimes referred to as *white blood cells*, are not often prepared from whole blood, as the apheresis collection technique results in a much higher number of granulocytes per collection. When a granulocyte component is prepared from whole blood, it is done by isolating the buffy coat. Hydroxyethel starch (HES), a precipitating agent, is added to the whole blood and the bag is left to settle by gravity. The plasma and the buffy coat layer are extracted into a satellite container using a manual or semi-automated press. The satellite container is centrifuged using a hard spin to concentrate the granulocytes and the majority of plasma is expressed using a plasma press. A granulocyte component prepared from whole blood generally contains 1.25×10^9 granulocytes and has a hematocrit of about 0.04 (4%).[2]

COLLECTION OF BLOOD COMPONENTS BY APHERESIS

Apheresis collections use a machine to draw whole blood from a donor, separate the blood, collect only the components that are required from that donor, and return the remainder to the donor, usually through the same collection line. The entire process occurs in a closed system. Figure 10-9 ■ shows photographs of one type of apheresis machine collecting from a donor.

Most apheresis machines use centrifugation to separate the various whole blood components. The collection set, which usually contains some type of centrifuge bowl or cone, is loaded into the machine and the donor is attached to the collection set through phlebotomy. As the machine rotates the centrifuge bowl, whole blood is drawn into the bowl and is mixed with ACD anticoagulant. When the centrifuge bowl reaches capacity, the machine increases the rate of rotation to optimal centrifugation speed and separates the whole blood into components. The selected component is drawn into a collection container and

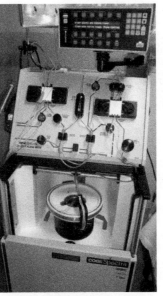
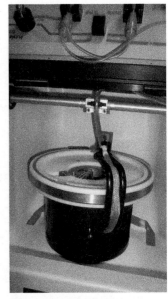

(a) Single use collection set loaded into an apheresis machine

(b) Centrifugation bowl

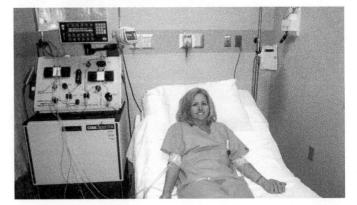

(c) Collection set is attached to the donor's circulation through one or two venipuncture sites (depending on the type of pheresis and instrument)

■ **FIGURE 10-9** Equipment for Collecting Components by Apheresis

Source: Janet Young.

✱ **TABLE 10-5** Blood Components Collected by Apheresis[2, 4]

Component Name	Product Characteristics
Plasma apheresis	• Volumes vary based on the weight of the donor, but the maximum is 600 mL • Plasma may be used as FFP or as plasma for manufacture • May be collected together with an apheresis platelet donation
Platelets apheresis	• Minimum acceptable platelet count is 3×10^{11} per component • Volume can vary from 100 to 500 mL • One platelet apheresis is equivalent to one adult dose of platelets • A high-yield apheresis platelet collection can be divided into more than one platelet apheresis component, as long as each component contains a minimum of 3×10^{11} platelets
Red blood cells apheresis	• Very similar to red blood cell components prepared from whole blood • Normally contain about 60 g of hemoglobin per component • May be collected together with an apheresis platelet and/or an apheresis plasma • Two red blood cell apheresis components can be collected from one donor if the donor meets eligibility requirements and no other apheresis components are collected during the same donation
Granulocytes apheresis	• Donors may be given drugs, such as corticosteroids or growth factors (G-CSF), or precipitating agents, such as hydroxyethyl starch (HES), to increase the number of granulocytes that can be collected • The minimum number of granulocytes per component is 1×10^{10}

the remainder of the donation is returned to the donor. This is often achieved by reversing the rotation of the centrifuge bowl. More than one collection and return cycle is normally required to complete a collection.

Apheresis can be used to collect plasma, platelet, red blood cell, and granulocyte components. Table 10-5 ✱ provides information about the types of components that can be collected.

CASE IN POINT (continued)

Currently you purchase both apheresis platelet products and whole blood–derived platelets (PRP method) from your blood supplier. The new blood supplier does not manufacture whole blood–derived platelets and will only provide apheresis platelet products.

6. What is the difference between a PRP platelet and an apheresis platelet based on volume and minimum platelet count?

7. How many units of PRP platelets are generally pooled to make one dose of platelets?

8. How many units of apheresis platelets make up one dose of platelets?

BLOOD COMPONENT LABELING

Blood component labeling is a critical control point in blood component production. Labeling is the stage where all donation, production, and testing records are reviewed and acceptable components are released to inventory to be made available for transfusion. Blood components that are unacceptable for any reason are removed from inventory.

The label on a blood component provides all of the information necessary to handle the product appropriately. It also creates a link, through the donation identification number, back to the original donor of the component. Information must be present in an eye-readable format. A barcode containing the same information may also be present. Barcode scanners are used to electronically transfer

the data to information systems. In addition to the product label, blood agencies are required to provide a **circular of information** to anyone involved in blood transfusion. The circular provides critical information about each blood component and how it is to be used.[2]

International Society for Blood Transfusion 128 Labeling

Until recently, each blood agency developed its own product labels in accordance with regulations and standards. This meant that the format of the information provided was not standardized and that the codes that were used to communicate critical information, such as blood group or component type, were not consistent. This lack of standardization increased the risk of error when hospitals received blood components from different blood suppliers.

In 2006, the AABB moved toward adopting the **ISBT 128** global standard for blood component labeling. The ISBT 128 standard was developed in 1994 by the International Society for Blood Transfusion (ISBT) and provides standards for the information that must be present on the blood component label. It also defines the structure of the barcodes used to code the information for computer systems. This standardized approach eliminates any duplication of identification numbers around the world and ensures traceability of blood components back to the original donor. It also ensures that critical information, such as product code and blood group, is communicated in a standard format to reduce the risk of error.

At minimum, the following critical pieces of information must be present on the ISBT 128 component label[7]:

• *Donation identification number.* This unique identifier is assigned at the time of donation and is carried through on every component that is produced from the donation. The donation identification number provides traceability back to the original donor and includes, as part of the number, a unique facility identification code. The facility identification code provides traceability back to the collection/production facility.

• *The blood group of the donor.* The blood group must consist of the ABO group and, for cellular components, the Rh type.

Unit identification number

Blood supplier name
City, State

Optional information; commonly:

• Blood supplier licensure information
• Unit donation date
• Reference to Circular of Information

Volunteer Donor

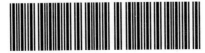

Product Code

Storage information

ABO

Rh(D) Type

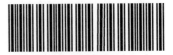

Expiration date

Special testing results

 FIGURE 10-10   Mock-up of an ISBT 128 Blood Component Label

• *The product code and description.* The product code communicates exactly what the component contains. This includes the anticoagulant used and the volume of the component and/or the target whole blood collection volume.

• *The expiration date.* The expiration time is incorporated if the component expires at any time other than midnight on the date of expiry.

• *Special testing.* This may include any red blood cell phenotyping that has been done and results of cytomegalovirus (CMV) testing.

Figure 10-10 ▦ provides a mock-up of a standard ISBT 128 label with the minimum required information.

☑ CHECKPOINT 10-7

How does the ISBT 128 labeling system improve the safety of the blood supply?

CASE IN POINT *(continued)*

The new blood center has provided samples of their blood labels for you to test with your blood bank computer system. Both blood suppliers label using the ISBT 128 format.

9. What information must be on the blood product label?

STORAGE OF BLOOD COMPONENTS

In order to understand how the optimal storage of blood components is determined, as noted in Table 10-5 later in this section, a discussion of the adverse effects of blood component storage and the moderating of these adverse effects is necessary.

Adverse Effects of Blood Component Storage

As soon as blood is removed from the human body, it starts to undergo changes that influence how its components function. The longer that blood is outside of the body, the more significant the effects become. Some changes are reversible following transfusion whereas others are not.[8] Changes associated with red blood cells, platelets, plasma proteins, and bacteria, followed by a discussion on moderating the adverse effects of storage, are detailed in the following sections.

Red Blood Cells

Changes specific to red blood cells are often referred to as **red cell storage lesions**. Hemolysis is the most obvious impact of storage on red blood cells. When whole blood is collected, it contains red blood cells of various ages. Over time, older red blood cells undergo **apoptosis**, also known as preprogrammed cell death. When red blood cells die, their membranes rupture and free hemoglobin is released into the storage fluid.[8]

Stored red blood cells maintain metabolic activity. In addition, anaerobic storage conditions cause cellular hemoglobin to release oxygen. Metabolic activity and oxygen release combine to reduce levels of adenine triphosphate (ATP) and 2,3-diphosphoglycerate (2,3-DPG) in stored red blood cells.[2, 8] Reduction in ATP levels leads to changes in the cell membrane, reducing flexibility and increasing removal from circulation when transfused. Membrane changes also cause intracellular potassium to leak into the extracellular storage fluid. Reduction in 2,3-DPG levels leads to impaired oxygen release by the red blood cells following transfusion.[8]

Many of these changes are reversible after transfusion, with intracellular potassium levels returning to normal within a few hours of transfusion.[8] Levels of ATP and 2,3-DPG are slower to return to normal; 2,3-DPG levels usually recover in 12–24 hours.[2] Membrane changes due to reduced levels of ATP may be irreversible, depending on storage conditions.[9]

> ## ☑ CHECKPOINT 10-8
>
> Which storage lesion change is quickly reversed after transfusion? Which one may be irreversible?

Platelets

Platelets are very fragile and sensitive cells. They can be adversely affected by temperature, forces applied during centrifugation, and other conditions that may be experienced through collection, production, and storage. Stressors result in changes to the platelet cytoskeleton and impaired ability to aggregate. These changes are reversible early in the storage period, but storage over several days results in platelet degranulation and irreversible membrane changes.[8]

Platelets have high levels of metabolic activity during storage. Lactic acid is produced through glucose metabolism and carbon dioxide is produced through fatty acid metabolism.[2] Oxygen is consumed during these activities, while pH falls and carbon dioxide levels rise. Prolonged storage in this type of environment eventually leads to cell death.

White Blood Cells

Granulocytes and other white blood cells are fragile and deteriorate very quickly after removal from the body.[2] Rapid deterioration of white blood cells can have serious consequences for other components prepared from whole blood. When white blood cells break down, they release many active substances, including cytokines and intracellular enzymes, which accelerate cell death in red blood cells and platelets. These substances can also cause serious reactions in patients when the components are transfused.[8]

Plasma Proteins

Most of the plasma proteins of interest in transfusion medicine are very stable in a wide range of storage conditions. However, coagulation factors V and VIII break down rapidly when plasma components are stored at temperatures above freezing.[2]

Bacteria

Although every step of blood collection and production is done aseptically and in a closed system in order to reduce the risk of bacterial contamination, there is a chance that minute numbers of bacteria may enter the system. Bacteria can flourish in blood components under ideal conditions. Bacterial metabolism accelerates the destruction of red blood cells, white blood cells, and platelets. Bacteria can also cause severe reactions in patients if the components are transfused.[10]

Moderating the Adverse Effects of Storage

Cellular blood components are the most susceptible to storage lesion. In order to be effective at the time of transfusion, cells must remain intact and metabolically active. Metabolic activity, however, is a primary cause of the changes that occur during storage. Storage conditions for blood components should ideally maintain cellular function while minimizing the storage lesion.

Collection and Storage Containers

Minimizing the storage lesion begins at the moment blood is removed from the body. Two features of the collection container contribute to improving blood component conditions during storage.

First, the plastics used in collection and storage containers affect cell function. The polyvinylchloride (PVC) plastic used in most collection sets and storage bags contains plasticizers that leach into blood components and have been shown to stabilize the red blood cell membrane. The non-PVC plastics used in platelet storage containers have high gas permeability and promote exchange of oxygen and carbon dioxide, providing oxygen for platelet metabolism and reducing build-up of carbon dioxide.[8]

Second, anticoagulant preservative solutions play a very significant role in reducing the storage lesion. Citric acid slows the breakdown of glucose during cell metabolism, dextrose provides a source of sugar to feed metabolism, monobasic sodium phosphate acts as a buffer to maintain a physiologic pH, and adenine helps to sustain ATP levels.

Storage Conditions

The condition under which prepared components are stored is an important determinant of component function at the time of transfusion. Storage conditions are defined by the temperature and the length of time of storage.

Reducing storage temperature tends to prolong storage time by slowing cell metabolism and the breakdown of proteins. Reducing storage temperature also inhibits the growth of any bacteria that may be present. Generally, the colder the storage temperature, the longer a component may be stored. However, the cellular components are very sensitive to temperature and reducing temperature below certain points adversely affects cell function and structure. Exposing red blood cells to temperatures below 33.8° F (1° C) can cause cell membrane rupture and hemolysis. Storing platelets below 68° F (20° C) prevents cell metabolism and results in loss of platelet function. Since plasma components have no functional cells, it is possible to freeze and store them for extended periods.[2]

The sensitivity of platelets necessitates special handling during storage. Providing continuous agitation to platelet components is important.[2] Agitation facilitates the transfer of oxygen and carbon dioxide through the gas-permeable storage container. Agitation also assists the buffering capacity of the anticoagulant, mixing the metabolically produced lactic acid with the phosphate buffer. The requirement to store platelets above 68° F (20° C) increases the risk that any bacteria in the system will proliferate. The risk of bacterial contamination is reduced through bacterial detection testing of components prior to transfusion[2] and a short expiration timeframe (5 days in Canada and the United States and 7 days in Europe).

☑ **CHECKPOINT 10-9**

How does refrigeration at 33.8–42.8° F (1–6° C) enhance the shelf life of red blood cell components?

Additive Solutions

Additive solutions have been shown to prolong the storage time for cellular components. At this time, only additive solutions for red blood cells have been approved for use in the United States. Red blood cell additive solutions provide glucose for cell metabolism, adenine, and phosphate to maintain ATP levels; some also contain mannitol to help maintain the cell membrane. These ingredients are suspended in a saline solution. Red blood cells (RBCs) stored in additive solutions demonstrate better maintenance of ATP levels over the storage period. Additive solutions also reduce hematocrit, which has been shown to reduce hemolysis during storage.[11] There are three red blood cell additive solutions currently licensed for use in the United States, all of which have been designed to preserve stored RBCs for 42 days: AS-1, AS-3, and AS-5, which are marketed under the trade names Adsol, Nutricel, and Optisol. All three additives contain varying amounts of dextrose, adenine, and sodium chloride. AS-1 and AS-5 both also possess mannitol. The presence of monobasic sodium phosphate, sodium citrate, and citric acid distinguish AS-3 from AS-1 and AS-5. They differ slightly in their composition, but all prolong the shelf life of the RBCs up to 42 days or roughly two times the shelf life before the usage of additive solutions (Table 10-6 ✳).

Additive solutions for platelet components have been used for many years in Europe. These solutions replace plasma as the storage medium. Current formulations use acetate and glucose suspended in saline as metabolic nutrients with phosphate to buffer the pH. Recently it was discovered that adding potassium, magnesium, and L-carnitine significantly improved platelet viability during storage.[12] Table 10-7 ✳ provides a summary of storage conditions for various blood components.

TRANSPORTATION OF BLOOD COMPONENTS

Transportation is a critical step in component production at all stages. Blood that is collected in a donor clinic must be transported to a production laboratory for separation into components and prepared components must be transported to hospitals for use in transfusion.

The most important feature of a transportation system is the ability to maintain the appropriate temperature range for the component(s) being shipped. In general, products that must be stored at 33.8–42.8° F (1–6° C) must maintain a shipping temperature of 33.8–50° F (1–10° C), while platelets and granulocytes must maintain a shipping temperature of 68–75.2° F (20–24° C). Frozen components are not as susceptible to temperature fluctuations as components shipped in a liquid state. Dry ice is normally used to keep frozen components below freezing temperature.[2] The traditional shipping container used for transporting blood components consists of a cardboard outer container with a foam insert to provide insulation.

Recently, a great deal of work has been done to find a packing system that provides better temperature maintenance while keeping the system relatively lightweight. These newer systems use **phase-change materials** to maintain temperatures for much longer periods of time. A phase-change material is a compound that shifts between a solid and a liquid state at a very specific temperature. It is able to store and release large amounts of energy in the form of heat and can act as an interceptor of heat energy in the shipping container. Shipping containers that incorporate phase-change materials can protect blood components through a wider range of external temperature variations over a longer period of time.[13]

It is important that blood products are maintained at the appropriate temperature during shipping, especially RBC units. Blood transportation systems must be validated to ensure that the system is capable of maintaining the appropriate temperature. In addition, transport temperatures may be monitored by one of a variety of reusable or disposable devices, including data loggers, recording thermometers, and reversible or nonreversible temperature monitors.

BLOOD COMPONENT MODIFICATION

Blood components may be modified after production to increase the safety of the product, to customize the product to meet specific patient needs, or to increase the amount of time that a product may be stored or used. Some modifications affect the storage conditions and expiration times of the component whereas others do not.

Leukoreduction

Leukoreduction is a process that removes white blood cells from whole blood or blood components. It is done to reduce the undesirable effects that white blood cells have on stored blood components and to reduce the risk of adverse reactions in patients receiving blood components.

✳ **TABLE 10-6** Content of Additive Solutions in mg/100mL (g/L)[4]

Additive Solution (mg/100 mL)	Dextrose	Adenine	Monobasic Sodium Phosphate	Mannitol	Sodium Chloride	Sodium Citrate	Citric Acid	Shelf Life
AS-1 (Adsol)	2200 (22)	27	0	750	900	0	0	42 days
AS-3 (Nutricel)	1100 (11)	30	276	0	410	588	42	42 days
AS-5 (Optisol)	900 (9)	30	0	525	877	0	0	42 days

★ **TABLE 10-7** Storage Conditions for Blood Components[2, 12]

Component	Storage Temperature	Expiration Time (from collection, except as noted)
Whole blood ACD/CPD/CP2D anticoagulant	33.8–42.8° F (1–6° C)	21 days
Whole blood CPDA-1 anticoagulant	33.8–42.8° F (1–6° C)	35 days
Red blood cells ACD/CPD/CP2D anticoagulant	33.8–42.8° F (1–6° C)	21 days
Red blood cells CPDA-1 anticoagulant	33.8–42.8° F (1–6° C)	35 days
Red blood cells additive solution	33.8–42.8° F (1–6° C)	42 days
Platelets	68–75.2° F (20–24° C) continuous gentle agitation	24 hours to 5 days
Platelets additive solution (not approved in U.S.)	68–75.2° F (20–24° C) continuous gentle agitation	Up to 7 days (not approved in U.S.)
Granulocytes	68–75.2° F (20–24° C) no agitation	24 hours
Fresh frozen plasma or Plasma frozen within 24 hours of phlebotomy	≤−0.4° F (≤−18° C)	12 months
Fresh frozen plasma or Plasma frozen within 24 hours of phlebotomy (after thawing)	33.8–42.8° F (1–6° C)	24 hours
Thawed plasma	33.8–42.8° F (1–6° C)	5 days from thawing
Liquid Plasma	33.8–42.8° F (1–6° C)	5 days after expiration of whole blood
Cryoprecipitated AHF	≤−0.4° F (≤−18° C)	12 months
Cryoprecipitated AHF thawed	68–75.2° F (20–24° C)	6 hours
Plasma cryoprecipitate reduced	≤−0.4° F (≤−18° C)	12 months
Plasma cryoprecipitate reduced thawed	33.8–42.8° F (1–6° C)	5 days from thawing

Prestorage leukoreduction is done at the time of component production and can be achieved in one of two ways. Whole blood may be centrifuged using a hard spin and the white blood cells can be removed by extracting out the buffy coat layer. Leukoreduction can also be achieved through the use of a specialized filter that traps white blood cells in a matrix that separates cells by size and by affinity for the filter material. Both methods remove the majority of granulocytes and monocytes, but some lymphocytes remain in the final leukoreduced components. The acceptable number of leukocytes that can remain is 5×10^6 per component in the United States and Canada and 1.0×10^6 per component in Europe.[2]

Pathogen Inactivation

Pathogen inactivation is a process that inactivates viruses and bacteria in prepared blood components. The technology is very new, but a number of manufacturers have developed processes and equipment to achieve inactivation. The methods that have been shown to be effective for treating plasma involve adding methylene blue, psoralen, or riboflavin to the component in a closed system, then exposing the component to light at specific wavelengths. All methods cause some reduction in plasma clotting factors after treatment. A similar process has been developed for platelets using psoralen or riboflavin, but both methods have shown some adverse effects on platelet function.[14] No successful commercial methods for treating red blood cell components have been developed to date.

Aliquoting

Aliquoting is normally done to prepare a product for low-volume transfusion, usually to neonatal or pediatric patients. Components may be aliquoted into syringes or transfer satellite containers. Aliquoting can be done in a closed system or an **open system**. An open system involves exposure to the outside environment and thus creates an increased risk of bacterial contamination. Products prepared in an open system must therefore be used within a very short time after modification. To maintain a closed system, aliquot containers must be attached to the original component bag with a sterile docking device.

Pooling

Pooling components may be done to reduce the number of bags that have to be accessed at the time of transfusion. Pooling is commonly done with PRP platelets or cryoprecipitated AHF to create a single treatment dose. Red blood cells may also be pooled with thawed plasma to recreate most of the constituents of whole blood for transfusion. As with aliquoting, pooling may be done in an open or closed system.

Volume Reduction

Volume reduction is done to remove plasma or additive solution from components. It is done by centrifuging cellular components and removing supernatant fluid, usually with a plasma press. The process may be done in an open or a closed system. However, either method of removing additive solution or plasma will affect the survival time of the RBCs or platelets. Volume reduction reduces the risk of circulatory overload and removal of excess plasma reduces the risk of adverse reactions related to transfusion of certain plasma proteins.

Irradiation

Cellular blood components may contain active T lymphocytes that can cause transfusion-associated graft versus host disease (GVHD) in susceptible individuals. Exposing blood components to gamma or x-ray radiation inactivates T lymphocytes with no adverse effect on platelet or red blood cell function. Specific equipment designed to deliver appropriate doses of radiation to blood components are commercially available. The acceptable dose of radiation delivered to the center of the component is a minimum of 25 Gy and a maximum of 50 Gy. Radiation exposure at these levels has no impact on platelet function or viability. Irradiation of red blood cells has some impact on the cell membrane and irradiated red blood cells demonstrate increased potassium leakage into the storage fluid.[2] Therefore, the expiration date for RBCs must be changed to 28 days or the original expiration date, whichever is shorter.

Washing

Washing of red blood cell or platelet components is done to remove plasma proteins that can cause severe reactions in certain patient populations. Washing is done with sterile normal saline and may be done manually or in an automated cell washer. Washing usually occurs in an open system, which again results in a shortened expiration date. Closed systems have also been developed.

Freezing, Thawing, and Deglycerolizing Red Blood Cells

It is advantageous to be able to store red blood cells with rare phenotypes for a long period of time and the best way to do this is to freeze them. However, red blood cells normally undergo cell lysis when they are frozen and then thawed. It is possible to reduce red blood cell damage during frozen storage by using a cryoprotective agent such as glycerol. Glycerol limits the formation of ice crystals within red blood cells, reducing damage to the cell membrane.[2]

Glycerol is added to the red blood cell component and the component is allowed to equilibrate before freezing. The equilibration phase allows time for the glycerol to enter the red blood cells. Once equilibration is complete, the glycerolized red blood cell component is frozen and stored at either $\leq-85°$ F ($\leq-65°$ C) or $\leq-112°$ F ($\leq-80°$ C), depending on the method used to freeze the component.[2] The freezing process may be done in an open system or in an automated closed system.

Red blood cells that have been frozen in glycerol are thawed at 98.6° F (37° C) and the glycerol must be removed prior to transfusion. Deglycerolization is achieved by washing the thawed component with successive concentration changes of sterile saline solution, starting with hypertonic saline. Deglycerolization can be done in an automated closed system if the component was originally frozen in the closed system. In all other cases, deglycerolization is done in an open system (see Table 10-8 ✳ for expiration intervals).[2]

Rejuvenation

Rejuvenation is a method used to reverse some of the adverse effects of storage on red blood cells. Rejuvenating solutions contain pyruvate, inosine, phosphate, and adenine, which have the ability to return 2,3-DPG and ATP levels to normal levels in stored red blood cell components. The process can be done up to 3 days after a RBC unit expires. Rejuvenated red blood cells must be washed prior to transfusion to remove the rejuvenating solution. Rejuvenation may also be done to improve the condition of red blood cells prior to freezing in glycerol.[2] Table 10-8 shows the impact of blood component modifications on storage conditions and expiry time (expiration date).

> ☑ **CHECKPOINT 10-10**
>
> Which blood component modification prevents graft versus host disease (GVHD)?

PLASMA FRACTIONATION

Plasma that is not used for transfusion can be shipped to large manufacturing facilities that are able to separate out specific proteins and package them to meet specific patient needs. Separation is achieved by pooling plasma from up to 10,000 donors, adding ethanol, and then manipulating the pH and the temperature of the solution. This process causes individual proteins to precipitate out at specific temperature and pH levels. Because the proteins precipitate out in fractions, the process is referred to as *plasma fractionation* (Chapter 11). The three major categories of proteins that are fractionated from pooled plasma are albumin, immune globulins, and coagulation proteins. Figure 10-11 ■ shows a schematic of the fractionation process.

The fractionation process also includes steps designed to increase the safety of the final products. For many products, the plasma pool undergoes solvent/detergent treatment to inactivate lipid-enveloped viruses. Plasma may also be filtered through a nanofilter, which has an extremely small pore size and is able to trap bacteria and viruses. Because of these additional steps, fractionated plasma protein products are generally considered to be safer than fresh blood components.

★ **TABLE 10-8** Storage Conditions for Modified Blood Components[2]

Modified Component	Storage Conditions and Expiry
Leukocyte-reduced components	No change to original storage conditions or expiry (expiration date)
Pathogen-inactivated components	No change to original storage conditions or expiry
Aliquoted red blood cell or thawed plasma—closed system into sterile transfer packs	No change to original storage conditions or expiry
Aliquoted red blood cells—syringes	Store at 33.8–42.8° F (1–6° C) for up to 4 hours from transfer into syringe
Aliquoted platelets	Transfuse as soon as possible
Pooled platelets—open system	Store at 68–75.2° F (20–24° C) for up to 4 hours after opening the system
Pooled platelets—closed system	Store at 68–75.2° F (20–24° C) for up to 5 days from whole blood collection; pool expires with the oldest platelet component in the pool
Pooled cryoprecipitate—open system	Store at 68–75.2° F (20–24° C) for up to 4 hours
Reconstituted whole blood (red blood cells pooled with thawed FFP)—closed system	Store at 33.8–42.8° F (1–6° C) until the earliest expiry date of either pooled component
Reconstituted whole blood (red blood cells pooled with thawed FFP)—open system	Store at 33.8–42.8° F (1–6° C) for no more than 24 hours from time of pooling or until the earliest expiry date of either pooled component
Volume reduced platelets—open system or closed system	Store at 68–75.2° F (20–24° C) for no more than 4 hours (open system). In either case, transfuse as soon as possible due to minimal plasma remaining in the component
Irradiated red blood cells	Store at 33.8–42.8° F (1–6° C) for up to 28 days after irradiation or to the original component expiry date, whichever comes first
Irradiated platelets	No change to original storage conditions or expiry
Washed red blood cells—open system	Store at 33.8–42.8° F (1–6° C) for up to 24 hours
Washed platelets—open system	Store at 68–75.2° F (20–24° C) for up to 4 hours
Frozen red blood cells—open or closed system	Store at ≤−85° F (≤−65° C) or ≤−112° F (≤−80° C) for up to 10 years
Deglycerolized red blood cells—open system	Store at 33.8–42.8° F (1–6° C) for up to 24 hours
Deglycerolized red blood cells—closed system	Store at 33.8–42.8° F (1–6° C) for up to 14 days
Rejuvenated red blood cells	Store at 33.8–42.8° F (1–6° C) for up to 24 hours or freeze with glycerol

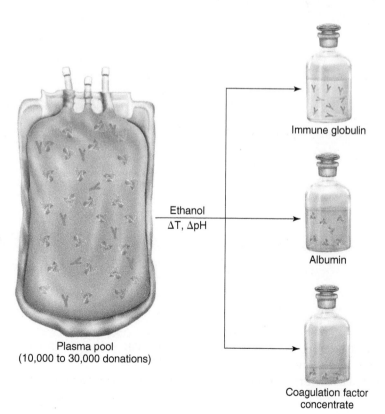

■ **FIGURE 10-11** Plasma Fractionation

CASE IN POINT (continued)

When comparing the red blood cell products that each blood center provides, you note that the current blood center only provides red blood cells in CPDA-1 anticoagulant whereas the new blood center provides both CPDA-1 red blood cells and AS-3 red blood cells. Both blood centers provide leukocyte-reduced blood products.

10. What is the difference in expiration date between the two anticoagulants?
11. What are leukocyte-reduced blood products?
12. What is the maximum number of white blood cells that can remain in a blood product labeled as leukocyte reduced?

You have a large oncology population at your hospital. These patients are often immunocompromised and require irradiated blood products.

13. What is blood product irradiation and why is it performed?
14. On which blood products is irradiation performed?

Albumin

Albumin was the first protein to be isolated and fractionated from human plasma. Albumin is the most plentiful of all proteins in plasma and fractionation of 1,000 kg of plasma can yield approximately 26 kg of albumin. Albumin is usually packaged and distributed as a liquid in 5% or 25% concentration.

Immune Globulins

Immune globulins are fractionated from the gamma globulin portion of plasma. Immune globulins may be specific or nonspecific. Specific immune globulin contains antibodies, primarily IgG, to a specific antigen; examples include Rh(D)-immune globulin and hepatitis B-immune globulin. Nonspecific immune globulin contains predominantly IgG antibodies that are directed against a wide variety of antigens. Nonspecific immune globulin is most commonly provided as an intravenous solution and is referred to as intravenous immune globulin (IVIG). Fractionation of 1,000 kg of plasma will yield approximately 4 kg of IVIG.

Coagulation Proteins

Most of the proteins involved in the coagulation cascade can be fractionated from pools of donor plasma. These individual proteins are normally provided in a lyophilized form and must be reconstituted prior to use. Some common commercially available coagulation proteins include Factor VIII, Factor IX, fibrinogen, anti-thrombin III, and protein C. There are also many commercially available combinations of coagulation proteins, including von Willebrand factor combined with Factor VIII and prothrombin complexes that contain Factors II, VII, IX, and X, with or without protein C.

RECOMBINANT PROTEIN PRODUCTION

Recent advances in the field of genetic engineering have led to the development of recombinant proteins. Recombinant proteins are produced by inserting the genetic information that codes for a specific human protein into the DNA of plant or animal cells. The cells are cultured in a bioreactor that contains nutrients and oxygen. As the cells metabolize, they excrete the protein that was coded into their DNA. Once the reaction is complete, the protein can be extracted, purified, and packaged for patient use. Recombinant technology has been used to manufacture coagulation proteins that were previously only available through plasma fractionation. Currently, much of the Factor VIII and Factor IX in use is recombinant rather than plasma-derived.

Recombinant proteins have a number of advantages over fractionated proteins:

1. Production does not rely on the availability of donor plasma, so supply is theoretically unlimited.
2. Manufacturers are moving toward methods that use no human or animal derived proteins during production, reducing the risk of transmitting human- or animal-borne illnesses.
3. The entire process, including the input, is completely within the manufacturer's control, so output is consistent and predictable.

Review of the Main Points

- The most significant historical events that have contributed to the progress of blood component production include the discovery of anticoagulants, the development of the fractionation process, the invention of the plastic blood bag, and the development of apheresis technology.
- Blood bank anticoagulants contain constituents that prevent blood clotting and prolong storage time.
- Whole blood can be separated into red blood cell, platelet, and plasma components.

- Cryoprecipitated AHF is prepared from fresh frozen plasma. Cryoprecipitated AHF contains coagulation proteins that precipitate out of plasma in the cold. These proteins are Factor VIII, fibrinogen, Factor XIII, von Willebrand factor, and fibronectin.
- There are two methods for preparing platelet components from whole blood. The platelet-rich plasma method first uses a soft spin to extract the platelets from whole blood, then a hard spin to concentrate the platelets. The buffy coat

method first uses a hard spin to extract platelets from whole blood; buffy coats from four to six donors are pooled and a soft spin is used to remove red blood cells from the pooled component.
- Apheresis is a process that allows the collection of specific components from a blood donor. The remainder of the donation is returned to the donor. Apheresis can be used to collect red blood cell, plasma, platelet, and granulocyte components.
- The ISBT 128 labeling standard defines the format and information that must be provided on a blood component label, ensuring traceability back to the original donor and a standard method for transferring critical information about the component.
- Blood component labels that meet the ISBT 128 standard must include, at minimum:
  - The donation number
  - The donor blood group
  - The product code and description
  - The expiration date
  - Any special testing
- Blood components show signs of deterioration during storage as a result of cell metabolism and protein breakdown. The adverse effects of storage are referred to as the storage lesion.
- With prolonged storage, red blood cells show signs of hemolysis, membrane damage, and reduced levels of ATP and 2,3-DPG. Platelets show changes in the cytoskeleton, degranulation, and impaired aggregation. These effects can be aggravated by the breakdown of leukocytes in the component or through the introduction of bacteria into the system.

- The adverse effects of storage are moderated through
  - The plastics used for storage of components
  - By the use of anticoagulants and additive solutions that support cell metabolism and control pH
  - By maintaining an appropriate storage temperature
- Transportation systems for blood components maintain appropriate temperatures for the components being transported.
- Phase-change materials are useful in maintaining appropriate transportation temperatures for a wide range of external temperature variations over long periods of time.
- Blood components may be modified after production to increase safety, to meet specific patient needs, or to extend the product expiry. Leukoreduction and pathogen inactivation increase product safety; aliquoting, pooling, volume reducing, irradiating, and washing help to meet specific patient needs; freezing and rejuvenating can extend product expiry.
- Component modifications may be done in open or closed systems. Because of the risk of bacterial contamination, components prepared in open systems have very short expiry times.
- Specific proteins can be fractionated from plasma using ethanol along with variations in temperature and pH. The three major categories of proteins that can be fractionated from plasma are albumin, immune globulins, and coagulation proteins.
- Recombinant technology can be used to manufacture proteins that were previously available only through plasma fractionation.

Review Questions

1. Which of the following components is *not* prepared from whole blood? (Objective #3)
   A. Red blood cells
   B. Fresh frozen plasma
   C. Cryoprecipitate
   D. Platelets apheresis

2. One unit of cryoprecipitated AHF prepared from whole blood contains a minimum of how many international units (IU) of Factor VIII? (Objective #6)
   A. 40
   B. 80
   C. 120
   D. 160

3. ISBT 128 blood component labeling guidelines require all of the following except: (Objective #10)
   A. Donor identification number
   B. Blood type
   C. Product expiration date
   D. Recipient name

4. Which of the following statements regarding blood storage conditions is *incorrect*? (Objective #15)
   A. CPDA-1 red blood cells are stored for 35 days at 33.8–42.8° F (1–6° C).
   B. Platelets are stored for 5 days at 33.8–42.8° F (1–6° C) with gentle agitation.
   C. Cryoprecipitated AHF is stored for one year at −0.4° F (−18° C).
   D. Granulocytes are stored for 24 hours at 68–75.2° F (20–24° C) with no agitation.

5. The primary populations that benefit from aliquoting blood products are: (Objective #18)

   A. Fetuses and neonates

   B. Neonatal and pediatric patients

   C. Pediatric and adolescent patients

   D. Adolescents and adults

6. The acceptable number of residual WBCs in a leukoreduced blood product is no greater than: (Objective #18)

   A. 5.0×10^6/L

   B. 5.0×10^{10}/L

   C. 1.0×10^6/L

   D. 1.0×10^{10}/L

7. To prevent engraftment of donor lymphocytes, cellular blood products should be: (Objective #18)

   A. Washed

   B. Volume-reduced

   C. Irradiated

   D. Pooled

8. The first protein to be isolated and fractionated from human plasma was: (Objective #22)

   A. Albumin

   B. Immune globulin

   C. Coagulation protein

   D. Prothrombin complex

9. Components that may be collected by apheresis include: (Objective #9)

   A. Red blood cells

   B. Platelets

   C. Granulocytes

   D. All of the above

10. The most important consideration for the transport of blood components between sites is: (Objective #16)

    A. Use of disposable devices

    B. Shipping temperature

    C. Shipping container

    D. Insulation of the transport vehicle

11. Which of the following preservative constituents serves to maintain ATP levels during blood storage? (Objective #2)

    A. Citric acid

    B. Dextrose

    C. Adenine

    D. Sodium phosphate

12. Which of the following production methods for preparing platelet components from whole blood is recommended for pediatric transfusion? (Objective #7)

    A. Buffy coat (B/C)

    B. Platelet-rich plasma (PRP)

    C. Soft spin

    D. Hard spin

13. Biochemical changes that occur during blood storage include: (Objective #13)

    A. Increase in plasma hemoglobin level

    B. Increase in pH level

    C. Increase in ATP level

    D. Increase in 2,3-DPG level

14. How much residual plasma remains in a component of cryoprecipitated AHF that is prepared from whole blood? (Objective #5)

    A. 100 mL

    B. 70 mL

    C. 35 mL

    D. 15 mL

15. Separation of blood components during apheresis is achieved through: (Objective #8)

    A. Washing

    B. Aliquoting

    C. Centrifugation

    D. Dilution

16. Decreased levels of _____ during blood storage results in impaired oxygen release by red blood cells after the blood is transfused. (Objective #13)

    A. Potassium

    B. Sodium

    C. 2,3-DPG

    D. Hemoglobin F

17. The blood component expiration date must *always* be changed to 24 hours when using which of the following blood component modification procedures? (Objective #20)

    A. Aliquoting red blood cells using a sterile connecting device

    B. Washing red blood cells in an open system

    C. Pooling platelets

    D. Leukoreduction of whole blood

18. Which of the following statements regarding transfusable plasma is true? (Objective #4)

A. FFP is processed within 8 hours of collection and contains both stable and labile proteins.

B. FP24 is processed within 8 hours of collection and contains both stable and labile proteins.

C. Liquid plasma is processed within 24 hours of collection and contains only stable proteins.

D. Thawed plasma is prepared from FFP, thawed at 33.8–42.8° F (1–6° C) and contains only stable proteins.

19. All of the following assist with the precipitation of proteins during plasma fractionation *except:* (Objective # 21)

A. Addition of ethanol

B. Regulation of pH

C. Temperature change

D. Solvent detergent treatment

20. The use of recombinant proteins includes all of the following advantages *except:* (Objective #24)

A. Availability

B. Predictability

C. Affordability

D. Risk reduction

References

1. AABB. *Highlights of Transfusion Medicine History* [Internet]. Bethesda, MD: AABB; c 2009 [updated 2006 Apr 12; cited 2009 Sept 2]. Available from: http://www.aabb.org/Content/About_Blood/Highlights_of_Transfusion_Medicine_History/highlights.htm
2. Roback JD, et al. *Technical Manual,* 17th ed. Bethesda (MD): AABB; 2011.
3. Spinella PC. Warm fresh whole blood transfusion for severe hemorrhage: U.S. military and potential civilian applicatons. *Crit Care Med* 2008; 36 (7 suppl): S340–5.
4. *Circular of Information for the Use of Human Blood and Blood Components.* Bethesda (MD): AABB; July 2009.
5. Filip DJ, Aster RH. Relative hemostatic effectiveness of human platelets stored at 4 degrees and 22 degrees C. *J Lab Clin Med* 1978; 91: 618–24.
6. Circular of Information for the Use of Human Blood and Blood Components. Canadian Blood Services; 2011.
7. Ashford P, ed. *ISBT 128 An Introduction* [Internet]. York (PA): ICCBBA; 2006 [cited 2 Sept 2009]. Available from: http://iccbba.org/ISBT128introbooklet.pdf
8. Solheim BG, et al. Clinical implications of red blood cell and platelet storage lesions: an overview. *Transfusion and Apheresis Science* 2004; 31: 185–189.
9. Palek J, Liu PA, Liu C. Polymerisation of red cell membrane protein contributes to spheroechinocyte shape irreversibility. *Nature* 1978; 274: 505–507.
10. Brecher M, Hay S. Bacterial contamination of blood components. *Clin Microbiol Rev* 2005; 18: 195–204.
11. Hess JR, et al. The effects of phosphate, pH, and AS volume on RBCs stored in saline-adenine-glucose-mannitol solutions. *Transfusion* 2002; 40: 1000–1006.
12. van der Meer PS. Platelet additive solutions: a future perspective. *Transfusion Clinique et Biologique* 2007; 14: 522–525.
13. Rentas FJ, et al. New insulation technology provides next-generation containers for "iceless" and lightweight transport of RBCs at 1 to 10 C in extreme temperatures for over 78 hours. *Transfusion* 2004; 44: 210–216.
14. Solheim BG. Pathogen reduction of blood components. *Transfusion and Apheresis Science* 2008; 39: 75–82.

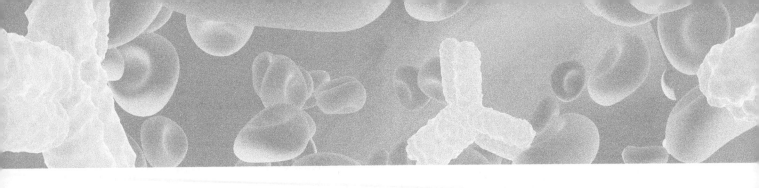

11 Component Therapy and Massive Transfusion

LARISA KAY MARISTANY

Chapter Objectives

Upon completion of this chapter, the student will be able to:

1. Identify the two main goals of transfusion therapy.
2. Cite five common laboratory tests used to assess the need for transfusion.
3. List indications for the transfusion of each blood component.
4. State the purpose of using a blood warming device during transfusion of blood products.
5. List contraindications for the transfusion of each blood component.
6. Define autologous donation and explain its role in clinical practice.
7. Describe directed donation, its role in clinical practice, and unit modifications that may be required in transfusion therapy.
8. List common modifications of cellular blood components.
9. Describe common reasons for cellular component modification.
10. Define and state four types of complications of massive transfusion.
11. Discuss common blood component administration practices.
12. Describe the process of preoperative autologous donation (PAD).
13. Describe the process of acute normovolemic hemodilution (ANH).
14. Describe the process of intraoperative blood salvage.
15. Discuss the use of coagulation factor concentrates and other fractionation products.
16. Describe the use of pharmaceuticals to reduce blood transfusion requirements.
17. State the advantages and disadvantages of the following human progenitor cell (HPC) collection processes: peripheral blood stem cells (PBSC) and bone marrow collection.

Key Terms

Acute normovolemic hemodilution (ANH)
Apheresis
Colloid solution(s)
Community directed donation(s)
Crystalloid solution(s)
Deglycerolization
Direct transfusion(s)
Directed donation(s)
Hemostasis

Intraoperative blood salvage

Massive transfusion

Myeloablative

Plasma fractionation

Preoperative autologous
  donation(s) (PAD)

Refractory

Tachyphylaxis

Transfusion trigger(s)

Xenotransfusion(s)

CASE IN POINT

RA is a 52-year-old man. His car broke down on a foggy morning while he was driving to work. He pulled to the side of the road to access equipment in the trunk. The driver of a passing car became confused in the fog and followed RA's car's taillights off the road. The driver hit RA's car at 45 miles per hour (70 kilometers per hour) and pinned him between the two vehicles. The accident occurred on a rural road more than 40 miles from the nearest hospital. Helicopters were grounded due to the fog. For these reasons, it took rescue personnel nearly 2 hours to transport RA to a trauma center.

What's Ahead?

Transfusion medicine staff members play a vital role in ensuring patients have the best possible outcomes. A thorough understanding of blood components—including indications, contraindications, risks, and expected response—aids clinical and laboratory personnel in choosing the right component or product.

This chapter addresses the following questions:

1. What blood components and blood transfusion therapies are currently available?
2. What are the common indications and contraindications for various blood component therapies?
3. What are the unique challenges presented by patients who require massive transfusion support?

HISTORICAL BACKGROUND

The practice of blood transfusion can be reliably traced back over 300 years. William Harvey changed medicine with his description of the circulatory system in 1616. This new understanding ushered in years of experiments to elucidate new therapies based on his revolutionary theory.

Subsequent experiments with **xenotransfusion**, which is transfusion across species lines, produced mostly poor clinical outcomes. By the mid-1800s, transfusion was almost exclusively human to human. Transfusion was accomplished by using an apparatus that would directly connect the donor's artery to the recipient's vein.

The discovery of the ABO blood group system (Chapter 4) reduced the incidence of immediate hemolytic transfusion reactions. The introduction of anticoagulants and preservatives (Chapter 10) allowed donor blood to be stored and transported. Together, these discoveries ushered in the era of modern blood transfusion.

The development of high-speed centrifugation, large-capacity refrigeration, and freezing all advanced the development of component therapy. Today, discrete portions of the whole blood collection are used to treat specific conditions, with the result that one donation may treat three or more patients. Additionally, advances in *apheresis* technology permit the efficient collection of double red blood cell units, platelets, granulocytes, and hematopoietic progenitor cells from the donor's peripheral circulation.

GOALS OF TRANSFUSION THERAPY

The need for transfusion is often a direct result of abnormalities in the hematologic or coagulation systems, whether congenital or acquired. The common goals of transfusion are to increase tissue oxygenation and/or restore **hemostasis**, which is the ability to stop bleeding. The complete blood count (CBC)—including hemoglobin, hematocrit, and platelet count—and common coagulation screening tests—including activated partial thromboplastin time (aPTT), prothrombin time (PT), international normalized ratio (INR), and fibrinogen—are often the first laboratory tests used to assess the need for transfusion. Table 11-1 ✳ lists common laboratory-based *transfusion triggers* and expected transfusion dose–response rates.

CATEGORIES OF BLOOD PRODUCTS

Blood components can be broadly classified into four major categories:

- Cellular components, which include whole blood, red blood cells, and granulocytes.
- Plasma components, which include platelet products, cryoprecipitate, fresh frozen plasma, and other transfusable plasma components.
- Hematopoietic progenitor cell (HPC) products, which include bone marrow, peripheral blood stem cell, and cord blood preparations.
- Plasma fractionation products, which are also called plasma protein products or manufactured products, and which include albumin, various immune globulins, and various coagulation factor concentrates.

☑ CHECKPOINT 11-1

Which blood products are considered cellular components?

✳ **TABLE 11-1** Laboratory Indices

Component	Common Transfusion Triggers*	Common Adult Dose	Expected Response per Dose**
Red blood cells	Hemoglobin <7 g/dL (70 g/L) Higher if there are underlying cardiac or pulmonary diseases	1 unit	Hemoglobin ↑ 1 g/dL (10 g/L)
Fresh frozen plasma	aPTT and/or PTT increased ≥ 1.5 times the upper limit of the normal range or INR > 2.0	10–20 mL/kg body weight Often 2 whole blood–derived units or 1 apheresis unit	Factor levels are ↑ by approximately 25%, resulting in shortened PTT/INR or aPTT. Results in the normal range are often not achieved by transfusion and are not necessary to prevent bleeding.
Platelets	Platelet count <10 × 10³/μL (10 × 10⁹/L) Platelet count may be normal if bleeding is due to dysfunctional platelets	1 apheresis unit or 4–6 pooled whole blood–derived units	1 hour post-transfusion ↑ of 30–50 × 10³/μL (30–50 × 10⁹/L)
Cryoprecipitate	Fibrinogen <100 mg/dL (<2.94 μmol/L)	10 units or 1 unit/10 kg body weight Can calculate amount based on current fibrinogen level, desired fibrinogen level and blood volume as estimated by body weight	14 units of cryoprecipitate = fibrinogen ↑ 50 mg/dL (1.47 μmol/L)
Granulocytes	Documented sepsis unresponsive to antimicrobial therapy	1 unit	Usually no demonstrable rise in neutrophil count

* Laboratory results should be correlated with clinical condition and should not be used as the sole reason for transfusion; ** In an average, nonbleeding, 70 kg adult; aPTT, activated partial thromboplastin time; PTT, prothrombin time; INR, international normalized ratio.

ADMINISTRATION OF BLOOD PRODUCTS

The following considerations must be taken into account in order to ensure proper administration of blood products: infusion rate, infusion sets and filters, needles, rapid infusers and blood warmers, infusion pumps, and infusion solutions. The description and suggested protocol notes for each consideration, as appropriate, are addressed in the next sections.

Infusion Rate

The infusion of all blood components should occur in less than 4 hours. This ensures the product will deliver the most therapeutic impact with minimal risk of bacterial contamination. Bacteria may be present in the unit, but undetected at the time of distribution. Refrigerated storage is known to inhibit the growth of bacteria. If small numbers of bacteria are present and still viable, extended storage at room temperature in a nutrient-rich environment such as blood could allow the bacteria to proliferate.

The infusion rate may be adjusted to allow for individual patient circumstances but should fall within the 4-hour limit. The infusion rate should be documented as part of the order to transfuse (Chapter 10).

The 4-hour limit does not necessarily apply to infusion of fractionation products. Manufacturers often specify administration instructions, including maximum infusion rates. As with blood component therapy, the infusion rate for each specific patient should be documented in the order to transfuse.

CASE IN POINT (continued)

The trauma physician ordered 4 units of red blood cells to be in the emergency department (ED) awaiting RA's arrival. The admitting personnel assigned RA an alias because his name and other identifiers were unavailable at the time.

The transfusion service has a policy to issue blood products in a cooler when more than 1 unit is issued at one time. Four red blood cell units were issued using RA's assigned alias and transported to the emergency room in a cooler. RA's blood type and antibody status were unknown at the time of issue.

1. What is the primary goal of red blood cell transfusion?
2. What group and type of red blood cells should be issued in this situation?
3. Why would the transfusion service have a policy to use a cooler when issuing more than 1 unit at a time? (Hint: Refer to the section, "Infusion Rate.")

Infusion Sets and Filters

There are several types of sets used to infuse blood products. Depending on the institution, these may be dispensed from the transfusion service when the unit is released or stocked on the floor where the patient is located. Policies that indicate how often infusion sets should be changed vary among institutions and is often dependent on the type of infusion set being used. Policies are usually based on a time limit or a maximum number of units or a combination.

The basic infusion set incorporates flexible plastic tubing and a standard inline blood filter with a pore size of 170–260 microns, which serves to trap larger cellular debris that might accumulate during the storage of blood units. More sophisticated infusion sets are used in certain situations.

Microaggregate filters may be used for red blood cell transfusions. Degenerating platelets, white blood cell fragments, and small strands of fibrin are among the debris these filters reduce. The screen or filter is effective for particle sizes as small as 20–40 microns, but the small pore size slows the rate of transfusion.

Leukocyte reduction filters are used to reduce the number of white blood cells in red blood cell or platelet components to less than 5×10^6 white blood cells per unit. These filters use multiple layers of synthetic fibers to trap white blood cells as the blood flows through the filter. The filters used for red blood cell components are not interchangeable with the filters designed for platelet components. Failure to strictly follow the manufacturer's instructions—for example, adhering to the specified flow rate—may make the filters ineffective.[1] Leukocyte reduction may happen prestorage while components are being prepared (Chapter 10) or just before transfusion, often at the bedside.

☑ CHECKPOINT 11-2

What is the pore size of the standard blood filter?

Needles

Using a needle with too small a bore diameter may cause hemolysis when transfusing red blood cells, especially if combined with rapid infusion. As with other transfusion parameters, needle size may vary with patient conditions. For example, smaller needles may be used for neonatal or pediatric patients. Typically, 18 gauge or larger needles are used for blood transfusion. However, needles as small as 23 gauge may occasionally be used.[2] The infusion rate should be slowed when using smaller needles to prevent hemolysis. On the other hand, needles with a large-bore diameter should be used when rapidly transfusing red blood cells.

Rapid Infusers and Blood Warmers

Rapid infusers resemble pressure cuffs that surround the entire bag of blood; pressure is exerted more uniformly than squeezing the blood bag by hand. Rapid infusers should not be inflated to 300 mm Hg or above because this level of pressure may cause the bag to rupture.

Massive rapid infusion or infusion into a central venous catheter carries a higher risk of hypothermia. Hypothermia can cause arrhythmia and can be fatal. Blood warmers can be used to prevent hypothermia. Blood warmers may occasionally be used when transfusing red blood cell components to patients with severe cold agglutinin disease, where the patient's condition increases the risk of hemolysis.

Blood warmers must be carefully maintained and monitored so the blood never reaches a temperature that could cause hemolysis. Depending on the facility, the transfusion service or biomedical engineers may be responsible for blood warmer maintenance and quality control.

Infusion Pumps

Mechanical pumps can be used to regulate the blood flow into the patient. These are often used in neonates where small shifts in volume may drastically affect the infant (Chapter 14). Very small volumes of blood are used in these settings and mechanical pumps are easily adapted to syringes with the small lumen needles necessary in such tiny patients. Mechanical pumps can be used in adults when rate control is indicated.

Only infusion pumps that have been tested and approved for use with blood products should be used for transfusion. Other infusion pumps may exert too much pressure on the red blood cells, causing hemolysis. Whereas in the past, few pumps were approved for use with blood products, the majority of new pumps have undergone the testing and approval process. Consequently, some facilities now use infusion pumps routinely for transfusion rather than in selected cases.

Infusion Solutions

Normal saline, 0.9% sodium chloride (USP), may be added to most blood components. In the past, saline was often added to increase flow rates of red blood cell units that did not contain additive solutions and therefore had higher hematocrits. Generally, medications and other intravenous solutions should not be added to blood components as they may cause clotting or hemolysis. Only substances that have regulatory approval, which in the United States would be from the U.S. Food and Drug Administration (FDA), or that have been documented to not affect blood products may be added to blood components.[3] Some examples of substances that meet these requirements and are safe to add to red blood cell units include ABO-compatible plasma, 5% albumin, and Plasma-Lyte®. Ringer's lactate solution should not be added to blood components because the high calcium content inactivates the anticoagulant, causing clots to form. When infusing fractionation products, the manufacturers' instructions should be checked. Solutions that are compatible with blood components may not be compatible with certain fractionation products.

CASE IN POINT (continued)

RA arrives in the ED and all 4 red blood cell units are immediately transfused via a rapid infuser.

4. What are two factors that the transfusionist probably considered when transfusing RA?
5. Why are these factors important?

WHOLE BLOOD

Whole blood consists of red blood cells, white blood cells, platelets, and plasma and is used as the starting point for component preparation (Chapter 10). Table 11-2 ✱ lists the cellular blood components available. Whole blood was used in the past for the dual purposes of volume replacement by the plasma and oxygen-carrying capacity by the red blood cells. The platelets in stored whole blood are usually

⋆ **TABLE 11-2** Cellular Blood Components

Component	Benefits	Major Indications	Contraindications	Risks
Whole blood	• Improves tissue oxygenation, • Replaces fluid, • Replaces nonlabile coagulation factors	• Presurgical autologous donation • Normovolemic hemodilution • Intraoperative blood salvage	Has largely been replaced by component therapy except in rare circumstances, but symptomatic anemia combined with volume loss, such as seen in massive hemorrhage, is an appropriate indication.	• Acute hemolytic transfusion reaction if not ABO identical • Delayed hemolytic transfusion reaction • Febrile nonhemolytic transfusion reaction • Allergic reactions • Bacterial, viral, or parasitic infection • Alloimmunization to red blood cell antigens • Circulatory overload • Iron overload • Nonimmunogenic hemolysis • Blood nearing its expiration date may have reduced capacity to off load oxygen to tissues
Red blood cell	Improves tissue oxygenation	Symptomatic anemia: • Acute anemia as seen with trauma, surgical blood loss, or medical conditions causing bleeding • Chronic anemia as seen with various hematological and other medical conditions	• Compensated anemia with no symptoms • Anemia that can be treated by alternatives, such as supplementation with iron, vitamin B_{12}, folic acid, and/or erythropoietin • Blood volume expansion	• Acute hemolytic transfusion reaction if ABO incompatible • Less risk of circulatory overload than with whole blood but still a risk, especially in select patient populations such as neonates and the elderly • Otherwise, same risks as whole blood
Granulocyte	Improves cellular immune function	• Neutropenia and infection that is unresponsive to usual therapy • Congenital neutrophil function defects	Infection that is responding to antibiotic or antifungal therapy	• Transfusion-associated graft versus host disease (TA-GVHD) if not irradiated • Allergic reactions to sedimentation agents • Hazards common to human source blood products, such as transmission of infectious agents

nonfunctional due to the refrigerated storage temperature. Today, volume depletion is usually treated with **crystalloid solutions**—which are aqueous solutions of water-soluble molecules such as normal saline, dextrose, or Ringer's lactate solutions—or **colloid solutions**—which are solutions containing larger insoluble molecules such as gelatin or starch. These solutions do not carry the risk of infectious diseases associated with products made from human blood. Component therapy, such as the use of red blood cell components to improve oxygen-carrying capacity, has largely replaced the use of whole blood.

Today, fresh whole blood may be used in specific circumstances, such as under battlefield conditions,[4] but for the most part it has been replaced by specific component therapy. If whole blood is used, it should be ABO identical and should be crossmatched (Chapter 7).

Preoperative Autologous Donation

Stored whole blood may also be used in **preoperative autologous donation (PAD)** programs, when a patient donates one or more units of blood 1–3 weeks before a scheduled surgery. In PAD, collected units are often held as whole blood to eliminate the costs involved in component preparation and storage. Overall, very little of this blood is given after surgery and some PAD programs have out-date rates as high as 50%. Therefore, the processing of whole blood into separate red blood cell and fresh frozen plasma (FFP) units is not generally cost-effective. Systems must be in place to ensure the use of autologous blood prior to the infusion of allogeneic blood products.

Acute Normovolemic Hemodilution

Another alternative to allogeneic transfusion that uses whole blood is **acute normovolemic hemodilution (ANH)**; just before surgery begins, whole blood is removed from a patient while simultaneously replacing the volume with crystalloid and/or colloid solutions. The main goal of ANH is to reduce the volume of red blood cells that are lost during a surgical procedure by decreasing the patient's hematocrit. Additionally, the collected blood is returned when the patient needs it most.

Blood is withdrawn using standard whole blood collection bags on collection tilt-rockers, which will automatically clamp off when a designated volume is reached. As the blood is being removed, crystalloid and/or colloid solutions are infused to maintain blood volume and cardiac output. The resultant lowering of the patient's hematocrit means that proportionally less red blood cells will be lost if the same volume of bleed occurs. Proportions generally used are crystalloid-to-blood ratios of 3:1 and colloid-to-blood ratios of 1:1.

After the major blood loss has subsided or sooner, if needed, the withdrawn blood is reinfused. If more than 1 unit was withdrawn, the units should be reinfused in reverse order. The first unit collected and the last reinfused will contain the largest amounts of fresh coagulation factors and platelets, thus providing the best therapy likely to stop continued bleeding. Because ANH occurs in the operating room, ANH programs are usually administered by operating room personnel. Collected products should be labeled appropriately and reinfused prior to the patient leaving the operating suite. As with any blood processing, accurate and clear labeling requirements must be followed.[5] Reinfusion guidelines must be established, practiced, and audited for quality assurance. ANH programs may be acceptable to some patients who refuse other blood transfusions for religious reasons.

What are two differences between preoperative autologous donation and acute normovolemic hemodilution?

Intraoperative Blood Salvage

Another form of autologous blood collection is **intraoperative blood salvage**, when blood is collected from the surgical site during or after surgery and reinfused. Blood salvage may involve whole blood or packed cells. Blood salvage may reduce allogeneic blood use during surgical procedures where large blood loss is experienced or expected (e.g., vascular aneurism repair or liver transplantation).

Any blood lost may be collected by suction, mixed with anticoagulant, and washed in a machine designed for this use. Figure 11-1 shows one example of a blood salvage instrument. The salvaged red blood cells are then reinfused. A second method filters salvaged blood instead of washing it and returns it to the patient as whole blood. A third method, called **direct transfusion**, takes the patient's blood used in cardiopulmonary bypass machines and transfuses it back to the patient as whole blood.

Contraindications for intraoperative blood salvage include the presence of infection or cancer cells at the site of surgery. As with other blood processing programs, clear policies for collection, labeling, and reinfusing should be established and implemented.

RED BLOOD CELL COMPONENTS

Red blood cell components, which are often called *packed cells* or *packed red blood cells*, are commonly used to treat anemia due to a variety of diseases or clinical situations. Red blood cells are unique

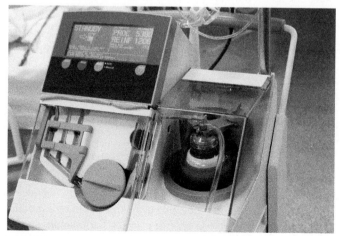

FIGURE 11-1 Cell Salvage Machine
Source: beerkoff/Shutterstock.

in their oxygen transport function. Both whole blood and red blood cell components can improve oxygen transport; however, red blood cell components can accomplish the same effect with a smaller volume transfusion and without the ABO-compatibility restrictions associated with the plasma portion of whole blood. Red blood cell components do not necessarily need to be ABO identical between donor and recipient, but they must be ABO compatible (Chapter 4). The donor red blood cells transfused must lack all ABO antigens that correspond to all ABO antibodies present in the recipient's plasma. Red blood cell components should be crossmatched prior to infusion (Chapter 7). Facilities must have policies governing transfusion of uncrossmatched red blood cell units.

Patients with anemia generally fall into two categories. The anemia may develop over time and may be hemodynamically compensated; that is, the patient does not have adequate oxygenation of tissues but does have adequate blood volume. Or the anemia may be a result of an acute blood loss due to trauma, surgery, or severe bleeding caused by underlying medical conditions, for example, a gastrointestinal bleed. These patients often need to be treated for both volume depletion and anemia.

Transfusion Triggers

Patients rarely need red blood cell transfusions if the hemoglobin concentration is above 10 g/dL (100 g/L). Below 7 g/dL (70 g/L), many patients experience symptoms of poor oxygenation and benefit from red blood cell transfusions. Between 7 and 10 g/dL (70 and 100 g/L), the patient's clinical presentation and the particular problem being treated exert more influence on the decision to transfuse. Hemoglobin and hematocrit are very useful diagnostic parameters. Guidelines such as those outlined above are often called **transfusion triggers**. However, the decision to transfuse should not be based only on laboratory findings. The clinician needs to consider the overall clinical picture of the patient, especially to determine if symptoms of oxygen carrying deficiency are present or not. The clinician should also consider any underlying disease when choosing to treat anemia with transfusion.[6]

Directed Donation

In preparing for elective surgical procedures, patients and their families often have concerns about transfusion-associated disease transmission. One strategy that may address this fear is the use of **directed donation**, when blood from a specific donor is drawn and set aside for a specific recipient. In directed donation, trusted family members and close friends of the patient donate samples for blood typing. Those with blood types compatible with the intended recipient donate whole blood at the hospital or local blood center. The blood is labeled with the information of the intended recipient and shipped to the hospital where the procedure is to be performed. Importantly, if the donation is from a first-degree family member, this unit must be irradiated prior to infusion in order to prevent transfusion-associated graft versus host disease (TA-GVHD). These units are screened for infectious diseases in the same manner as community donors. Directed units are processed into packed red blood cell units. Plasma portions of these units are usually placed in the main donor supply and not designated for the recipient of the directed donation.

If the red blood cell unit is not transfused to the intended recipient, it may cross over into the main donor supply because directed donors meet all of the same screening requirements as community donors. However, policies vary among facilities and some may choose to discard directed donor units if they are not transfused to the intended recipient.

Several social issues impact the use of directed donation. Donors may feel pressured to donate for the ill family member. Some donors may have confidential reasons not to donate. Under this social pressure, they may falsify responses to screening questions designed to identify high-risk behavior. The confidential exclusion process for donors can be helpful in addressing this specific risk.

Directed donation programs help family members feel included in the care of their loved one. Directed donors may respond to a positive donation experience by becoming donors for the general, community blood supply. Transfusion services should have systems in place that ensure that autologous units are used first, followed by any directed donation units, before units from community donors are transfused.[1]

Directed donations may be the norm in some developing countries that have not yet established strong community-based donor programs.

Community Directed Donations

One newer application of the directed donor paradigm is becoming more widely used in the treatment of hemoglobinopathies. Patients with sickle cell anemia and thalassemias often require large numbers of transfusions in the treatment of their disease (Chapter 17). Transfusion of red blood cells phenotypically matched for several common antigens is recommended for these patients. Traditionally, community donors tend to be of European ethnicity, whereas sickle cell anemia and thalassemia occur more frequently in people of African and Mediterranean ethnicity, respectively. This can make it difficult to support a phenotype matching program or to find compatible red blood cells for patients who have already made antibodies.

Known as **community directed donations**, these programs aim to increase the number of donors of African ethnicity.[7] Treating these as directed donations where several donors are linked to a specific, chronically transfused patient has been shown to increase donor participation. The use of phenotypically matched red blood cells decreases the risk of alloimmunization in the patient. An additional benefit of these community directed donation programs are fewer donor exposures for the recipient.

> ### ☑ CHECKPOINT 11-4
> What is the difference between a directed donation and a community directed donation?

GRANULOCYTES

Granulocyte units are collected by **apheresis** (a procedure in which whole blood is removed from the body, a specific component removed—in this case granuloctyes—and the remainder of the blood

is returned to the donor) and are used to treat neutropenic patients who have bacterial and/or fungal sepsis that has been shown to be resistant to antimicrobial therapy.

Granulocyte transfusion is used primarily as interim therapy for patients who are expected to recover neutrophil production. Patients with congenital abnormalities in neutrophil function may benefit from this component also. Granulocyte therapy is not generally a first-line therapy for patients with bacterial or fungal sepsis. Neutropenia due to a documented bacterial or fungal infection is usually first treated with antibiotics or antifungal medication. Continued neutropenia may be treated with granulocyte colony-stimulating factor (G-CSF) to try to stimulate the patient's own neutrophil production. After a poor response to G-CSF, donor granulocyte transfusion may then be considered. Generally an increase in neutrophils is not seen immediately after granulocyte therapy; however, the infection may improve as the infused granulocytes engulf and destroy the bacteria or fungal cells. The patient should be reassessed after 4–7 consecutive days of granulocyte transfusion.

Recombinant growth-stimulating hormones, usually G-CSF, may be used to mobilize the donor's bone marrow to release larger numbers of granulocytes and produce a higher yield of granulocytes in the apheresis product. If G-CSF is not used, sometimes a sedimenting agent, such as hydroxyethyl starch, can be used to help increase product yield. Granulocyte units should be transfused as soon as possible, and must be transfused within 24 hours of collection, to obtain the most viable cell dose. Granulocyte units should always be irradiated to prevent TA-GVHD. They should not be infused with microaggregate or leukoreduction filters. These filters trap white blood cells and therefore would obviously make the transfusion ineffective. The donor and recipient should be both Rh and human leukocyte antigen (HLA) compatible. A crossmatch should be performed if more than 2 mL of red blood cells are present in the granulocyte unit.[3]

HEMATOPOIETIC PROGENITOR CELLS

Hematopoietic progenitor cell (HPC) transplants are paired with high-dose chemotherapy or radiation to treat a number of disorders. HPC transplants may use cells collected from cord samples, bone marrow, or peripheral circulation. Table 11-3 ✳ lists common HPC components. HPC transplants can be either autologous or allogeneic depending on the disease being treated.

> ### ☑ CHECKPOINT 11-5
> What are two diseases that may be treated with a hematopoietic progenitor cell transplant?

Types of Hematopoietic Progenitor Cells

Hematopoietic stem cells are primitive cells that have the capacity for both self-renewal and maturation into different cell lineages. In response to specific hormones and chemokines, stem cells produce red blood cells, white blood cells, or platelets. For example, anemia stimulates the kidneys to produce erythropoietin, which signals the bone marrow to mature stem cells into the erythroid lineage,

✴ TABLE 11-3 Hematopoietic Progenitor Cells

Components	Benefits	Major Indications	Risks
HPC-Aphereis HPC-Marrow HPC-Cord	Transfusion of CD34+/lin− cells	• Leukemia, lymphomas, severe aplastic anemias, some other hematologic malignancies with poor prognostic indicators such as myeloproliferative neoplasms or myelodysplastic syndromes • Multiple myeloma • Severe combined immunodeficiency syndrome (SCIDS) • Some hemoglobinopathies • Some solid tumors • Some metabolic disorders	• Graft versus host disease (GVHD) except if autologous transplant • DMSO toxicity if using frozen product • Hazards common to human source blood products
T cells	Transfusion of CD3+ cells	Donor lymphocyte infusion (DLI) following HPC transplant to enhance graft versus disease effect	Hazards common to human source blood products

HPC, hematopoietic progenitor cells; DMSO, dimethyl sulfoxide.

resulting in more red blood cells to address the need for increased tissue oxygenation. Once differentiated into a blood cell lineage, the stem cells lose their capability for self-renewal and are referred to as hematopoietic progenitor cells. In common usage, both cell types are often referred to as HPCs. The majority of HPCs reside in the bone marrow, attached to the stromal lining. However, HPC can also be found in the peripheral circulation; usually less than 1% of circulating white blood cells can be classified by flow cytometric analysis as HPC. After migration from the bone marrow to the peripheral blood, these cells may be referred to as peripheral blood stem cells (PBSC).

Hematopoietic Progenitor Cell Products

HPCs were initially collected only by surgical aspiration of bone marrow directly from the donor's pelvis. In the 1980s, the successful manufacture of recombinant growth factors, which are also called colony-stimulating factors (CSF), allowed for the collection of what is now termed *"mobilized"* PBSC. Colony-stimulating factors induce the bone marrow to release early progenitor cells to the peripheral blood, where they develop into certain cell lines. Stimulation can increase the number of HPC to 1–5% of the white blood cells in the peripheral circulation. The HPCs circulating in the blood are collected using an apheresis machine, which collects the HPC from the mononuclear white blood cell layer when the whole blood is centrifuged.

Today, bone marrow is still collected for transplantation, but collection of PBSC is more common. There are differences to the recipient as well as the donor between using bone marrow and peripheral cells as the transplant source. PBSC have a shorter time to engraftment, but generally have higher rates of graft versus host disease (GVHD). Conversely, bone marrow takes a few days longer to engraft, but GVHD is often less severe. Bone marrow collection carries a greater risk for the donor from the surgical procedure and anesthesia. PBSC collection often requires a catheter placement, which carries a risk of infection and bleeding. The risks and benefits for both donor and recipient are considered before a specific product type is requested.

The HPCs used for transplantation have some identifying antigens; most significantly, they express cluster designation 34 (CD34) and lack lineage specific markers (lin-). This characteristic is used

to quantify the number of HPCs present in the product. Generally, $2.5-5.0 \times 10^6$ CD34+/lin− cells per kg recipient weight are given to achieve durable engraftment of the donor's white blood cell, red blood cell, and platelet cell lines.

An alternate source of stem cells is cord blood. Cord blood is collected from the umbilical cord and placenta immediately after birth and has a high number of HPCs. Cord blood cells are stored for future use in one of two types of facilities. Autologous cord cell storage is available in private cord cell banks, which, for a fee, will test, freeze, and store these products in the unlikely event that the infant needs a transplant later in life. Cord cells can also be donated for use as an allogeneic source of stem cells. These cells are stored in public cord banks for use by anyone matching the HLA type of the cord. The mother who agrees to an allogeneic cord blood donation provides an extensive medical history and is tested for infectious diseases. The collected cord blood is tested for ABO/Rh, HLA type, and CD34 content. Data is entered into national and global databases. The cord blood is then immediately available for a donor who has an emergent need and who is an HLA match.[8] Cord blood is cryopreserved using dimethyl sulfoxide (DMSO) and stored frozen.

Autologous Hematopoietic Progenitor Cell Transplants

Autologous HPCs are collected from the patient's bone marrow or peripheral blood after lower doses of chemotherapy and cryopreserved using 10% DMSO. After collection and freezing of adequate numbers of HPCs, the patient is treated with extremely high doses of chemotherapy and/or radiation to attempt to kill any remaining cancer cells. These doses are so high that the patient's marrow is damaged extensively and the ability of the HPCs for self-renewal and differentiation is severely impaired or completely destroyed. The patient's cryopreserved HPCs are then thawed and reinfused, restoring hematopoietic function, hopefully with minimal residual or no cancer cells remaining. This strategy is currently used for diseases such as Hodgkin's lymphoma, non-Hodgkin's lymphoma, multiple myeloma, testicular cancer, and neuroblastoma, where the patient's disease has proven resistant to first-line chemotherapy and irradiation. If the higher-dose therapy does not cure the malignancy, the therapeutic goal is to extend the amount of time the patient has with less extensive disease.

Allogeneic Hematopoietic Progenitor Cell Transplants

If the malignancy is centered within the HPC line itself, autologous transplantation obviously cannot be expected to give a complete remission from the disease. In these cases, HPCs transplanted from another person can be used to rescue the patient from high-dose chemotherapy or radiation treatment. In allogeneic transplants, the goal is the remission or cure of the patient's malignancy and replacement of their HPCs with cells from a healthy donor. Cells can be used from HLA-matched related donors or from HLA-matched unrelated donors. After treatment and transplant, recipients of an allogeneic transplant initially require immunosuppressive therapy to prevent GVHD. Allogeneic HPC transplantation is best utilized for patients with acute myelogenous leukemia (AML), high-risk cytogenetic acute lymphocytic leukemia (ALL), aplastic anemia (AA), high-risk cytogenetic myelodysplastic syndrome (MDS), late-stage or imatinib-resistant chronic myelogenous leukemia (CML), some of the hemoglobinopathies, and inherited immunological deficiencies. In the United States, imatinib is marketed under the trade name Gleevac®. Allogeneic transplant is used in certain patients after failure of an autologous transplant.

HLA-matched sibling transplants are often the best source for allogeneic transplants. For those patients who do not have an HLA-matched sibling, an HLA-matched unrelated donor must be located. The blood samples from many thousands of volunteer donors are tested (Chapter 18) and the data is listed in a large database for possible matching to a recipient in need. This information is maintained by the National Marrow Donor Program (NMDP) in the United States. Other national and international databases also exist and are searchable by any transplant center, which then requests a product when a patient has a match to a registered donor in any of the registries. The donor is then asked to participate in an HPC donation. If he or she agrees to donate, the donation is collected at a donor center near to the donor and the product is transported to the recipient. The product is infused after **myeloablative**, which means complete destruction of the bone marrow, treatment. Donations remain anonymous for at least 1 year, but may be kept anonymous forever if the donor chooses.

Allogeneic transplants are based on matching the HLA antigens of recipient and donor. HLA genes are inherited on the short arm of chromosome 6 (Chapter 18). A patient's best HLA match for an allogeneic transplant may be incompatible for ABO and Rh antigens. The task of providing blood products for patients who receive an ABO- and/or Rh-incompatible HPC transplant can be complex. Transfusions of red blood cell and plasma-containing products must be compatible with both the recipient and donor for the immediate post-transplant period (Chapter 4).

Donor Lymphocyte Infusion

After an HLA-matched allogeneic transplant, some patients experience a relapse of their original disease. One treatment often used in these cases is an infusion with additional T-cell lymphocytes from the original HPC donor. This is called a *donor lymphocyte infusion (DLI).*

The goal is to induce a graft versus leukemia (GvL) effect; the grafted T-cells play a part in the destruction of malignant blood cells in the recipient. The dose to be transfused is based on number of lymphocytes per kilogram recipient weight. The T-cell lymphocytes in the product are identified by the CD3 marker. Flow cytometry can be used to count the number of CD3(+) cells in a sample of product. This number can then be used to estimate the number of T-cells in the entire product.

☑ CHECKPOINT 11-6

What laboratory technology can be used to identify the quantity of a certain cell type—for example, CD3(+) or CD34(+)—in a sample?

MODIFICATION OF CELLULAR COMPONENTS

Table 11-4 ✳ lists the common modifications made to cellular components: leukocyte reduction, irradiation, washing, and freezing. Both red blood cell and platelet units can be washed. Freezing is generally used only for red blood cells with rare antigen phenotypes. Products with reduced risk for cytomegalovirus (CMV) may also be requested by clinicians.

Leukoreduction

Leukoreduction helps to prevent the formation of antibodies to HLA antigens because white blood cells carry HLA antigens. Patients who would be most adversely affected by alloimmunization to HLA antigens, such as those awaiting a HPC transplant, should receive leuko-reduced cellular blood products. HLA alloimmunization has been associated with febrile nonhemolytic transfusion reactions, transfusion-related acute lung injury (Chapter 12), refractoriness to platelet transfusion (Chapter 16), and rejection of transplanted organs.

Transfused white blood cells are also believed to be responsible for transfusion-associated immunomodulatory effect (TRIM). Transfusion may be associated with an increased incidence of bacterial infections and malignancy recurrence, with stronger correlations in certain patient populations and little or no correlation in other populations.[9] Conversely, allogeneic transfusion is also associated with a decreased rate of kidney transplant rejection.[10] The cause of TRIM is not yet proven, but several white blood cell–mediated mechanisms, which lead to immunosuppression and/or inflammation, may be involved.[11] It is likely that several mechanisms are involved in TRIM.

Certain viruses, such as CMV, human T-cell lymphotropic virus (HTLV-I), and Epstein-Barr virus (EBV), are known to reside in white blood cells and disease transmission can occur with transfusion of infected white blood cells in the donor product.[6] Leukoreduction decreases the viral load in the product and therefore can decrease the incidence of transfusion-related transmission of these viruses.

There are leukocyte reduction filters that can be used with whole blood, red blood cell, or platelet units. The filters are not interchangeable between products. Leukocyte reduction filters remove 95–99%

✳ **TABLE 11-4** Component Modification

Modification	Components	Benefits	Precautions
Leukoreduction*	Red blood cells, platelets	Potential prevention of • Febrile, nonhemolytic transfusion reaction • CMV infection • HLA immunization • Immunomodulatory effects	Hypotensive reactions in recipients taking ACE inhibitors may occur more frequently with bedside filtration and certain filters than when leukoreduction is done at the time of collection or in the lab.
Irradiation	Mandatory: Granulocytes Optional/selected situations: Red blood cells, platelets	Prevention of TA-GVHD	Shorten expiration date of irradiated red blood cell units to 28 days from date of irradiation if before original expiration date. Irradiated red blood cells experience increased potassium leakage.
Tested for anti-CMV	Red blood cells, platelets, granulocytes, hematopoietic progenitor cells	Prevention of CMV infection, especially in • Immunocompromised patients • Premature and low birth weight neonates • Fetuses receiving intrauterine transfusion • HPC transplant recipients • Solid organ transplant recipients	CMV seronegative units may provide the least risk of CMV transmission. In areas with endemic CMV rates, leukoreduction can be used as the next best alternative.
Washing	Red blood cells, platelets	Removes plasma. Indications include transfusion to • IgA-deficient recipients with anti-IgA when IgA-deficient products are not available • Recipients with repeated, severe anaphylactic reactions following transfusion	If washing is performed using an open system, red blood cell units expire within 24 hours of the start of washing and platelet units expire within 4 hours of the start of washing. Open systems may increase the risk of bacterial contamination.
Freezing and deglycerolization	Red blood cells with rare phenotypes or from IgA-deficient donors	• Prevention of hemolytic transfusion reactions in recipients with multiple antibodies or an antibody to a high-incidence antigen • Prevention of anaphylactic reactions in IgA-deficient recipients with anti-IgA	If glycerolization and/or deglycerolization used an open system, the red blood cell units expire 24 hours from the start of the thaw or wash cycle. Open systems may increase the risk of bacterial contamination.

* Leukoreduction may occur prestorage or at the time of transfusion; CMV, cytomegalovirus; HLA, human leukocyte antigens; ACE, angiotensin converting enzyme; TA-GVHD, transfusion associated graft versus host disease; HPC, hematopoietic progenitor cells.

of the white blood cells. No more than 15% of the unit's red blood cells should be lost during filtration.[3]

Single-donor platelets can be collected by an apheresis machine in a manner that renders the product leukodepleted during the collection process itself. The apheresis machine must be validated as producing units low in white blood cells, before the products can be labeled as leukoreduced.[11] A number of products are also tested periodically to ensure the leukoreduction procedure is still adequate.[3]

☑ **CHECKPOINT 11-7**

What are two risks of transfusion that can potentially be reduced by using leukocyte reduction?

Irradiation

Irradiation is used to prevent TA-GVHD (transfusion-associated graft versus host disease). Red blood cell, granulocyte, and platelet units contain white blood cells. TA-GVHD occurs when viable transfused lymphocytes replicate in the recipient, recognize the recipient as foreign, and mount a destructive immune response against the recipient's body. TA-GVHD produces a pancytopenia within days of the transfusion and is almost uniformly fatal.

Gamma irradiation disrupts the DNA in the white blood cell nuclei, which destroys the white blood cells' ability to replicate. To prevent TA-GVHD the blood component should receive a radiation dose of 25 Gy (2500 cGY) delivered to the midplane and 15 Gy (1500 cGy) to all parts of the bag (Chapter 10).[3]

Because immunocompromised patients are most susceptible to TA-GVHD, they commonly receive irradiated red blood cell and platelet units. Products that are from a first-degree relative of the recipient must be irradiated, as the recipient would be at high risk for TA-GVHD. Fresh frozen plasma (FFP), detailed later in this chapter, does not need to be irradiated because it seldom contains viable white blood cells.[6]

Cytomegalovirus (CMV) Prevention

Cytomagalovirus (CMV) infection is often asymptomatic in a person with a robust immune system (Chapter 13). In immune-suppressed individuals, CMV infection can cause debilitating effects and even death. Patient populations where transfusion-transmitted CMV infection can cause significant morbidity and mortality include low-birth-weight infants (<1500g), CMV-seronegative HPC transplant recipients or potential recipients, CMV-seronegative antepartum women, fetuses receiving intrauterine transfusion, and HIV-infected patients and children born to HIV-positive mothers. Each facility should have clearly communicated guidelines that list the at-risk patient populations applicable to the facility and that outlines the methods the facility uses to decrease the risk of transfusion-associated CMV transmission.

There are two methods to decrease the risk of transfusion-associated CMV transmission. Leukoreduction is the first method, while testing blood donors for antibodies to CMV is the second method. Controversy exists over the best strategy to use when transfusing susceptible populations.[12,13]

CMV infects white blood cells; therefore, leukoreduction can reduce the viral load in blood components. In order to reduce CMV transmission and HLA alloimmunization, some countries have converted their blood supply to prestorage, universal leukoreduced, which ensures that all cellular blood products have reduced numbers of white blood cells.[14,15]

CMV serologic testing is not technically a modification, but it is not performed on every donor. If the donor is tested and is found to be seronegative, the components may be labeled as CMV negative or anti-CMV negative. The incidence of CMV infection in the general population varies and can be quite high. In regions with a high prevalence of CMV, it is difficult to maintain a large inventory of red blood cell and platelet components from CMV-seronegative donors.

Neither leukoreduction nor CMV seronegativity may confer complete protection from transmission of CMV, and perhaps the combination is most effective in preventing CMV infection in susceptible populations.[16]

☑ CHECKPOINT 11-8

What are two methods for reducing the risk of transfusion-transmitted cytomegalovirus infection?

Washing

Washing of red blood cell and platelet units is indicated in only a few clinical situations. Not all transfusion services have the equipment needed to wash components. The procedure uses centrifugation most often in an open system, which markedly reduces the allowable storage period of the washed product. An open system means that the seal of the component has been breached. Washed red blood cell units expire in 24 hours from the time of washing, platelets in 4 hours.[3] Washing of red blood cell units eliminates approximately 85% of the white blood cells, about 15% of red blood cell mass, and virtually 99% of the plasma.

Due to the tremendous reduction of plasma, washed red blood cell and platelet components can be transfused to IgA-deficient patients who have antibodies to IgA. IgA-deficient blood products are not readily available, making washed products a useful alternative. Washing may also be indicated in patients who have severe allergic reactions to blood products. The labor-intensive process should not be routinely ordered and consultation with the medical director is generally required. The high efficiency of leukoreduction filters is more effective and less costly than washing; therefore, washing should not be used as a means to reduce white blood cells.

Freezing

Blood from donors with rare red blood cell phenotypes may be stored frozen for up to 10 years and used for autologous or allogeneic transfusion. Many countries maintain a national rare blood registry, which may be accessed by any transfusion center when there is a need for a rare phenotype. Each unit is phenotyped extensively prior to freezing using a cryoprotective agent, such as 20% or 40% glycerol. When the unit is to be transfused the cryoprotective agent must be washed, a process called **deglycerolization** (Chapter 10). The expiration date of the deglycerolized red blood cell components is 24 hours for open systems or 2 weeks for closed systems.[3]

Cryopreservation of platelets is not widely available. DMSO is the most common cryopreservative used for frozen platelet storage.[17] Multiple methods have been described. In all cases, platelet recovery is low, with as few as one-third of the original platelets remaining at the time of transfusion. As well, the freezing and thawing processes are time-consuming and expensive. Frozen platelet products can be stored for 2 years.[18] The product is thawed and to decrease toxicity, the DMSO is reduced before transfusion. Indications for using frozen platelets are even fewer than for frozen red blood cell components due to the lack of availability and the large loss of platelet numbers.[1]

☑ CHECKPOINT 11-9

What is the common cryoprotective agent used when freezing red blood cells?

TRANSFUSION TREATMENT OF COAGULOPATHIES

Several components are used to treat deficiencies in and abnormalities of coagulation proteins. Fresh frozen plasma (FFP), platelet products, and cryoprecipitate are three types of plasma-derived products commonly used. Table 11-5 ✳ identifies and compares these plasma products.

✳ **TABLE 11-5** Plasma Products

Components	Benefits	Major Indications	Contraindications	Risks
Fresh frozen plasma (FFP) Fresh frozen plasma, apheresis Fresh frozen plasma, quarantined	Improves hemostasis; provides all coagulation factors	To treat or prevent bleeding due to coagulopathy: • When multiple coagulation factors are deficient • In massively transfused patients • In patients with a coagulation factor deficiency if no specific factor concentrate is available • When rapid reversal of warfarin is required To provide functioning proteins: • In patients with TTP • In patients with rare, specific protein deficiencies Replacement fluid in therapeutic plasma exchange	• If specific factor concentrates can be used as an alternative • To reverse warfarin therapy if there is time to try vitamin K therapy as an alternative • As a volume expander without the need to correct coagulopathy	• Positive direct antiglobulin test and/or hemolysis if donor plasma contains an antibody and recipient red blood cells carry the corresponding antigen • Hazards common to human source blood products
Plasma frozen within 24 hours Plasma, cryoprecipitate reduced Liquid plasma Thawed plasma	Improves hemostasis; provides all coagulation factors except Factors V and VIII	Similar to FFP Plasma, cryoprecipitate reduced may provide additional benefit for treatment of TTP.	Similar to FFP	Similar to FFP
Platelets Platelets, pooled Platelets, apheresis	Improve hemostasis; provide functional platelets	To treat or prevent bleeding in thrombocytopenic patients or patients with dysfunctional platelets	Bleeding unrelated to platelet deficiencies, either in number or function TTP or ITP unless there is life-threatening bleeding	• Alloimmunization to HLA and/or HPA • Bacterial contamination occurs more often with platelet components because of the storage temperature • Hazards common to human source blood products
Cryoprecipitate	Provides Factors VIII, XIII, von Willebrand factor, fibrinogen, fibronectin	Replacement of fibrinogen or less often Factor VIII or von Willebrand factor Also used prior to surgery when patient is known to have dysfibrinogenemia	• If specific factor concentrates can be used as an alternative • When specific factor deficiencies are not documented	• Positive direct antigobulin test if ABO-incompatible cryoprecipitate is transfused • Hazards common to human source blood products

FFP, fresh frozen plasma; TTP, thrombocytic thrombocytopenic purpura; ITP, immune thrombocytopenic purpura; HLA, human leukocyte antigens; HPA, human platelet antigens.

TRANSFUSABLE PLASMA COMPONENTS

Fresh frozen plasma (FFP) is primarily used to replace dysfunctional or deficient coagulation proteins when specific coagulation factor concentrates are not routinely available or when multiple coagulation factors must be rapidly replaced to control bleeding. Coagulation factor deficiencies are usually caused by congenital diseases such as hemophilia A or B, which are deficiencies of Factor VIII and IX, respectively. Inhibitors or antibodies to coagulation factors will make the coagulation process ineffective and may result in bleeding.

Multiple coagulation deficiencies are often present in patients with liver damage or failure because the liver produces many of the coagulation proteins. Plasma transfusion may also be used to rapidly reverse the effects of vitamin K antagonists like warfarin, which is commonly known by the trade name Coumadin®. Vitamin K antagonists or deficiencies of vitamin K affect multiple coagulation factors.

Therapeutic plasma exchange is used to treat certain conditions by removing abnormal substances, often while simultaneously providing functional plasma components. Plasma, which will provide functional proteins, is one of several substances that can be used as the replacement fluid during a therapeutic plasma exchange.

FFP should not be used to dilute red blood cell units for faster infusion; crystalloids can be used and will not expose the patient to another donor. Specific coagulation factor concentrates have largely replaced FFP as the treatment of choice for people with congenital factor abnormalities. Factor concentrates carry less risk of infectious disease transmission as compared to blood components. FFP is usually only used if no factor concentrate is available.

The supernatant remaining after the manufacture of cryoprecipitate is refrozen and labeled as "plasma, cryoprecipitate reduced," which is sometimes called cryo-poor plasma. Plasma, cryoprecipitate reduced is often the product of choice for treating patients with thrombotic thrombocytopenic purpura (Chapter 17).

The decision to treat patients with FFP should not be based solely on laboratory values, such as coagulation screening tests, but should take into consideration the patient's underlying disease and clinical status.

PLATELET COMPONENTS

Platelet components may be manufactured from whole blood or may be collected using apheresis (Chapter 10). Platelet transfusion is indicated in a variety of clinical situations where decreased platelet production, increased platelet destruction, or platelet dysfunction may lead to bleeding.

Certain thrombocytopenic patients may benefit from prophylactic platelet transfusion to reduce bleeding risk. A platelet count of less than $10 \times 10^3/\mu L$ $(10 \times 10^9/L)$ is often used as a trigger to initiate prophylactic platelet transfusions to prevent intracranial hemorrhage. Common patient groups with low platelet counts that are treated prophylactically include premature neonates, cancer patients receiving chemotherapy, and transplant patients, both solid organ and HPC. Prophylactic platelet transfusions may occur at higher platelet counts such as $100 \times 10^3/\mu L$ $(100 \times 10^9/L)$, when the patient has additional risk factors that may lead to bleeding; for example, if the patient has already suffered an intracranial hemorrhage, if the patient is scheduled for neurosurgery, or if the patient is at increased risk for pulmonary or ophthalmic bleeding.[2]

Platelet transfusions are also used to treat patients who have dysfunctional platelets and who are bleeding. In these cases, the patient's platelet count may be within the normal range. There are congenital platelet abnormalities, such as Glanzmann's thrombasthenia; or platelet dysfunction can also be acquired. For example, many drugs can reversibly or irreversibly alter platelet function. Acetylsalicylic acid (ASA or aspirin) has been joined by newer medications on the list of drugs that interfere with platelet function.

Many donor centers primarily collect apheresis platelet products, which are also called single-donor platelets. Although the time involved for the donor is increased with apheresis collections, there are benefits to the recipients. For adults, the usual dose per transfusion is one apheresis platelet or 6 whole blood–derived platelets. Typical dosage of whole blood–derived platelets can vary among facilities from 4 to 10 units per dose. Therefore, use of apheresis platelets can dramatically reduce the number of donors that a recipient is exposed to, decreasing the risk of transfusion-transmitted disease. For pediatric and neonatal patients, a sterile connection device may be used to aseptically split the platelet unit into smaller doses.[19] If frequent transfusions are expected, the same unit can supply multiple infusions over its shelf life.

Apheresis platelets where the donor and recipient are matched for certain antigens, may be transfused when a recipient becomes **refractory** to platelet transfusions. Refractory means the patient does not exhibit the expected increase in platelet numbers after infusion of a platelet product (Chapter 16). A common cause of platelet refractoriness is alloimmunization from repeated transfusions and the formation of antibodies to HLA or platelet antigens.

☑ CHECKPOINT 11-10

What is the purpose of platelet transfusion?

CRYOPRECIPITATE

Cryoprecipitate is manufactured from FFP (Chapter 10). It contains Factor VIII, fibrinogen, von Willebrand factor (vWF), Factor XIII, and fibronectin.

Historically, the major use of cryoprecipitate, which is often labeled cryoprecipitated AHF, was to treat hemophilia A. AHF is an acronym for antihemophiliac factor. Hemophilia A is a congenital deficiency of Factor VIII (Chapter 17). In the late 1970s, specific factor concentrates became available and replaced cryoprecipitate as the treatment of choice for hemophilia A and von Willebrand disease (vWD).

Currently, the major use of cryoprecipitate is as a source of fibrinogen. Deficiencies of fibrinogen are seen in massive transfusion and disorders involving activation of the coagulation system. Cryoprecipitate can also be used to treat congenital deficiencies or dysfunctions of fibrinogen. Human fibrinogen (Riastap™) was approved by the U.S. Food and Drug Administration (FDA) in 2009 to treat patients with a congenital fibrinogen deficiency. A recombinant human fibrinogen product is available in Europe and may eventually replace the use of cryoprecipitate as fibrinogen replacement. Recombinant products have a reduced risk of infectious disease transmission compared to products manufactured from human plasma.

CASE IN POINT (continued)

The first 4 units of red blood cells are transfused to RA in less than 10 minutes. The treating physician immediately called the transfusion service to initiate the massive transfusion protocol and ordered an additional 6 red blood cell units and 6 plasma units. The patient's first CBC and INR results were a hemoglobin level of 12 g/dL (120 g/L), a hematocrit of 36% (0.36), and an INR of 1.3.

6. What is the purpose for transfusing plasma?
7. Why would the physician order plasma even before he saw the laboratory results in this case?

FIBRIN GLUE AND PLATELET GEL

Commercial preparations of fibrin glue are used as a sealant in surgical procedures in order to produce tight closure of the wound. Cryoprecipitate combined with bovine thrombin and calcium chloride can be used for this purpose as well,[20] but the commercial preparations are easy to store and administer and have had extra treatment to decrease the risk of infectious disease transmission.

Platelet gel is the intraoperative combination of autologous platelet and white blood cell–rich plasma, calcium chloride, and thrombin in a wound in order to stimulate coagulation and healing. This application of hemostatic mechanisms could theoretically be used in topical wound applications and as a component of grafting procedures. Clinical investigations of potential applications for fibrin sealants and platelet gel are ongoing.[21]

PLASMA FRACTIONATION PRODUCTS

Plasma fractionation methodologies have resulted in targeted therapies for a large number of diseases and coagulopathies. In the United States, the FDA and the Plasma Protein Therapeutics Association provide oversight and accreditation of **plasma fractionation** (a term referring to the general processes required to separate plasma components for subsequent transfusion) facilities (Chapter 20). Plasma fractionation products may be distributed by the transfusion service or by the pharmacy according to each facility's policies. While not entirely free of infectious diseases, improved processing methods and testing have increased the safety of these products dramatically (Chapter 10).

Albumin

Albumin is the protein that is present in the largest amount in human plasma. It contributes to fluid balance both within the blood vessels and throughout the body. It is most commonly used as a volume replacement in trauma, shock, burns, and therapeutic plasma exchange.

Rh-Immune Globulin

Rh-immune globulin (RhIg) is administered to prevent immunization to the D antigen. Anti-D is of major concern in women of childbearing age as it can cause serious hemolytic disease of the fetus and newborn (Chapter 14).

Common indications for the administration of RhIg include Rh(D)-negative mothers in the 28th week of pregnancy and following delivery of an Rh(D)-positive infant. Pregnant Rh(D)-negative women who are at increased risk for a feto–maternal hemorrhage in the perinatal period are also often given RhIg (Chapter 14), for example, following amniocentesis or abdominal trauma.

RhIg administration is also considered when transfusing Rh(D)-positive platelets to an Rh(D)-negative woman of childbearing age. Platelets do not carry the Rh antigens, but platelet components may be contaminated with red blood cells. Apheresis platelet units carry a low risk of Rh immunization because they usually have very low levels of red blood cell contamination.[22] Each facility should have a policy regarding the use of RhIg following transfusion of Rh nonidentical platelets and/or red blood cell components.

RhIg is often administered intramuscularly when given in the perinatal or postnatal period. Many RhIg preparations can only be given intramuscularly; at this time one product can be given either intramuscularly or intravenously. The route chosen for post-transfusion RhIg administration is often dependent on the dose of RhIg that will be given. If administering large doses of RhIg, a rate of administration that will reduce the risk of acute hemolysis should be specified.

RhIg can be used in some cases as an alternative to *intravenous immune globulin (IVIG)*, a product described in the next section, for the treatment of immune thrombocytopenia (ITP). RhIg is only effective in nonsplenectomized, Rh(D)-positive patients. The RhIg must be given intravenously; therefore, only certain RhIg preparations can be used. Patients receiving this treatment should be monitored for increased levels of hemolysis.[23]

Intravenous Immune Globulin (IVIG)

Isolation of the IgG portion in the plasma fractionation process yields a product composed of IgG antibodies directed at many antigens (Chapter 10). This product, called *intravenous immune globulin (IVIG)*, has been used to treat a variety of diseases, some of which are listed in Table 11.6 ✳. There are several different formulations from different manufacturers; differences among the formulations may include concentration (5 or 10%), stabilizers (usually one or more sugars), level of IgA, or form (liquid or lyophilized). A subcutaneous formulation of immune globulin received FDA approval in 2006; this product is commonly self-administered at home by patients with hypogammaglobulinemia.

Hyperimmune Globulins

Preparations of specific immune globulins, sometimes called *hyperimmune globulins*, are also available. These are made from donor plasmas that have high titers of the desired immune globulin and are used as passive immunity for patients exposed to infectious diseases. Some examples include rabies, rubella, cytomegalovirus, tetanus, varicella zoster, vaccinia, respiratory syncytial, and hepatitis B.[2, 6] Product availability varies among countries and changes over time as new products are approved or older products are replaced or removed from distribution.

> ☑ **CHECKPOINT 11-11**
>
> What are two examples of hyperimmune globulins?

Coagulation Factor Concentrates

Coagulation factor concentrates are used to prevent or to treat bleeding episodes in patients with coagulation deficiencies. The number and type of concentrates available is constantly changing; availability varies from country to country and is dependent on approval from the appropriate regulatory body(ies). Many countries also have a mechanism that allows the rare use of unapproved products in exceptional circumstances. Patients may also receive unapproved products as part of a research study. Research and approval protocols for fractionated products are very similar to those used for pharmaceutical products.

Patients with congenital factor deficiencies or with acquired factor inhibitors receive targeted therapy with the appropriate factor concentrate. Hemophilia patients are especially prone to developing

✳ **TABLE 11-6** Intravenous Immune Globulin (IVIG) Treatment

Indication Category	Category of Disorder	Example Diseases
Approved indications	Primary immune deficiencies	Hypogammaglobulinemia/aggamaglobulinemia Common variable immunodeficiency Severe combined immunodeficiencies Wiskott-Aldrich syndrome Hyper IgM syndromes
	Acquired immune deficiencies	Pediatric HIV with recurrent bacterial infections Postallogeneic bone marrow transplantation Chronic lymphocytic leukemia
	Immune cytopenias	Immune thrombocytopenia purpura
	Autoimmune disorders	Kawasaki's disease Chronic inflammatory demyelinating polyneuropathy
Commonly accepted indications	Hematology	Pure red blood cell aplasia Neonatal alloimmune thrombocytopenia Hemolytic disease of the fetus and newborn Post-transfusion purpura
	Neurology	Guillain-Barré syndrome Myasthenia gravis Multifocal motor neuropathy
	Rheumatology	Dermatomyositis Polymyositis
	Infectious disease	Staphylococcal toxic shock syndrome Necrotizing fasciitis

inhibitors (Chapter 17). Factor concentrates are easier to transfuse and safer for the patient than broad-spectrum treatment with FFP transfusion. Factor concentrates have a smaller volume and have less risk of disease transmission because of the viral inactivation steps used in the manufacturing process. Several factor concentrates are now made in a recombinant form (Chapter 10) and contain no human plasma-derived products, reducing the risk of infectious disease transmission theoretically to zero.

Plasma-derived coagulation factor concentrates include Factor VIII, Factor IX, Factor XIII, Factor VII, and fibrinogen. Some products contain a combination of coagulation factors (Chapter 10). Other plasma-derived protein concentrates include antithrombin, protein C, and C1-esterase inhibitor. Some recombinant products include Factor VIII, Factor IX, activated Factor VII, and antithrombin.

PHARMACEUTICALS

There are several drug strategies used to reduce or prevent bleeding. Most medications are dispensed by the pharmacy but because of their impact on blood product usage, the transfusion service may dispense certain pharmaceuticals.

Desmopressin

Desmopressin acetate is a synthetic peptide, 1-deamino-8-D-arginine vasopressin (DDAVP). It is used as a presurgical prophylaxis to reduce or prevent bleeding in patients with mild hemophilia A or type I von Willebrand disease. DDAVP causes the release of Factor VIII and von Willebrand factor (vWF) from vascular endothelial cells. In mild cases of these two disorders, factor levels are low but not absent. Residual vWF released from the patient's reserves helps platelets adhere to the vascular endothelium and the additional Factor VIII promotes

clot formation. DDAVP only works for the first few doses but is then ineffectual until the depleted reserves are replenished. This is sometimes referred to as **tachyphylaxis**, which means a rapidly decreasing response to a drug after administration of a few doses. DDAVP must be used with caution in patients susceptible to high blood pressure. The use of DDAVP in type II von Willebrand disease or any disorder with abnormal platelet function is controversial and may be contraindicated.[8, 21] DDAVP is also not used for patients with type III von Willebrand disease as there is too little vWF to be clinically helpful.

Vitamin K

Vitamin K can be used to reverse the effect of oral anticoagulants; for example, to treat warfarin overdose or to prepare patients for surgery. Reversal of anticoagulation may be indicated for catheter insertion or other invasive procedures. Vitamin K takes 10–12 hours to reverse oral anticoagulation and should be used in nonemergent clinical situations. The infusion of prothrombin complex concentrates (Chapter 10) or FFP is a faster method of reversing warfarin-induced coagulopathy and can be used when the coagulopathy must be quickly addressed.[24]

Erythropoietin

Erythropoietin (EPO) is produced by the kidneys and stimulates erythropoiesis, the production and release of red blood cells by the bone marrow. Recombinant EPO (such as epoetin alfa [Procrit®] or darbepoetin alfa [Aranesp®]) is primarily used to treat anemia in patients with renal failure, who therefore have decreased production of endogenous EPO. EPO treatment can reduce the frequency and number of transfusions these patients require, which leads to an improved quality of life. Perioperative autologous donation and bloodless surgery programs may prescribe EPO with iron supplementation to their patients prior to donation or surgery. EPO is contraindicated in several situations, including patients with certain impairments of cardiac function or with hematological disorders such as sickle cell disease.[25] EPO has been used by athletes as a performance enhancing drug and is banned by some sports regulatory bodies.

Thrombopoietin

Thrombopoietin (TPO) is the chemokine responsible for stimulating maturation of platelets from megakaryocytes. It is naturally produced by the liver and kidneys and to a lesser extent by the spleen, bone marrow, testes, muscles, and brain. In response to low numbers of circulating platelets, TPO production is increased and platelets are released from megakaryocytes. Recombinant TPO can be used to stimulate platelet production in patients suffering from bone marrow suppression that has caused thrombocytopenia.[8] Thrombopoietin receptor agonist is another class of biologic agents used to stimulate platelet production; romiplostim (Nplate®) and eltrombopag (Promacta®) are examples of this class of platelet stimulator approved for use in patients with idiopathic thrombocytopenic purpura (ITP).

Colony-Stimulating Factors

Granulocyte colony-stimulating factor (G-CSF) and granulocyte macrophage colony-stimulating factor (GM-CSF) are two naturally occurring chemokines that have also been manufactured as recombinant therapies. Hematopoietic progenitor cell (HPC) donors routinely receive colony-stimulating factor(s) prior to donation to increase the number of HPCs in the collection. Another widespread use is for treatment of neutropenia after chemotherapy in cancer patients. Neutropenic days are reduced significantly, resulting in decreased numbers of infections. G-CSF can be used alone but GM-CSF tends to work better when used in conjunction with G-CSF. Examples of recombinant human G-CSF are filgrastim (Neupogen®) and pegfilgrastim (Neulasta™), a longer-acting form of G-CSF; sargramostim (Leukine®) is a GM-CSF.

Plerixafor

Plerixafor, which is also sometimes called AMD 3100 and is currently distributed under the trade name Mozobil™, is the first CXCR4 chemokine receptor inhibitor approved by the FDA. It blocks binding of the ligand stromal derived Factor-1-alpha (SDF-1α) to the CXCR4 receptor. Its usefulness as a stem cell mobilizer was incidentally discovered when it was given to prevent the entrance of HIV-1 and HIV-2 into cells through the co-receptor CXCR4. It was found that CD34+ hematopoietic stem cell counts in the peripheral blood increased rapidly, in 4–5 hours as compared to the few days required by G-CSF. This new therapeutic class of drug has been useful for patients who were unable to produce sufficient amounts of autologous HPC for collection when treated with G-CSF alone. The two medications are generally given together and few side effects have been noted. Plerixafor is currently used for patients with non-Hodgkin's lymphoma or multiple myeloma.[26]

Antifibrinolytics

Antifibrinolytics, as the name implies, inhibit fibrinolysis. Fibrinolysis normally increases during cardiopulmonary bypass. Antifibrinolytics may be administered during cardiac surgery to reduce bleeding due to the increased fibrinolysis.[27]

In 2011, the two most common antifibrinolytics are analogues of the amino acid lysine, which inhibit plasmin and plasminogen activators. Aprotinin, a serine protease inhibitor, has been discontinued in many countries due to safety concerns. Currently on the market are Σ-aminocaproic acid, marketed under the trade name Amicar®, and tranexamic acid, marketed under the trade name Cyklokapron®. As with all pharmaceuticals, the availability varies among countries depending on regulatory approval. Both medications are water-soluble; 80–90% of the drug is excreted by the kidneys within 12 hours of administration. Antifibrinolytic therapy is contraindicated in disseminated intravascular coagulation (DIC).

Recombinant Factor VIIa

The FDA approved on-label indications for recombinant human Factor VIIa (NovoSeven®), include supplementing low Factor VII levels in patients with a Factor VII deficiency and treating or preventing hemorrhage in hemophilia A or B patients who have inhibitors or in patients with acquired hemophilia.[28] However, recombinant Factor VIIa has been used off-label in a variety of trauma cases. Activated Factor VII initiates deposition of fibrin on platelets and induces platelet aggregation at the site of bleeding. In order for treatment with recombinant Factor VIIa to be effective the patient must have adequate platelet and fibrin levels. Therefore, it is common in trauma and massively transfused patients either to measure fibrinogen or to transfuse cryoprecipitate prior to giving the VIIa product. While the coagulation precipitated by activated Factor VII tends to be localized to the site of bleeding, the most common adverse event of treatment with recombinant Factor VIIa is undesired thrombosis. Research continues, especially in the hematology and surgical settings, in determining the risks and benefits of using recombinant Factor VIIa.

CASE IN POINT (continued)

RA was taken to the operating room to repair crush injuries to his lower pelvis and for bilateral leg amputation. The patient continued to bleed throughout surgery and was transfused multiple blood products. The results from the last set of specimens sent to the laboratory from the operating room included:

- Hemoglobin = 8 g/dL (80 g/L)
- Hematocrit = 24% (0.24)
- Platelet count = 104 × 10³/μL (104 × 10⁹/L)
- INR = 1.4
- Fibrinogen = 70 mg/dL (2.06 μmol/L)

8. What blood product may be indicated based on the above laboratory results?
9. The physician also ordered a dose of recombinant Factor VIIa. What is the purpose of the Factor VIIa infusion?
10. Which laboratory values are commonly checked before Factor VIIa is given and why?

TRANSFUSION PROCESS

The transfusion process is an intricate set of steps involving multiple entities. Measures that increase both donor (Chapter 9) and recipient (Chapter 7) safety are built into each step from vein to vein. The blood bank and the transfusion service need processes that will prevent errors prospectively, detect errors when they occur, and retroactively identify root causes and improvement opportunities. In massive transfusion situations, a great risk to the recipient is delays in obtaining blood products. Therefore, some abbreviated processes may be substituted for the usual processes. These shortened processes must still ensure that critical safety points are met.

Examples of massive transfusion-related processes include:

- Process for identifying patients in emergency situations when the patient's identity is unknown.
- Process to allow for transfusion in the absence of informed consent when the patient is unable to give consent.
- Issue of uncrossmatched red blood cell units when no testing or not all testing is completed.
- Deletion of the serological crossmatch if a serological crossmatch is usually performed and if the patient's antibody screen is negative.
- Switching to ABO-identical donor red blood cell units following transfusion of multiple ABO-compatible, nonidentical red blood cell units. Commonly this becomes a concern when multiple-group O donor units are issued and transfused as uncrossmatched blood.
- Alternately, if shortages occur, identify acceptable switches to nonidentical blood components for both the ABO and Rh groups.
- Process to link results once a previously unidentified patient is identified.

MASSIVE TRANSFUSION

Massive transfusion, which is defined as replacement of a patient's total blood volume with donor components within 24 hours, occurs in a variety of situations. Table 11-7 ✷ lists some common conditions that may result in massive transfusion. An average-size adult has a blood volume of approximately 5L. Generally speaking, most facilities define massive transfusion as more than 10 red blood cell units transfused in 24 hours or less.

> ### ☑ CHECKPOINT 11-12
>
> What is the definition of *massive transfusion*?

The medical response to massive blood loss follows certain principles. The first step is establishing intravenous access. Once access is established, crystalloid solutions such as normal saline or lactated Ringer's solution are used to restore circulating systemic volume to avoid circulatory collapse. Crystalloid infusion is the usual first-line treatment,[29] but it may be followed by colloid infusion if there is a continued need to maintain blood volume.[1] Colloids include dextran and various starch-based solutions.

After restoration of cardiac function, oxygen delivery must be enhanced or preserved to prevent tissue and end organ ischemia. Red blood cell units are the blood component of choice for this purpose. Then, the source of bleeding must be surgically repaired or medically reversed.

Often a massively transfused patient develops coagulopathy from the dilution effects of large-volume infusions of crystalloid solutions, colloid solutions, and red blood cell units. An additional complication may be the loss of coagulation factors and platelets from blood loss or clotting. Infusion of FFP, platelets, and cryoprecipitate can aid in restoring hemostatic function. In some cases, this process is quickly effective, the bleeding is stopped, and the patient recovers. In other cases end-organ and tissue damage from prolonged blood loss results in further complications for the patient. Patients who begin bleeding due to underlying diseases are often difficult to manage and the blood product usage rate may be very high.

Recent research has raised the issue of transfusing FFP early in the resuscitation efforts of massively bleeding patients.[30] The premise of using a 1:1 ratio of red blood cell and plasma units is controversial.[31] However, it may be of benefit, especially in cases of penetrating trauma, as seen during military combat.[32] Therefore, some facilities have adopted the use of trauma packs for massive transfusion. The trauma pack components vary among institutions but usually contain a standard number of red blood cell and plasma units with or without a standard number of platelet units.

Coagulopathy is not the only complication of massive transfusion. Patients who are massively transfused are at risk for the same complications that affect other transfusion recipients, namely, febrile reactions, allergic reactions, volume overload, sepsis, viral infection, transfusion-related acute lung injury (TRALI), alloimmunization, and hemolytic reactions (Chapters 12 and 13). Some transfusion complications occur more frequently in massive transfusion situations because of the speed and volume of the transfusion, namely, anticoagulant toxicity, hyperkalemia, and hypothermia. Coagulopathy, hypothermia, and acidosis are of particular concern in exsanguinating patients, as they are major contributors to mortality.[33]

Massive transfusion is one indication for the use of blood warmers because the risk of hypothermia increases with rapid infusion of blood and other intravenous fluids. Rapid infusers are also commonly used in massive transfusion situations.

Clear and frequent communication with the patient care area helps the transfusion service to efficiently prioritize product requests and replenish inventory in a timely fashion. Inventory management is a fluid, complex set of decision-making opportunities (Chapter 7). Each transfusion service must establish guidelines for routine blood product supply and for extraordinary situations, whether relatively common such as massive transfusion or relatively rare such as mass casualty or implementation of other emergency preparedness plans.

Massive transfusion situations require that the clinical status of the patient and the inventory of the transfusion service be assessed at regular intervals because both are usually changing rapidly. Table 11-8 ✷ lists some common questions that may arise during a massive transfusion situation. While laboratory values may be used to monitor patients experiencing either acute or chronic blood loss or coagulopathy, the laboratory values alone should not be used to assess the status of the patient; clinical signs and symptoms must always be considered. This is especially true in massively bleeding and/or massively transfused patients where the laboratory values may be affected by fluid resuscitation treatment and the patient's physiological responses to acute blood loss.[29]

✳ **TABLE 11-7** Common Causes of Massive Transfusion

Category	Examples	Monitoring Tests
Trauma	• Motor vehicle accident • Gunshot wounds • Stabbings • Other penetrating trauma • Other blunt-force trauma	Common laboratory tests*
	• Other crush injuries	Common laboratory tests plus fibrin degradation products (FDP) as disseminated intravascular coagulation (DIC) is a common sequela
Obstetrics	• HELLP (hemolysis with elevated liver enzymes and low platelets) syndrome • Abruption • Other prenatal or postnatal bleeding	Common laboratory tests
	• Disseminated intravascular coagulation (DIC)	Common laboratory tests plus FDP, lactate dehydrogenase (LDH), haptoglobin
Surgery	• Liver transplant • Heart transplant • Coronary artery bypass graft replacement • Cardiac valve replacement • Other surgical bleeding	Common laboratory tests
Gastrointestinal bleeding	• Upper • Lower	Common laboratory tests
Aneurysm	• Aortic • Abdominal • Repair	Common laboratory tests
Exchange therapies	• Plasma exchange in thrombocytic thrombocytopenic purpura (TTP) or hemolytic uremic syndrome (HUS) • Red blood cell exchange in sickle cell anemia or hemolytic disease of the fetus and newborn	• Common laboratory tests plus manual white blood cell differential to look for schistocytes, lactate dehydrogenase (LDH), haptoglobin, urea, creatinine • Common laboratory tests plus hemoglobin electrophoresis or hemoglobin S level if treating sickle cell anemia
Extracorporeal membrane oxygenation	• Meconium aspiration • Other treatable condition with compromise of heart or heart/lung function; often in neonates • Less often, pediatric or adult patients with compromise of heart or heart/lung function	Common laboratory tests
Bleeding with coagulation factor deficiency	• Hemophilia A • Hemophilia B • Hemophilia A or B with inhibitors • Other congenital coagulation factor deficiencies • Acquired coagulation factor deficiencies	Common laboratory tests plus specific factor deficiency assays, Bethesda titers if inhibitors are suspected

* Common laboratory tests used to monitor transfusion therapy in massive transfusion: hemoglobin, hematocrit, platelet count, fibrinogen, activated partial thromboplastin time (aPTT), prothrombin time (PT), and/or international normalized ratio (INR).

✳ **TABLE 11-8** Common Questions in Massive Transfusion Situations

Question	Possible Answer(s)
When should plasma, platelets, and/or cryoprecipitate be transfused?	• Traditionally, after 10 red blood cell units are transfused, coagulation factor and platelet replacement therapy should be considered. • Newer evidence is leaning toward earlier transfusion of plasma and/or platelets, such as the use of trauma packs.
What do the laboratory indices mean if the patient is bleeding?	• Hemoglobin and hematocrit levels in the acute phase of trauma may not reflect the extent of blood loss. • If the patient has received crystalloids, the sample may be diluted. Postoperative values may be diluted. • Samples obtained from central venous catheters or temporary ports might be contaminated with anticoagulant. If this is suspected, requesting a recollection might be appropriate.

(Continued)

✳ **TABLE 11-8** *Continued*

Question	Possible Answer(s)
When should blood be ordered from the supplier?	As soon as minimum inventory levels are being approached. • Consider the time needed for transport. • Larger orders often take longer to pack. • Weather may play a role in product transport. • Increase the lead time if delays are expected, multiple patients are bleeding, or the transfusion service is minimally staffed (e.g., on off shifts, weekends, or holidays).
When should supervisors or medical directors be informed?	• Clear communication policies should be developed. • Staff members should feel comfortable asking for help whenever they are overwhelmed or uncertain of the correct actions to take.
When should the transfusion service suggest monitoring of laboratory indices to the clinician?	• Policies for pre- and post-transfusion laboratory monitoring should be developed. • Policies for severely bleeding patients should be developed. These often include exceptions for pretransfusion laboratory tests (e.g., the normal policy is to assess a fibrinogen level before issuing any cryoprecipitate). However, if the patient is bleeding it is common to give the requested blood products and then monitor values once the patient has stabilized. Common situations: • The patient is postoperative. • A large portion of the inventory is requested for a nonbleeding patient. • Many products have been used with no laboratory measurements.
What happens if no pretransfusion sample is available for testing?	Policies should be developed: • Identification of recipients whose identity cannot be immediately determined. • Issuing blood in the absence of pretransfusion testing. • The acceptable ABO group for red blood cell, plasma, and platelet units when the recipient's blood group is unknown or cannot be determined. • The acceptable Rh(D) type for red blood cell and platelet units when the recipient's blood group is unknown or cannot be determined. • Collection, testing, and notification of results for transfusion service samples collected after emergency transfusion. Generally speaking, the process is usually: • Issue the requested units stat. • Obtain and test a pretransfusion testing sample as soon as possible. • Notify the attending physician and medical director if there are testing results that indicate that the emergency-released blood products may cause hemolysis (e.g., the antibody screen is positive and uncrossmatched red blood cells have already been transfused).
When can ABO or Rh nonidentical units be transfused?	Policies should be developed: • Acceptable ABO group for red blood cell, plasma, and platelet units when the inventory of the identical ABO group is low. • Criteria for when ABO identical red blood cells can be transfused following transfusion of ABO nonidentical red blood cell, platelet, or cryoprecipitate units. • Acceptable Rh(D) type for red blood cell and platelet units when the inventory of the identical Rh(D) type is low.

CASE IN POINT (continued)

The transfusion service has a policy that the medical director reviews all cases of emergency release of blood products and/or massive transfusion. While you were preparing the paperwork for medical director review, you noted that the patient's initial laboratory values were nearly normal: hemoglobin of 12 g/dL (120 g/L) and hematocrit of 36% (0.36). Yet the physician transfused multiple blood products.

11. Why might a transfusion service have a policy of medical director review of emergency release of blood products?

12. Why might a transfusion service have a policy of medical director review of massive transfusion?

13. Why did the physician order blood products for a patient who had near normal laboratory values?

TRANSFUSION COMMITTEE

The transfusion committee may consist of members representing both the laboratory and clinical areas. Depending on the terms of reference, the committee may be responsible for review of all of the elements required by Standards or the responsibility for the required elements may be split among several individuals or committees. Elements requiring review commonly include[3]:

• Ordering practices, including informed consent and follow-up of verbal orders

• Patient identification, including patients who are not immediately identified by name

• Sample collection and labeling, and therefore specimen rejection rates and causes

• Infectious and noninfectious adverse events

- Near-miss events, usually as captured in an occurrence management system
- Usage and discard of blood components and products
- Appropriateness of use, which may focus on problematic components such as platelets or a new fractionation product where there is no clear consensus on clinical guidelines for off-label use
- Blood administration policies
- Ability to meet patient needs
- Compliance with meeting recommendations identified through external and internal assessments

Cases of massive transfusion are often reviewed by transfusion committees because they can include elements of patient identification, inventory management, appropriate blood usage, and ability to meet patient needs. The transfusion committee may also be involved in drafting or reviewing emergency preparedness plans, especially if the committee has cross-functional membership. Some emergency preparedness plans—for example, external disasters and mass casualties—will contain processes for massive transfusion.

Review of the Main Points

- Red blood cells deliver oxygen from the lungs to the peripheral organs and tissues.
- Hemostasis is the balance of coagulation and fibrinolysis.
- Coagulation factors and platelets are integral to the coagulation process.
- Common laboratory tests that aid the transfusion service include hemoglobin, hematocrit, platelet count, activated partial thromboplastin time (aPTT), prothrombin time/international normalized ratio (PT/INR), and fibrinogen.
- Cellular blood components include whole blood, red blood cell, granulocyte, and hematopoietic progenitor cell units.
- Policies should be developed that ensure that infusion rates, sets, filters, and needles are appropriate for the patient's condition.
- Plasma components include fresh frozen plasma, other transfusable plasma products, cryoprecipitate, and platelet units.
- Whole blood is usually divided into components, but may be used in certain circumstances such as preoperative autologous donation, acute normovolemic hemodilution, and intraoperative blood salvage.
- Directed donations are when a specific donor's blood component will be transfused to a specific patient.
- Directed donations may involve family or friends of a presurgical patient.
- Directed donations may also be used to pair phenotypically similar community donors with specific recipients when required, such as for chronic transfusion in sickle cell disease or transfusion in patients who are platelet refractory.
- Red blood cells are used to treat symptomatic acute or chronic anemia.
- Plasma products are used to correct coagulopathy or to replace other plasma proteins.
- Nonhuman-source products should be used to treat volume depletion.
- Specific factor concentrates, some of which are now available in recombinant form, should be used to treat conditions where coagulation factors are absent, reduced, or dysfunctional.
- Platelets are used to prevent or control bleeding when platelet counts are low or when platelets are not functioning.
- Cryoprecipitate is usually used to treat low levels of fibrinogen or dysfunction of fibrinogen.
- Hematopoietic progenitor cell (HPC) transplants are used to treat an increasing number of diseases.
- Fractionation products include albumin, used for volume expansion; immune globulins used to provide passive immunity and coagulation factors used to replace specific factor or factors when a congenital or acquired deficiency occurs.
- Preoperative autologous donation (PAD) is the use of whole blood donated prior to an elective surgery that is transfused back to the same donor/recipient during or after surgery.
- Acute normovolemic hemodilution (ANH) is the removal of whole blood in the operating room with fluid replacement, resulting in a lowered hematocrit during surgery. The collected autologous blood is transfused back to the same donor/recipient when required.
- Intraoperative blood salvage uses a variety of instruments to collect and modify bloodshed during an operation so that it can be safely transfused back to the same donor/recipient.
- Modifications to cellular components include leukoreduction, irradiation, washing, and freezing.
- Leukoreduction reduces alloimmunization to white blood cell antigens, febrile nonhemolytic transfusion reactions, and white blood cell–mediated viral transmission.
- The risk of transfusion-associated cytomegalovirus transmission can be reduced with the use of leukoreduced products or products from seronegative donors.
- Irradiation prevents transfusion-associated graft versus host disease (TA-GVHD).
- Graft versus host disease occurs when the recipient's white blood cells engraft and mount an immune response to the donor's tissues.
- Washing is used to remove plasma components, which may cause anaphylactic transfusion reactions.
- Red blood cells of rare phenotypes may be frozen, which extends their shelf life up to 10 years.

- Pharmaceuticals that increase release of specific cell types from the bone marrow or that limit fibrinolysis may reduce the need for transfusion in specific patient conditions.
- Massive transfusion is defined as the transfusion of at least one blood volume within 24 hours.
- Massive transfusion may be associated with trauma, obstetrical complications, surgery, certain conditions, and some transfusion therapies.

- Complications of massive transfusion include coagulopathy, hypothermia, hyperkalemia, and anticoagulant toxicity.
- The transfusion committee conducts retroactive reviews to identify trends and opportunities for process improvements.

Review Questions

1. Select the appropriate blood product for each clinical situation: (Objective #3)

    ____Patient with mucosal bleeding, platelet count 5 × 10³/ul.

    ____History of anemia, Hgb 6.0 g/dL

    ____Bleeding, fibrinogen level 50mg/dL

    ____Neutropenic patient with sepsis, unresponsive to antibiotics

    ____Trauma patient, elevated PT and aPTT, INR = 2.5

    A. Fresh frozen plasma

    B. Platelets

    C. Red blood cells

    D. Granulocytes

    E. Cryoprecipitate

2. In order for a blood product to be designated as leukoreduced, the product must have less than _____ white blood cells per unit. (Objective #8)

    A. 1.0×10^{10}

    B. 5.5×10^{10}

    C. 5.0×10^{6}

    D. 3.0×10^{11}

3. The use of a blood warming device for transfusion of blood components is beneficial in which of the following situations? (Objective #4)

    A. Trauma patient, massive transfusion

    B. Patient with cold agglutinin disease

    C. Blood product infusion through a central venous catheter

    D. Pediatric patient, packed red blood cell transfusion

4. Select the substances that will NOT have an adverse effect on blood components when they are infused during a blood transfusion. (Objective #11)

    A. ____Penicillin

    B. ____0.9% Sodium chloride

    C. ____5% Albumin

    D. ____Dextrose

    E. ____Ringer's lactate

    F. ____ABO-compatible plasma

5. Contraindications to transfusion include: (Objective #5)

    A. RBC transfusion for a mild iron deficiency

    B. Cryoprecipitate for fibrinogen deficiency

    C. Granulocyte transfusion for an infection responsive to antibiotics

    D. FFP for volume expansion

6. A patient donates two units of autologous blood 3 weeks prior to a scheduled surgical procedure. This type of donation is called: (Objective #12)

    A. Double apheresis

    B. Hemodilution

    C. Preoperative donation

    D. Postoperative salvage

7. Select the statements that are associated with the process of acute normovolemic hemodilution (ANH): (Objective #13)

    A. Blood units should be reinfused in the same order they were collected.

    B. Transfusions are typically administered by operating room staff.

    C. The first donor unit collected will likely contain the largest amount of fresh coagulation factors.

    D. The last unit reinfused is least likely to stop bleeding problems as a result of low platelet count.

8. Choose the types of directed donor blood units that require irradiation prior to transfusion: (Objective #7)

   A. Nick C. donates a unit of packed red blood cells to his friend who is a cardiac patient.

   B. Mary L. donates a unit of packed red blood cells to her mother who is scheduled for hip surgery in 2 weeks.

   C. Joan Y. donates a unit of packed red blood cells to her husband John who is scheduled for a routine procedure.

   D. Anthony M. donates a unit of packed red blood cells to his mother-in-law who is having knee-replacement surgery.

9. Specific requirements for transfusion of a unit of granulocytes include: (Objective #8)

   A. HLA compatibility

   B. Leukofiltration

   C. Irradiation

   D. Transfusion within 24 hours of collection

10. Which of the following statements is *true* regarding the benefits and risks of peripheral blood stem cell (PBSC) collection and bone marrow collection? (Objective # 17)

    A. PBSC requires insertion of a catheter, which reduces risk of infection.

    B. Bone marrow collection has a shorter engraftment period than PBSC.

    C. Bone marrow collection carries a lower risk for the donor.

    D. PBSC carries a higher incidence of graft versus host disease (GVHD).

11. Select the patients who are at risk for transfusion-transmitted CMV. (Objective #9)

    A. Adult patient with agammaglobulinemia

    B. Premature newborn

    C. Fetus with intrauterine transfusion

    D. Bone marrow transplant recipient

12. Choose the expiration date for each modified blood product: (Objective #8)

    _____ Washed red blood cells (open system)

    _____ Frozen, deglycerolized red blood cells (open system)

    _____ Directed donor red blood cells, irradiated

    _____ CPD red blood cells, leukoreduced

    A. 24 hours

    B. 21 days

    C. 28 days

13. The appropriate blood product for a patient with mild hemophilia is: (Objective #3)

    A. Red blood cells

    B. Fresh frozen plasma

    C. Cryoprecipitate

    D. Platelets

14. Prevention of Rh immunization is achieved through transfusion of which of the following products? (Objective #15)

    A. RhIg

    B. Plateletpheresis

    C. 22% Albumin

    D. IVIG

15. Complications of massive transfusion often include: (Objective #10)

    A. Depletion of coagulation factors

    B. High incidence of transfusion reaction

    C. Anticoagulant toxicity

    D. Hyperglobulinemia

References

1. Roback JD, Grossman BJ, Harris T, Hillyer CD, eds. *Technical manual*, 17th ed. Bethesda (MD): AABB Press; 2011.

2. Petrides M, Stack G. *Practical guide to transfusion medicine*. Bethesda (MD): AABB Press; 2001.

3. AABB. *Standards for blood banks and transfusion services*, 27th ed. Bethesda (MD): AABB Press; 2011.

4. Spinella PC. Warm fresh whole blood transfusion for severe hemorrhage: U.S. military and potential civilian applications. *Crit Care Med* 2008; 36(S7): S340–5.

5. AABB. *Standards for perioperative autologous blood collection and administration*, 4th ed. Bethesda (MD): AABB Press; 2009.

6. McCullough J. *Transfusion medicine*, 2nd ed. Philadelphia (PA): Elsevier; 2005.

7. American Red Cross Missouri Illinois Blood Services Region [Internet]. St. Louis (IL): Special program The Charles Drew community blood donation campaign; [cited 2009 Sept 30]. Available from: http://mir.bloodisneeded .org/GiveBlood/SpecialPrograms.aspx

8. Anstee DJ, Klein HG. *Mollison's blood transfusion in clinical medicine*. Malden (MA): Blackwell Publishing; 2005.

9. Blajchman MA. Transfusion immunomodulation or TRIM: What does it mean clinically? *Hematology* 2005; 10(S1): 208–14.

10. Opelz G, Sengar DP, Mickey MR, Terasaki PI. Effect of blood transfusions on subsequent kidney transplants. *Transplant Proc* 1973; 5: 253–9.

11. Hillyer CD, Silberstein LE, Ness PM, Anderson KC, Roush KS. *Blood banking and transfusion medicine: Basic principles and practice*. Philadelphia (PA): Churchill Livingstone; 2003.

12. Bowden RA, Slichter SJ, Sayers M, Weisdorf D, Cays M, Schoch G, Banaji M, Haake R, Welk K, Fisher L, McCullough J, Miller W. A comparison of filtered leukocyte-reduced and cytomegalovirus (CMV) seronegative blood products for the prevention of transfusion-associated CMV infection after bone marrow transplant. *Blood* 1995: 86(9); 3596–603.

13. Nichols WG, Price TH, Gooley T, Corey L, Boechkh M. Transfusion-transmitted cytomegalovirus infection after receipt of leukoreduced blood products. *Blood* 2003: 101(10): 5195–200.

14. Hébert PC, Fegusson DA. Evaluation of a universal leukoreduction program in Canada. *Vox Sang* 2002: 83(S1); 207–9.

15. Pietersz RN. Universal leukoreduction in The Netherlands. *Transfus Apher Sci* 2001: 25(3); 209–10.

16. Blajchman MA, Goldman M, Freedman JJ, Sher GD. Proceedings of a consensus conference: Prevention of post-transfusion CMV in the era of universal leukoreduction. *Transfus Med Rev* 2001: 15(1); 1–20.

17. Valeri CR, Feingold H, Marchionni LD. A simple method for freezing human platelets using 6 per cent dimethylsulfoxide and storage at -80 degrees C. *Blood* 1974: 43(1); 131–6.

18. Melaragno AJ, Carciero R, Feingold H, Talarico L, Weintraub L, Valeri CR. Cryopreservation of human platelets using 6% dimethyl sulfoxide at -80 degrees C. Effects of 2 years of frozen storage at -80 degrees C and transportation in dry ice. *Vox Sang* 1985: 49(4); 245–58.

19. FDA Guidance: Use of sterile connection devices in blood bank practice, November 2002.

20. Brennan M. Fibrin glue. *Blood Rev* 1991: 5(4); 240–4.

21. Spiess BD, Spence RK, Shander A. *Perioperative Transfusion Medicine*, 2nd ed. Philadelphia (PA): Lippincott, Williams & Wilkins; 2006.

22. Bartley AN, Carpenter JB, Berg MP. D+ platelet transfusions in D− patients: cause for concern? *Immunohematology* 2009: 25(1); 5–8.

23. Gaines AR. Acute onset hemoglobinemia and/or hemogobinuria and sequelae following Rh$_o$(D) immune globulin intravenous administration in immune thrombocytopenic purpura patients. *Blood* 2000; 95(8): 2523–9.

24. Simon TL, Dzink WH, Snyder EL, Stowell CP, Strauss RG. *Rossi's principles of transfusion medicine*. Philadelphia (PA): Lippincott, Williams & Wilkins; 2002.

25. Epogen® [Prescribing information]. Thousand Oaks (CA): Amegen Manufacturing; 2009.

26. Mozobil™ [Product insert]. Cambridge (MA): Genzyme Corporation; 2008.

27. Carless HD, Fergusson D, Laupacis A. The safety of aprotinin and lysine-derived antifibrinolytic drugs in cardiac surgery: A meta-analysis. *CMAJ* 2009; 180(2): 183–93.

28. NovoSeven® [Product insert]. Princeton (NJ): Novo Nordisk Incorporated; 2006.

29. Gutierrez G, Reines HD, Wulf-Guiierrez ME. Clinical review: Hemorrhagic shock. *Critical Care* 2004; 8: 373 –81.

30. Gonzalez EA, Moore FA, Holcomb JB, Miller CC, Kozar RA, Todd SR, Cocanour CS, Balldin BC, McKinley BA. Fresh frozen plasma should be given earlier to patients requiring massive transfusion. *J Trauma* 2007; 62(1): 112–9.

31. Kashuk JL, Moore EE, Johnson JL, Haenei J, Wilson M, Moore JB, Cothren CC, Biffl WL, Banerjee A, Sauaia A. Postinjury life threatening coagulopathy: Is 1:1 fresh frozen plasma: Packed red blood cells the answer? *J Trauma* 2008; 65(2): 261–70.

32. Spinella PC, Perkins J, Grathwohl KW, Beekley AC, Niles SE, McLaughlin DF, Wade CE, Holcomb JB. Effect of plasma and red blood cell transfusions on survival in patients with combat related traumatic injuries. *J Trauma* 2008; 64(2S): S69–77.

33. Mitchell KJ, Moncure KE, Onyeije C, Siram S. Evaluation of massive volume replacement in the penetrating trauma patient. *J Natl Med Assoc* 1994; 86(12): 926–9.

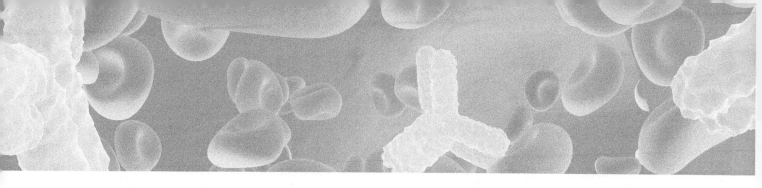

12 Adverse Reactions to Transfusion

DEANNA C. FANG, SUSAN CONFORTI, AND COLLEEN YOUNG

Chapter Objectives

Upon completion of this chapter, the student will be able to:

1. Define adverse transfusion reaction.
2. Recognize the difference between an acute and a delayed transfusion reaction.
3. Identify the reporting requirements for transfusion-related fatalities in the United States.
4. Discuss the rationale for transfusion reaction reporting and outline the benefits of a national surveillance system for transfusion reactions.
5. For each type of transfusion reaction covered in this chapter, identify, describe, and compare and contrast the following *pertinent* aspects:
   - Incidence
   - Pathophysiology, including theoretical mechanisms
   - Clinical presentation
   - Differential diagnosis and clinical work-up
   - Treatment and prevention strategies
6. Identify the component modification performed to reduce the risk of transfusion associated graft versus host disease
7. Identify the initial steps taken when investigating an adverse transfusion-reaction.
8. Discuss key diagnostic tests that may be used to differentiate transfusion reactions with similar symptoms.

Key Terms

Acute reaction(s)
Anaphylactoid
Delayed reaction(s)
Disseminated intravascular coagulation (DIC)
Hemoglobinemia
Hemoglobinuria
Hyperhemolysis
Hypoxemia
Pruritus
Pyrogen(s)
Surveillance network(s)
Urticaria

(continued)

CASE IN POINT

PH is a 42-year-old woman who is undergoing chemo-therapy for non-Hodgkin's lymphoma. She receives regular transfusions in the outpatient clinic. She presents today with a hemoglobin level of 6.8 g/dL (68 g/L) and a platelet count of $7.0 \times 10^3/\mu L$ ($7.0 \times 10^9/L$). Her physician orders transfusion of 2 units of red blood cells and 1 unit of apheresis platelets. The transfusion service tests the crossmatch specimen drawn today and prepares the requested blood products. PH's test results are the following: O Rh(D) positive with a negative antibody screen.

What's Ahead?

Since the latter quarter of the 20th century, the safety of transfusion has been of great interest to medical practitioners and the general public alike. A great deal of attention has been focused on transfusion-transmitted viral infections, particularly the human immunodeficiency (HIV), hepatitis B, and hepatitis C viruses. Safety measures implemented to address these concerns have resulted in transfusion being a much safer medical intervention than in previous decades. However, there remain several risks to transfusion that can result in serious consequences to patients.

This chapter addresses the following questions:

1. What are the known risks of transfusion that are unrelated to the transmission of blood-borne pathogens?
2. What are the causes of adverse transfusion events?
3. What are the various types of transfusion reactions and how do they compare in terms of incidence, pathophysiology/theoretical mechanism(s), clinical presentation, differential diagnoses and clinical work-up, and treatment and prevention strategies?
4. What can be done to prevent or manage adverse transfusion events?

DEFINITIONS

An *adverse transfusion reaction* can be broadly defined as a negative unintended consequence of transfusion. Generally, the term is not used to describe transfusion-transmitted bacterial, viral, prion, or parasitic infections (Chapter 13). All other unintended adverse events are normally described under the umbrella of transfusion reactions.

Adverse transfusion reactions may occur during or very close to the time of transfusion, in which case they are referred to as immediate or **acute reactions**. Reactions are commonly classed as acute if they occur within 24 hours of transfusion. Symptoms of other reactions may take a significant time to appear, in which case they are referred to as **delayed reactions**. Delayed reactions may present anywhere from 1 day to 2 or more weeks after transfusion. Table 12-1 ✶ lists adverse transfusion reactions characterized by time to presentation of symptoms.

TRANSFUSION REACTION SURVEILLANCE

One important aspect of transfusion safety is the reporting and surveillance of adverse transfusion events. Within hospitals, review of transfusion reaction reports is an important part of transfusion practice oversight. These reviews are used to monitor adverse events and, where possible, develop preventative measures within each facility (Chapter 21).[1]

Many developed countries have implemented **surveillance networks** to track and monitor adverse events on a larger, often national, scale. The two oldest and most well established are the Serious Hazards of Transfusion (SHOT)—a voluntary reporting scheme in the United Kingdom—and the Haemovigilance Network of the Agence Française de Sécurité des Produits de Santé (AFSSAPS)—a mandatory reporting scheme in France. National surveillance systems allow for aggregate data, which can identify systemic problems much earlier

✴ TABLE 12-1 Acute and Delayed Adverse Transfusion Reactions

Acute	Delayed
Acute hemolytic	Delayed hemolytic
Air embolus	Hemosiderosis
Allergic	Post-transfusion purpura (PTP)
Anaphylactic/anaphylactoid	Transfusion-associated graft versus host disease (TA-GVHD)
Citrate toxicity	
Febrile nonhemolytic	
Hypotensive	
Hypothermia	
Nonimmune hemolysis	
Transfusion-associated circulatory overload (TACO)	
Transfusion-associated dyspnea (TAD)	
Transfusion-related acute lung injury (TRALI)	

than may be seen within individual facilities. The success of these types of systems is illustrated by SHOT, which published, in 13 years of reporting, that the total number of reports increased while simultaneously the number of patients experiencing serious adverse events significantly decreased.[2] SHOT and other hemovigilance systems have been instrumental in identifying emerging trends in transfusion-related adverse events, including sepsis associated with platelet transfusion and transfusion-related acute lung injury (TRALI).[3]

A biovigilance system was first proposed in the United States in 2006. The United States model is a collaborative effort involving both public and private organizations. The national hemovigilance program, which is one of the four components that will make up the complete system, was launched in 2010.

In the United States, the Food and Drug Administration (FDA) has a guidance document that outlines the steps for notifying the agency of any fatalities related to blood collection or transfusion. There are no requirements to report all adverse transfusion reactions, but any transfusion-associated fatalities are required to be reported to the Centre for Biologics Evaluation and Research (CBER) as soon as possible, with a full written report required within 7 days. As per the guidance document, details related to patient demographics, suspected cause of death, the nature and type of blood components transfused, and the circumstances surrounding the death are requested in order to allow the FDA to assess these fatalities from a public health perspective.[4]

☑ CHECKPOINT 12-1

In the United States, what government agency needs to be notified if a death is associated with a transfusion?

IMMUNE-MEDIATED HEMOLYTIC TRANSFUSION REACTIONS

Immune-mediated hemolytic transfusion reactions are among the best known and most completely characterized adverse events in transfusion medicine. These reactions are most commonly associated with patient antibodies that are directed against antigens present on the transfused red blood cells. However, there have also

been case reports where red blood cell antibodies present in the plasma of transfused components react with recipient red blood cells and cause a hemolytic transfusion reaction.[5]

Immune hemolytic transfusion reactions can be divided into two categories. Acute hemolytic reactions tend to occur almost immediately after exposure to the transfused component, often during the transfusion, and are associated with complement-mediated intravascular hemolysis, where the red blood cells are destroyed within the circulation (Chapter 1). Delayed hemolytic reactions may occur days to weeks after transfusion and are associated with extravascular hemolysis, where antibody and/or complement-coated red blood cells are cleared through phagocytosis by macrophages in the spleen, liver, and bone marrow (Chapter 1).

Pretransfusion testing and patient identification procedures have been designed primarily to prevent immune-mediated hemolytic transfusion reactions (Chapter 7). In most cases, it is a failure or a limitation in these processes that gives rise to this type of adverse event. The most serious acute hemolytic reactions occur as a result of patients receiving ABO-incompatible red blood cells, either through misidentification of the patient, the specimen, or the blood component or through errors in pretransfusion testing.[6]

Delayed hemolytic reactions are most often due to the presence of patient antibodies to non-ABO red blood cell antigens. Although a delayed hemolytic reaction may occur as a result of a misidentification or testing error, in many cases antibodies to non-ABO red blood cell antigens may not be present at detectable levels at the time of pretransfusion testing. It is only upon reexposure to these antigens during transfusion that the antibodies reach a significant level, resulting in a delayed hemolytic reaction. The rapid rise in antibody levels when a patient is exposed to the same antigen after the first exposure is called an anamnestic, or memory, response (Chapter 1).[7]

ACUTE HEMOLYTIC TRANSFUSION REACTIONS

Incidence

As with many other types of adverse transfusion events, it is difficult to determine the exact frequency of acute hemolytic reactions. Major contributing factors to this difficulty are that these incidents are often underreported or incorrectly diagnosed. In 2005, the UK SHOT scheme estimated the incidence of ABO-incompatible transfusions to be 1 in 100,000 components transfused.[6] American estimates put the incidence at around 1 in 77,000 components transfused,[5] with the resulting patient death estimated to occur in 1 in 500,000 to 1 in 1,000,000 transfusions.[7] The most common blood component implicated in acute hemolytic reactions is red blood cell units.

Pathophysiology and Clinical Presentation

Acute hemolytic transfusion reactions occur when antibodies react with antigens on red blood cells and initiate complement activation (Chapter 1). Complement activation leads to intravascular hemolysis and **hemoglobinemia**, which is free hemoglobin circulating in the recipient's plasma. Box 12-1 lists the signs and symptoms of an acute hemolytic transfusion reaction. Because ABO antibodies are predominantly IgM, and IgM antibodies tend to be strong activators of complement, most ABO-incompatible red blood cell transfusions will result in acute hemolytic reactions (Chapter 4).

☑ CHECKPOINT 12-2

What blood group incompatibility is most commonly associated with acute hemolytic transfusion reactions?

BOX 12-1   Clinical Presentation of an Acute Hemolytic Transfusion Reaction

Signs and Symptoms of Acute Hemolytic Transfusion Reaction

Most common:
Fever with or without chills
Hemoglobinuria (hemoglobin in the urine)

Variability in occurrence:
Hemoglobinemia (free hemoglobin in the plasma)
Positive direct antiglobulin test (DAT)
Pain at the intravenous site
Abdominal, chest, flank, or back pain
Nausea or vomiting
Hypotension, sometimes progressing to shock
Dyspnea (difficulty breathing)
Disseminated intravascular bleeding (DIC)
Renal failure

Once complement activation and intravascular hemolysis has occurred, a cascade of immune-mediated consequences follows. Activated C3a and C5a are potent anaphylatoxins and stimulate the release of histamine and serotonin from mast cells, resulting in vasodilation and smooth muscle contraction. The antigen–antibody complex itself causes the release of bradykinin and norepinepherine. The net results of these reactions are symptoms that may include infusion site pain, hypotension, wheezing, chest pain, flushing, and gastrointestinal symptoms.

Acute hemolytic reactions are also characterized by associated coagulation abnormalities. Antibody–antigen complexes can activate Factor XII in the coagulation cascade, triggering the intrinsic pathway, while activated complement can increase expression of the tissue factor

(Factor III) expressed on leukocytes and endothelial cells, activating Factor VII and triggering the extrinsic coagulation pathway. This process leads to the development of **disseminated intravascular coagulation (DIC)**, where microvascular thrombi form, causing organ and tissue damage due to blockage of capillaries and uncontrolled bleeding due to consumption of coagulation factors and platelets.[5]

Renal damage is a significant risk for patients experiencing an acute hemolytic reaction. This may be partially due to free hemoglobin being excreted through the kidneys; however, reduced renal blood flow and the deposition of antigen–antibody complexes are thought to be of more significant consequence.[5]

Differential Diagnosis and Clinical Work-Up

Immune-mediated acute hemolytic reactions share many of the same symptoms as other types of immune-mediated adverse transfusion events. In addition, the underlying condition of the patient may complicate recognition of an acute hemolytic reaction. One characterizing feature is **hemoglobinuria**, the presence of hemoglobin in the urine. An acute hemolytic reaction results in free hemoglobin in the circulation, some of which is excreted through the kidneys. Acute hemolysis may also be associated with nonimmune mechanisms.

The laboratory investigation is key to correctly diagnosing an acute hemolytic transfusion reaction, particularly a clerical check to identify any errors in patient or blood component identification. In most cases, the post-transfusion direct antiglobulin test (DAT) will be positive; however, a negative DAT should not rule out the diagnosis of acute hemolytic transfusion reaction because all antibody-coated red blood cells may be destroyed during the initial phase of the reaction. Depending on the volume of incompatible red blood cells transfused, hemolysis may be seen upon visual inspection of the plasma in a post-transfusion specimen. Figure 12-1 ■ illustrates visible hemolysis in plasma specimens.

Treatment

The most important first step when a patient, nurse, or physician becomes aware of any adverse symptoms that may be related to the transfusion is to stop the transfusion. Specifically in the case of an

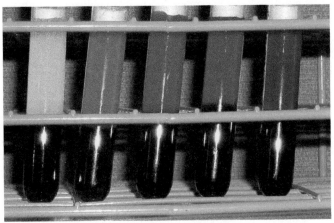

| Normal | Slight hemolysis | Moderate hemolysis | Moderate hemolysis | Gross hemolysis |

■ **FIGURE 12-1**   Normal and Hemolyzed Plasma Specimens
Source: Lisa Denesiuk.

ABO-incompatible transfusion, early intervention can prevent serious consequences because the severity of the reaction is directly proportional to the amount of incompatible blood transfused.[5]

Treatment of acute hemolytic reactions depends on the amount of incompatible blood transfused and the severity of the patient's symptoms. If the symptoms are mild and the patient is otherwise stable, observation may be the only follow-up required. Venous access should be maintained with a saline infusion, which also assists in treating hypotension and maintaining renal blood flow. Furosemide (trade name Lasix°), a diuretic, may be used to increase urine output and improve blood flow to the kidneys. Because of the risk of DIC, it is critical that the patient be kept hemodynamically stable. This may necessitate the administration of platelets, plasma, and/or cryoprecipitate.[7]

CASE IN POINT (continued)

PH is transfused one apheresis platelet without incident. The nurse begins the first red blood cell transfusion. Pretransfusion vital signs are normal:

- Blood pressure 127/76 mm Hg
- Pulse 89 beats/minute
- Temperature 98.2° F (36.8° C)
- Respirations 18 breaths/minute

One hour into the red blood cell transfusion, PH says, "I am colder than I have ever been in my life." The nurse goes to retrieve a blanket for the patient. When she returns, the patient is experiencing chills.

1. Is it possible that PH is experiencing a transfusion reaction?
2. What is the first thing that the nurse should do?
3. Would this be considered an immediate or delayed transfusion reaction? Why?

Prevention

The most common cause of an acute hemolytic transfusion reaction is a patient receiving the incorrect blood component. Clerical errors in patient or specimen identification at the time of collection for pretransfusion testing, and in patient and blood component identification at the time of transfusion, are the most common causes of patients receiving incorrect blood components. Laboratory testing errors can also contribute to the risk of this type of incident. The 2005 UK SHOT summary notes that the risk of a patient receiving an incorrect blood component is 1 in 15,000 blood components transfused.[6] While not every patient who receives an incorrect blood component will experience an acute hemolytic transfusion reaction, the potential exists every time this error occurs.

The most important tool in preventing an acute hemolytic reaction is strict adherence to policies and procedures. Table 12-2 ✱ lists the policies and procedures that have significant impact on preventing acute hemolytic reactions. Historically, many of these processes have been subject to a high degree of human error. More recently, technology has helped to reduce the risk of error. Barcode scanners

✱ **TABLE 12-2** Information to Prevent Acute Hemolytic Reactions

Document Type	Document Subject
Policy	Identification of patients
Procedure	Identification of patients for laboratory testing and/or Identification of patients for pretransfusion testing and/or Collection of pretransfusion testing specimens
Policy	Specimen acceptance/rejection
Procedure	Pretransfusion testing and/or ABO test
Procedure	Tagging/reserving/issuing red blood cell components
Procedure	Infusing blood components
Policy	Monitoring of patients during a blood transfusion

and radio frequency identification chips have the ability to improve patient, specimen, and blood component identification. Increased automation and the use of laboratory information systems can reduce laboratory testing errors by removing the requirement to manually interpret test results, preventing release of anomalous results, and providing a source of historical test results to which current results can be compared.

DELAYED HEMOLYTIC TRANSFUSION REACTIONS

Incidence

There is wide variability in reported rates of delayed hemolytic transfusion reactions. As with acute hemolytic reactions, these events are often unrecognized and frequently go unreported. Delayed hemolytic reactions are known to occur with much greater frequency than acute hemolytic reactions, with estimates ranging from 1 in 2,339 to 1 in 5,405 components transfused.[5]

Pathophysiology and Clinical Presentation

Delayed hemolytic reactions begin much the same way as acute hemolytic reactions. Antibodies directed against red blood cell antigens bind to the red blood cell membrane; however, complement activation is not initiated or is incomplete, so immediate intravascular hemolysis does not occur. Instead, antibody-bound and/or complement-coated red blood cells remain in circulation where they are eventually cleared by phagocytes in the spleen, liver, and bone marrow.

Because the mechanism of clearance involves minimal complement activation and no immediate release of free hemoglobin, delayed hemolytic reactions tend to be less severe than acute hemolytic reactions. Patients may present with fever and anemia days to weeks after transfusion and may also demonstrate other signs of extravascular hemolysis, including jaundice, leukocytosis, and hemoglobinuria.[7]

Hyperhemolysis

In some patients, a delayed hemolytic transfusion reaction can progress to **hyperhemolysis**, where the patient's red blood cells are destroyed in addition to the transfused donor cells. This is most often seen in multiply transfused patients with sickle cell disease or thalassemia. It has been hypothesized that the destruction of the patient's red blood cells may be due to complement activation occurring during the destruction of donor red blood cells, or it could possibly be due to transfusion-related immunomodulation that results in the production of self-directed autoantibodies. Hyperhemolysis involves both intravascular and extravascular hemolysis and is a potentially life-threatening condition.[8]

Differential Diagnosis and Clinical Work-Up

As with acute hemolytic reactions, laboratory follow-up is key to diagnosing delayed hemolytic transfusion reactions. The post-transfusion DAT will usually be positive, unless all antibody-coated red blood cells have been cleared from circulation. Regardless of whether antibodies were detected in the pretransfusion specimen, the post-transfusion specimen will typically show evidence of one or more previously undetected or unidentified antibodies to red blood cell antigen. Retrospective antigen typing of the transfused red blood cells will normally demonstrate that at least one of the components was positive for a corresponding red blood cell antigen. Other laboratory tests that may be used in the differential diagnosis include bilirubin and lactate dehydrogenase, both of which are strong indicators of increased red blood cell destruction.

> ☑ **CHECKPOINT 12-3**
>
> What are two transfusion medicine laboratory tests that are commonly performed to confirm a delayed hemolytic transfusion reaction?

Treatment

Delayed hemolytic reactions are often relatively mild, so treatment generally consists of observation and supportive care. If the resulting anemia necessitates additional transfusions, red blood cells negative for the antigen(s) against which the patient's antibody(ies) is directed must be selected in order to prevent further hemolysis.[7] For patients who progress to hyperhemolysis, treatment with immunosuppressive agents may be required and for those patients who remain unresponsive a splenectomy may be indicated.[8]

Prevention

As previously discussed, delayed hemolytic transfusion reactions may occur as a result of an error in patient, specimen, or blood component identification, or due to a laboratory testing error. These types of errors are mitigated by strict adherence to all policies and procedures around pretransfusion testing and blood component administration. Use of technology and automation can also reduce the risk of human error.

In some patients with a history of exposure to foreign red blood cell antigens, antibodies implicated in delayed hemolytic transfusion reactions may not be detectable at the time of pretransfusion testing. A complete patient history, that includes if a patient has been transfused before, has been a transplant recipient, has been pregnant, and/or has been identified as having antibodies to red blood cell antigens can often help identify patients that are at an increased risk for delayed hemolytic transfusion reactions. Patients with a history of red blood cell antibodies known to cause hemolysis must receive red blood cells that are negative for the corresponding antigen, regardless of whether the antibody is detectable at the time of pretransfusion testing. This will prevent the patient from experiencing an anamnestic response to the antigen and a subsequent delayed hemolytic transfusion reaction. Antibodies to a number of different red blood cell antigen systems have a strong association with this type of behavior, particularly Kidd, Duffy, Kell, and MNS (Chapter 6).[7]

Patients who have been recently transfused or are pregnant may be stimulated by foreign red blood cell antigens that may not have reached detectable levels at the time of pretransfusion testing. For this reason, testing for recently transfused or pregnant patients must be performed with samples drawn no more than 3 days before planned transfusion (Chapter 7). This will maximize the ability of the laboratory to detect any newly formed red blood cell antibodies.

FEBRILE NONHEMOLYTIC TRANSFUSION REACTIONS (FNHTR)

Incidence

Febrile nonhemolytic transfusion (FNHTR) and simple allergic reactions are the most commonly reported complications associated with transfusion. Although varying definitions of a febrile transfusion reaction exist, it is typical that the reaction involves an increase in body temperature of at least 1.8° F (1° C) either during or shortly after the transfusion. The occurrence of chills or rigor, even in the absence of fever, is also considered an FNHTR. The febrile reaction occurs most frequently among people who have been multiply transfused or previously pregnant. Recurrences are common after an initial reaction is reported. Although the patient may experience discomfort, the reaction is generally mild and not considered to be life-threatening.

Pathophysiology and Clinical Presentation

The FNHTR is a leukocyte-mediated reaction. Two mechanisms are known to exist:

- The recipient has been alloimmunized to human leukocyte antigens (HLA) because of exposure to foreign white blood cells during a prior pregnancy, transfusion, or transplant. The recipient's HLA antibody attacks the transfused leukocytes that possess the concurrent antigen.

- Cytokine substances are released from leukocytes during blood product storage. The cytokines are passively transfused to the recipient and initiate an inflammatory response.

Both mechanisms result in the release of **pyrogens**, which are substances that cause fever. FNHTR is known to occur after transfusion of leukocyte-containing blood products such as red blood cell products and platelets. The cytokine-mediated reaction is most often associated with the transfusion of platelet products.[7] FNTR can occur when leukoreduced products are transfused, although the more widespread use of prestorage, leukoreduced products has reduced the incidence of FNTR.[9]

The onset of symptoms of FNHTR occurs during or up to 4 hours after transfusion. The definitive symptoms are fever $> 100.4°$ F ($38°$ C) oral or equivalent with a change of $\geq 1.8°$ F ($1°$ C) from pretransfusion value or occurrence of chills/rigors even in the absence of fever.[10] Other symptoms that may be present include respiratory distress (wheezing, coughing, dyspnea), hypertension or hypotension, headache, or vomiting.

☑ CHECKPOINT 12-4

What are the two defining symptoms of a febrile, nonhemolytic transfusion reaction (FNHTR)?

Differential Diagnosis and Clinical Work-Up

Although FNHTR is not life-threatening, the differential diagnosis requires careful consideration because the onset of fever during or immediately after transfusion is an initial symptom of other severe and life-threatening transfusion reactions including transfusion-related acute lung injury (TRALI), acute hemolysis, or bacterial contamination (Chapter 13). Preexisting conditions or infection may also cause fever.

Because varying definitions of the FNHTR exist, the criteria for diagnosis and follow-up testing are determined by each facility. Follow-up tests that may be performed to rule out other types of transfusion reactions and conditions typically include:

- Direct antiglobulin test to rule out hemolysis.
- Blood culture on patient to rule out sepsis.
- Blood culture on residual blood component to rule out bacterial contamination of the donor unit.

CASE IN POINT (continued)

Over the next 10 minutes, PH complains of shortness of breath and nausea. The nurse notes that the patient is now breathing rapidly and seems uncomfortable. Her vital signs are shown in the chart below. Acetaminophen (trade name Tylenol®) is administered to treat the fever and chills.

Vital Sign	Pretransfusion	Post-Transfusion
Blood pressure (mm Hg)	127/76	138/65
Pulse (beats/minute)	89	123
Respirations (breaths/minute)	18	29
Temperature	98.2° F (36.8° C)	101.4° F (38.6° C)

4. What conditions should be considered in the differential diagnosis?
5. Hospital policy requires the transfusionist to perform a clerical check immediately when a transfusion reaction is suspected. Why is this important?

Treatment

If symptoms of fever, chills, or rigor appear during a transfusion, the transfusion should be immediately discontinued. An antipyretic, such as acetaminophen, can be administered to reduce fever and alleviate patient discomfort. In certain circumstances, when it is likely that the fever is due to a FNHTR and not one of the life-threatening reactions, the transfusion may be restarted at a slower pace so long as the transfusion is completed within the required 4-hour timeframe. More frequent monitoring of the patient's vital signs is often performed in these situations.

Prevention

Recurrence of FNHTR is common after an initial reaction. An effective method of prevention is prestorage removal of leukocytes from blood products, which reduces the likelihood of the formation of antigen–antibody complexes as well as the release of cytokine substances. Although bedside filtration meets the standard of reducing leukocyte counts in a red blood cell unit to $<5.0 \times 10^6$, prestorage filtration is more effective in reducing the cytokine-mediated response and has been effective in reducing reported incidence of FNHTR. Alternatively, patients who are known to be susceptible to FNHTR are sometimes given an antipyretic prior to subsequent transfusions.

ALLERGIC TRANSFUSION REACTIONS

Incidence

Allergic responses to blood products are common nonhemolytic transfusion reactions that occur in 1–5% of the transfused population. Allergic responses are frequently encountered during the transfusion of plasma products, and can be identified in combination with febrile transfusion reactions. Most allergic reactions to transfusion are mild and occur within a few minutes of exposure to the allergen in the transfused product. Mild allergic reactions involve no immediate risk to the life of the recipient and respond well to treatment. Confirmation of allergic transfusion reactions requires the rule out of other types of environmental, drug, or dietary causes.

Pathophysiology and Clinical Presentation

Allergic transfusion reactions are caused by protein-based allergens that react with preformed plasma antibodies. The specific mechanism of allergic transfusion reactions is not fully understood; however, the antibodies can originate in either the donor or the recipient. The preformed antibodies that respond to the allergens are primarily of the IgG or IgE immunoglobulin class. The antibody binds to the allergen; this activates mast cells and causes the release of histamine and heparin, which stimulate vasodilation and an influx of fluids to the tissues with subsequent edema.

☑ CHECKPOINT 12-5

What two classes of antibodies are commonly associated with allergic transfusion reactions?

Symptoms of mild allergic reactions are not life-threatening and usually occur during the transfusion, but may occur 1 or 2 hours after transfusion. Symptoms are mucocutaneous and initially present as **urticaria**, which means hives or rash that appear on the surface of the skin. A morbilliform or measles-like rash can occur with or without **pruritus**, which is defined as itching. Flushing of the skin and localized edema, which is fluid accumulation beneath the surface of the skin, can occur particularly on the lips, tongue, uvula, and the periorbital area around the eyes. The signs and symptoms of allergic reactions are summarized in Table 12-3 ✳. At least two symptoms must be observed in order for the allergic reaction to be confirmed.

Differential Diagnosis and Clinical Work-Up

When symptoms of an allergic reaction appear, the transfusion should be stopped immediately. If the symptoms are strictly mucocutaneous, a detailed laboratory investigation is usually not necessary. No reliable laboratory tests exist for the confirmation of allergenic agents with respect to allergic transfusion reactions. Consequently, the identification of specific allergens in allergic transfusion reactions is typically not performed. Screening of blood donors or recipients for the presence of allergenic agents or allergic symptom–causing plasma antibodies is not routinely performed as part of either the blood donation process or recipient pretransfusion testing.

Treatment

The transfusion should be stopped immediately and intravenous access should be maintained. An antihistamine such as diphenhydramine (trade name Benadryl®) can be given orally or intramuscularly to reduce the symptoms and recipient discomfort. The transfusion can be resumed once the symptoms resolve and if the reaction was mild, such as a rash covering less than two-thirds of the body surface area with no respiratory symptoms.

Prevention

Allergic transfusion reactions are not completely preventable. Recipients that have a confirmed history of at least one previous allergic reaction can be medicated with an antihistamine approximately 30 minutes prior to the transfusion. Washing cellular products to remove plasma and therefore any allergens is rarely performed, but may be considered if the recipient has experienced recurrent or severe allergic reactions to previous transfusions.

ANAPHYLACTIC/ANAPHYLACTOID TRANSFUSION REACTIONS

Incidence

Anaphylactic transfusion reactions are rare allergic responses to plasma-containing blood products that are severe and life-threatening. Anaphylactic reactions are nonhemolytic, type I hypersensitivity reactions that occur within minutes of exposure, typically after the infusion of a few milliliters of blood.

Pathophysiology and Clinical Presentation

Anaphylactic transfusion reactions, like simple allergic reactions, are caused by the reaction between a protein allergen in the transfused product and its corresponding antibody, which is either in the recipient's plasma or in the donated blood component. Attachment of the antigen–antibody complex to mast cells causes activation of the cells. Release of histamine and other mediators from mast cells cause immediate observable symptoms in the recipient.

When reactions to plasma proteins result in the production of non-IgE-class antibodies with non-IgE-mediated release of mast cell mediators, they are defined as **anaphylactoid**.[7] Anaphylactoid transfusion reactions are severe and life-threatening. Anaphylactoid reactions have the potential to occur in IgA-deficient individuals when they have made antibody to IgA after exposure to IgA through a previous transfusion or pregnancy. When these individuals are subsequently transfused with plasma-containing blood products, the IgA in the blood product initiates the response. Although IgA deficiency is found in approximately 1:700 people, with the highest incidence in people of European ethnicity, the incidence of development of anti-IgA with subsequent risk of IgA-mediated anaphylactoid reactions is very rare.

☑ **CHECKPOINT 12-6**

What is the incidence of IgA deficiency?

✳ **TABLE 12-3** Clinical Presentation of Allergic and Anaphylactic Transfusion Reaction[10]

Allergic Reaction	Anaphylactic Reaction
At least two of the following signs or symptoms, occurring during or within 2 hours of transfusion: • Rash • Urticaria (hives) • Pruritis (itching) • Generalized flushing • Edema of lips, tongue, and/or uvula • Erythema (redness of the skin) and edema in the periorbital area • Conjunctival edema	In addition to any one or more of the symptoms of an allergic reaction, at least one of the following signs or symptoms: • Symptoms of a constricted airway: tightness of the throat, dysphagia (difficulty swallowing), dysphonia (difficulty speaking), hoarseness, stridor (high-pitched respiratory sounds) • Pulmonary symptoms: dyspnea (labored breathing), cough, wheezing, bronchospasm, hypoxemia (deficient oxygenation of the blood as demonstrated, for example, by blue-tinged lips or extremities or low pulse oximetry readings) • Hypotension (low blood pressure) • Hypotonia (decreased muscle tone) • Syncope (fainting)

The symptoms of anaphylactic and anaphylactoid reactions are clinically indistinguishable. The absence of fever is a key feature that distinguishes these reactions from others that have similar clinical presentations. Observable symptoms include immediate and severe respiratory problems or hypotension, in addition to at least two of the mucocutaneous symptoms that are observed in the mild allergic transfusion reaction. Respiratory symptoms may be laryngeal, which include tightness of the throat, difficulty swallowing (dysphagia), weak voice (dysphonia), hoarseness, or a high-pitched sound when breathing (stridor). Pulmonary symptoms include shortness of breath (dyspnea), coughing, wheezing, and bronchial spasms.

Differential Diagnosis and Clinical Work-Up

The confirmation of anaphylactic transfusion reactions must include the rule out of other environmental, drug, or dietary allergenic sources. Because anaphylactic and anaphylactoid reactions are similar in presentation, it is not necessary to distinguish between them clinically. When IgA deficiency is suspected as the cause of the transfusion reaction, the recipient should be tested for IgA levels. If IgA levels are low, then a test for anti-IgA can be performed. It is recommended that the specimen for IgA level be drawn a minimum of 10 days after the transfusion reaction because testing performed on serum that is drawn immediately after a transfusion reaction may be falsely negative.[11] Similarly, transfused IgA may deplete anti-IgA levels. Therefore, it is preferable to test for anti-IgA on a pretransfusion specimen.

Anaphylactic/anaphylactoid transfusion reactions must be distinguished from other reactions that have similar symptoms.[7] Reactions that include respiratory distress, shock, or unconsciousness can mimic the anaphylactic response but have different treatment protocols. Transfusion-related acute lung injury presents with respiratory symptoms similar to those that are observed in the anaphylactic transfusion reaction; however, the mucocutaneous symptoms (e.g., itching and hives) found during an allergic reaction are notably absent. Hypotensive and anaphylactic/anaphylactoid reactions share a drop in blood pressure and possible loss of consciousness as common symptoms. However, hypotensive reactions do not usually display any respiratory or mucocutaneous symptoms.

Treatment

If an anaphylactic or anaphylactoid reaction is suspected, the transfusion must be stopped immediately. The transfusion is never resumed even if immediate symptoms are resolved. Treatment is based on the severity of symptoms and is determined by a physician at the time of the reaction. Immediate medical intervention usually requires monitoring the airway, blood volume, and blood pressure. The intravenous line should be kept open so that epinephrine and steroids, such as prednisone, can be administered. Oxygen therapy is given to maintain respiratory function. Intubation of the patient may be necessary.

Prevention

Prevention of an anaphylactic transfusion reaction is based on previous history of either a suspected or confirmed severe reaction to a plasma-containing blood product. The following transfusion options are available for individuals at risk of anaphylactic/anaphylactoid transfusion reactions:

- Washed red blood cell or platelet units.
- Autologous donation of blood and/or plasma.
- Products from an IgA-deficient donor, especially if plasma is required or if anti-IgA is suspected or confirmed as the likely cause of the reaction. Rare donor registries include known IgA-deficient donors.
- Deglycerolized rejuvenated red blood cell units.

TRANSFUSION-RELATED ACUTE LUNG INJURY (TRALI)

Incidence

Before the term *transfusion-related acute lung injury (TRALI)* was coined in 1985, terms in the earlier literature that probably referred to TRALI include *noncardiogenic pulmonary edema, allergic pulmonary edema, leukoagglutinin transfusion reaction,* and *hypersensitivity reaction.*[5] The true incidence of TRALI is unknown and in the past was thought to be underreported for several reasons[12]:

- Lack of a uniformly accepted definition of TRALI.
- TRALI can be difficult to distinguish from fluid overload and the diagnosis can be complicated if the patient has other possible causes of acute lung injury.
- Clinicians may not feel a need to report TRALI because there is no difference in the treatment between TRALI and other forms of acute lung injury (ALI).
- The antibody work-up is expensive and time-consuming, and the potential loss of donors through a positive finding can be prohibitive to making a diagnosis of TRALI.

Reported incidences of TRALI range from as many as 1 in 1,300 transfusions to as few as 1 in 100,000, depending on the source. Higher reported incidences are probably a result of a clearer definition of TRALI and an increase in recognition of TRALI rather than an actual increase in incidence. A widely accepted definition of TRALI was developed at an international consensus conference held in 2004.[13] TRALI is the leading cause of transfusion-associated fatalities, comprising 48% of mortalities reported to the U.S. Food and Drug Administration (FDA) between 2005 and 2009.[14]

TRALI can occur with any plasma-containing blood component but is associated more frequently with plasma-rich products from female donors, who are more likely to make alloantibodies because of exposure through pregnancies. Fresh frozen plasma (FFP) was the most likely blood component in cases reported to the FDA between 2005 and 2006.[14] Recommendations to reduce TRALI were published in the United States in 2007 and included minimization of the use of female donors for the production of plasma and platelet components.[15] Since the implementations of these recommendations, FFP involvement in reported cases of TRALI in the United States has decreased; red blood cell units and apheresis platelet units are now equally likely culprits. Other countries have followed the lead of first the United Kingdom and later the United States, and predominantly use donations from male donors to make transfusable plasma components. Donations from females are used to make plasma-poor components such as red blood cells, with diversion of the donated plasma to make fractionation products.

Pathophysiology and Clinical Presentation

TRALI is an acute adverse reaction that occurs within 6 hours of transfusion. It is characterized by the onset of acute **hypoxemia** in the absence of cardiac involvement. Hypoxemia is inadequate oxygenation of the blood. Visible pulmonary infiltrates are observed on x-rays of the lungs. No evidence of lung injury or predisposing risk factor exists prior to the transfusion.

The exact mechanism of TRALI, and why the lungs are the affected organs, is still under investigation. No matter the mechanism, it is generally agreed that neutrophils are involved with the ultimate result of damage to the pulmonary capillaries and subsequent pulmonary edema. Both immune and nonimmune processes have been identified to explain this type of response to transfusion. Because this reaction is exclusive to the pulmonary microvasculature, it is proposed that TRALI is actually a two-step event. First, a preexisting condition such as recent surgery, stress, sepsis, cytokine therapy, or massive transfusion causes the neutrophils to congregate in the lining of the lungs. Then an immune or nonimmune process results in the onset of symptoms.

The immune response or antibody-mediated reaction involves antibodies that are directed against HLA Class I, HLA Class II, or human neutrophil antigens (HNA). In the majority of cases, the alloantibodies are made by the donor and therefore are in the transfused unit.[16] Donor antibodies are presumed to arise from exposure to alloantigens via pregnancy or previous transfusion. Once transfused, the antibodies bind to the patient's neutrophils and it is believed the antibody-coated neutrophils localize to the pulmonary microvasculature. The complement system is then activated, which triggers a cascade that ultimately leads to destruction of capillaries in the lungs. Fluid is released into the alveolar sacs with resulting edema.

The nonimmune mechanism for TRALI is explained by the presence of biologic response modifiers, which are naturally produced substances that can build up in cellular blood components during product storage.[7] Biologic response modifiers cause nonspecific activation of primed neutrophils, which then release the contents of their granules. When an underlying condition has caused primed neutrophils to aggregate in the lung lining, the end result is endothelial damage and pulmonary edema.

Transfusion recipients can also possess neutrophil antibodies directed against antigens on the donor leukocytes; however, in these instances there is less risk of TRALI because fewer leukocytes exist in the donor product.

The signs and symptoms of TRALI are listed in Box 12-2. Observable symptoms may also include chills, cough, fever, and hypotension. The defining characteristic is the presence of pulmonary edema in the absence of cardiac involvement, notably circulatory overload, which is another transfusion complication. The severity of symptoms varies from mild to fatal. Most cases resolve in hours to days with supportive care. Although most cases resolve without long-lasting complications, TRALI is identified as the leading cause of transfusion-associated death.

BOX 12-2   Clinical Presentation of Transfusion-Related Acute Lung Injury (TRALI)[10]

Signs and Symptoms

- No evidence of acute lung injury (ALI) prior to the transfusion
- Acute onset of ALI during or within 6 hours of transfusion
- Hypoxemia ($\downarrow$ O_2) defined by:
  - PaO_2/FiO_2 <300 mm Hg or
  - Oxygen saturation of <90% on room air or
  - Other clinical evidence
- No evidence of left atrial hypertension
- No alternative risk factor for ALI during or within 6 hours of completion of transfusion
- Bilateral infiltrates on chest radiograph

CHECKPOINT 12-7

What is the usual finding when a chest x-ray is performed on a patient experiencing a transfusion-related acute lung injury (TRALI)?

Differential Diagnosis and Clinical Work-Up

The diagnosis of TRALI is complicated by other risk factors for acute lung injury (ALI). These risk factors are listed in Table 12-4 ✱. In order for a differential diagnosis to be made, no other risk factor for ALI must exist either before or within 6 hours of the transfusion. Furthermore, TRALI must be distinguished from transfusion-associated circulatory overload (TACO) and anaphylactic transfusion reactions because these reactions present with similar respiratory symptoms but respond to different treatments.

The clinical work-up for diagnosis should include a chest x-ray, which will show pulmonary infiltrates if a TRALI has occurred. A complete blood count (CBC) may show a decrease in circulating neutrophils, or neutropenia. Visual inspection of the patient's specimen for hemolysis and a DAT should be performed to rule out a hemolytic event. The identification of antibodies to HLA or HNA can be performed to support the diagnosis, but is not used to determine treatment of the patient. Supportive treatment of the patient is the same regardless of the antibody identified and often needs to

---

✱ **TABLE 12-4** Risk Factors for Acute Lung Injury (ALI)

Direct Lung Injury	Indirect Lung Injury
• Aspiration	• Severe sepsis
• Pneumonia	• Shock
• Toxic inhalation	• Multiple trauma
• Lung contusion	• Burns
• Near drowning	• Acute pancreatitis
	• Cardiopulmonary bypass
	• Drug overdose

occur before an antibody identification can take place, especially since antibody detection for HLA or HNA is time-consuming and often occurs only at referral laboratories.

Treatment

When symptoms of TRALI are evident, the transfusion must be stopped immediately. The bags of all units transfused within the last 6 hours should be returned to the laboratory and the unit that was the last to be transfused should be identified.[12]

There is no specific treatment for TRALI; rather, supportive therapy, especially for respiratory distress, is provided as needed. Patients experiencing TRALI tend to require supplemental oxygen, but the need for intubation varies depending on the severity of the patient's symptoms. Vasopressors can be used to manage hypotension if present. Diuretics either have no effect or can worsen the symptoms and should be avoided. If TACO is initially suspected, but diuretic therapy has no effect, TRALI should be investigated. In most patients experiencing TRALI, symptoms resolve after a few days with no further complications.

Prevention

Because, in most cases, the culprit of TRALI arises from donor antibodies in a blood component, the patient does not have to go through any work-up to prevent future reactions. Subsequent transfusions from a different donor are typically acceptable. Screening of blood donors for antibodies to HLA and HNA antigens is not recommended. As a precautionary measure, blood collection facilities have implemented the practice of selecting plasma from predominantly male donors for transfusion because these collections are less likely to contain antibodies to neutrophils, which have often been implicated in cases of TRALI. Plasma from female donors may be diverted to other purposes, such as further manufacturing into products such as albumin and intravenous immune globulin (IVIG).

TRANSFUSION-ASSOCIATED CIRCULATORY OVERLOAD (TACO)

Incidence

Transfusion-associated circulatory overload (TACO) is a rarely reported adverse reaction. It is believed that the actual incidence is much higher because the reaction is underreported. The FDA summary report on transfusion fatalities for the years 2005–2009 indicates that TACO comprises 8% of transfusion-related fatalities.[13]

All transfusion recipients are susceptible to TACO; however, increased frequency is observed among the elderly, infants, people with small blood volumes, and those with cardiac or pulmonary disease. Individuals with chronic anemia are also at increased risk.

Pathophysiology and Clinical Presentation

Rapid rate of infusion of blood products is the most common cause of TACO. Excess fluid volume in the circulation can result in acute pulmonary edema and/or chronic heart failure; either condition requires immediate medical intervention.

Symptoms of TACO manifest either during the transfusion or shortly after the transfusion is ended. To definitively diagnose TACO, at least three of the following symptoms must occur within 6 hours of transfusion[10]:

- Acute respiratory distress; for example, dyspnea, orthopnea (difficulty breathing except when sitting upright), cough
- Evidence of positive fluid balance
- Elevated brain natriuretic peptide (BNP)
- X-ray evidence of pulmonary edema
- Evidence of left heart failure
- Elevated central venous pressure (CVP)

Differential Diagnosis and Clinical Work-Up

Causes of blood volume expansion that are not related to the transfusion, including infusions of medications and intravenous solutions, must be excluded in order to diagnose TACO. Preexisting cardiac and pulmonary insufficiencies that are not related to the transfusion must also be excluded. The clinical work-up for suspected cases of TACO typically include electrocardiogram, pulmonary function tests, chest x-ray, monitoring of central venous pressure, and vital signs.

Adverse reactions to transfusion that present with similar symptoms, particularly those that include pulmonary edema, can make the diagnosis of TACO difficult. TRALI is often confused with TACO; Table 12-5 ✳ compares the symptoms that are the same and that are different between TACO and TRALI. Testing for brain natriuretic peptide (BNP) levels has been suggested as a noninvasive way to differentiate TACO and TRALI because BNP is elevated in TACO. However, BNP testing is of limited value in critically ill patients, as the levels are elevated following an episode of hypoxemia regardless of the cause of the hypoxia.[17]

✳ **TABLE 12-5** Differential Diagnosis of Transfusion-Associated Circulatory Overload (TACO) and Transfusion-Related Acute Lung Injury (TRALI)

Signs and Symptoms That Occur in . . .		
Both TACO and TRALI	**TACO Only**	**TRALI Only**
• Respiratory distress • Radiographic evidence of pulmonary edema	• Left arterial hypertension • Elevated brain natriuretic peptide (controversial) • Responds to diuretics	• Fever commonly occurs

---

☑ CHECKPOINT 12-8

In transfusion medicine, what does the acronym TACO stand for?

Treatment

If TACO is suspected, the transfusion should either be stopped immediately or the rate of transfusion significantly slowed if the transfusion is vital. Patients may be placed in an upright position to help with respiratory distress and supportive treatment often includes oxygen therapy. Diuretics may be given to increase urinary output and reduce blood volume. If severe symptoms persist, therapeutic phlebotomy can be used to rapidly reduce blood volume.

Prevention

TACO is prevented by identifying patients in high-risk groups and taking appropriate measures to limit the rapid expansion of blood volume during transfusion. The most common preventions used include transfusing each blood product slowly over the allowed 4 hours with time between additional transfusions; splitting the blood product and transfusing each aliquot over the allowable 4-hour limit; and/or treating the patient with diuretics before and possibly also after transfusion. Washed or frozen red blood cells that have lesser amounts of plasma than packed red blood cells can alternatively be used, but may carry additional risks related to their preparation. For example, if prepared in an open system there is an increased risk of bacterial contamination. Whole blood products for patients at risk should be avoided. Vital signs should be carefully monitored during the transfusion.

TRANSFUSION-ASSOCIATED DYSPNEA (TAD)

Transfusion-associated dyspnea (TAD) is a term used by many hemovigilance networks and increasingly used in literature that captures transfusion reactions when the patient experienced respiratory distress but when TRALI, TACO, and other causes have been ruled out.[10]

HYPOTENSIVE TRANSFUSION REACTIONS

Incidence

Hypotensive transfusion reactions are identified as a drop in blood pressure (systolic or diastolic) of >30 mm Hg that occurs during or within 1 hour after the transfusion. The diagnosis of these reactions is often difficult because many adverse reactions to transfusion include symptoms of hypotension. If other symptoms occur in addition to hypotension and these symptoms suggest a particular type of reaction—for example, anaphylactic, TRALI, hemolytic, or bacterial sepsis—then the reaction should be categorized as the particular reaction type and should not be reported as a hypotensive reaction.[10] True hypotensive transfusion reactions are very rare.

Platelet units are the most common blood component implicated in hypotensive transfusion reactions. To a lesser extent, hypotensive reactions have been reported during the transfusion of whole blood and packed red blood cell units.

Pathophysiology and Clinical Presentation

Hypotensive reactions are related to bradykinin function and metabolism. Bradykinin is a peptide produced naturally in the body by the kinin–kallikrein system of blood proteins. Bradykinin causes vasodilation and subsequent lowering of blood pressure.

Over half the hypotensive transfusion reactions reported have been associated with angiotensin-converting enzyme (ACE) inhibitor treatment.[5] ACE is the enzyme most responsible for naturally breaking bradykinin down into its degradation products. To lower blood pressure and stabilize cardiac function, ACE inhibitors are sometimes prescribed during hypertensive episodes. Because the drug inhibits ACE, patients taking ACE inhibitors have less ability to break down bradykinin. Bradykinin causes vasodilation; therefore, an increase in bradykinin levels lowers blood pressure. Figure 12-2 ■ diagrams the interactions involved in hypotensive reactions.

If a transfusion increases bradykinin levels in a patient who has an impaired ability to degrade bradykinin, the patient's blood pressure can drop rapidly. Use of negatively charged bedside leukoreduction filters[18] or negatively charged apheresis kits can cause an increase in bradykinin because the negatively charged surface activates coagulation Factor XII. Activated Factor XII releases kallikrein from high-molecular-weight kininogen, to which it is normally bound. Kallikrein, in turn, generates bradykinin by cleaving high-molecular-weight kininogen.[19]

ACE inhibitor–related hypotensive reactions have also been reported in liver transplant recipients.[20] There is a genetic polymorphism that causes decreased bradykinin degradation; this might explain some of the hypotensive reactions that occur in people who are not on ACE inhibitors.[21]

The main symptom of the hypotensive transfusion reaction is a rapid decrease in blood pressure of >30 mm Hg. This change can occur either during the transfusion or up to 1 hour after the transfusion is complete. In rare circumstances, other symptoms such as flushing of the face, dyspnea, and cramping may occur.

Differential Diagnosis and Clinical Work-Up

In order to diagnose a hypotensive transfusion reaction, it is essential that other adverse reactions characterized by symptoms of hypotension are excluded. Follow-up testing should be ordered in accordance with patient symptoms to rule out other types of reactions, including hemolytic reactions, which can cause a decrease in blood pressure. The patient should have no preexisting condition that can explain the decrease in blood pressure. Patient history, including current and previous medications, should be obtained by the clinician prior to diagnosis.

Treatment

When hypotensive transfusion reactions are suspected, the transfusion must be discontinued immediately. Treatment, including vasopressors to increase blood pressure, can be administered to offset symptoms. The response to treatment in hypotensive transfusion reactions is often rapid and occurs within a few minutes of the administration of medications to increase blood pressure. When response to treatment does not occur within minutes, other conditions should be suspected by the clinician.

☑ CHECKPOINT 12-9

What type of medication is commonly used to treat a hypotensive reaction?

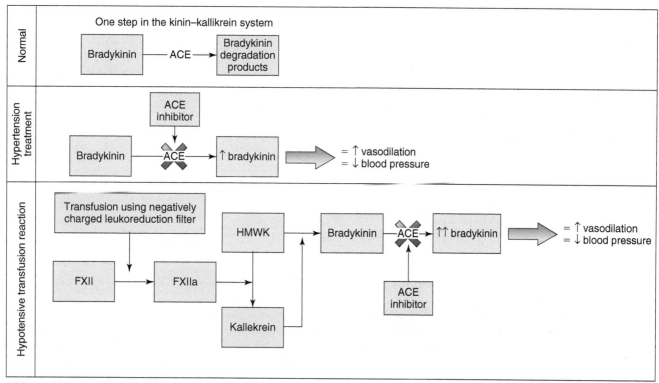

ACE = angiotensin-converting enzyme
FXII = coagulation Factor XII
FXIIa = acitvated coagulation Factor XII
HMWK = high-molecular-weight kininogen

FIGURE 12-2 Simplified Diagram of Bradykinin, Angiotensin-Converting Enzyme (ACE), and ACE Inhibitor Interactions

Prevention

Hypotensive transfusion reactions can be prevented by discontinuing ACE inhibitor treatment for a period of time before blood transfusion is administered. ACE inhibitor treatment should not be administered to the patient at the time of transfusion. A different class of antihypertensive medications can be used to treat patients who require transfusion.

The elimination of bedside leukoreduction filters is also recommended. Blood products that are leukoreduced at the time of collection or during laboratory storage are preferred. For patients with known or suspected history of hypotensive transfusion reactions, vital signs should be closely monitored during the transfusion.

TRANSFUSION-ASSOCIATED GRAFT VERSUS HOST DISEASE (TA-GVHD)

Incidence

Transfusion-associated graft versus host disease (TA-GVHD) is a rare complication of transfusion, but the mortality rate is approximately 90%. Death from TA-GVHD occurs rapidly, within 1–3 weeks of onset.

Pathophysiology and Clinical Presentation

TA-GVHD is caused by donor T-cell lymphocytes from transfused blood products that are able to recognize the host (or recipient) cells as a result of differences in human leukocyte antigens (HLA). The donor T-cell lymphocytes attack the host's tissues that carry the different HLA. While a small number of donor lymphocytes may enter a patient's circulation during transfusion, in most circumstances, recipient lymphocytes recognize the donor lymphocytes as nonself and eliminate the donor lymphocytes shortly after they enter the circulation.

Certain immunodeficient states that interfere with the recipient's ability to eliminate the donor lymphocytes will predispose transfusion recipients to developing TA-GVHD. Table 12-6 ✳ lists some of the patients usually considered at a higher risk for developing TA-GVHD. Interestingly, human immunodeficiency virus infection/ acquired immunodeficiency syndrome (HIV/AIDS) does not seem to be a risk factor and theories to explain this phenomenon are still being investigated.

Immunocompetent patients may be at risk for TA-GVH if transfused cellular products from a donor who shares a high degree of similarity in HLA type (Chapter 18); for example, a donor who is homozygous HLA A1/A1 and a recipient who is heterozygous HLA A1/A2.

Even with a fully functional immune system, the patient's lymphocytes may not recognize the donor's lymphocytes because they share the HLA A1 antigen. However, the donor lymphocytes may recognize the patient's HLA A2 as nonself and can attack the recipient's tissues. The risk of a homozygous donor sharing a haplotype with a heterozygous recipient in the general population is very low, but is greatly increased if the donor is a blood relative.

Symptoms of TA-GVHD typically occur within a few days to approximately 6 weeks after transfusion. The symptoms of

★ TABLE 12-6 Patients at Greater Risk for Transfusion-Associated Graft versus Host Disease (TA-GVHD)[22]

High Degree of Consensus	More Controversial
• Fetuses • Neonates who received an intrauterine transfusion previously • Patients with congenital cellular immunodeficiencies such as severe combined immunodeficiency, di George syndrome, Wiskott-Aldrich syndrome, purine nucleoside phosphorylase deficiency • Patients with Hodgkin's disease • Patients treated currently or anytime previously with purine analogs such as fludarabine, cladribine, or deoxycoformycin • Hematopoietic stem cell transplant recipients (both autologous and allogeneic) • Patients receiving transfusion from donor with a high degree of HLA similarity such as granulocyte transfusions, HLA-matched platelet transfusions, and cellular product transfusions from blood relatives	• Premature, low-birth-weight neonates • Patients with hematologic disease other than Hodgkin's who do not meet any other risk factor • Patients with solid organ tumors • Solid organ transplant recipients

TA-GVHD include fever, body rash, enlarged liver, and diarrhea. Other nonspecific symptoms may be present such as anorexia, nausea, and vomiting.[5] The pancytopenia that develops within 3–4 weeks after transfusion leads to further complications such as infection or bleeding. Box 12-3 lists the laboratory signs of graft versus host disease.

BOX 12-3   Definitive Diagnosis of Graft versus Host Disease (GVHD)[10]

Laboratory and Radiological Results

Evidence of liver dysfunction such as elevated liver enzymes and/or elevated bilirubin

Pancytopenia

White blood cell chimerism (when two white blood cell populations are in circulation) in the absence of alternative diagnosis

Characteristic histological appearance of skin or liver biopsy

Bone marrow abnormalities such as hypoplasia, aplasia, or presence of infiltrates

---

Differential Diagnosis and Clinical Work-Up

The diagnosis of TA-GVHD may not always be immediately evident because of its rarity, the delay from transfusion to onset of symptoms, and that the general symptoms of rash and diarrhea are not necessarily specific to TA-GVHD. Drug reactions and infections may sometimes be confused with TA-GVHD.

Histologic evaluation of skin, liver, and bone marrow biopsies can aid in the diagnosis. Skin biopsies show epidermal basal layer degeneration and vacuolization, separation of epidermis from underlying dermis (seen as a blister/bulla with the naked eye), perivascular lymphocytic infiltrate, and hyperkeratosis with apoptotic keratinocytes. While drug eruptions are often characterized by the presence of eosinophils, they cannot always be distinguished from TA-GVHD on biopsy.[23] Liver biopsies show bile duct damage with lymphocytic infiltration of the portal tracts.[24] Bone marrow aspirates and biopsies show hypoplasia or aplasia.

Chimerism studies can help definitively diagnose TA-GVHD, but the test is not universally available. However, a diagnosis of TA-GVHD can often still be made in the absence of chimerism study results based on the clinical context and other signs and symptoms. Molecular testing of the HLA antigens can distinguish donor and host lymphocytes if the donor has HLA antigens different from the recipient's. HLA testing will not be useful when the donor is homozygous for HLA antigens shared by the host/recipient. In these cases, chimerism can still be evaluated by testing for short tandem repeat (STR) or polymorphic microsatellite markers since these should be different in two individuals even if they share the same HLA haplotype.[25, 26] Fluorescent in situ hybridization (FISH) can provide rapid evaluation if the donor and host are of different genders by comparing female XX cells to male XY cells.[27]

Treatment

Currently, there is no standard therapy for TA-GVHD. Spontaneous resolution has been reported but is rare.[28] With a 90% mortality rate, prevention becomes the key issue in dealing with TA-GVHD. Attempted treatment modalities have included steroids, intravenous immune globulin, cyclophosphamide, cyclosporine, antithymocyte globulin, methotrexate, azathioprine, and T-cell monoclonal antibodies.

Extracorporeal phototherapy may be used as treatment. This process involves removing white blood cells and mononuclear cells from the circulation, treating the cells with psoralen and ultraviolet light while outside the body, and then returning the cells to the patient. This therapy regimen has shown promise in treating patients with GVHD.[29, 30, 31]

There is a case report of using hematopoietic progenitor cell (HPC) transplantation to successfully treat TA-GVHD.[32] HPC transplants are unlikely to become a routine treatment for TA-GVHD. The hypoplasia associated with TA-GVHD is likely to cause most autologous transplants to fail. If allogeneic transplant was considered, the time interval between patient presentation and death is often shorter than the time that would be needed to diagnosis TA-GVHD, find a suitable HPC donor, and complete all testing.

Prevention

The minimum number of leukocytes required to cause TA-GVHD is not known, in part because the variability of a patient's immune state is a contributing factor.[33] Leukoreduction decreases the number of donor lymphocytes transfused and therefore can reduce the incidence of TA-GVHD.[34] However, TA-GVHD has occurred when only leukoreduced products were transfused.[35, 36]

Gamma irradiation is effective in preventing TA-GVHD and acts by inactivation of donor lymphocytes, inhibiting their ability to proliferate in the host. Irradiation destroys any nucleated cells present while non-nucleated red blood cells and platelets remain virtually unaffected. Typical radiation dose requirements include a minimal delivery of 25 Gy to the center of a cellular blood component, with no less than 15 Gy delivered to the rest of the unit.[37] X-ray irradiation may be a substitute to gamma irradiation.[38] Patients at increased risk for TA-GVHD should be transfused only with irradiated cellular blood products.

☑ CHECKPOINT 12-10

How can transfusion-associated graft versus host disease (TA-GVHD) be prevented?

HEMOSIDEROSIS

Incidence

Hemosiderosis, or iron overload, is an adverse response to multiple (usually >100) red blood cell transfusions. Hemosiderosis is a concern in chronically transfused patients, particularly those that may need long-term or even life-long transfusion support. This includes most commonly patients with sickle cell disease or thalassemia, but patients with less commonly occurring hereditary hemolytic anemias and hemoglobinopathies are also at risk. Although the overall incidence of hemosiderosis is low, it is essential to monitor patients who may be at risk because the complications of iron toxicity can be fatal.

Pathophysiology and Clinical Presentation

Dietary intake of iron is essential for the production of hemoglobin. Most iron that is absorbed from the diet is incorporated into hemoglobin synthesis. Approximately 1 mg of iron is excreted per day; the rest is stored, recycled, and used to make new hemoglobin.

One red blood cell unit contains approximately 250 mg of iron. When a patient is receiving chronic transfusion support, excess iron begins to accumulate and deposit in tissues of the body because iron is not readily excreted. Iron deposits interfere with major organ function and lead to significant injury and infection.

The physical symptoms of hemosiderosis include weakness and fatigue. Laboratory findings of jaundice, anemia, and cardiac arrhythmia are often present. Untreated hemosiderosis can lead to liver and/or heart failure.

Differential Diagnosis and Clinical Work-Up

Hemosiderosis is suspected when multiply transfused patients present with symptoms that indicate iron toxicity. Blood ferritin levels and total iron binding capacity (TIBC) should be determined to confirm the diagnosis. Special stains for the presence of iron deposits in the tissues should be performed to confirm organ involvement.

Treatment

Iron toxicity can be prevented, delayed, or treated with iron chelation therapy. The chelating agent forms a complex with iron that facilitates its excretion through urine or feces. Desferrioxamine (trade name Desferal®) was the first FDA-approved iron chelator and is administered parenterally via injection. Patient compliance was historically low with this treatment because of the inconvenience and discomfort of the injection route. The first oral iron chelator, deferiprone (trade name Ferriprox™), received European approval in 1999. It has shown increased patient compliance but may be less effective than the desferrioxamine. Defersirox (trade name Exjade®) is an oral iron chelator that received FDA approval in 2005. As with all medications, each of the iron chelation therapies has side effects. Combination therapy with both desferrioxamine and deferiprone has also been used to treat hemosiderosis.[39, 40]

Prevention

Prevention of hemosiderosis is best achieved by limiting transfusion of red blood cell products. The transfusion of neocytes, or young red blood cells, can be effective in reducing iron toxicity by increasing the time between transfusions because these cells have a longer lifespan.[41] Donor red blood cell products must be further manipulated to isolate the neocytes; this is not commonly performed in North America.

POST-TRANSFUSION PURPURA (PTP)

Incidence

Post-transfusion purpura (PTP) is a rare complication of transfusion that presents as a severe and life-threatening thrombocytopenia. The majority of cases of PTP are identified in females over the age of 60. Cerebral hemorrhage is the main cause of death. Transfusion of leukoreduced blood products has decreased the incidence of PTP over the past several years.[34]

Pathophysiology and Clinical Presentation

The mechanism of thrombocytopenia is thought to be an anamnestic response of preexisting alloantibodies in recipient plasma against donor platelet antigens that result in platelet destruction by the reticuloendothelial system (RES). The majority of cases involve antigen-negative patients who develop alloantibodies after exposure to platelet antigens through pregnancy or transfusion. Female:male ratio of patients experiencing PTP is 5:1.[5] The classic patient is the multiparous female, who develops profound thrombocytopenia 5–12 days following a transfusion.

The transfused blood products most often associated with PTP are red blood cells and whole blood; however, PTP can occur after the transfusion of any cellular blood product. Leukoreduction decreases the amount of donor platelets present in red blood cell and whole blood units and can reduce the incidence of PTP.[34]

Anti-HPA-1a is the most commonly identified antibody in cases of PTP, accounting for more than 75% of cases.[34] The antibody target is the human platelet antigen 1a (HPA-1a) on glycoprotein IIIa

(GPIIIa). This polymorphism of GPIIIa is also known as Pl^{A1}, Zw^a, and CD61[42] and is present in 98% of the population, leaving 2% of the general population with the potential to develop the antibody if exposed to the antigen. Alloantibodies against other platelet antigens and human leukocyte antigens (HLA) have also been associated with PTP.

While alloantibodies explain the destruction of donor platelets, antigen-negative recipient platelets are also paradoxically destroyed. The mechanism for the concurrent autologous platelet destruction is unknown, but three main theories have been proposed:[5]

- Soluble antigen (e.g., soluble HPA-1a) that exists in the donor plasma form antigen–antibody immune complexes with the recipient's antibody. These complexes bind to the Fc receptor on recipient platelets, causing platelet destruction.

- Soluble antigen in the donor plasma adsorbs onto the surface of recipient platelets. In this way, the formerly antigen-negative patient platelets are converted into antigen-positive platelets that react with the antibody, leading to platelet destruction.

- Exposure to the donor antigen induces an autoantibody to develop. This autoantibody binds to both donor and recipient platelets, causing their destruction.

CHECKPOINT 12-11

What is the most common antibody implicated in post-transfusion purpura (PTP)?

Wet purpura is the classic presentation for PTP. This includes a speckled purple-red rash as a result of hemorrhages in the skin and bleeding from the mucous membranes, gastrointestinal tract, urinary tract, and nose. The clinical features of PTP are listed in Box 12-4. Platelet count levels in PTP are usually less than $10 \times 10^3/\mu L$ (10×10^9/L), falling to this level in approximately 80% of cases.[5]

BOX 12-4   Clinical Presentation of Post-Transfusion Purpura (PTP)[10]

Definitive Diagnosis

Platelet level is < 20% of pretransfusion level

Platelet drop occurs 5–12 days post-transfusion

Alloantibodies in the patient directed against platelet-specific antigens are detected at or after the development of the reaction (most common is anti-HPA-1a)

PTP is usually a self-limiting disease, meaning that it tends to resolve on its own. However, reported mortality rates have ranged from 0 to 12.8%, with intracranial hemorrhage as the main cause of death.[5]

Differential Diagnosis and Clinical Work-Up

Laboratory tests that help to distinguish PTP from other conditions that cause thrombocytopenia are listed in Table 12-7 ✷. Differential diagnosis can be difficult to elucidate in patients that have multiple health issues.

Thrombocytopenic patients who have had prior exposure to platelet antigens through transfusion or pregnancy may have anti-platelet antibodies that do not necessarily cause PTP. An antibody titration should be performed whenever it is important to distinguish PTP-induced thrombocytopenia from other causes of thrombocytopenia. The antibody titer in a PTP patient will be high, whereas the titer will remain low with other causes of thrombocytopenia.

Treatment

Treatment methods for managing PTP include intravenous immune globulin, plasmapheresis, high-dose steroids, and splenectomy. Intravenous immune globulin is currently considered the treatment of choice. Response to treatment is generally not immediate and takes days to weeks to be observed. Sometimes it is difficult to determine if the response is caused by the treatment itself or is part of the natural resolution of the condition. Platelet transfusions are not recommended for treatment of PTP because the transfused platelets will be destroyed.

Prevention

The increase in transfusion of leukodepleted blood products has resulted in a significant decrease in the incidence of PTP.[34] Routine screening for platelet antibodies or transfusion with antigen-matched platelets for the average patient is not recommended. Although recurrence of PTP is rare even for those patients with a confirmed history, antigen-negative platelets are recommended for future transfusions. Because of the high incidence of the HPA-1a antigen in the population, antigen-negative platelets are acquired through autologous donation, family members (siblings), or from identified blood donors.

REACTIONS ASSOCIATED WITH MASSIVE TRANSFUSION

The following transfusion reactions are most commonly associated with rapid transfusion of large amounts of blood products:

- Citrate toxicity (hypocalcemia and/or hypomagnesemia and/or metabolic acidosis)
- Hypothermia
- Dilutional coagulopathy

Citrate Toxicity

Plasma citrate levels increase during transfusion of blood products, but the rise is usually transient because the liver metabolizes excess citrate. Citrate toxicity can occur if rapid, massive transfusion overwhelms the liver's capacity to metabolize the citrate or if liver dysfunction prevents excess citrate from being metabolized. Citrate toxicity is of concern during exchange transfusion in newborns and for patients undergoing massive transfusion, particularly those who have liver dysfunction.

✴ **TABLE 12-7** Laboratory Tests in the Differential Diagnosis of Post-Transfusion Purpura (PTP)

Laboratory Test	Usual Result in Post-Transfusion Pupura (PTP)	Usual Result in Other Conditions
Platelet antibody screen/identification (anti-HPA)	Present with a high titer	Absent in all of the following: Idiopathic thrombocytopenia purpura (ITP) Sepsis Disseminated intravascular coagulation (DIC) Thrombocytic thrombocytopenic purpura (TTP) Heparin-induced thrombocytopenia Bone marrow failure
Blood culture	Negative	Positive in sepsis
D-Dimer	Negative	Positive in ITP
Red blood cell morphology	Normal	Schistocytes present in the following: DIC TTP
Heparin antibodies	Absent	Present in heparin-induced thrombocytopenia
Bone marrow biopsy	Normal	Decreased megakaryocytes in bone marrow failure

Citrate binds calcium and magnesium. Hypocalcemia, or low blood calcium level, is the main consequence of elevated citrate levels in transfusion recipients. Symptoms of hypocalcemia include tingling, spasm, muscle tremors, and electrocardiogram changes. Hypomagnesium, or low blood magnesium level, can also occur. Citrate toxicity can cause a metabolic acidosis because bicarbonate, which lowers blood pH, is a byproduct of citrate metabolism.

✓ **CHECKPOINT 12-12**

What two plasma ions are bound by citrate?

Hypothermia

Hypothermia occurs when body temperature drops below 95° F (35° C). Hypothermia related to transfusion is mainly attributed to rapid infusion of large volumes of cold-temperature blood products, particularly plasma products that require thawing prior to transfusion. Symptoms of hypothermia include body temperature $<95°$ F ($<35°$ C), lactic acidosis, and ventricular arrhythmia. Immune system function is inhibited. Hypothermia can be prevented through the use of blood warming devices when large volumes of product are being transfused.

Dilutional Coagulopathy

Massive transfusions of red blood cell products can result in the dilution of platelets and coagulation factors. The use of fluids including crystalloids and colloids may have a similar dilutional effect.

OTHER REACTIONS
Nonimmune Hemolysis

Several conditions, both physical and chemical in origin, can cause red blood cells to hemolyze prior to transfusion. Symptoms of nonimmune hemolysis may be subtle but typically include chills, hypotension, hemoglobinuria, and shortness of breath. Absence of fever is

a common finding in both physical and chemical types of hemolysis. Table 12-8 ✴ lists the physical and chemical inducers of hemolysis.

The differential diagnosis of nonimmune hemolysis requires the initial rule out of immune hemolytic transfusion reaction (either immediate or delayed) or intrinsic defects in either the donor or recipient red blood cell membrane. When non-immune hemolysis is suspected, the transfusion should be stopped and the intravenous line kept open. Cardiac and respiratory function should be monitored.

Nonimmune hemolysis is best prevented through adherence to written protocols and standards. Only equipment and solutions approved by the regulatory body should be used for all transfusions; the regulatory body in the United States is the Food and Drug Administration (FDA). Equipment function must be regularly assessed.

Hyperkalemia

Hyperkalemia, or excess potassium in the blood, is a serious adverse reaction that, if not immediately treated, can result in respiratory failure and death. Hyperkalemia is caused by the buildup of extracellular potassium in a red blood cell containing product that is subsequently transferred to the patient during transfusion.

Red blood cells release potassium as they age during storage, thus older blood products typically contain higher potassium levels and are more often implicated in causing hyperkalemia. Irradiation of red blood cell products increases the leakage of potassium through the red blood cell membrane, hence the maximum expiration date for irradiated red blood cell products is shortened to 28 days from the date of irradiation or the original expiry date, whichever is first. Patients at increased risk for complications from increased potassium in transfused blood include premature neonates and those with renal or cardiac dysfunction. Treatment with exchange transfusion should be considered, particularly in neonates, when plasma potassium levels reach 8 mEq/L (8 mmmol/L).

Hypokalemia

Hypokalemia, or low potassium level in the blood, is caused by transfusion of products that contain low potassium levels, such as washed red blood cells and deglycerolized red blood cells. Hypokalemia

✷ **TABLE 12-8** Physical and Chemical Causes of Hemolysis

Inducer	Example Cause(s)	Prevention
Heat	Improper use of blood warmer Improper storage, exposure to high temperatures	Blood warmers must be validated and maintained. Blood warmers should have an audible alarm that signals if a unit is overheating. Maintain proper storage conditions for blood products at all times.
Freezing temperatures	Inadequate glycerolization prior to freezing Inadequate deglycerolization after thawing Improper storage, exposure to freezing temperatures	Proper glycerolization and deglycerolization of red blood cells, if rare cells are to be stored frozen. Maintain proper storage conditions for blood products at all times.
Mechanical	Excess pressure from roller pumps Use of small bore needles during rapid transfusion	Only use pumps that have been approved for use with red blood cell products. Infusion pumps must be properly maintained. Use a larger-bore needle if transfusion is to occur quickly.
Osmotic lysis	Addition of hypotonic or hypertonic solutions	No solutions should be added to infusion line or red blood cell product except 0.9% normal sodium chloride or other solution that is approved for use with red blood cell transfusions.
Chemically induced	Drugs cause cellular changes that result in swelling or lysis	No medications should be added to infusion line or blood product.

causes mainly cardiac disturbances. Premature infants and patients with renal disease are at the most risk for complications of depleted potassium.

Air Embolus

An *air embolus*, or air bubble formation, is a rare adverse reaction of blood transfusion. An embolus can occur when a leak or crack permits the entry of air into the infusion site. The consequence of an air bubble in the blood vessel is circulatory obstruction. Symptoms of air embolus include cough, chest pain, and dyspnea. In the past, air embolism was of concern because glass and rubber tubing were used during transfusion and were more likely to allow air entry. With the introduction of plastic administration sets, the risk of air embolus is now minimal. Prevention of air embolus includes expelling air from blood tubing before starting the transfusion and when changing bags and inspecting tubing for leaks or cracks.

TRANSFUSION-RELATED IMMUNOMODULATION (TRIM)

Transfusion-related immunomodulation (TRIM) refers to the transient immune suppression that appears to occur following transfusion of allogeneic blood products. TRIM was first recognized in renal transplant recipients, when patients receiving transfusions experienced a lower incidence of graft rejection. While this is a beneficial effect of TRIM, deleterious effects have also been proposed, particularly an increased recurrence of cancer and increased occurrence of infection. The effects of TRIM have been difficult to prove.[43] Likewise, the cause of TRIM remains unproven. It is likely that transfused leukocytes account for some of the effects of TRIM and leukoreduction may reduce transfusion-associated immune suppression. Pro-inflammatory effects of transfused soluble bioactive factors have also been proposed as a mechanism of TRIM.

INITIAL LABORATORY INVESTIGATION OF SUSPECTED TRANSFUSION REACTIONS

Because many types of transfusion reactions demonstrate similar symptoms, it is critical that a complete follow-up and investigation be performed on every reported reaction. This will ensure that the patient receives appropriate treatment and may prevent the patient from experiencing reactions during future transfusions. When investigating a transfusion reaction, both the clinical evaluation and the laboratory work-up are critical to correctly diagnosing the etiology of the reaction. Table 12-9 ✷ summarizes the transfusion reaction types to be considered based on the primary presenting symptom(s).

Upon suspicion of a transfusion reaction, the transfusion services laboratory should be contacted for direction. In most cases, the laboratory will have a standard form with instructions for following up a transfusion reaction. Depending on the symptoms and the patient history, the laboratory may request that any remaining blood component, along with the infusion tubing, be forwarded to the laboratory along with a post-transfusion blood sample for investigation. It is critical that any identifying labels and tags remain on the component being forwarded. The post-transfusion specimen should be collected following the same stringent patient identification procedures used for pretransfusion sample collection. The laboratory may also request a urine specimen for evaluation of hemoglobinuria.

Initial laboratory investigation includes a clerical check for errors on the pretransfusion specimen label, initial laboratory requisition, other paperwork, pretransfusion testing results, component tags and labels, and the post-transfusion specimen label. If any errors are identified in the clerical check, possible companion errors due to mix-ups in blood specimens or component labels should be investigated in order to prevent adverse effects in other transfusion recipients.[7]

TABLE 12-9 Differential Diagnoses Based on Primary Presenting Symptom[21]

Symptom	Possible Reaction Type
Fever	Acute hemolytic
	Bacterial sepsis
	Febrile, nonhemolytic
Dyspnea	Transfusion-associated circulatory overload (TACO)
	Transfusion-related acute lung injury (TRALI)
	Anaphylaxis/anaphylactoid
	Transfusion-associated dyspnea (TAD)
Rash	Anaphylaxis/anaphylactoid
	Minor allergic
	Transfusion-associated graft versus host disease (TA-GVHD)
Hypotension	TRALI
	Acute hemolytic
	Anaphylaxis/anaphylactoid
	Bradykinin-mediated hypotensive
Hemolysis	Acute hemolytic
	Delayed hemolytic
	Nonimmune hemolysis
Cytopenia	TA-GVHD
	Post-transfusion purpura (PTP)

Standard initial laboratory testing includes ABO testing of the post-transfusion sample and may include retesting of the pretransfusion sample. The pre- and post-transfusion samples are visually inspected for signs of hemolysis, although low levels in free hemoglobin may not be visible to the naked eye, and a DAT is performed on the post-transfusion sample.

CASE IN POINT *(continued)*

The bedside clerical checks do not reveal any errors. The nurse reports the transfusion reaction to the transfusion service. She sends the empty platelet bag, the remainder of the red blood cell unit, the blood tubing and fluids used during both transfusions, and a postreaction specimen to the laboratory. The transfusion service performs an initial transfusion reaction investigation and obtains the following results:

Result	Pretransfusion	Post-transfusion
Clerical check	Negative	Negative
Visible hemolysis check	Negative	Negative
Visual inspection of blood product, tubing, and fluids	N/A	Nothing abnormal noted
ABO/Rh	O Rh (D) positive	O Rh(D) positive
Direct antiglobulin test	Negative	Negative
Antibody screen	Negative	Negative

6. Given the initial investigation results, is a hemolytic reaction likely? Why?

☑ **CHECKPOINT 12-13**

What are three standard tests initially performed on a post-transfusion specimen when a transfusion reaction is suspected?

FOLLOW-UP TESTING

Any further testing that is done is determined by the results of initial testing and the patient's symptoms. Table 12-10 summarizes the initial and follow-up testing that may be performed when different types of reactions are suspected. Testing may be used to rule in (confirm) or rule out (exclude) different types of reactions.

CASE IN POINT *(continued)*

Due to the increase in PH's temperature, the transfusion service medical director requests gram stains and cultures on the platelet and red blood cell bags, as well as a blood culture on the patient.

7. Why is it important to culture the patient's blood and the blood products?

No bacteria are seen on the gram stains. PH is placed on broad-spectrum antibiotics for 5 days as prophylaxis because she is immunosupprsssed and experienced a high fever. Her fever and chills subside within the next hour. She refuses the transfusion of the second unit of red blood cells. After discussion with her physician, PH decides that she will have a complete blood count drawn and tested in 3 days and that she will receive transfusions then if required. Her physician writes an order that until PH finishes chemotherapy, she will receive acetaminophen 30 minutes prior to transfusion and will be transfused with cellular products that are leukodepleted. Five days later all of the cultures of the units and PH's blood are reported as no growth. *Note:* Some laboratories will culture specimens related to transfusion reactions for longer to check for the growth of fastidious organisms.

8. What is the most likely type of transfusion reaction that PH experienced?
9. Why is this type of reaction more common in people who have received multiple transfusions?

✴ **TABLE 12-10** Follow-Up Testing for Transfusion Reaction Investigation[10]

Suspected Reaction Type	Clinical Presentation	Diagnostic Testing
Acute hemolytic	Chills, fever, hemoglobinuria, hypotension, renal failure with oliguria, disseminated intravascular coagulation (oozing from intravenous sites, petechia), back pain, pain along infusion vein, anxiety	• Clerical check • Direct antiglobulin test (DAT) • Visual inspection of plasma for free hemoglobin (or plasma hemoglobin quantitation) • Repeat patient ABO on pre- and post-transfusion specimen • Further tests as indicated to define possible incompatibility • Further tests as indicated to detect hemolysis (e.g., bilirubin, lactate dehydrogenase) • Further tests as indicated to detect or monitor disseminated intravascular coagulation (e.g., D-dimer, fibrin degradation products, blood smear for schistocytes) • Further tests as indicated to detect or monitor renal failure (e.g., creatinine)
Delayed hemolytic	Fever, anemia, new positive antibody screening test or new additional identified antibody, jaundice	• Antibody screen • DAT • Tests for evidence of hemolysis (e.g., bilirubin, plasma hemoglobin, lactate dehydrogenase, urine hemosiderin)
Febrile, nonhemolytic	Fever, chills/rigors, headache, vomiting	• Rule out hemolysis (DAT, inspect for hemoglobinemia, repeat patient ABO) • Rule out bacterial contamination (component culture, patient blood culture)
Allergic/urticarial	Urticaria, pruritus, flushing	• Rule out hemolysis (DAT, inspect for hemoglobinemia, repeat patient ABO)
Anaphylactic/anaphylactoid	Hypotension, urticaria, bronchospasm (respiratory distress, wheezing), local edema, anxiety	• Rule out hemolysis (DAT, inspect for hemoglobinemia, repeat patient ABO) • IgA quantitation • Anti-IgA screen
Transfusion-related acute lung injury (TRALI)	Hypoxemia, respiratory failure, hypotension, fever, bilateral pulmonary edema	• Rule out hemolysis (DAT, inspect for hemoglobinemia, repeat patient ABO) • Rule out cardiogenic pulmonary edema (arterial or venous pressure monitoring; brain natriuretic peptide level) • Chest x-ray • Human leukocyte antigen (HLA) antibody screen in donor and recipient. If positive, antigen typing may be indicated.
Transfusion-associated circulatory overload (TACO)	Dyspnea, orthopnea, cough, tachycardia, hypertension, headache	• Rule in cardiogenic pulmonary edema (arterial or venous pressure monitoring; brain natriuretic peptide level) • Chest x-ray
Hypotensive	Flushing, hypotension	• Rule out hemolysis (DAT, inspect for hemoglobinemia, repeat patient ABO) • Medication history (use of angiotensin-converting enzyme inhibitors)
Transfusion-associated graft versus host disease (TA-GVHD)	Erythroderma, maculopapular rash, anorexia, nausea, vomiting, diarrhea, hepatitis, pancytopenia, fever	• Skin biopsy • HLA typing • Molecular analysis for chimerism
Hemosiderosis	Diabetes, cirrhosis, cardiomyopathy	• Serum ferritin level • Liver enzyme levels • Endocrine function tests
Post-transfusion purpura (PTP)	Thrombocytopenic purpura and bleeding 5–12 days after transfusion	• Platelet antibody screen and identification
Citrate toxicity/hypocalcemia	Paresthesia (tingling), tetany, arrhythmia	• Ionized calcium level • Prolonged Q-T interval on electrocardiogram
Nonimmune hemolysis	Hemoglobinuria, hemoglobinemia	• Rule out immune-mediated hemolysis (DAT, repeat patient ABO) • Test red blood cell component for hemolysis
Hypothermia	Cardiac arrhythmia	• Central body temperature
Air embolus	Sudden shortness of breath, acute cyanosis, pain, cough, hypotension, cardiac arrhythmia	• X-ray for intravascular air

Review of the Main Points

- Adverse transfusion reactions are negative unintended consequences of transfusion that do not involve transmission of blood-borne bacteria, viruses, parasites, or prions.

- Acute reactions occur during or within 24 hours of a transfusion event.

- Delayed reactions occur days to weeks after a transfusion event.

- The U.S. Food and Drug Administration requires that transfusion-related fatalities be reported in writing within 7 days of the fatality.

- Transfusion reaction reporting provides an opportunity for facilities to identify systemic issues and implement preventive strategies.

- National surveillance systems use aggregate data and are often able to recognize systemic issues sooner than individual facilities might.

- Acute hemolytic transfusion reactions are associated with intravascular hemolysis and complement activation.

- Symptoms of acute hemolytic transfusion reactions include fever, pain at the infusion site, hypotension, wheezing, chest pain, flushing, and gastrointestinal symptoms. Severe reactions may proceed to disseminated intravascular coagulation and renal damage.

- The most common causes of acute hemolytic transfusion reactions are clerical errors related to patient or specimen or component identification, followed by laboratory testing errors.

- Symptoms of a delayed hemolytic reaction include fever, anemia, and/or jaundice occurring days to weeks after transfusion.

- Red blood cell destruction during acute hemolytic reactions involves complement activation resulting in intravascular hemolysis compared to extravascular hemolysis in delayed hemolytic reactions where antibody- or complement-coated cells are removed by phagocytes in the spleen, liver, and bone marrow.

- Anamnestic response refers to a fast rise in antibody titer after a second or subsequent exposure to an antigen.

- Anamnestic antibody response is common in delayed hemolytic reactions where the antibody titer might have fallen to undetectable levels prior to the transfusion.

- Febrile nonhemolytic transfusion reactions are a common type of reaction, exhibiting generally mild symptoms, most commonly fever and/or chills.

- Serious adverse reactions must be ruled out before diagnosing a febrile nonhemolytic transfusion reaction because some symptoms, such as fever, are common to many reactions.

- Anaphylactoid reactions occur when an IgA-deficient recipient who has made an anti-IgA is exposed to IgA in plasma-containing blood products.

- Patients who are known to be IgA deficient with anti-IgA must receive plasma components collected from IgA-deficient donors. Cellular components may be washed to remove residual plasma.

- Transfusion-related acute lung injury (TRALI) results in bilateral pulmonary edema.

- One proposed mechanism of TRALI is based on donor antibodies directed against human leukocyte antigens (HLA) or human neutrophil antigens (HNA) reacting with patient neutrophils that have congregated in the lungs.

- A second proposed mechanism of TRALI involves transfused biologic response modifiers activating neutrophils that have congregated in the patient's lungs because of an underlying condition.

- Using predominantly male plasma components for transfusion significantly reduces the risk of TRALI because multiparous donors are more likely to have made the white blood cell–related antibodies.

- Transfusion-associated graft versus host disease (TA-GVHD) occurs when donor lymphocytes present in transfused components proliferate in the patient and mount an immune response against the patient's tissues.

- Patients who are immunocompromised are at increased risk of transfusion-associated graft versus host disease (TA-GVHD) because they cannot mount an immune response to destroy transfused donor lymphocytes.

- Gamma irradiation of cellular blood components inactivates donor lymphocytes and prevents TA-GVHD.

- Initial investigation of suspected transfusion reactions should include clerical checks and the following tests on a post-transfusion specimen: visual check for hemolysis, direct antiglobulin test (DAT), and ABO group.

- Key diagnostic tests for differential diagnosis of serious adverse reactions include:

  - Direct antiglobulin test—positive result is evidence of immune-mediated hemolysis

  - Antibody screen—new positive result or additional identified antibody suggests a delayed hemolytic transfusion reaction

  - Urinalysis, serum bilirubin, or lactate dehydrogenase levels—hemoglobinuria, increased bilirubin, and/or increased lactate dehydrogenase can indicate hemolysis

  - Chest x-ray—bilateral pulmonary infiltrates support a diagnosis of transfusion-related acute lung injury

  - IgA and anti-IgA—IgA deficiency and presence of anti-IgA supports a diagnosis of anaphylactoid reaction

  - Skin or liver biopsy—characteristic histological changes indicate graft versus host disease.

Review Questions

1. A serious acute hemolytic transfusion reaction can occur as a result of which of the following situations? (Objective #2)

   A. Packed red blood cell product labeled as blood type B transfused to a group O patient

   B. Error in patient identification at the time of specimen draw for pretransfusion testing

   C. Misidentification of the patient at the bedside at the time of transfusion

   D. Computer entry error during reporting of pretransfusion test result

2. From the following list, select the signs and symptoms of an acute hemolytic transfusion reaction. (Objective #2)

   A. Hemoglobinuria

   B. DIC

   C. Increased renal blood flow

   D. Hypotension

   E. Negative DAT

   F. Pain at site of infusion

3. A full written report of a transfusion-associated fatality must be reported to the Centre for Biologics Evaluation and Research (CBER) within _____ days of the incident. (Objective #3)

   A. 3

   B. 7

   C. 10

   D. 14

4. Patient John Smith is receiving a transfusion of 1 unit of red blood cells for an anemic condition. Upon taking vital signs, his nurse suspects he might be having an adverse reaction to the transfusion. What is her first course of action? (Objective #7)

   A. Elevate the patient to a sitting position

   B. Inform his next of kin

   C. Administer IV furosemide STAT

   D. Discontinue the transfusion

5. Select the mode of prevention for each of the adverse transfusion reactions: (Objective #5)

   _____ Febrile

   _____ Allergic

   _____ Transfusion-associated GVHD

   _____ TACO

   _____ Anaphylactic

   _____ TRALI

   (a) Washed red blood cells

   (b) Transfusion of small aliquots

   (c) Leukoreduced red blood cells

   (d) Pretransfusion administration of antihistimine

   (e) Transfusion of plasma from male donors

   (f) Irradiation of blood products

6. Choose two specific mechanisms of a FNHTR. (Objective #5)

   A. HLA antibodies

   B. IgA antibodies

   C. Release of cytokine substances

   D. Bradykinin production

7. How can anaphylactic and anaphylactoid transfusion reactions be distinguished from other reactions with a similar clinical presentation? (Objective #8)

   A. Absence of IgA

   B. Absence of fever

   C. Presence of respiratory distress

   D. Shock

8. Which of the following clinical findings best differentiates TRALI from TACO? (Objective #8)

   A. X-ray evidence of pulmonary edema

   B. Brain natriuretic peptide (BNP) level

   C. Central venous pressure (CVP) level

   D. Presence of hypoxia

9. Select the transfusion recipients who are at increased risk for TACO. (Objective #5)

   A. Immunocomprimised patient

   B. Elderly patient

   C. Cardiac patient

   D. Anemic patient

   E. Leukemic patient

   F. Newborn infant

   G. Septic patient

   H. Trauma patient

10. Which blood product is most commonly implicated in hypotensive transfusion reactions? (Objective #5)

    A. Platelets

    B. Whole blood

    C. Packed red blood cells

    D. Fresh frozen plasma

11. How does gamma irradiation of blood products prevent TA-GVHD? (Objective #5)

   A. It reduces the number of donor lymphocytes in the transfused product.

   B. It destroys non-nucleated cells such as red blood cells and platelets.

   C. It inhibits the proliferative capability of donor lymphocytes.

   D. It increases HLA compatibility between donor and recipient.

12. Hemosiderosis is caused by excessive exposure to _____. (Objective #5)

   A. Citrate

   B. Calcium

   C. Potassium

   D. Iron

13. Select the laboratory findings that aid in the differential diagnosis of PTP. (Objective #5)

   A. Presence of platelet-specific antibody

   B. Negative D-Dimer

   C. Abnormal bone marrow biopsy

   D. Positive blood culture

14. What is the *main* consequence of elevated citrate levels in transfusion recipients? (Objective #5)

   A. Hypocalcemia

   B. Hypoproteinemia

   C. Hypokalemia

   D. Hypomagnesium

15. What is the first step in the initial blood bank laboratory investigation of a suspected transfusion reaction? (Objective #7)

   A. Repeat ABO testing

   B. Visual inspection for hemolysis

   C. DAT

   D. Clerical check

References

1. Saxena S, Shulman I, eds. *The Transfusion Committee: Putting Patient Safety First*. Bethesda (MD): AABB Press; 2006.

2. Serious hazards of transfusion [Internet]. Annual report 2009. Manchester; c 2010. [cited 16 Nov 2010]. Available from: http://www.shotuk.org/wp-content/uploads/2010/07/SHOT2009.pdf.

3. Stainsby D, Jones H, Asher D, Atterbury C, Boncinelli A, Brant L, Chapman CE, Davison K, Gerrard R, Gray A, Knowles S, Love EM, Milkins C, McClelland DB, Norfolk DR, Soldan K, Taylor C, Revill J, Williamson LM, Cohen H; SHOT Steering Group. Serious hazards of transfusion: A decade of hemovigilance in the UK. *Trans Med Rev* 2006; 20: 273–82.

4. Food and Drug Administration [Internet]. Guidance for industry: Notifying FDA of fatalities related to blood collection or transfusion. Final Guidance. (September 22, 2003). Rockville, MD; c2003. [cited 16 Nov 2010]. Available from: http://www.fda.gov/downloads/BiologicsBloodVaccines/GuidanceComplianceRegulatoryInformation/Guidances/Blood/ucm062897.pdf.

5. Popovsky MA, ed. *Transfusion Reactions*, 3rd ed. AABB Press: Bethesda, MD; 2007.

6. Stainsby D. ABO incompatible transfusions – experience from the UK Serious Hazards of Transfusion (SHOT) scheme Transfusions of ABO incompatible. *Transf Clin Biol* 2005; 12: 385–8.

7. Roback JD, ed. *Technical Manual*, 16th ed. Bethesda (MD): AABB Press; 2008.

8. Hannema S, Brand A, van Meurs A, Smiers F. Delayed hemolytic transfusion reaction with hyperhemolysis after first red cell transfusion in child with β-thalassemia: challenges in treatment. *Transfusion* 2010; 50: 429–32.

9. Heddle N. Universal leukoreduction and acute transfusion reactions: putting the puzzle together. *Transfusion* 2004; 44: 1–4.

10. Centers for Disease Control and Prevention. The National Healthcare Safety Network (NHSN) Manual, Biovigilance Component. Atlanta (GA): Centers for Disease Control and Prevention; 2010.

11. Mayo Clinic [Internet]. Mayo Medical Laboratories Test Catalog. Unit code 8154. Anti-IgA Antibodies, IgG Class, Serum; c1995-2011 [cited 30 Aug 2010]. Available from: http://mayomedicallaboratories.com/test-catalog/Specimen/8154.

12. Toy P, Lowell C. TRALI-definition, mechanisms, incidence and clinical relevance. *Best Pract Res Clin Anaestheiol* 2007; 21: 183–93.

13. Kleinman S, Caulfield T, Chan P, Davenport R, McFarland J, McPhedron S, Meade M, Morrison D, Pinsent T, Robillard P, Slinger P. Toward an understanding of transfusion-related acute lung injury: Statement of a consensus panel. *Transfusion* 2004; 44: 1774–89.

14. Center for Biologics Evaluation and Research [Internet]. Fatalities Reported to FDA Following Blood Collection and Transfusion. Annual Summary for Fiscal Year 2009. Silver Springs, MD. [updated 2010 Mar 03; cited 23 Feb 2010.] Available from: http://www.fda.gov/BiologicsBloodVaccines/SafetyAvailability/ReportaProblem/TransfusionDonationFatalities/ucm204763.htm.

15. AABB. Association Bulletin #06-07 Re Transfusion-Related Acute Lung Injury. 2006.

16. Middleburg RA, van Stein D, Briët E, van der Bom JG. The role of donor antibodies in the pathogenesis of transfusion-related acute lung injury: A systematic review. *Transfusion* 2008; 48: 2167–76.

17. Li G, Daniels C, Kojicic M, Krpata T, Wilson GA, Winters J, Breanndan Moore S, Gajic O. The accuracy of natriuretic peptides (brain natriuretic peptide and N-terminal pro-brain natriuretic) in the differentiation between transfusion-related acute lung injury and transfusion-related circulatory overload in the critically ill. *Transfusion* 2009; 49:13–20.

18. Lavee J, Yoav P. Hypotensive reactions associated with transfusion of bedside leukocyte-reduction filtered blood products in heart transplanted patients. *J Heart Lung Transplant* 2001; 20: 759–61.

19. Bruno DS, Herman JH. Acute hypotensive transfusion reactions. *Lab Medicine*. 2006; 37: 542–5.

20. Doria C, Elia ES, Kang Y, Adam A, Desormeaux A, Ramirez C, Frank A, diFrancesco F, Herman JH. Acute hypotensive transfusion reaction during liver transplantation in a patient on angiotensin converting enzyme inhibitors from low aminopeptidase P activity. *Liver Transpl* 2008; 14: 684–7.

21. Callum JL. *Bloody Easy 2; Blood Transfusions, Blood alternatives and Transfusion Reactions; A Guide to Transfusion Medicine*, 2nd ed. Toronto (ON): Sunnybrook and Women's College Health Sciences Centre; 2006.

22. Schroeder ML. Transfusion-associated graft-versus-host disease. *Brit J Haemotol* 2002; 117: 275–87.

23. Rapini RP. *Practical Dermatopathology.* Philadelphia (PA): Elsevier Mosby; 2005.

24. Scheuer PJ, Lefkowitch JH. *Liver Biopsy Interpretation,* 7th ed. Philadelphia (PA): Elsevier Mosby; 2006.

25. Wang L, Juji T, Tokunaga , Takahashi K, Kuwata S, Uchida S, Tadokoro K, Takai K. Brief report: polymorphic microsatellite markers for the diagnosis of graft-versus-host disease. *N Eng J Med* 1994; 330: 398–401.

26. Sage D, Stanworth S, Turner D, Navarrete C. Diagnosis of transfusion-associated graft vs.-host disease: The importance of short tandem repeat analysis. *Transfus Med* 2005; 15: 481–5.

27. Akay MO, Temiz G, Teke HU, Gunduz E, Acikalin MF, Isiksoy S, Durak B, Gulbas Z. Rapid molecular cytogenetic diagnosis of transfusion associated graft-versus-host disease by fluorescent in situ hybridization (FISH). *Transfus Apher Sci* 2008; 38: 189–92.

28. Mori S, Matsushita H, Ozaki K, Ishida A, Tokuhira M, Nakajima H, Kizaki M, Sugiura H, Kikuchi A, Handa M, Kawai Y, Yamamori S, Ikeda Y. Spontaneous resolution of transfusion-associated graft-versus-host disease. *Transfusion* 1995; 35: 431–5.

29. Perotti C, Del Fante C, Tinelli C, Viarengo G, Scudeller L, Zecca M, Locatelli F, Salvaneschi L. Extracorporeal photochemotherapy in graft-versus-host disease: A longitudinal study on factors influencing the response and survival in pediatric patients. *Transfusion* 2010; 50: 1359–69.

30. Garban F, Drillat P, Makowski C, Jacob MC, Richard MJ, Favrot M, Sotto JJ, Bensa JC, Cahn JY. Extracorporeal chemophototherapy for the treatment of graft-versus-host disease: Hematologic consequences of short-term, intensive courses. *Haematologica* 2005; 90: 1096–101.

31. Grass JA, Wafa T, Reames A, Wages D, Corash L, Ferrara JL, Lin L. Prevention of transfusion-associated graft-versus-host disease by photochemical treatment. *Blood* 1999; 93: 3140–7.

32. Hutchinson K, Kopko PM, Muto KN, Tuscano J, O'Donnell RT, Holland PV, Richman C, Paglieroni TG, Wun T. Early Diagnosis and successful treatment of a patient with transfusion-associated GVHD with autologous peripheral blood progenitor cell transplantation. *Transfusion* 2002; 42: 1567–72.

33. Shroeder ML. Transfusion-associated graft-versus-host disease. *Br J Haematol* 2002; 117: 275–87.

34. Williamson LM, Stainsby D, Jones H, Love E, Chapman CE, Navarrete C, Lucas G, Beatty C, Casbard A, Cohen H; Serious Hazards of Transfusion Steering Group. The impact of universal leukodepletion of the blood supply on hemovigilance reports of posttransfusion purpura and transfusion-associated graft-versus-host disease. *Transfusion* 2007; 47: 1455–67.

35. Akahoshi M, Takanashi M, Masuda H, Yamashita H, Hidano A, Hasegawa K, Shimizu M, Mitoji T, Oshimi K, Mizoguchi H. A case of transfusion-associated graft-versus-host disease not prevented by white cell-reduction filters. *Transfusion* 1992; 32: 169–72.

36. Hayashi H, Nishiuchi T, Takenda K. Transfusion-associated graft-versus-host disease caused by leukocyte-filtered stored blood. *Aneshesiology* 1993; 79: 1419–21.

37. AABB. *Standards for blood banks and transfusion services,* 27th ed. Bethesda (MD): AABB Press; 2011.

38. Janatpour K, Denning L, Nelson K, Betlach B, Mackenzie M, Holland P. Comparison of X-ray vs. gamma irradiation of CPDA-1 red cells. *Vox Sang* 2005; 89: 215–9.

39. Telfer PT, Warburton F, Christou S, Hadjigavriel M, Sitarou M, Kolnagou A, Angastiniotis M. Improved survival in thalassemia major patients on switching from desferrioxamine to combined chelation therapy with desferrioxamine and deferiprone. *Haematologica* 2009; 94: 1777–8.

40. Daar S, Pathare AV. Combined therapy with desferrioxamine and deferiprone in beta thalassemia major patients with transfusional iron overload. *Ann Hematol* 2006; 85: 315–9.

41. Spanos T, Ladis V, Palamidou F, Papassotiriou I, Banagi A, Premetis E, Kattamis C. The impact of neocyte transfusion in the management of thalassaemia. *Vox Sang* 1996; 70: 217–23.

42. Metcalfe P, Watkins NA, Ouwehand WH, Kaplan C, Newman P, Kekomaki R, De Haas M, Aster R, Shibata Y, Smith J, Kiefel V, Santoso S. Nomenclature of human platelet antigens. *Vox Sang* 2003; 85: 240–5.

43. Hellings S, Blajchman MA. Transfusion-related immunosuppression. *Anaesthesia and Intensive Care Medicine* 2009; 10: 231–4.

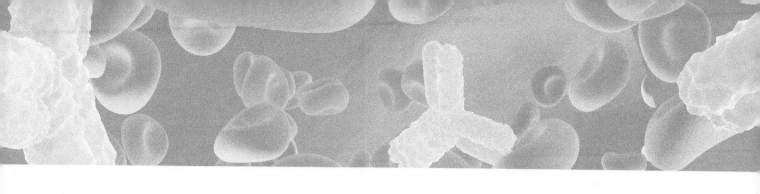

13 Transfusion-Transmitted Infections

SUSAN CONFORTI

Chapter Objectives

Upon completion of this chapter, the student will be able to:

1. List the transmissible disease tests that are performed on donated blood.
2. Compare and contrast the hepatitis viruses A, B, C, D, E, and G in terms of their structure, pathology, and modes of transmission.
3. State the transfusion risks for hepatitis A, hepatitis B, and hepatitis C.
4. Name the immunological markers in hepatitis B infection in order of their occurrence.
5. Describe the structure, pathology, and modes of transmission for the retroviruses: HIV I and II and HTLV I and II.
6. List the immunological markers that can be identified in HIV infection and when they are detectable.
7. State the current transfusion risks in the United States for HIV I/II and HTLV I/II.
8. Discuss the disease manifestation after transfusion transmission of the following viruses: parvovirus, Epstein-Barr virus, cytomegalovirus, and West Nile virus.
9. Name three viral agents that are not routinely tested for as part of the transmissible disease panel for donated blood.
10. Define the term prion.
11. Compare and contrast the pathophysiology and modes of transmission for Creutzfeldt-Jakob disease and variant Creutzfeldt-Jakob disease.
12. Discuss the two most frequent causes of bacterial contamination of donor blood, including implicated products, modes of transmission, detection, follow-up treatment, etc.
13. Discuss the etiologic agents for syphilis and Lyme disease, including organisms involved, transmission, etc.
14. Describe the pathology, modes of transmission, and treatment for the following transfusion-transmitted parasitic infections: babesiosis, malaria, Chagas disease, leishmaniasis, and toxoplasmosis.
15. List the infectious agents that have the highest infectivity rate in the leukocytes.
16. Discuss the benefits of using leukoreduced blood products to reduce the risk of transfusion-transmitted infections.

(continued)

Chapter Objectives (continued)

17. Name one pathogen inactivation procedure that is currently available for plasma products.
18. State two limitations for pathogen inactivation of donor blood.

Key Terms

Acquired immunodeficiency syndrome (AIDS)
Adult T-cell leukemia/lymphoma (ATL)
Aplastic crisis
Babesiosis
Chagas disease
Creutzfeldt-Jakob disease (CJD)
Cytomegalovirus (CMV)
Epstein-Barr virus (EBV)
Hepatitis A virus (HAV)
Hepatitis B virus (HBV)
Hepatitis C virus (HCV)
Hepatitis D virus (HDV)
Hepatitis E virus (HEV)
Hepatitis G virus (HGV)
Human herpes virus 8 (HHV-8)
Human immunodeficiency virus (HIV)
Human T-cell lymphotrophic virus (HTLV)

Incubation period
Infectious mononucleosis
Leishmaniasis
Lyme disease
Malaria
Parenterally
Parvovirus B19
Pathogen inactivation
Prion(s)
Retrovirus(es)
Sepsis
Syphilis
Toxoplasmosis
Transmissible spongiform encephalopathy(ies) (TSE)
Trypanosomiasis
variant Creutzfeldt-Jakob disease (vCJD)
Vertically
West Nile virus (WNV)
Window period
Yersinia enterocolitica

CASE IN POINT

GW is a 98-year-old female who was admitted to the ER last night. She was a relatively healthy woman who lived on her own until 3 months ago when she fell while walking her dog and broke her tibia. She was admitted to the hospital where medical staff surgically set her tibial fracture. She was given 2 units of blood during the surgery for anemia and discharged to a long-term care facility for rehabilitation.

Two days ago, she spiked a fever and became unresponsive. The long-term care facility ordered a battery of lab tests and noted her hemoglobin and hematocrit were 6.8 mg/dL and 20%. The laboratory also noted "inclusion bodies consistent with *Babesia spp.*" on her blood smear. Her family decided to bring her to the hospital for treatment.

Upon arrival in the ED, the physician described the patient as having been moribund. ED staff was able to collect specimens for another CBC and a chemistry panel, which suggested a hemolytic process was taking place. Unfortunately, ED staff members were unsuccessful in accessing a venous line. The patient had an advanced directive in place and her family decided to stop all medical care.

What's Ahead?

Pathogens that can contaminate the human blood supply are divided into four main categories: viruses, prions, bacteria, and parasites. For the past two decades, efforts to reduce transfusion risks from infectious agents have been very successful. The blood supply is extremely safe. Although the risk of acquiring a transfusion-transmitted infection is minimal, it is necessary to identify existing and emerging pathogens that have the potential to threaten the future safety of the blood supply. Identifying and assessing the risk factors for emerging pathogens can be particularly complex when they are first identified in developing countries that have insufficient resources for disease tracking. This chapter investigates both existing and emerging pathogens that affect the safety of the blood supply by answering the following questions:

1. Which infectious agents can be identified in transmissible disease screening of donor blood?
2. What is the structure, pathology, mode of transmission, prevalence, and blood transfusion risk for each of the following hepatitis viruses: hepatitis A, hepatitis B, hepatitis C, hepatitis D, hepatitis E, hepatitis G?
3. How does the chronic carrier status of hepatitis B differ from that of hepatitis C?
4. What is the structure, pathology, mode of transmission, prevalence, and blood transfusion risk for the retroviruses: HIV I, HIV II, HTLV I, HTLV II?
5. What is the structure, pathology, mode of transmission, and blood transfusion risk for other known viruses: parvovirus, Epstein-Barr virus, cytomegalovirus, West Nile virus?
6. What is a prion?
7. How do the prion diseases, Creutzfeldt-Jakob disease and variant Creutzfeldt-Jakob disease differ, with respect to their ability to be transfusion transmitted?
8. How does bacterial contamination of blood products occur?
9. What complications are likely to result from transfusion of bacterially contaminated blood products?
10. Which blood products are most likely to cause transfusion-transmitted bacteremia?
11. What is the disease manifestation and mode of transmission for syphilis and Lyme disease?
12. What is the name of the etiologic agent, pathology, mode of transmission, regional prevalence, and blood transfusion risk for each of the following parasitic infections: babesiosis, Chagas disease, malaria, leishmaniasis, and toxoplasmosis?
13. Which blood products are most effectively treated with solvent detergent?
14. What pathogen inactivation procedure is currently under development?
15. Why is pathogen inactivation of red blood cell products particularly difficult to achieve?

HEPATITIS VIRUSES

There are six categories of hepatitis pertinent to this discussion. These categories are differentiated by placing the appropriate capital letter after the term *hepatitis*. A description of each of these hepatitis categories (A–E and G) is located in the sections that follow.

Hepatitis A (HAV)

Hepatitis A virus (HAV) is a small, nonenveloped RNA virus in the *Picornaviridae* family. HAV is transmitted when unsanitary conditions result in contaminated food or water, which is then ingested (Table 13-1 ✳). HAV is the most common of all the hepatitis viruses (Table 13-2 ✳) and is transmitted mainly through the fecal–oral route (Table 13-1). Lack of available clean food and water and inaccessibility to vaccination are major reasons for the significantly higher prevalence of HAV in developing countries. The **incubation period**, which is the time between primary infection and onset of symptoms, is about 4 weeks for HAV. Symptoms include fatigue, fever, jaundice, and vomiting. Approximately 25% of persons infected with HAV are asymptomatic. The period of active infection for HAV usually lasts less than 2 months and there is no known chronic carrier state. Rare fatalities from HAV have been documented, mainly in the elderly or those with preexisting liver disease. Gestational complications and preterm labor can occur in pregnant women with an acute HAV infection. The prevalence of HAV in the United States is rapidly decreasing as a result of a vaccine that has been available since 1995.

HAV is transmissible through blood transfusion. Although viremia occurs early in infection and can persist for several weeks after onset of symptoms, blood-borne transmission of HAV is uncommon. Most donors in the acute stage of infection will exhibit symptoms and will be excluded through donor history review. Serologic assays for the detection of both IgM and IgG HAV antibodies are available but are not routinely performed. Because transfusion-transmitted HAV is rare, blood donor screening for HAV is not currently recommended.

HAV is resistant to *pathogen inactivation* procedures because the virus, like parvovirus B19, does not have an envelope. **Pathogen inactivation** is the process by which blood and blood products are treated to remove or inactivate infectious agents. Pathogen

inactivation is discussed in more detail at the end of this chapter and whenever possible multiple methods of pathogen inactivation are utilized.

Hepatitis B (HBV)

Hepatitis B virus (HBV) is an enveloped DNA virus in the *Hepadnaviridae* family. The prevalence of HBV in the United States has also decreased during the last couple decades as a result of available vaccination. Each year, however, there are over 200,000 new infections, with approximately 1.25 million chronic carriers.[1] HBV can be transmitted sexually; **parenterally**, which means by injection through a route other than the gastrointestinal tract; and **vertically**, which means from a mother to her fetus through the placenta. Intravenous (IV) drug users sharing contaminated needles can result in transmission of blood-borne viruses including HBV; for this reason some countries provide clean needles to IV drug abusers. Percutaneous transmission of HBV can occur by breaking the skin with contaminated sharp objects such as surgical instruments and phlebotomy needles and is worrisome for health care workers and emergency personnel. An additional concern is that the virus can survive and be infective in dried blood for up to 1 week.

Approximately 95% of people with HBV have an acute infection only. Five percent of people with HBV progress to a long-term carrier state, which can persist for 10 years or longer. Acute HBV infection is often asymptomatic. When symptoms occur, they include flu-like symptoms, jaundice, and elevated liver enzymes and present after a 2- to 6-month incubation period. A small percentage of long-term carriers of HBV will progress to chronic disease. Complications of chronic infection include cirrhosis of the liver and hepatocellular carcinoma, which together cause most of the fatalities associated with HBV.

The structure of HBV includes an inner protein core antigen (HBc) and a hepatitis Be antigen (HBe) surrounded by an outer surface antigen (HBsAg) (Figure 13-1 ■). Before it was known that hepatitis B is caused by a virus, it became clear that hepatitis B was infectious and the unknown agent responsible was called the Dane particle. Baruch Blomberg won the Nobel Prize in Medicine in 1976 for the discovery of the virus causing hepatitis B.

✳ **TABLE 13-1** Summary of Hepatitis Viruses

Virus	Mode of Transmission	Transfusion Transmitted	Acute or Chronic	Long-Term Complications
Hepatitis A	Fecal/oral	Rare; only if donor is in active state of infection	Acute illness only	None
Hepatitis B	Parenteral including IV drug use, sexual, vertical from mother to fetus	Yes	Acute, with 5% becoming chronic carriers	In chronic cases, cirrhosis and hepatocellular carcinoma
Hepatitis C	Parenteral including IV drug use, sexual, vertical from mother to fetus	Yes	Acute, with 80% becoming chronic carriers	In chronic cases, cirrhosis and hepatocellular carcinoma
Hepatitis D	Parenteral, sexual	Rare; requires simultaneous transmission of hepatitis B	Severe acute illness; rare chronic carriers	In chronic cases, cirrhosis and hepatocellular carcinoma
Hepatitis E	Fecal/oral	Rare; few cases reported outside the U.S.	Mild acute illness; rare chronic carriers	Rare fatalities reported
Hepatitis G	Parenteral, sexual	Yes, but no disease association	Mainly asymptomatic	None

✳ **TABLE 13-2** Summary of Transfusion Risk of Hepatitis Viruses in the United States

Virus	Incidence in the Population	Risk of Transfusion Transmission (per number of units transfused)
Hepatitis A	30%	Rare
Hepatitis B	1.25 million chronic carriers	1:220,000
Hepatitis C	3 million chronic carriers	1:2 million
Hepatitis D	Unknown; co-infection with HBV	Unknown
Hepatitis E	2%	No reports in the United States, but reports in other countries
Hepatitis G	2%	No disease association identified

After initial infection, antigens appear in the serum of the infected person in the following order: HBsAg, HBc, and HBe (Figure 13-1). Common laboratory test methods can detect HBsAg and HBe antigens. The HBsAg is the first to appear about 1 month after exposure and 1 month before symptoms may appear. HBe antigen marker is associated with a high level of infectivity, but this test is not generally done on donors. These antigens usually disappear after 4–6 weeks. In chronic carriers, the HBsAg will remain detectable. Young children

and babies infected intrauterine are most likely to be chronic carriers and to have bad outcomes such as cirrhosis and hepatocellular carcinoma. Hepatitis B DNA is detectable slightly later than the HBsAg and nucleic acid testing of donors for HBV is currently optional.

The next markers to appear are the antibodies: (1) anti-HBc, (2) anti-HBe, and (3) anti-HBs (Figure 13-1). Anti-HBc IgM and IgG are used to detect HBV infection during the window period when HBsAg has declined and anti-HBs has not appeared yet. Anti-HBc

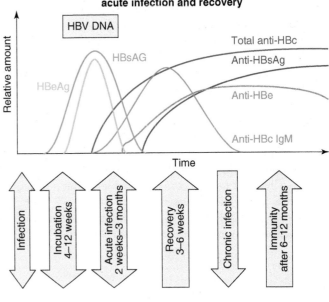

Antigen and antibody concentrations—acute infection and recovery

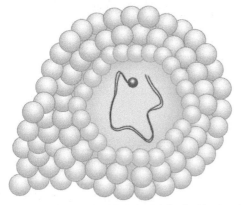

Simplified schematic of the hepatitis B virus structure

Red = DNA polymerase and partially double-stranded DNA which is inside the nucleocapsid

Green = Nucleocapsid containing the core antigen (HBcAg) and the Be antigen (HBeAg)

Blue = Viral envelope including the lipids and proteins that make up the surface antigen (HBsAg), which can form a tail and also shed off the virus

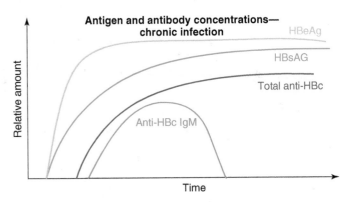

Antigen and antibody concentrations—chronic infection

DNA, deoxyribonucleic acid

■ **FIGURE 13-1** Immunologic Markers in Hepatitis B Virus Infection

can be falsely positive in some people. Both anti-HBc and anti-HBs can persist for years. Anti-HBs is also expressed in persons who respond to vaccination.

Transfusion-transmitted HBV infections peaked between 1975 and 1985 among hemophiliacs who were dependent on transfusion of pooled coagulation factors. Transfusion-transmitted infections have declined in the last decades due to deferral of high-risk donors, confidential self-exclusion,[2] transmissible disease testing, and vaccine use. HBV is a plasma-borne virus that is easily transmitted through all blood components and most products. The risk of transmission is highest when plasma is pooled for the manufacture of plasma products and derivatives. An assay for the detection of HBsAg became available in 1971. Transmissible disease testing for HBV among blood donors that included testing for both HBsAg and anti-HBc by enzyme-linked immunosorbent assay (ELISA) was implemented in 1976 (Box 13-1). A nucleic acid test (NAT) for HBV is currently available; however, this method may not be used as part of the transmissible disease test panel or may be run in pooled batches because it is not considered cost-effective to test each donor singly. The current risk in the United States of HBV infection from a single-unit blood transfusion is 1:220,000.[2]

☑ CHECKPOINT 13-1

What percentage of people infected with hepatitis B become chronic carriers?

BOX 13-1   Blood Donor Screening Tests in the United States as of 2012

Syphilis antibody
Hepatitis B surface antigen (HBsAg)
Hepatitis B core antibody (anti-HBc)
Hepatitis C antibody (anti-HCV)
HIV-I and II antibody
HTLV-I and II antibody
NAT for HIV, HCV, and WNV
NAT for HBV*
Trypanosoma cruzi IgG antibody (one time)

*Not required but usually performed

Hepatitis C (HCV)

Hepatitis C virus (HCV) is a small enveloped RNA virus in the *Flaviviridae* family (Figure 13-2 ■). HCV was first identified as the cause of non-A, non-B hepatitis (NANBH) in the 1980s. HCV is prevalent in the United States, with more than 20,000 new cases each year and 3 million chronic carriers.[3] HCV is transmitted parenterally, particularly through contaminated sharp objects such as infected needles. Intravenous drug use and sharing of needles between partners are the

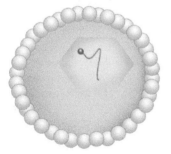

Simplified schematic of the hepatitis C virus structure

Purple = Tegument (vial matrix or core) composed of proteins
Red = Single stranded RNA, which is inside the nucleocapsid
Green = Nucleocapsid containing the viral RNA
Blue = Viral envelope composed of lipids and proteins

RNA, ribonucleic acid

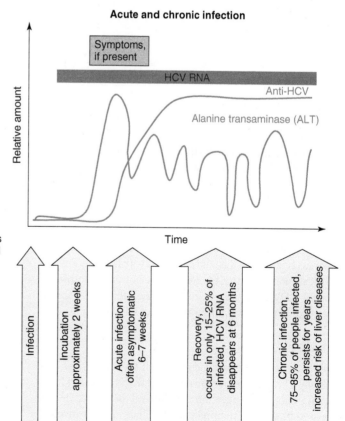

■ **FIGURE 13-2** Immunologic and Enzyme Markers in Hepatitis C Virus Infection

most common sources of transmission. Sexual and placental transmissions are possible; however, they are uncommon.

Most acute HCV infections are asymptomatic. When symptoms occur they usually include jaundice and elevated liver enzymes that indicate changes in liver function. Unlike HBV where most infections are resolved, approximately 80% of persons infected with HCV become chronic carriers. The long-term risk of chronic carrier status includes cirrhosis of the liver and hepatocellular carcinoma. These disease manifestations are more likely to develop in chronic carriers of HCV compared to chronic carriers of HBV.

Transfusion-transmitted HCV has been a concern for decades and was responsible for hepatitis in as many as one out of 10 recipients of blood products in the 1970s. It was known as "hepatitis non-A, non-B" for many years. The first serologic test for HCV antibody in blood donors was implemented in the United States in 1990. In 1999, a NAT assay for HCV was added to the panel of transmissible disease tests, which greatly reduced the time between infection and detection (Figure 13-2). In the United States, it was estimated that an additional 56 transfusion-related HCV infections were prevented each year because of the NAT testing implementation.[4] This subsequently reduced the transfusion risk of HCV to 1:2,000,000. Testing for elevated liver enzymes such as alanine aminotransferase (ALT) was helpful in the past in identifying hepatitis C infections before the advent of HCV antibody and NAT testing, but is not in use today.

☑ CHECKPOINT 13-2

What year was the first serologic test for HCV implemented for donor blood in the United States?

Hepatitis D (HDV)

Hepatitis D virus (HDV) is a small RNA virus that is sometimes referred to as the "delta hepatitis" virus. HDV is the only virus in the genus *Deltavirus*. HDV is not classified into a viral family because it is a unique virus dependent on HBV. HDV infection can only occur as a co-infection with HBV or with a preexisting HBV infection. The envelope of HDV particles contains the hepatitis B surface antigen (HBsAg) and the production and transmission of HDV is entirely dependent on HBV to provide HBsAg for HDV replication. HDV is transmitted mainly through parenteral and sexual routes, but only in the presence of HBV. People with hepatitis B and hepatitis D co-infection experience a more severe, acute illness than those infected with hepatitis B alone. Assays to detect antibodies to HDV are available; however, blood donor screening for HDV is not recommended because the elimination of hepatitis B–positive donors eliminates the risk of HDV transmission.

Hepatitis E (HEV)

Hepatitis E virus (HEV) is a nonenveloped RNA virus in the *Hepeviridae* family. The mode of transmission for HEV is similar to HAV because it is transmitted mainly through the fecal–oral route. HEV is not known to be sexually transmitted. HEV illness usually involves a mild form of hepatitis and few fatalities have been reported from complications of liver disease. Most cases of HEV are acute and do not proceed to a chronic illness. Rare transfusion transmission of HEV from infected donors has been reported in countries outside of the United States. A recent report in Japan confirmed a case of transfusion-transmitted HEV from a platelet donor that was infected through contaminated food, most likely pork.[5] Serologic tests for HEV are available; however, blood donor screening for HEV is not recommended because transmission in the United States is unsubstantiated.

Hepatitis G (HGV)

Hepatitis G virus (HGV), which is also called GB virus (GBV), is an enveloped RNA virus in the *Flaviviridae* family. HGV has three known species, one of which (HGV-C or GBV-C) is found in humans and is related to the hepatitis C virus. HGV is parenterally and sexually transmitted. Although HGV is transmitted through blood transfusion, the virus does not appear to cause disease in humans. HGV does not cause hepatitis-like illness. Although assays for the identification of HGV are available, blood donor screening for HGV is not recommended because of the lack of an associated disease state.

☑ CHECKPOINT 13-3

Name two hepatitis viruses that are transmitted mainly through the fecal-oral route.

RETROVIRUSES

Two groups of viruses comprise the retroviruses of interest in this discussion: human immunodeficiency viruses (HIVs) and human T-cell lymphotrophic viruses (HTLVs). Each group has two members, noted as I and II. These two groups of viruses are described next.

Human Immunodeficiency Virus (HIV) I and II

Human immunodeficiency virus (HIV) is an enveloped virus in the *Retroviridae* family. HIV is composed of an outer envelope of proteins around an inner core of RNA and reverse-transcriptase enzyme. **Retroviruses**, such as HIV, use reverse transcriptase to convert their viral single-stranded RNA into double-stranded DNA that is then inserted into the host genome and replicated. Two main types of HIV have been identified, HIV-I and HIV-II, each having several subtypes. The subtypes of HIV-I and II share up to 50% of their genetic sequence; this creates the potential for cross reactivity during testing. HIV-I is prevalent worldwide and HIV-II is endemic in western Africa. HIV group O (for outlier) is found in several African countries and some HIV tests do not detect HIV group O. For donor centers using tests that cannot detect HIV group O, questions pertaining to travel/living in these African countries and sexual contacts or blood transfusions while there must be added to the Donor History Questionnaire.

Both HIV-I and II are the causative agents of **acquired immunodeficiency syndrome (AIDS)**, which was first reported as an infectious disease in 1981. After the disease was identified, reports of HIV transmission increased significantly, with approximately 1.5 million people infected in the United States by the year 2000. HIV is considered a global epidemic, with an estimated 38.6 million cases in 2005.[5] HIV is transmitted parenterally, sexually, vertically, and through breast milk. Approximately 40% of people that are infected with HIV exhibit flu-like symptoms, with the remainder of infections being asymptomatic for 10 years or longer. End-stage HIV infection or clinical AIDS is identified when the immune system is depressed and complications such as malignancy and opportunistic infections arise. Modern treatments have increased the life expectancy for people with AIDS. As a result, the number of reported fatalities has decreased throughout the last decade.

Transfusion transmission of HIV was first reported in the early 1980s. Concerns regarding HIV transmission and the overall safety of the blood supply led to detailed donor history requirements in 1983 and subsequent implementation of transmissible disease testing for the HIV-I antibody in 1985. Confirmatory tests for HIV infection include the Western blot and immunofluorescence assay. A combined test for antibodies to both HIV-I and HIV-II was implemented for blood donor screening in 1992. Although the risk of transfusion transmission significantly decreased after implementation of the combined antibody test, a small number of transmissions of HIV were still being reported. These rare cases were a direct result of donors that were recently infected but were seronegative, which is a length of time defined as the **window period**. The window period is the time between infection and detection of serological markers.

For HIV, the window period is 22 days. In 1996, the test for HIV-1p24 antigen was added to the panel of transmissible disease tests performed on blood donor samples. HIV-1p24 testing reduced the window period to approximately 16 days. The marker for the p24 antigen in newly infected persons is detectable several days earlier than the antibodies (Figure 13-3 ■). The test for HIV-1p24 antigen

was discontinued after NAT for HIV was implemented in 2002. The increased sensitivity of NAT testing further reduced the window period to 12 days, which is the equivalent of reducing the number of transmissions of HIV by approximately five cases per year in the United States.[6] The combined strategies of high-risk donor deferral, confidential self-exclusion, and transmissible disease testing have reduced the overall risk of transfusion-transmitted HIV I/II to 1:2,000,000.

☑ **CHECKPOINT 13-4**

What are the modes of transmission for HIV-I and HIV-II?

Human T-Cell Lymphotrophic Virus (HTLV) I and II

Human T-cell lymphotrophic virus (HTLV) types I and II are delta retroviruses. The incidence of HTLV in the population is less than 10%. HTLV type I is endemic in certain parts of Japan, South America, the Caribbean, and Africa and HTLV II makes up about 50% of the positive test results in the United States, particularly among drug abusers. The modes of transmission for HTLV I and II are parenteral and sexual. HTLV is also transmitted through breast milk. Active infection is usually asymptomatic and infection is life-long. After a lag period of 20–30 years, a very small percentage of HTLV-infected people develop either a rare leukemia in HTLV-infected patients known as **adult T-cell leukemia/lymphoma (ATL)**, a demyelinating neurologic disorder known as HTLV-associated myelopathy (HAM), or tropical spastic paraparesis.

HTLV is transmissible through blood transfusion and is capable of inducing active infection in a recipient. HTLV is a cell-associated virus that is highly concentrated in leukocytes. This differs from the HIV retrovirus, which is mainly concentrated in the plasma. HTLV is rarely present in plasma product derivatives, which are not considered sources of transmission. Refrigeration and storage of red blood cell products for more than 10 days results in degradation of the lymphocytes and a drop in viral load that subsequently reduces the likelihood of transmission. Serologic testing of all blood donors for HTLV I began in the United States in 1988. A combined ELISA test for HTLV I/II was implemented in 1994 and has been successful in reducing the risk of transfusion-transmitted HTLV I/II to 1:2,993,000 in the United States. Leukocyte reduction of red blood cell products is also recommended to minimize the incidence of transfusion-transmitted HTLV. Leukocyte reduction of blood products may be achieved through prestorage leukocyte reduction, bedside filtration, or washing (Chapter 11).

OTHER VIRUSES

A variety of viruses make up the "other viruses" category and include parvovirus B19, Epstein-Barr, cytomegalovirus, West Nile, human herpes virus 6 and 8, a virus known as SEN, and torque teno virus. A brief description of each of these viruses is in the sections that follow.

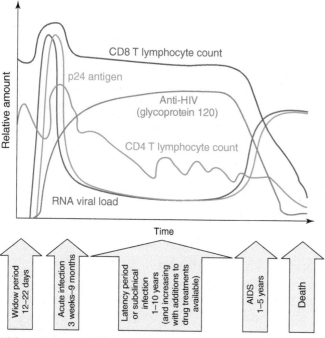

AIDS, acquired immunodeficiency syndrome
RNA, ribonucleic acid

■ **FIGURE 13-3** Immunologic Markers and Lymphocyte Counts in Human Immunodeficiency Virus Infection

Parvovirus B19

Parvovirus B19 is the only known pathogenic human parvovirus. It is a nonenveloped single-stranded DNA virus. It infects red blood cells and therefore is classified as an erythrovirus. Parvovirus is mainly transmitted through the respiratory route by way of aerosols. Parvovirus causes a common childhood illness called *erythema infectiosum* or *fifth disease*. In young children, fifth disease is usually a self-resolving illness that presents with a fever followed by a "slapped cheek" or lacy rash on the face. Approximately 50% of adults have been exposed to parvovirus with no complications. Persons at risk for complications from parvovirus include immunocompromised patients, pregnant women, and people with reduced RBC lifespan such as in sickle cell disease or other hemoglobinopathies. RBC production in the bone marrow is temporarily decreased or arrested in all people infected with parvovirus B19, but infection may cause an **aplastic crisis** (defined as a type of anemia that results from bone marrow disorders in which red blood cell production is deficient) with transfusion dependence in patients who already have chronic anemia. If the virus is transmitted in pregnancy up through around 20 weeks of gestation, parvovirus can cause severe fetal anemia and lead to hydrops fetalis and miscarriage or stillbirth.

Parvovirus is transmitted mainly in plasma products and to a lesser extent, red blood cell products. Because parvovirus is a nonenveloped virus like hepatitis A, it is also resistant to common methods of pathogen inactivation, including heat treatment and solvent detergent. In the investigation of the inactivation of viruses in Factor VIII products, parvovirus was determined to be susceptible to a dry-heat treatment procedure at 176° F (80° C) for 72 hours.[7] There is currently no screening protocol for parvovirus among blood donors. For all seronegative recipients in high-risk categories, it is recommended that products be screened for parvovirus through PCR analysis before they are used for transfusion. Nucleic acid testing (NAT) in pools is also used by plasma manufacturers to screen out high-risk parvovirus-positive donors.

Epstein-Barr Virus (EBV)

Epstein-Barr virus (EBV) was first identified in 1964 as a member of the *Herpesviridae* family. In the United States, approximately 95% of the adult population over age 40 has been exposed to EBV. Exposure to EBV is common among teens and young adults in the developed countries. EBV is mainly acquired through contact with infected saliva, thus it is often referred to as the kissing disease. EBV is the causative agent of **infectious mononucleosis**. EBV infection can be asymptomatic but can demonstrate symptoms of sore throat, enlarged lymph nodes, fever, lethargy, and malaise. EBV infects B lymphocytes, which can result in latent infection that lasts throughout life. Most cases of infectious mononucleosis are self-resolving, with the recommended treatment consisting of bed rest and increased fluid intake to prevent dehydration. Immunocompromised people are at an increased risk for complications from EBV infection and several lymphomas have a correlation with EBV infection. In some parts of Africa, EBV infection in young children is strongly associated with an aggressive form of Burkitt leukemia/lymphoma.

A few cases of transfusion-transmitted EBV have been reported. Because of the high prevalence of EBV exposure in the adult population, there is currently no screening protocol for EBV detection among blood donors. Studies have reported that leukocyte reduction of red blood cell products is helpful in preventing the transmission of EBV from donor to recipient.[8] To prevent complications from transfusion-transmitted EBV, it is recommended that seronegative individuals that are immunocompromised receive leukocyte-reduced blood products. Some transfusion facilities will also test donors of products for immunocompromised seronegative recipients for EBV antibodies. IgM viral capsid antigen (VCA) is the earliest antibody present and IgG VCA and IgG Epstein-Barr virus nuclear antigen (EBNA) both persist after infection (Figure 13-4 ■).

> ☑ **CHECKPOINT 13-5**
>
> What is the mode of transmission for Epstein-Barr virus?

Cytomegalovirus (CMV)

Cytomegalovirus (CMV) is a DNA virus that is a member of the *Betaherpesvirinae* subfamily. Exposure rates to CMV among adults in the United States range between 50% and 85%.[9] The mode of transmission of CMV is through direct contact of blood and body fluids with infected leukocytes. CMV can be transfusion transmitted. CMV can also be transmitted vertically, from mother to fetus.

CMV infection, in most cases, causes a mild or asymptomatic illness in healthy individuals. After the initial infection, CMV can remain latent for several years and become reactive later in life. CMV can cause severe and potentially life-threatening complications in high-risk groups. Individuals who are at risk for complications from CMV infection include those who are immunosuppressed, including low-birth-weight neonates and cellular or solid organ transplant recipients.

CMV is detectable through immunological techniques including ELISA, fluorescence assay, hemagglutination, and latex agglutination. Blood donors are not routinely screened for CMV as a result of the high prevalence of past CMV exposure in the adult population of the United States.[10] As with HTLV and EBV, blood recipients that are at increased risk for complications from CMV should receive leukocyte-reduced products. Although it is not possible to completely eliminate the incidence of transfusion-transmitted CMV, leukocyte reduction has significantly reduced the number of reported cases. Transfusing products from seronegative donors may add an additional layer of safety, but this remains controversial. As the seropositivity rate can vary geographically, the decision of whether to use CMV-safe (i.e., leukoreduced) or anti-CMV-negative cellular products often depends on the availability of seronegative donors.

West Nile Virus (WNV)

West Nile virus (WNV) was first identified as an emerging threat in the United States in 1999. Outbreaks of the virus had occurred previously in other parts of the world, most frequently in Middle Eastern countries, hence the name of the virus. However, the outbreak that began in New York State was the first instance of WNV being transmitted in North America. The virus has since spread across the continent and is endemic in some geographic areas at certain times of the year.

Simplified schematic of the Epstein-Barr virus structure

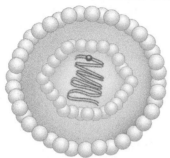

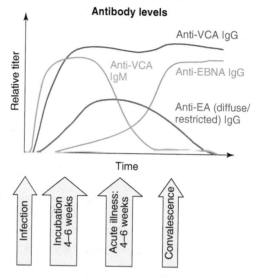

Antibody levels

Purple = Tegument (viral matrix or core) composed of proteins
Red = Double stranded DNA, which is inside the nucleocapsid (EA = early antigen is part of the DNA polymerase protein)
Green = Nucleocapsid composed of proteins (EBNA = Epstein Barr nuclear antigen) and containing the viral DNA
Blue = Viral envelope composed of lipids and proteins (VCA = viral capsid antigen)

Simplified schematic of the Epstein-Barr virus life cycle

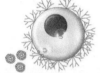

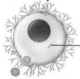

Early antigen (EA) is produced prior to structural proteins

Infection of a B lymphocyte:
• Viral protein binds with MHC class II molecule.
• Virus is encapsulated and taken into the cell.
• Viral capsid dissolves and viral genome is transported to cell nucleus.

Latent infection:
• Viral DNA remains in the cell nucleus, but not all viral genes are expressed.
• Therefore no viruses are produced.

Reactivation:
• Viral DNA changes from a circular configuration to linear.
• All viral genes are expressed.
• Viruses are assembled.
• Lymphocyte buds and viruses are shed from the cell.

Recovery: no virus present
or
Latent infection: viral DNA dormant in cells; no virus and no symptoms
or
Reactivation: dormant DNA is reactivated; virus and symptoms reappear
or
Chronic infection: symptoms persist

DNA, deoxyribonucleic acid

FIGURE 13-4   Immunologic Markers of Epstein-Barr Virus Infection

WNV is an enveloped single-stranded RNA virus of the *Flaviviridae* family. The virus is found primarily in bird species but can also be found in other animals, including horses and cattle. WNV is transmitted to humans through infected mosquitoes. Peak times of transmission of the virus are in late summer and early fall when mosquitoes are abundant. It is difficult to accurately identify the total number of people that have been infected with the virus because approximately 80% of humans infected with WNV are asymptomatic. It is estimated, however, that between 1 and 2 million people in the United States have been infected with West Nile since 1999. In 2008, there were 1,338 symptomatic cases of WNV reported by state and local health departments.[11]

People with symptomatic infection, called WNV fever, develop flu-like symptoms that include fever, rash, headache, and vomiting. Symptoms usually last from 3 to 6 days and only supportive care is needed. Rare complications, in as few as 0.7% of WNV infections, include encephalitis and meningitis. In people over age 50, there is an increased risk of long-term neurological symptoms. Fatalities from WNV infection have been reported each year since 2002 and include both elderly and immunocompromised individuals. Recommendations to prevent WNV infection include use of mosquito repellent during the peak season and to remain indoors in the early morning and evening when mosquitoes are most active.

WNV is transmissible through blood products. In the United States in 2002 more than 20 cases of transfusion-transmitted WNV

were reported. The response of the North American blood system to the emerging threat of WNV was very rapid. By 2003, a screening test that used NAT technology was developed and added to blood donor testing. Improved Donor History Questionnaires in addition to testing for the virus have significantly reduced the number of cases of transfusion-transmitted WNV to the point that they are now rarely reported. Rare transmissions are still encountered from recently infected blood donors that are reported as seronegative at the time of donation. The window period for WNV is typically 2 weeks. Research is presently being conducted to develop a vaccine for WNV.

☑ **CHECKPOINT 13-6**

List two risk factors for complications with a West Nile virus infection.

Human Herpes Virus 6 (HHV6) and 8 (HHV8)

Human herpes virus 6 (HHV-6) is the viral agent that causes roseola infantum or sixth disease. HHV-6 is a common childhood illness that is transmitted mainly through the respiratory route. HHV-6 is prevalent in the general population and most adults have had previous exposure to the virus. HHV-6 is not known to be transmissible through blood transfusion.

In contrast, **human herpes virus 8 (HHV-8)** is associated with Kaposi's sarcoma and is not a common virus in the general population. HHV-8 is a gamma herpes virus that is transmitted parenterally and is present in blood, saliva, and semen. Approximately 3–5% of blood donors in the United States are seropositive for HHV-8.[8] A historical study of cardiac surgery patients provided evidence that was consistent with transfusion transmission of HHV-8 infection in two of 406 blood recipients.[12] HHV-8 transmission may be a concern in immunosuppressed patients who are at an increased risk for developing complications from infection. At the present time testing for HHV-8 among blood donors is not recommended.

SEN Virus

SEN virus (SEN-V) is a newly discovered nonenveloped DNA virus in the *Circoviridae* family. The prevalence of SEN-V varies worldwide. SEN-V is found in 3% of United States blood donors. There is a high prevalence of SEN-V among transfusion recipients and the virus is known to be transmitted through blood transfusion. Although SEN-V is a transfusion-transmitted virus, there is no known disease association. Screening of blood donors for SEN-V is not currently recommended.

Torque Teno Virus (TTV)

Torque teno virus (TTV) was first identified in 1997. TTV is a DNA virus with two identified genetic subgroups. TTV is found in the general population and it has been identified in approximately 10% of blood donors in the United States. Although TTV is known to be transmitted through blood and body fluids, no disease association for TTV has been established. Screening of blood donors for TTV is not currently recommended.

PRIONS

Prions are a relatively new discovery and refer to infectious self-regulating proteins that convert normal proteins into abnormal structures. The group of diseases caused by prions is called **transmissible spongiform encephalopathies (TSE)**, with different disease names being applied to different species of affected animals

✳ **TABLE 13-3** Prion Diseases

Animal	Prion Disease(s)
Human	Creutzfeld-Jakob disease (CJD)
	variant Creutzfeld-Jakob disease (vCJD)
	Kuru
	Gerstmann–Straussler–Scheinker syndrome (GSS)
	Fatal familial insomnia (FFI)
Cattle	Bovine spongiform encephalopathy (BSE), also known as mad cow disease
Sheep/goat	Scrapie
Deer/elk	Chronic wasting disease (CWD)
Greater kudu/nyala	Exotic ungulate encephalopathy (EUE)
Mink	Transmissible mink encephalopathy (TME)
Cat	Feline spongiform encephalopathy (FSE)

(Table 13-3 ✳). Prion diseases typically affect brain and neurologic function when abnormal protein aggregates cause sponge-like lesions in brain tissue. Most of these diseases are specific to one species of animal, but potentially could cross to other species if meat contaminated with the brain and spinal cord of an infected animal is ingested. Two diseases associated with Creutzfeldt-Jakob resulting from the action of prions are discussed in the following sections.

Creutzfeldt-Jakob Disease (CJD)

Creutzfeldt-Jakob disease (CJD) was first identified in 1920. CJD can be transmitted through human growth hormone products from human pituitary glands (no longer allowed), intravenous immune globulin (IVIG), infected electrodes for EEGs, cannibalism, and some transplant materials (corneas and dura mater). There is also a known hereditary component, which is rare, and sometimes the etiology remains unknown, especially given the long incubation period.

The incubation period of CJD can last anywhere from 4 to 20 years and very few patients exhibit symptoms before age 50. The onset of symptoms in CJD is sudden and often includes rapidly progressing dementia, poor coordination, visual problems, and involuntary movements. All cases of CJD are eventually fatal, with death usually occurring within 1 year of the onset of symptoms. CJD is only confirmed by a postmortem biopsy of the brain and cerebral spinal fluid may be tested for the Tau protein and protein 14.3.3, which may be done before death. With respect to blood transfusion, there have been no confirmed cases of transmission of CJD through blood products.[13] Blood donor screening for CJD is not currently recommended.

variant Creutzfeldt-Jakob Disease (vCJD)

Both classic and **variant Creutzfeldt-Jakob disease (vCJD)** are fatal neurological diseases with similar symptoms and both are believed to be caused by prions; however, the progression of the diseases are different.

In 1996, vCJD was first identified in the United Kingdom. While the symptoms were similar to classic CJD, the incidence was higher and the population affected was of a younger age. Patients with vCJD are usually younger than 40 years old, whereas classic CJD is primarily a disease of the elderly. The outbreak of this new disease, which appears to have peaked at about 160 cases in the United Kingdom, has been linked to the eating of infected beef after a change in the disinfectant used to clean slaughter houses. Since the initial reports of the disease, cases of vCJD have also been confirmed in France and other European countries.

In contrast to classic CJD, vCJD is transmissible through blood transfusion (Table 13-4 ✳). The first case of transfusion-transmitted vCJD was reported in the United Kingdom in 2004. The blood donor was asymptomatic at the time of the donation. Because the disease is eventually fatal, several strategies have been implemented in the United States and other countries to reduce the risk of transmission of vCJD through infected blood products. Blood donors from the United Kingdom or certain European countries or people who spent a significant amount of time there, such as businesspeople or military personnel, are permanently deferred from donating blood in the United States.

✱ **TABLE 13-4** Comparison of Classic Creutzfeld-Jakob Disease (CJD) and variant Creutzfeld-Jakob Disease (vCJD)

	Classic Creutzfeldt-Jakob Disease (CJD)	Variant Creutzfeldt-Jakob disease (vCJD)
Mode of transmission	Human growth hormone, IVIG, transplant material, EEG electrodes (reused without adequate processing), many cases unknown etiology	Ingestion of meat from infected cattle
Median age at onset of symptoms	50	Under age 40
Symptoms	Dementia, poor coordination, visual problems, involuntary movements; delayed onset after exposure	Dementia, poor coordination, visual problems, involuntary movements; rapid onset after exposure
Transfusion transmitted	No	Yes, red blood cell–containing products

Because the highest concentration of infectivity is in the leukocytes, leukocyte reduction has been recommended as a strategy for reducing the risk of transmitting prions via transfusion. Research has indicated, however, that leukocyte reduction of donor blood is not completely effective in eliminating the overall number of infected products.

Additional strategies to reduce the risk of transfusion-transmitted vCJD are still experimental. New methods of *pathogen inactivation* (a concept described later) are under investigation because the current available methods of inactivation are ineffective against prions. The development of a screening test for the detection of vCJD through the identification of a marker named PRP^TSE is promising. Tests implemented as part of the blood donor screening panel need to be both practical and cost-effective. Plasma products and plasma derivatives do not appear to transmit vCJD; a study of 20,000 hemophilia patients reported that no cases of CJD or vCJD occurred among patients who received plasma derivatives.[14]

☑ CHECKPOINT 13-7

Which prion agent is documented as transmissible through transfusion of blood products?

BACTERIAL CONTAMINATION OF BLOOD PRODUCTS

Bacterial contamination of donor blood is a rare occurrence. Reports of transfusion-transmitted bacteremia indicate that most blood component contamination occurs during venipuncture at time of collection or during the manufacture and handling of blood components. The most frequently identified causes of contamination are poor disinfection of the venipuncture site or improper handling of an open product, for example, if the bag or vial has a crack or a broken seal. In rare cases, transfusion-transmitted bacteremia is a result of asymptomatic infection in the blood donor at the time of the donation.

Regardless of the cause, bacterial contamination of blood products is associated with a high incidence of morbidity and mortality and therefore poses a serious health threat. Transfusion of bacterially contaminated blood components causes an infection in the blood known as **sepsis** in the recipient. The clinical symptoms of sepsis include high fever, tachycardia, disseminated intravascular coagulation, low back pain, and shock. Immediate antibiotic treatment is necessary to avoid life-threatening complications.

Platelet products are most frequently implicated in transfusion-transmitted bacteremia. Room temperature storage at 68–75.2° F (20–24° C) is required to maintain optimal platelet function, but this temperature combined with a high-protein medium, such as human plasma, is also optimal for microorganism growth. **Yersinia enterocolitica** has been reported as one of the most common bacteria[15] identified in contaminated donor red blood cell components and can actually grow in refrigerated RBC products; most other bacteria die or fail to thrive in refrigeration. While donors may have no symptoms or only minor symptoms and a low bacteremia, patients can have severe transfusion reactions (sometimes fatal) to the bacteria and endotoxin present within blood products at the time of transfusion. *Pseudomonas, Staphylococcus, Serratia, Bacillus,* and *Salmonella* species have also been identified in blood products.

Several measures are in place to reduce the likelihood of transfusion-transmitted bacteremia. AABB Standards define strict requirements for maintaining sterility during the blood collection process that include proper skin disinfection to reduce contamination during the phlebotomy procedure.[16] Regulations and standards also include best practices designed to reduce the chance of contamination occurring during manufacture, handling, and storage of blood components. Blood donor exclusion criteria in many countries include deferrals aimed at reducing the incidence of donors with asymptomatic bacteremia. For example, in the United States donors with increased body temperature or recently recovering from minor surgeries are temporarily deferred. In 2004, screening of platelet products for bacteria was implemented. Although bacterial screening is effective, there are still rare reports of transfusion-transmitted infections being attributed to platelet products that had negative screening results. Two bacterial diseases with a known history of being transmitted through blood products are syphilis and Lyme disease.

☑ CHECKPOINT 13-8

State two ways donor blood can become contaminated with bacteria.

Syphilis

Syphilis is an infection caused by the spirochete *Treponema pallidum*. Syphilis is most commonly spread through sexual contact. In the 1940s, syphilis was the most widely recognized transfusion-transmitted disease. Transfusion-transmitted syphilis is now rare as a result of strategies that have improved the blood donor screening process, transmissible disease testing, and available antibiotic therapies. The incubation period for infected persons is from 4 weeks to 5 months. Active infection is readily treated with antibiotics. The spirochete is not transmissible through stored blood when it is refrigerated for more than 72 hours at temperatures of 33.8–42.8° F (1–6° C). It is also not transmitted through plasma derivatives prepared by fractionation of pooled human plasma such as IVIG.

The screening test for syphilis was the first transmissible disease test to be required of blood donors; it was implemented in the 1950s. The number of reported cases of transfusion-transmitted syphilis has been significantly reduced as a result of careful blood donor selection and the exclusion of high-risk blood donors. Donors with a positive test for syphilis are deferred from donating blood for 12 months.

Lyme Disease

Lyme disease is a bacterial illness that is spread by a tick bite. The causative agent is the spirochete *Borrelia burgdorferi*. In the United States, no cases of transfusion-transmitted Lyme disease have been reported, but the disease is present in the general population and in the donor population. Blood donors who have a history of Lyme disease can donate if they have no visible symptoms, have completed a full course of antibiotics, and have been cleared to donate by a physician. Screening of blood donors for Lyme disease as part of the transmissible disease test process is not currently recommended.

PARASITIC INFECTIONS

Parasitic infections where the parasite is present in the bloodstream of infected people include babesiosis, Chagas disease, trypanosomiasis, malaria, leishmaniasis, and toxoplasmosis (Table 13-5 ✱). Each condition is described in the sections that follow.

Babesiosis

Babesiosis is a parasitic infection caused by the protozoan *Babesia microti*. The parasite is transmitted to humans through tick bites, specifically from the *Ixodes* tick, which is also called the deer tick. Babesiosis is common in the United States, particularly in the Northeast during warm-weather seasons when ticks are likely to be abundant. The organism enters the host through the bloodstream and infects the red blood cells. Although many cases of babesiosis are asymptomatic, a symptomatic person will experience fever, chills, lethargy, and, in some cases, hemolytic anemia. In rare cases the disease may be fatal. The infection is typically treated with antibiotics. At the present time there is no specific test for babesiosis. The organism is visible on a Wright-stained blood smear and is often identified as part of a WBC differential examination with accompanying morphological examination of the red blood cells.

Transfusion-transmitted babesiosis has been reported in the United States, including rare fatalities among elderly and immunosuppressed individuals.[17] Because the incubation period for babesiosis is 1–8 weeks, many transfusion-transmitted infections are not identified until several weeks after the transfusion. *B. microti* can survive for up to 5 weeks in refrigerated blood products. Because there is no blood donor screening test for babesiosis, prevention of transmission depends on exclusion of high-risk donors. Blood centers in endemic areas may question donors around activities that would increase their exposure to ticks. Donors that are feeling unwell are temporarily deferred. Donors that have been diagnosed with babesiosis are indefinitely deferred, even if they were successfully treated.

> ### CASE IN POINT (continued)
>
> The next day, the hematopathologist confirmed *Babesia spp.* on the patient's blood slide and immediately notified the blood bank.
>
> 1. What is the normal route of transmission of *Babesia spp.*?
> 2. What events in the patient's history suggest that she acquired her Babesia infection via blood transfusion?
> 3. What patient characteristic makes her more susceptible to a *Babesia spp.* infection?

Chagas Disease and Trypanosomiasis

Chagas disease is a parasitic infection caused by the flagellate protozoan, *Trypanosoma cruzi*. *T. cruzi* is transmitted to humans when a reduviid bug defecates during a blood meal on an unsuspecting human. The motile parasites migrate from the insect feces into the

✱ **TABLE 13-5** Summary of Blood-Borne Parasites

Parasite	Disease	Vector	Endemic Areas
Babesia microti	Babesiosis	*Ixodes* tick	Northeast United States
Trypanosoma cruzi	Chagas disease	Reduviid bug	Central and South America, Mexico
Plasmodium species	Malaria	*Anopheles* mosquito	Africa, Asia, Latin America
Leishmania species	Leishmaniasis	Sandfly	Middle East
Toxoplasma gondii	Toxoplasmosis	Undercooked meat; feces of farm animals and house pets	Anywhere meat is eaten undercooked or there are domesticated animals

bloodstream by entering the body at the site of the insect blood meal. Chagas disease is not common in the United States; however, it is prevalent in Central America, South America, and certain parts of Mexico. Approximately 20% of people infected with *T. cruzi* are asymptomatic in the early stages of the disease and many infections remain undetected. The long-term carrier rate for Chagas is very high and most individuals enter a latent stage of the disease that can last up to 40 years. If the disease is not properly treated, it may progress to an end stage, when cardiac problems and other complications can be fatal.

A few cases of transfusion- and transplant-transmitted Chagas disease have been reported in the United States. The parasite can be transmitted during the latent stage of the disease. Most cases of transfusion-transmitted infection are reported to have occurred in immunocompromised individuals. The parasite can survive in red blood cells and platelet products, and is resistant to refrigeration, cryopreservation procedures, and thawing.

Morphologic features of *T. cruzi* can be identified on a Wright- or Geimsa-stained blood smear during microscopic examination. The trypomastigote, which is the infectious life stage of the protozoa, can be identified on the smear during the acute stage of the infection. Alternatively, the infection can be confirmed through a test for detection of antibodies. Available methods for detection include indirect hemagglutination test (IHA), indirect immunofluorescence assay (IFA), and ELISA. More than one method of screening is recommended to confirm chronic infections, particularly in endemic regions.[18] Screening of blood donors for Chagas disease is recommended at least one time per donor, especially in endemic areas, because many carriers of *T. cruzi* are asymptomatic.

Trypanosomiasis can also be found in several sub-Saharan African countries, where it causes irreversible neurologic damage called *sleeping sickness* and death, if untreated. *T. brucei gambiense* and *T. brucei rhodesiense* are transmitted by the tsetse fly (genus *Glossina*) and may occur in epidemics.

Malaria

Malaria is the disease caused by the parasite *Plasmodium*. Malaria is a worldwide health problem, with over 247 million infections and approximately 880,000 deaths each year.[19] Malaria is found mainly in Africa, Asia, and Latin America. In the United States, malaria is found primarily among military personnel and individuals that have returned from travel to endemic areas.

The five species of malarial parasites affecting humans are *Plasmodium falciparum*, *Plasmodium vivax*, *Plasmodium ovale*, *Plasmodium malariae*, and *Plasmodium knowlesi*. The parasite is transmitted to humans through the bite of the *Anopheles* mosquito. *P. falciparum* and *P. vivax* are the most common species; *P. falciparum* is the most fatal. *P. knowlesi* is the rarest source of human infection and is more common in Southeast Asia than in other malarial endemic areas. Co-infection with more than one type of parasite can occur.

The parasite is transferred from the mosquito to the human bloodstream where it targets the red blood and liver cells. The symptoms of malaria include intermittent fevers, lethargy, and hemolysis of red blood cells with resulting anemia. Symptoms of malaria appear approximately 2 weeks after infection. Diagnosis is made through morphologic examination of thin and thick blood smears. Rapid antibody tests are also currently available. The treatment of malaria depends on the species causing the infection and the level of parasitemia. Prognosis is good if the infection is treated promptly. Resistance of the parasite to prophylactic and treatment protocols is a public health concern.

Only a few cases of transfusion-transmitted malaria are reported in the United States each year. These cases are associated with blood donors that were asymptomatic at the time of the donation. Malarial parasites remain viable during refrigeration and storage of red blood cell products and can survive in platelet products at room temperature. Malaria is resistant to cryopreservation and thawing procedures. Malaria is not transmitted in products that are free of red blood cells such as fresh frozen plasma or plasma derivatives.

Thin and thick smears and rapid antibody tests for malaria are not considered effective for blood donor screening. Instead, donor deferrals are used to reduce the risk of malarial infection of the blood supply. Donors are deferred for 1 year following travel to an area where malaria is endemic. Donors who have lived in a malarial endemic region or who have been treated for malaria are deferred for 3 years from the time that they left the endemic area or completed treatment.

Leishmaniasis

Leishmaniasis is an infection that is caused by the parasite *Leishmania*, which is transmitted to humans by the bite of an infected sandfly. The parasite is known to be transmitted in blood and body fluids as well as through blood transfusion. Rare cases of transfusion-transmitted *Leishmania* have been reported. Presently there is no recommended blood donor screening test for *Leishmania*.

Leishmaniasis is endemic in Middle Eastern countries. Although *Leishmania* is not prevalent in blood donors in the United States, temporary donor deferrals have been implemented because of increased travel to endemic areas, including increased numbers of American military personnel serving in endemic countries. Donors are deferred for 1 year following return from an endemic area.

Toxoplasmosis

Toxoplasmosis is a parasitic infection that is caused by the protozoan *Toxoplasma gondii*. The parasite can be transmitted to humans through undercooked meats and feces from farm animals and household pets, particularly cats after eating infected rodents. Many cases of toxoplasmosis are asymptomatic; however, symptoms and complications can occur in children and immunocompromised patients. Fetal demise can result in pregnant women infected early in the gestational period. The parasite invades white blood cells and remains viable for several weeks in stored blood. Rare transmissions of toxoplasmosis via blood transfusion have been reported. Blood donor screening is not currently recommended.

☑ CHECKPOINT 13-9

Name the parasitic infection that is caused by the bite of an infected sandfly.

CASE STUDY *(continued)*

The hospital decided to use this case study as a training opportunity for physicians and residents. They have asked you to attend the training as the blood bank representative.

4. The first statement that the moderator made was that viruses such as hepatitis, HIV, or HTLV remain the single biggest threat of transfusion-transmitted infection. What is the estimated risk of acquiring one of these viruses from a transfusion?

5. Assume the risk of a transfusion-transmitted bacterial infection is 1:75,000. Which is more prevalent, a viral or bacterial transmission?

After discussing the cases in detail, the floor was opened to audience questions. The first question that was asked was "Why wasn't the *Babesia spp.* caught during the initial testing of the blood product?"

6. How would you explain why the *Babesia spp.* was not seen during infectious disease testing of the donor?

RISK-REDUCTION STRATEGIES

The safety of the human blood supply has been greatly increased during the last two decades. Strategies that have been successful in reducing transfusion risks include enhanced regulatory oversight of the blood collection process, more stringent blood donor eligibility criteria, tracking of infection rates for emerging pathogens, new blood donor screening assays, and the development of pathogen inactivation methods.

Pathogen inactivation of blood products is an effective means of reducing transfusion risks. Pathogens can cause disease in a transfusion recipient even when screening test results are negative. Elimination of pathogenic agents is particularly beneficial for those transmissions that occur during the window period of infection and for those pathogens in which a screening test has not yet been developed.

Heat inactivation at 140° F (60° C), the first pathogen reduction method, was developed in 1948. This method is only effective against heat labile viruses such as HIV and HCV. Subsequent development of organic solvents as a means to inactivate pathogens has been effective against the nonlipid enveloped viruses such as HAV and parvovirus. These virus-inactivation techniques have been used extensively in the production of fractionated plasma products but not in blood components, where the desired component would also be destroyed by the process. Generally, two or more techniques are utilized for pathogen inactivation when feasible.

In the 1990s, solvent detergent treatment of plasma was implemented to eliminate lipid-enveloped viruses in plasma products. Solvent detergent–treated plasma products are currently available in European countries, but not in the United States. Use of solvent detergent–treated plasma was halted in the United States because of concerns about both the risk of liver disease from residual chemicals and cost-effectiveness.

Another proposed method of pathogen inactivation uses psoralens and ultraviolet (UV) light to destroy pathogens. In clinical trials, this method appears to be effective for both platelet and plasma products. Psoralen treatment is undergoing clinical trials for red blood cell–containing products to confirm whether UVA (long wavelength ultraviolet light) exposure is toxic to the red blood cells.

Concerns regarding red blood cell viability and cost-effectiveness have limited the development of pathogen-inactivation methods for red blood cell–containing products. Investigative efforts for pathogen inactivation of red blood cells include frangible anchor-linked effectors (FRALE) that are capable of inhibiting DNA and RNA activity; Inactine, which prevents replication; and riboflavin (vitamin B_{12}) light treatment.

☑ **CHECKPOINT 13-10**

List two pathogen-reduction methods that are effective against viruses.

Review of the Main Points

- The safety of the blood supply continues to improve.
- Four categories of pathogens within the blood supply are viruses, prions, bacteria, and parasites.
- The hepatitis viruses—HAV, HBV, and HCV—can be transmitted through transfusion.
- HDV is associated with HBV infection.
- No disease association has been discovered for HGV.
- Transfusion-transmitted HEV infection has been reported outside the United States.
- HIV and HTLV are retroviruses.
- HIV is the causative agent of AIDS.

- HTLV may cause adult T-cell leukemia/lymphoma (ATL), a demyelinating neurologic disorder known as HTLV-associated myelophathy (HAM), or tropical spastic paraparesis after long-term infection in a small number of infected people.
- WNV emerged as a threat to North American blood supplies with an outbreak in 1999. It has since spread throughout North America and is transmitted to humans by mosquitoes.
- Routine donor testing includes tests for HBV, HCV, HIV I and II, HTLV I/II, and WNV.
- EBV and CMV can be transmitted by transfusion but the high prevalence of previous infection in the general population makes donor screening impractical.

- Other viruses that are not routinely tested for in blood donors include parvovirus B19, HHV-6, HHV-8, SEN-V, and TTV.
- No reports of transfusion transmission of the prion disease classic CJD have been made. However, contaminated human growth hormone and transplant material have caused transmission of CJD.
- The first report of transfusion-transmitted vCJD occurred in 1996. Eating BSE-contaminated meat is believed to have caused the emergence of vCJD.
- The bacterium that causes syphilis is tested for as part of routine donor screening. The bacterium that causes Lyme disease is not currently tested for as part of the donor testing panel.

- Bacterial screening of platelet products has been implemented in many countries, including the United States.
- Parasitic infections associated with transfusion include babesiosis, Chagas disease, trypanosomiasis, malaria, leishmaniasis, and toxoplasmosis.
- Donor deferral is used to reduce the risk of parasitic infections. Deferrals are based on travel to endemic areas, diagnosis of the infection, and identification of common symptoms.
- Heat inactivation and solvent/detergent treatment are used during the manufacturer of plasma protein products to inactivate pathogens.
- Pathogen-inactivation methods that may be used with blood components are currently being researched.

Review Questions

1. Which of the following transmissible disease tests is required to be performed on all donated blood? (Objective #1)

   A. CMV antibody

   B. HCV antibody

   C. Sickle cell screen

   D. Toxoplasma antibody

2. How are the hepatitis B and hepatitis C viruses similar? (Objective #2)

   A. Both are DNA viruses.

   B. Neither virus contains an envelope.

   C. Neither virus has a chronic carrier state.

   D. Both viruses are transmitted parenterally.

3. The first marker to appear in a hepatitis B infection is: (Objective #4)

   A. Anti-HBc

   B. Anti-HBe

   C. HBsAg

   D. HevAg

4. Which transfusion-transmitted parasitic infection is caused by a tick bite? (Objective #14)

   A. Chagas disease

   B. Malaria

   C. Babesiosis

   D. Leishmania

5. Which two hepatitis viruses are transmitted through contaminated food products? (Objective #2)

   A. Hepatitis A and E

   B. Hepatitis B and D

   C. Hepatitis C and E

   D. Hepatitis B and C

6. Which of the following hepatitis viruses has the highest incidence of transfusion transmission in the United States? (Objective #3)

   A. Hepatitis A

   B. Hepatitis B

   C. Hepatitis C

   D. Hepatitis D

7. All of the following are retroviruses except: (Objective #5)

   A. HIV-1

   B. HTLV-1

   C. HIV-2

   D. HBV

8. The etiologic agent for syphilis is: (Objective #13)

   A. Borrelia burgdorferi

   B. Treponema pallidum

   C. Plasmodium vivax

   D. Babesia microti

9. Approximately 80% of humans that become infected with _____ remain asymptomatic. (Objective #8)

   A. HTLV

   B. Parvovirus

   C. Epstein-Barr virus

   D. West Nile virus

10. How are CJD and vCJD similar? (Objective #11)

    A. Both are transfusion transmitted.

    B. Their latent periods are identical.

    C. They present with identical symptoms.

    D. Their median age at onset of symptoms is equivalent.

11. Transfusion-transmitted sepsis occurs most frequently after the transfusion of which type of blood product? (Objective #12)

   A. Leukoreduced red blood cells

   B. Fresh frozen plasma

   C. Cryoprecipitate

   D. Platelet pheresis

12. Select the hepatitis virus that is associated with the highest chronic carrier rate: (Objective #2)

   A. Hepatitis A

   B. Hepatitis B

   C. Hepatitis C

   D. Hepatitis D

13. Infectivity of leukocytes is highest in which *three* infectious agents? (Objective #15)

   A. EBV

   B. CJD

   C. CMV

   D. HAV

14. Select the correct etiologic agent for each disease: (Objective #2, 11, 13, 14)

   _____Malaria

   _____variant CJD

   _____Lymes disease

   _____Hepatitis C

   A. Parasite

   B. Virus

   C. Bacteria

   D. Prion

15. Which organism causes Chagas disease? (Objective #14)

   A. *Treponema pallidum*

   B. *Borrelia burgdorferi*

   C. *Plasmodium vivax*

   D. *Trypanosoma cruzi*

References

1. Lin, K, Kirchner, J. Hepatitis B. *American Family Physician* 2004; 69(1): 75–82.

2. Busch M, Kleinman S, Nemo G. Current and emerging infectious risks of blood transfusions. *Journal of the American Medical Association* 2003; 289: 959–962.

3. Armstrong GL, et al. The prevalence of Hepatitis C virus infection in the United States, 1999 through 2002. *Annals of Internal Medicine* 2006; 144(10): 705–14.

4. Stramer S, et al. Detection of HIV-1 and HCV infections among antibody negative blood donors by nucleic acid-amplification testing. *New England Journal of Medicine* 2004; 351: 760–68.

5. Matsubayashi K, et al. A case of transfusion-transmitted hepatitis E caused by blood from a donor infected with hepatitis E virus via zoonotic foodborne route. *Transfusion* 2008; 48: 1368–75.

6. Joint United Nations Programme on HIV/AIDS [Internet]. 2006 Report on the Global AIDS epidemic. http://data.unaids.org/pub/GlobalReport/2006/2006_GR_CH02_en.pdf. Last accessed on 30June2009.

7. Roberts PL, El Hana C, Saldana J. Inactivation of parvovirus B19 and model viruses in factor VIII by dry heat treatment at 80° C. *Transfusion* 2006; 46: 1648–50.

8. Qu L, Xu S, Rowe D, Triulzi D. Efficacy of Epstein-Barr virus removal by leuko-reduction of red blood cells. *Transfusion* 2005; 45: 591–5.

9. Roback JD, Combs MR, Grossman BJ, Hillyer CD. *Technical Manual*, 16th ed. Bethesda (MD): AABB; 2008. pp. 252–3.

10. Qu Lirong, Jenkins F, Triulzi DJ, Human herpesvirus 8 genomes and sero-prevalence in United States blood donors. *Transfusion* 2010; 50: 1050–6.

11. Centre for Disease Control. West Nile Virus: Statistics, surveillance and control [Internet]. www.cdc.gov/ncidod/dvbid/westnile/surv&controlCaseCount08_detailed.htm. Last accessed March 1, 2009.

12. Dollard S, Nelson K, Ness P, Stambolis V, Kuehnert M, Pellett P, Cannon M. Possible transmission of human herpesvirus-8 by blood transfusion in a historical United States cohort. *Transfusion* 2005; 45: 500–3.

13. Zou S, Fang C, Schonberger L. Transfusion transmission of human prion diseases. *Transfusion Medicine Reviews* 2008; 22: 58–69.

14. Brown P. Creutzfeldt-Jakob disease: reflections on the risk from blood product therapy. *Haemophilia* 2007; 13: 33–40.

15. Depcik-Smith ND, Hay SN, Brecher ME. Bacterial contamination of blood products, *Journal of Clinical Apheresis* 2001; 16: 193.

16. AABB Standards. *Blood Banks and Transfusion Services*, 27th ed. Bethesda (MD): AABB; 2011.

17. Blue D, Graves V, McCarthy L, Cruz J, Gregurek S, Smith D. Fatal transfusion-transmitted Babesia microti in the Midwest. *Transfusion* 2008; 49: 8.

18. Pirard M, Iihoshi N, Boelaert M, Basanta P, Lopez F Van der Stuyft P. The validity of serologic tests for *Trypanosoma cruzi* and the effectiveness of transfusional screening strategies in a hyperendemic region. *Transfusion* 2005; 45: 554–61.

19. World Health Organization. Malaria [Internet]. Fact Sheet No. 94. www.who.int/mediacentre/factsheets/fs094/en/print/html. Last accessed March 1, 2009.

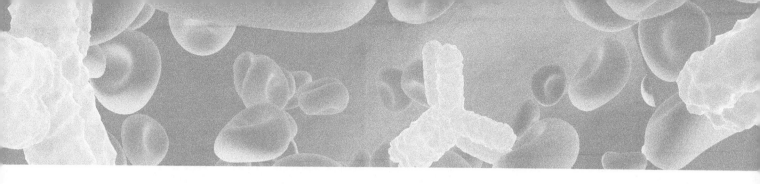

14 Perinatal and Neonatal Transfusion Issues

JANET L. VINCENT AND ELIZABETH A. HARTWELL

Chapter Objectives

Upon completion of this chapter, the student will be able to:

1. Describe the conditions that affect the stimulation of the immune system in HDFN: lack of maternal antigen, presence of fetal antigen, exposure to antigen, and production of antibody that has the ability to cross the placenta.
2. Identify the class of immunoglobulin implicated in HDFN.
3. Discuss the three categories of HDFN including antibody specificity, pathophysiology, incidence, treatment, and prevention.
4. Analyze the potential for HDFN given the mother and father's genetic information.
5. Justify the testing done on the mother's blood during the first trimester.
6. Discuss and evaluate the need for the weak D testing on mother's blood.
7. Describe the methods that can be used to predict HDFN, including levels of risk for both the mother and fetus.
8. Compare the use of amniocentesis and Doppler flow studies in determining the severity of HDFN.
9. Discuss the methods of plasma exchange and intrauterine transfusion in the antepartum treatment of anemia in HDFN.
10. List the indications for administration for Rh-immune globulin (RhIg).
11. Calculate the percent of fetal maternal hemorrhage and the amount of RhIg required to protect against the formation of anti-D.
12. Judge the necessity of performing ABO, Rh typing, DAT, and elution tests on the neonate.
13. Compare exchange transfusion to booster transfusion to neonates.
14. List the ways the neonate's physiology is different from an adult.
15. Discuss requirements and concerns when transfusing infants less than 4 months of age.
16. Indicate special considerations when transfusing platelets, plasma components, and granulocytes to infants.
17. Judge the need for blood and components in the ECMO procedure.
18. Given a case scenario with appropriate laboratory results, propose appropriate next steps.

Key Terms

Continuous exchange

Cordocentesis

Discontinuous exchange

Erythroblastosis fetalis

Erythropoietin (EPO)

Exchange transfusion

Extracorporeal membrane
  oxygenation (ECMO)

Fetomaternal hemorrhage
  (FMH)

Gravid

Gravida

Hemolytic disease of the fetus
  and newborn (HDFN)

Hepatosplenomegaly

Hydrops fetalis

Infant

Intrauterine transfusion (IUT)

Kernicterus

Liley graph

Neonate

Para

Percutaneous umbilical blood
  sampling (PUBS)

Perinatal

Phototherapy

Rh-immune globulin (RhIg)

Syncytiotrophoblast

CASE IN POINT

SC is a 28-year-old female who is pregnant with her second child. During her first pregnancy, she was involved in a car accident in which another driver ran a stop sign at 35 mph and t-boned her car. The impact ruptured her uterus and the baby was delivered at 34 weeks' gestation by emergency cesarean section. The patient was transfused 2 red blood cell units in the operating room.

What's Ahead?

Pregnancy, infants, and children present special issues for the transfusion service. The unique physiology of the fetus, newborn, and pediatric patient means they cannot be treated like adults when it comes to transfusion of blood and blood components. Transfusion service plays several roles, beginning with pregnancy and continuing through childhood. Typically, the first encounter occurs during the first trimester of pregnancy when the obstetrician orders an ABO, Rh, and antibody screen on the pregnant female. This may involve identification of antibodies in the pregnant female and how they might affect the fetus. The preparation of blood products specific for the mother, fetus, neonate, and child are additional responsibilities for transfusion service personnel. This chapter addresses the following relevant questions:

- What transfusion medicine tests are performed during pregnancy and in the postpartum period?
- What is hemolytic disease of the fetus and newborn (HDFN)? How is it diagnosed, treated, and in some cases prevented?
- What is Rh-immune globulin (RhIg) and how is it used?
- What are the special requirements for transfusion products used to treat neonatal and pediatric patients?

TERMINOLOGY

There is a set of distinctive terminology used during and after pregnancy. **Perinatal** refers to the period beginning as early as the 20th week of gestation or as late as the 28th week of pregnancy and ending 28 days after birth. So the discipline of perinatology includes study of the mother, the fetus, and the neonate. A **neonate** is defined as a newborn from birth to 4 weeks of age; an **infant** is defined as a baby during the first year of life.[1] Often the terms *neonate* and *infant* are used interchangeably, sometimes resulting in much confusion. For transfusion purposes, neonates are babies who are 4 months old or less and infants are babies over 4 months of age.[2]

When doing case studies, information may be present about a woman's pregnancy history, for example, gravida 2 para 1 (abbreviated G_2P_1). The term **gravid** means a pregnant woman; **gravida** expresses the number of pregnancies experienced by a woman regardless of whether they resulted in a birth or not.[1] **Para** refers to delivery of a live infant. When multiple infants from one pregnancy such as twins or triplets occur, that event is still considered to be a single parous event. Therefore, a G_2P_1 woman would have two pregnancies and one live birth. This may mean she is now pregnant with baby #2, or it may mean she has been pregnant twice, but lost one baby prior to birth. Sometimes the letter "A" is

present after the letter "P." This represents the word *abortus* and is used to indicate the number of pregnancies lost for any reason, including spontaneous or induced abortions or miscarriages. If the patient in the above example had a miscarriage previously, her obstetric history would be represented as $G_2P_1A_1$. Another system, the TPAL system, uses gravida with a digit and para with four digits after the "P." The first digit after "P" is the number of children delivered at term; the second is the number of premature babies; the third is for abortions, miscarriages, or ectopic pregnancies; and the last digit is for the number of living children. Thus G_6P_{3123} would indicate six pregnancies with three term births, one premature birth, two abortions or miscarriages, and three living children.

Since D antigen and anti-D are integral concepts involved in the content of this chapter, a review of the terminology associated with them is appropriate to address here. As previously stated in Chapter 5, historically, the terms D antigen, Rh factor, and anti-D were used to designate the various forms of "D". Since D antigen and anti-D are part of the Rh system and the term D antigen is synonymous with the term Rh factor, a more recent designation of D as Rh(D) and $Rh_0(D)$ evolved, particularly when referring to D antigen, D antibody, and result interpretation. The $Rh_0(D)$ designation is primarily used in this chapter. References to variations of $Rh_0(D)$, for example weak D, remain as is except when notating result interpretation such as weak $Rh_0(D)$ positive.

CASE IN POINT *(continued)*

The physician on duty took detailed notes on the patient's condition.

1. How would the physician abbreviate the pregnancy history of this patient?

HEMOLYTIC DISEASE OF THE FETUS AND NEWBORN (HDFN)

Hemolytic disease of the fetus and newborn (HDFN) is defined as the shortened lifespan of fetal or neonatal red blood cells caused by the action of maternal antibodies attaching to corresponding antigens on the baby's red blood cells. These antibodies are transferred from the circulation of the mother to the fetal circulation through the placenta. Hemolysis of fetal and/or newborn red blood cells occurs, resulting in anemia, accumulation of bilirubin, and an enlarged spleen and liver. If the hemolysis is severe enough, the anemia can result in heart failure and may be fatal. Likewise, hyperbilirubinemia can cause permanent sequelae or death. The hemolytic process begins during intrauterine life, affecting the fetus, and can continue into the first days and weeks of newborn life. Other conditions can also cause hemolysis or jaundice in the fetus and newborn and these should be kept in mind when evaluating the patient for HDFN.[3] Refer to Table 14-1 *.

Historically, Rh incompatibility was the number one cause of HDFN and still remains number one in some parts of the world. It generally occurred following exposure of an $Rh_0(D)$, formerly referred to as Rh or D,-negative mother to the red blood cells of her $Rh_0(D)$-positive fetus/newborn and the subsequent

pregnancies were affected. The advent of *Rh-immune globulin (RhIg)*, a prevention strategy defined in detail later, decreased the amount of $Rh_0(D)$-related HDFN tremendously. Today the most common cause of hemolytic disease of the newborn (HDN) in most countries is ABO incompatibility between the mother and the infant. Typically, this occurs in group A or B infants born to group O mothers who have the naturally occurring IgG anti-A,B antibody, which reacts to either A or B cells. Therefore, in contrast to HDFN caused by other clinically significant IgG antibodies, ABO HDN can occur with the first pregnancy. Severe hemolysis, however, does not generally occur with ABO incompatibility as the A and B antigens are not fully developed on red blood cells at birth. In the postnatal period, these babies are often asymptomatic; any hemolysis that occurs is usually mild or goes undetected.

☑ CHECKPOINT 14-1

List three causes of HDFN.

Pathophysiology of HDFN

There are four stages in the pathogenesis of HDFN: (1) exposure of the mother to fetal red blood cell antigens with subsequent production of (maternal) blood group antibodies (anti-A,B is an exception that does not require previous exposure to red blood cell antigens); (2) placental transfer of the maternal antibodies to the fetus with attachment to fetal red blood cell antigens; (3) subsequent immune destruction of the antibody-coated fetal red blood cells; and (4) clinical manifestations resulting from the destruction of these marked red blood cells (Table 14-2 *). It is important to realize the mother will not make an antibody against every "foreign" fetal red blood cell antigen, even though the fetal red blood cells enter her circulation during pregnancy. The "model" for HDFN is an $Rh_0(D)$ negative mother who makes anti-$Rh_0(D)$ directed against the $Rh_0(D)$ positive red blood cells of her fetus (Figure 14-1 ■). The mystery of maternal tolerance

---

★ TABLE 14-1 Conditions Causing Red Blood Cell Hemolysis in the Fetus or Newborn

Genetic red blood cell membrane defects, enzyme deficiencies, or hemoglobinopathies:
Glucose-6-phosphate dehydrogenase deficiency
Pyruvate kinase deficiency
Thalassemia
Hereditary spherocytosis
Hereditary elliptocytosis
Disorders of hemoglobin synthesis
Acquired defects of the red blood cells secondary to infection:
<u>T</u>oxoplasmosis, <u>R</u>ubella, <u>C</u>ytomegalovirus, <u>H</u>erpes simplex (TORCH)
Parvovirus B19
Syphilis

✶ **TABLE 14-2** Conditions Necessary for Maternal Antibody Formation in Hemolytic Disease of the Fetus and Newborn

1. The mother must lack the antigen present on the fetal red blood cells.
2. The fetal antigen must be well developed *in utero*.
3. The mother is exposed to the fetal antigen.
4. The mother produces an IgG antibody to the antigen, capable of crossing the placenta.

or intolerance to fetal antigens has been investigated for more than 50 years.[4] The immunogenicity of fetal antigens is due in part to the degree of maturity and the number of antigens present on the fetal red blood cells. Some blood groups such as ABO are poorly developed in the fetus and newborn, whereas others such as Rh are well developed prior to birth.

The immaturity of the fetal immune system requires the mother to actively pass antibodies across the placental barrier to provide protection for the fetus. The main immunoglobulins transferred to the fetus to protect against disease are IgG, because

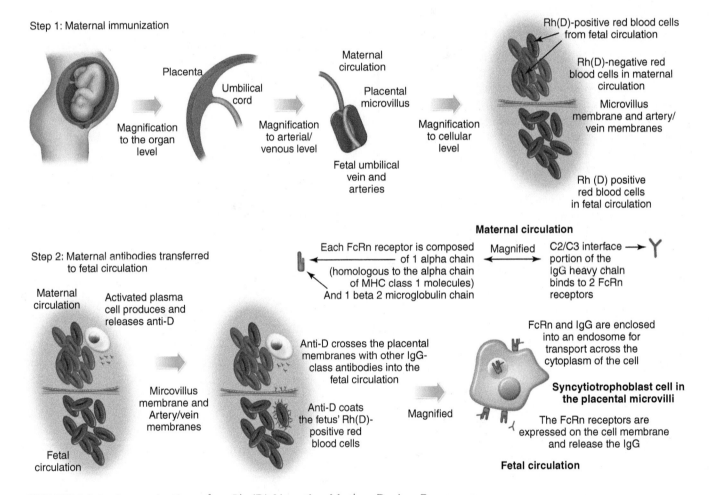

FIGURE 14-1   Immunization of an Rh_0(D)-Negative Mother During Pregnancy

Step 1:
  (a) Some Rh_0(D)-positive fetal cells move from the fetal circulation across the placental membrane and into the maternal circulation.
  (b) The maternal immune system recognizes the Rh_0(D) antigen as foreign and mounts an immune response, including differentiation of B lymphocytes into plasma cells that produce and excrete anti-Rh_0(D).

Step 2:
  (a) Maternal IgG is actively transported across the placental membrane and into the fetal circulation. Most of these antibodies are beneficial, being an important source of passive immunity to protect the fetus from infection both while *in utero* and in the first few weeks of life.
  (b) However, in the case of antibodies to red blood cell antigens that are on the baby's cells, there are negative effects. The antibodies coat the baby's red blood cells. Red blood cells coated in antibodies are destroyed, resulting in decreasing hemoglobin and increasing bilirubin, which lead to the physiological effects of hemolytic disease of the fetus and newborn.

Not drawn to scale.

they are monomers and are small enough to cross the placenta easily. A blood group IgG antibody can cross the placental barrier, enter the fetal circulation, and attach to the specific antigen on the fetal red blood cells. These red blood cells are then removed within the fetal spleen and liver via the macrophage Fc receptors for the constant region of the antibodies attached to fetal red blood cells. The subsequent degradation of the fetal red blood cells produces an increase in unconjugated bilirubin, also known as the indirect bilirubin fraction. The unconjugated bilirubin is transported across the placenta to the maternal circulation, where it is converted to the conjugated water-soluble form, or direct bilirubin fraction, and excreted by the mother. Figure 14-2 ■ illustrates the removal of antibody-coated RBC and the metabolism of hemoglobin.

As the red blood cells are destroyed, the fetus becomes more anemic. Erythropoiesis is increased and immature nucleated red blood cells are released into the fetal circulation from the bone marrow, which is known as **erythroblastosis fetalis**. As the demand for oxygen increases, extramedullary hematopoiesis or production

of blood cells outside of the bone marrow occurs in the liver and spleen. Both organs become enlarged, called **hepatosplenomegaly**, due to the need to produce red blood cells as well as to remove the sensitized red blood cells. While the blood cells are made in the liver *in utero*, by birth most of the blood cells are made in the bone marrow. Progressive anemia causes tissue hypoxia, triggering increased cardiac output, and the heart begins to beat rapidly with eventual heart failure. The hepatic involvement leads to portal hypertension with hepatocellular damage, producing hypoalbuminemia, ascites, and the serious complication of **hydrops fetalis**, a clinical condition involving significant fluid build-up characterized by respiratory and circulatory distress, hepatosplenomegaly, and cardiac decompensation. Death *in utero* or shortly after birth may occur.

At birth, affected newborns are anemic but not jaundiced, since the increased bilirubin produced during intrauterine life was processed and excreted by the mother's liver, as previously illustrated in Figure 14-2. After birth, the infant must take over the process of bilirubin metabolism. However, the neonatal liver cannot process high

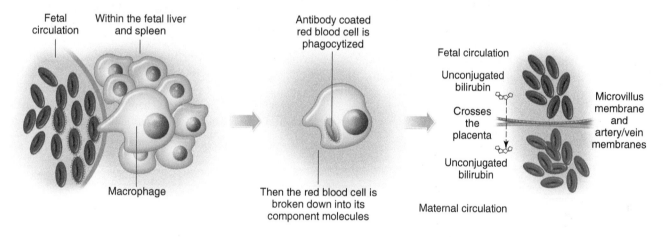

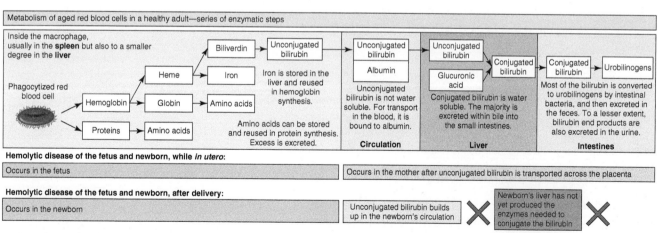

■ **FIGURE 14-2**   Removal of Antibody-Coated Red Blood Cells and Metabolism of Hemoglobin

In utero, the major symptom of hemolytic disease of the fetus and newborn is anemia because much of the bilirubin produced from the breakdown of antibody-coated red blood cells is transferred to the maternal circulation. The mother's liver conjugates the bilirubin and it is excreted.

After birth, the newborn will suffer from jaundice as well as anemia because the newborn's liver cannot conjugate the bilirubin. The unconjugated bilirubin cannot be excreted and will build up in the newborn's circulation.

Not drawn to scale.

levels of bilirubin adequately due to the lower levels in newborns of the enzyme uridine glucuronyl transferase, which converts unconjugated to conjugated bilirubin. When the level of unconjugated bilirubin exceeds the binding capacity of albumin, jaundice develops. At high enough levels, unconjugated bilirubin can be very toxic to the newborn. Since indirect bilirubin is lipid-soluble, it can cross the blood–brain barrier and become deposited in the cells of the basal ganglia and hippocampus, leading to cell death.[5] This condition, known as **kernicterus**, is characterized by seizures, poor feeding, hearing loss, and even death.[6] Infants who survive have permanent neurologic sequelae that may include the choreoathetoid (hyperkinetic) form of cerebral palsy, deafness, and impairment of vision.

☑ CHECKPOINT 14-2

What condition is described by fetal red blood cell destruction, anemia, and the release of immature nucleated red blood cells into the fetal circulation?

History of HDFN

The first written account of HDFN was by Plater in 1641 where he described the condition subsequently known as *hydrops fetalis*.[7] The pathogenesis of HDFN was elucidated after discovery of the Rh_0 antigen. Prevention started with the advent of Rh-immune globulin (RhIg) in 1968.[8] For a historical overview of the observation, treatment, and prevention phases of HDFN, see Table 14-3 ✳.

EVALUATION AND TESTING OF THE MOTHER

There are three areas of HDFN evaluation worthy of consideration in this discussion: sensitization, prenatal, and measurements of condition severity. Each area is described below along with corresponding testing that may be performed on the mother.

Sensitization

A mother may be sensitized to blood group antigens by previous pregnancies or from a transfusion of red blood cells. For sensitization to occur during pregnancy the mother must lack the antigen that the fetus has and the mother must respond to the foreign antigen by producing an antibody.

The transfer of oxygen, nutrients, and waste products between the mother and fetus occurs via a unique fetal–maternal communication system. The fetal blood vessels form the umbilical cord, which connects the developing fetus to the placenta. In the placenta, the fetal blood vessels branch into capillaries encased in small islands of tissue known as villi, as illustrated previously in Figure 14-1. The villi are surrounded by spaces containing maternal blood; they are separated from these spaces by a layer of cells called the **syncytiotrophoblast**. During a normal pregnancy, fetal red blood cells cross the placental barrier to enter the maternal circulation beginning in the first trimester.[9] In this manner, fetal red blood cells possessing a paternal antigen foreign to the mother can enter the maternal circulation. This is termed **fetomaternal hemorrhage (FMH)**. Usually the number of fetal red blood cells entering the maternal circulation is

---

✳ **TABLE 14-3** Major Historical Events for Hemolytic Disease of the Fetus and Newborn

Observation Phase[7, 8, 58]
1641—Plater gives the first written account of hydrops fetalis
1892—Ballantyne establishes criteria for the diagnosis of hydrops fetalis
1932—Diamond, Blackfan, and Baty recognize that hydrops fetalis, icterus gravis neonatorum, and anicteric anemia as all the same disease
1940—Landsteiner and Weiner discover the Rh factor as the cause of HDFN
1949—Officially called hemolytic disease of the newborn
Treatment Phase[7, 8, 58]
1946—Wallerstein is the first to suggest and perform exchange transfusion
1950—Allen, Diamond, and Vaughn treat 109 infants with exchange transfusion; they all survive
1954—Allen, Diamond, and Jones propose preterm delivery as a method of treatment
1956—Bevis determines the significance of bilirubin in amniotic fluid
1957—Kliehauer, Braun, and Betke develop the differential staining technique for fetal cells
1961—Liley suggests intrauterine transfusion
1963—Intraperitoneal transfusion of fetus takes place
Prevention Phase
1960—Freda, Gorman, and Pollack have the first meeting to discuss treatment
1964—First clinical trials of Rh-immune globulin (RhIg) occur
1968—Administration of RhIg postdelivery takes place
1984—RhIg is administered antenatally
1981—Intravascular fetal transfusion is performed using percutaneous cordocentesis
1993—Prenatal determination of fetal Rh(D) genotype by DNA amplification performed
1998—Noninvasive Doppler ultrasonography is used to determine fetal status

quite small; however, a larger degree of FMH can occur at delivery, after amniocentesis, spontaneous or induced abortion, chorionic villus sampling, rupture of an ectopic pregnancy, or blunt trauma to the abdomen.[2]

When fetal red blood cells pass into the maternal circulation, the mother's reticuloendothelial system (RES) will recognize the foreign antigen. The foreign antigen will be processed and antibody production may occur in those women who are responders and thus prone to making antibodies. Whether an antibody is produced is dependent on the mother's genetic makeup, the dose of antigen presented, the ability of the antigen to cause a response, how often the antigen is presented, and whether fetal red blood cells are ABO compatible with the maternal serum.

Large fetomaternal bleeds are more likely to occur at delivery when the placenta separates from the uterine wall; therefore, the primary antibody response would occur after the first delivery of an antigen-positive infant. Severe HDFN is rare in the first pregnancy because of the time factor of primary sensitization (Chapter 3). During the second or succeeding pregnancies with an antigen-positive fetus, even small amounts of fetal red blood cells entering the maternal circulation can cause a brisk secondary anamnestic antibody response. The sections that follow describe three sensitization-related aspects associated with laboratory testing of a mother suspected of having HDFN.

Antigens

All antigens are not considered equal in stimulating the immune system. Those antigens localized to the red blood cell membrane seem to be more antigenic than those also found in a wide variety of tissues[10] such as Fy^a and Fy^b. In addition, early maturation of the antigen seems to play a role in the severity of the HDFN. For example, the K1 antigen in the Kell blood group system is developed on red blood cells early in erythroid development. When anti-K1 crosses the placental barrier, depression of erythropoiesis and/or the destruction of erythroid precursors occurs as well as destruction of circulating K1-positive fetal red blood cells and may cause severe anemia of the fetus.[11, 12] The density of the antigen on the red blood cells also determines the severity of HDFN.[13] Because only the father passes on the gene for the antigen in question, the fetus is heterozygous and the fetal red blood cells will have a single dose of the antigen rather than a double dose present in genetically homozygous fetuses. There is some evidence that fetuses with the R$_2$r (cDE/cde) genotype are more likely to cause sensitization of their mothers to Rh$_0$(D) than are Rh-positive babies with other genotypes. Lastly, the structure of the antigen plays a role in the ability of the fetal macrophages to recognize the coated red blood cells. If the antigen is further away from the lipid bilayer of the red blood cell membrane, the macrophages recognize the coated cell more readily.[14] See Table 14-4 ✴ for a list of antigens known to cause HDFN.

> ☑ **CHECKPOINT 14-3**
>
> Which Rh antibody specificity is most frequently implicated in HDFN?

✴ **TABLE 14-4** Antibodies Implicated in Hemolytic Disease of the Fetus and Newborn

Blood Group System	Antibody	Usual Severity of HDFN*
ABO	A or B or A,B	Most cases mild Occasional moderate Very rare to see severe cases
RH	D	About 20% of cases are severe
	C, cE	Most cases mild Some moderate or severe
	E, C,Ce,C^w,e	Most cases mild Rare to see severe cases
Kell	K1	About equal distribution of severe, moderate, and mild cases
Duffy	Fy^a	About half of cases are severe Rest are moderate or mild
	Fy^b	Rare cause of mild HDFN
Kidd	Jk^a	Rare cause of severe HDFN
MNS	M	Rare cause of severe HDFN
	S	Most cases mild Rare severe case reported
	U	Most cases mild Rare severe case reported

*Hemolytic disease of the fetus and newborn definitions:

  Mild: no treatment required or phototherapy treatment only

  Moderate: Phototherapy required with or without neonatal exchange transfusion

  Severe: occurrence of hydrops fetalis or perinatal death; intrauterine transfusions can be required

Immunoglobulin Class

The immunoglobulin G (IgG) crosses from the mother's circulation to the fetal capillaries in the placenta via the cells of the syncytiotrophoblast layer. There are Fc receptors for IgG in the placenta; this Fc receptor is termed *neonatal Fc receptor (FcRn)*. The FcRn binds to the Fc portion or constant region of maternal IgG and actively transports the immunoglobulin from the mother's circulation to the fetal circulation.[15] Placental transfer of antibodies is illustrated in Figure 14-1. The FcRn has a dual role: transport of IgG from mother to fetus and homeostasis of IgG in circulation.[16] Maternal IgM antibodies are large pentamers and do not cross the placenta.

Maternal immunoglobulins are transferred to the fetus beginning early in the second trimester because the fetus/neonate does not make antibodies efficiently until 4–6 months after birth. When maternal and cord immunoglobulin levels are compared, there is more IgG1, IgG3, and IgG4 in the cord blood compared to the corresponding maternal blood, with IgG1 having the greatest difference and IgG4 having the least. Conversely, there is more IgG2 in the maternal rather than the cord samples.[17] Therefore, IgG1 is the most efficiently transported subclass and IgG2 is the least. At term, the total IgG levels in the fetus typically exceed the maternal level. The contribution of IgG subclasses to HDFN remains unclear. Some studies have shown that IgG3 anti-$Rh_0()$ is more destructive of $Rh_0(D)$ positive red blood cells than IgG1 anti-$Rh_0(D)$. Other studies have indicated the combination of IgG1 and IgG3 together causes red blood cell destruction, while others claim IgG1 causes the most damage.[18, 19]

Influence of ABO Group

The ABO group of the fetus can be an important factor in reducing the incidence of maternal formation of anti-$Rh_0(D)$. In group O $Rh_0(D)$ negative mothers who carry a group A or B $Rh_0(D)$ positive fetus, fetal red blood cells entering the maternal circulation are destroyed by the anti-A, anti-B, and/or anti-A,B before the fetal $Rh_0(D)$ positive antigen sites are recognized by the mother's antibody-producing cells.[10]

PRENATAL EVALUATION

There are four issues, each of which is detailed in the following sections that have proven useful to investigate when conducting a prenatal evaluation for the presence of HDFN: maternal history, serological studies, paternal phenotype, and typing of the fetus.

Maternal History

To evaluate the possibility of HDFN, the history of the pregnant female must be considered. This step is sometimes overlooked; however, the maternal history can be extremely important. Pertinent questions would be whether the mother had a previous infant affected by HDFN or an infant who required transfusion during the pregnancy or following birth. As a second step, the historical records in the blood bank should be reviewed and compared to the current results obtained during testing.[20] By checking past records, laboratory personnel will be able to better determine the likelihood of problems arising during this pregnancy.

Serological Studies

During the first trimester, the physician should request ABO, Rh, and antibody screen testing on the mother's blood. If the mother's red blood cells do not react at immediate spin with reagent anti-$Rh_0(D)$, then a weak D test is not required and she is considered $Rh_0(D)$ negative.[20, 21] Historically, all mothers' red blood cells were tested for weak D and some laboratories continue to do weak D testing (Chapter 5) on all pregnant women to avoid confusion when interpreting the screen for FMH. The current licensed anti-$Rh_0(D)$ reagents are sufficiently potent to detect most common weak D phenotypes using routine typing methods. These patients will be considered $Rh_0(D)$ positive and therefore not candidates for Rh-immune globulin (RhIg).[20] By not performing the test for weak D, a few women with weak D may be labeled as $Rh_0(D)$ negative and be considered candidates for RhIg. While not ideal, this generally would not result in clinically significant harm to either the mother or the fetus. On the other hand, a mother with the rare partial-D phenotype will likely type as $Rh_0(D)$ positive and not be considered a candidate for RhIg. Such individuals may form anti-$Rh_0(D)$ since the maternal red blood cells are missing a portion of the $Rh_0(D)$ antigen. This could cause clinically significant harm to subsequent $Rh_0(D)$-positive fetuses.[22]

If the antibody screen is positive, the transfusion service must determine the antibody specificity by performing a panel (Chapter 8). Once the antibody is identified, the mother's red blood cells are antigen-typed for the corresponding antigen to confirm that she is lacking the antigen to her antibody. For $Rh_0(D)$-negative women whose initial antibody screen is negative, a second antibody screen should be performed at 28 weeks' gestation prior to giving prophylactic RhIg. This is to detect immunization that might have occurred previously, but the anti-$Rh_0(D)$ became weak or appeared negative prior to reexposure with the current pregnancy.

The presence of an antibody does not indicate HDFN will occur.[11] The transfusion service must determine if antibodies classically considered IgM and, therefore, clinically insignificant because they do not cross the placenta are in fact IgM. Anti-P_1, anti-Le^a, and anti-Le^b are known to be IgM antibodies and have not been found to cause HDFN; in addition, the red blood cell antigens are poorly developed at birth. However, the antibody to the M antigen, which is usually an IgM antibody, has been shown to be IgG in some women and has been implicated (rarely) in HDFN.[11] Anti-M that reacts at 98.6° F (37° C) or at the antiglobulin phase of testing would be considered potentially clinically significant for causing HDFN.

Once a clinically significant IgG antibody is identified, antibody titrations can be used to determine the relative concentration of the antibody. The antibody titration does not predict the severity of HDFN; rather, it is a screening test that can help in decisions about performing invasive procedures. Titration should not be performed on IgM antibodies because these antibodies will not cross the placenta. As early as possible in the pregnancy, a baseline titer should be established. Each sample tested should be frozen to use for comparison when performing future titrations. When performing titrations, care must be taken to use the same technique, to use cells of the same red blood cell phenotype, and to test the current sample in parallel with a previously frozen sample, if available. There is some controversy as to selection of the phenotype of the red blood cells used in the titration. Some laboratories are adamant the red blood cells should possess the strongest expression of homozygous or double dose of the antigen; others select red blood cells of the same expected phenotype of the fetus, which would be heterozygous or single dose of the antigen. The most important aspect is to be consistent and to follow the procedure of the facility.

The titration technique validated by the facility should be used. Gel methodology or use of enhancement media such as LISS or PEG are not currently recommended.[2] Titration results are reported out as the reciprocal of the dilution giving the last 1+ reaction. The critical titer is one associated with a significant risk of HDFN and should be determined at each facility in conjunction with the obstetrical staff. Most critical antibody titers are between 8 and 32.[23] It is important to note that the American College of Obstetricians and Gynecologists (ACOG) does not recommend serial titers for the monitoring of a patient with a previous history of an affected fetus or neonate, nor do they consider titers appropriate for monitoring patients with an anti-K.[23] In these cases, the antibody is always considered clinically significant regardless of the titer.

☑ CHECKPOINT 14-4

Name the test procedure that can be used to determine the concentration of maternal antibody in HDFN.

Paternal Phenotype

Determining the phenotype of the red blood cells from the putative father can be helpful in predicting the likelihood that the fetus carries the antigen to which the mother has formed an antibody. Once the phenotype is obtained, calculations can be performed to determine the probability of the putative father carrying a single or double dose of the offending antigen. Knowing the likelihood of paternal antigen heterozygosity or homozygosity allows a prediction to be made as to the probability of the fetus inheriting the antigen. If the putative father is negative for the offending antigen, further assessment is typically unnecessary. However, the mother should be counseled in private to determine the likelihood of the putative father being the true biological father of the fetus. The maternal antibody may have been made following previous exposure to blood products or fetal red blood cells from a different father. Many institutions do not perform paternal blood testing when considering the possible effect of a maternal antibody on the fetus, as the father may not be known or available for testing. Not all women may be truthful about the identity of the father, particularly if the father is not the boyfriend or husband and there are other legal and ethical considerations involved in the issue of paternity (Chapter 19).

Obtaining a sample of blood from the putative father is helpful in cases where a maternal antibody to a low-frequency antigen is probable. The antibody to a low-frequency antigen may have been determined during a previous pregnancy, upon delivery, or picked up as an incompatible crossmatch with a rare red blood cell unit if the mother required blood. Suspect an antibody to a low-incidence antigen in the mother when the neonate's direct antiglobulin test is

positive, but the eluate is negative with both the antibody screen and panel cells.

Typing of the Fetus

Knowing the phenotype of the fetal red blood cells would be ideal in predicting HDFN. However, obtaining a sample of red blood cells from a fetus can present a risk to either the fetus and/or the mother. Amniocentesis, chorionic villus sampling, and the extraction of fetal blood in the umbilical cord with the assistance of advanced imaging ultrasound technology known as **percutaneous umbilical blood sampling (PUBS)** or **cordocentesis** are invasive methods used to obtain fetal cells. Amniocentesis is the procedure of choice to obtain amniotic cells containing fetal DNA.[23] Methods using a polymerase chain reaction (PCR) technique are available for molecular detection of many red blood cell polymorphisms, including *RHCE, RH(D), K, Fy,* and *Jk* genes.[24, 25]

Fetal DNA can also be isolated from the maternal plasma.[26, 27] Fetal DNA is present in maternal plasma in detectable quantities as early as 32 days' gestation.[24] Using a real-time fluorogenic PCR technique, the amount and type of fetal DNA can be determined. Research is ongoing to determine the accuracy and predictability of this technique.[28, 29, 30] It is not yet routinely available for DNA determination of genes other than fetal *Rh(D)* status,[24] but holds promise for predicting HDFN and treating complicated pregnancies in a non-invasive manner.

☑ CHECKPOINT 14-5

List three invasive methods of obtaining fetal red blood cells to assess the risk of HDFN.

CASE IN POINT (continued)

At her first prenatal appointment, SC's physician orders a type & screen. The laboratory reports that she is A Rh$_0$(D) negative with a positive antibody screen. The antibody identified is anti-C at a titer of 8.

2. When was SC likely sensitized to the C antigen?
3. What are the risks of HDFN to the fetus before birth?
4. What are the risks of HDFN to the neonate after birth?
5. Which factors influence whether a foreign red blood cell antigen will result in antibody formation in a pregnant woman?
6. The physician orders antigen typing for C and c on the father. Why may this be helpful?

MEASUREMENTS OF HDFN SEVERITY

The severity of HDFN is difficult to predict using laboratory assays alone. Interpretation of antibody titer results is complicated by the different techniques used in different laboratories; nonetheless, it is one of the first tests routinely performed. Cellular assays—such as the monocyte monolayer assay (MMA),[31] the antibody-dependent cell-mediated cytotoxicity assay (ADCC), and the chemiluminescence test (CLT)—have all been used to predict the clinical significance of antibodies. However, these assays are complex to perform and have not yet made their way into routine laboratory use.[32] The tests that are routinely done in laboratories today are described in the following sections.

Amniotic Fluid Analysis

The level of bilirubin pigment present in amniotic fluid has been shown to correlate with the degree of hemolysis of fetal red blood cells *in utero*. Historically, amniocentesis was usually performed in women who had a previous history of HDFN, resulting in a still-birth or a newborn requiring exchange transfusion or an antibody titer at or above a defined critical value. Complications of amniocentesis include miscarriage, cramping and vaginal bleeding, needle injury to the baby, leaking of amniotic fluid, Rh sensitization, and infection to the mother and/or the fetus. Since the advent of ultrasound-guidance for amniocentesis, the incidence of complications has declined but is still significant. This invasive, indirect technique has now largely been replaced by Doppler ultrasonography of the fetal middle cerebral artery to evaluate the degree of fetal anemia. Amniocentesis may still be done to collect fetal DNA or when the ultrasound findings are questionable or highly concerning for the safety of the fetus.[23, 24] Spectrophotometers are no longer commonly available in every laboratory to perform this analysis.

Amniocentesis can be performed as early as 15 weeks' gestation, although it is typically not performed until weeks 24–26. Using ultrasound guidance, a needle is inserted into the amniotic cavity and 20–50mL of fluid surrounding the fetus is removed and analyzed via spectrophotometry over certain wavelengths. Bilirubin has maximum absorbance at 450 nm wavelength, allowing the laboratory to calculate the ΔOD_{450}. This value can then be plotted on a **Liley graph**, which tracks the ΔOD_{450} versus gestational age. The Liley graph is separated into three zones and, based on the optical density (OD) value, predicts the severity of anemia of the fetus and whether intrauterine transfusion or early delivery may be indicated.[2] If the ΔOD_{450} is used to monitor a pregnancy, the amniocentesis is usually repeated every 1–3 weeks. Figure 14-3 ■ shows an example of a Liley graph.

Doppler Flow Studies

Doppler ultrasound is a noninvasive method of monitoring the presence of anemia in the fetus.[33] Brain tissue depends on oxygen for proper functioning and the middle cerebral artery (MCA) in the brain responds quickly to hypoxemia. By measuring the peak velocity of blood flow in the MCA, the degree of fetal anemia can be assessed.[23] The MCA is easily visualized in the fetus with little observer variability.[34, 35, 36] Oepkes et al. found Doppler ultrasonography of the middle cerebral artery was more sensitive and more accurate for assessing the degree of fetal anemia when compared to the measurement of amniotic fluid ΔOD_{450}.[34] Importantly, it carries no risk of injury or death to the fetus or mother.

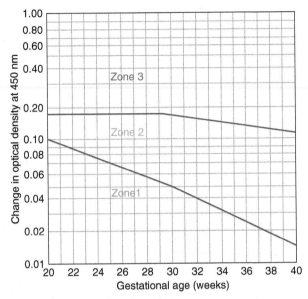

■ **FIGURE 14-3** Liley Graph

Zone 3: Fetus is likely suffering from a severe hemolytic disease of the fetus and newborn. Medical intervention, such as an intrauterine transfusion with $Rh_0(D)$-negative, irradiated donor red blood cells concentrated to have a high hematocrit is typically indicated.
Zone 2: Fetus is likely suffering from moderate hemolytic disease of the fetus and newborn. Medical intervention may or may not be required; continued monitoring of the level of hemolysis experienced by the fetus should occur.
Zone 1: Fetus has only mild or no hemolysis occurring; medical intervention is not required.

Fetal Blood Sampling

Percutaneous umbilical blood sampling (PUBS) or cordocentesis allows direct access to fetal blood and became feasible in the mid-1980s with the advance of ultrasound technology. Fetal blood sampling is the most accurate means of determining the severity of fetal hemolytic anemia and the need for treatment of the fetus. Using ultrasound guidance, a needle is inserted into an umbilical blood vessel close to its point of insertion into the placenta. It is important to determine that the blood obtained does indeed come from the fetus. Typically this can be easily done by performing a mean cell volume (MCV) on the sample. Fetal red blood cells will have a higher MCV (100–110 μm^3/100–110 fL) than those of the mother (80–95 μm^3/80–95 fL) and is even more elevated in anemic fetuses. Once it has been verified the blood sample is of fetal origin, the blood can be used in a variety of tests, including hematocrit, direct antiglobulin test, and fetal blood type.

This procedure is also not without hazards. PUBS carries a high risk of FMH and is associated with a 1–2% rate of fetal death.[2, 33] Therefore, its use is usually recommended only for patients with signs of severe fetal anemia by Doppler flow studies or high ΔOD_{450} values, or those with a previous newborn with severe HDFN. In such patients, the procurement of a fetal blood sample is often immediately followed by intrauterine transfusion of the fetus.

☑ CHECKPOINT 14-6

What is a Liley graph?

ANTEPARTUM TREATMENT OF HDFN

There are two strategies that may be used in the antepartum treatment of HDFN: plasma exchange and intrauterine transfusion. A description of each strategy is next.

Plasma Exchange

Plasma exchange can be safely performed in pregnant women, with the goal of removing maternal alloantibody. Typically, this procedure is reserved for those women with a previous history of a severely affected pregnancy. Plasma exchange should be considered early in the pregnancy prior to development of hydrops in the fetus.[37] In some instances, plasma exchange has been used in combination with the administration of intravenous immune globulin (IVIG) to the mother.[33, 38, 39] This approach has been successful in managing complicated pregnancies and may be repeated throughout the pregnancy or until intrauterine transfusions to the fetus can be performed.

Intrauterine Transfusion

Studies performed on the mother and fetus may indicate that infusion of red blood cells into the fetus *in utero*, known as **intrauterine transfusion (IUT)**, is necessary. The IUT may need to be performed several times until it is feasible to deliver the fetus with a reasonable chance for extrauterine survival. Before the ability to directly access the fetal circulation through the umbilical blood vessels, IUT was performed via the intraperitoneal route: red blood cells injected directly into the peritoneal cavity of the fetus, where they were adsorbed through the lymphatic vessels into the circulation. This adsorption process was relatively slow, with variable success rates, and has largely been replaced by intravascular transfusion via the umbilical blood vessels. Using the same PUBS technique as for sampling fetal red blood cells, direct intravascular fetal transfusion can be performed as early as the 20th week of gestation. In some hospitals, a combination of intraperitoneal and intravascular transfusion is utilized, allowing for a rapid infusion of red blood cells to the fetus, followed by the slower absorption of red blood cells in the peritoneal cavity.

The selection of red blood cell units for an IUT is important. Typically, group O Rh(D) negative red blood cell units lacking the offending antigen are used. It is preferable that the unit be relatively fresh, generally less than 7 to 10 days old, or washed. In addition, the red blood cell units should be leukocyte-reduced, CMV-reduced-risk, irradiated to prevent graft versus host disease (GVHD), and compatible with the mother's plasma.[5] It is usually also desirable to use red blood cell units lacking hemoglobin S. If antigen-negative red blood cell units are difficult to procure, the mother's red blood cells may be used to provide antigen-negative blood, providing she is able to tolerate the blood donation process. However, it is then extremely important the red blood cell unit is washed to remove the offending antibody and irradiated to avoid transfusion-associated GVHD, which is more common when blood from first-degree relatives is transfused. To minimize the chance of volume overload in the fetus, the smallest volume of red blood cells possible must be transfused; therefore, the red blood cell units are concentrated to a hematocrit of at least 75–85% (0.75–0.80). Based on the gestational age and hematocrit of the fetus, only 10–20mL of red blood cells may need to be transfused. The goal is to increase the fetal hematocrit to 40–50%

(0.40–0.50).[33] Transfusions will often need to be repeated every 2–3 weeks until delivery, depending on the degree of hemolysis occurring. See Table 14-5 ✳ for how to select red blood cell units for fetal transfusion, exchange transfusion, and small-volume transfusion.

CASE IN POINT *(continued)*

At 28 weeks' gestation, Doppler flow studies indicate that the baby is slightly anemic. The physician requests blood for intrauterine transfusion.

7. What factors should be considered when choosing blood for the IUT?

PREVENTION OF HDFN

Although HDFN has been associated with numerous blood group antibodies, only those cases due to anti-$Rh_0(D)$ have been successfully prevented. The use of a commercially prepared product consisting of purified anti-$Rh_0(D)$, known as **Rh-immune globulin (RhIg)**, has dramatically decreased the incidence of HDFN resulting from production of anti-$Rh_0(D)$ by an $Rh_0(D)$ negative mother. The following section provides a historical perspective, highlights of research using Rh_0Ig, and its mechanism of action and composition. Furthermore, because Rh_0Ig may be given both during and after pregnancy, there is a section dedicated to discussing its prophylactic use in each phase.

Rh-Immune Globulin (RhIg)

In the early 1960s, two research groups, one in the United States and the other in the United Kingdom, began looking at ways to prevent Rh immunization.[40] The U.S. group's theory was based on antibody-mediated immune suppression while the U.K. group's theory was based on the reduced incidence of Rh immunization occurring in ABO-incompatible pregnancies.

The U.S. research group injected prisoners with $Rh_0(D)$-positive blood on day one; on day three, the prisoners were then given an injection of human anti-$Rh_0(D)$.[41] The U.K. researchers used policemen as volunteers in a similar study.[42] These initial investigations were followed by clinical trials in $Rh_0(D)$ negative pregnant women, and by 1968 the first RhIg was produced and approved for administration in the United States. Ever since, RhIg has been effective in preventing anti-$Rh_0(D)$ HDFN without knowing exactly how it works. It is known that RhIg must be administered in a sufficient dose and given prior to the occurrence of Rh immunization for it to work.

The mechanism by which RhIg works to prevent sensitization to the D antigen has not been fully elucidated and animal models emulating Rh-mediated HDFN have not been found, so investigation remains problematic. The human studies performed in the

✳ **TABLE 14-5** RBC selection for Transfusion to Fetus and Neonates

Intrauterine Transfusion Components

Regardless of maternal or fetal ABO/Rh type:
Fresh or washed red blood cell units, leukocyte-reduced, irradiated, Volume-reduced to desired hematocrit, **AND**

Mother's IAT:

Positive	Group O $Rh_0(D)$ negative, IAT crossmatch compatible with mother's plasma and negative for antigens for which mother has antibody
Negative	Group O $Rh_0(D)$ negative, immediate spin or computer crossmatch compatible with mother

IAT, indirect antiglobulin test.

Exchange Transfusion Components

Regardless of maternal or fetal ABO/Rh type:
Red blood cell units less than 5 days old, reconstituted to desired hematocrit with FFP that is ABO compatible with newborn, **AND**

Mother's IAT	Mother's ABO*	Newborn's Rh*	
Negative	O	Positive	O $Rh_0(D)$ positive, immediate spin or computer crossmatch compatible with mother or newborn
		Negative	O $Rh_0(D)$ negative, immediate spin or computer crossmatch compatible with mother or newborn
	Non-O	Any	ABO/Rh and immediate spin or computer compatible with newborn
Positive	Any	Any	ABO compatible with both mother and newborn, Rh compatible with newborn, IAT crossmatch compatible with mother's plasma, negative for antigens for which mother has the antibody

*Regardless of mother's Rh type or newborn's ABO group.

Small-Volume Transfusion in Newborns

Mother's IAT	Mother's ABO*	Newborn's Rh*	Regardless of maternal or fetal ABO/Rh type: RBC up to expiry date AND
Negative	O	Positive	O $Rh_0(D)$ positive, immediate spin or computer crossmatch compatible with mother or newborn
		Negative	O $Rh_0(D)$ negative, immediate spin or computer crossmatch compatible with mother or newborn
	Non-O	Any	ABO/Rh and immediate spin or computer compatible with newborn
Positive	Any	Any	ABO compatible with both mother and newborn, Rh compatible with newborn, IAT crossmatch compatible with mother's plasma, negative for antigens for which mother has the antibody

*Regardless of mother's Rh type or newborn's ABO group.

1960s could not be performed in current times due to concerns about informed consent and coercion, especially when prisoners are used as study subjects. Theories as to how RhIg prevents immunization have been postulated. Antibody-mediated immune suppression is involved, but the exact mechanism is still unclear. A recent theory involves the production of specific cytokines that work to suppress a primary immune response in the mother to $Rh_0(D)$ positive fetal red blood cells.[43] It has been shown that RhIg does not coat all available antigen sites on the $Rh_0(D)$ positive red blood cell, leaving some antigen sites unoccupied. However, the degree of binding is sufficient to inhibit an immune response by the B-cells.[42] This inhibition is not long-lasting and RhIg must be administered with each pregnancy.

RhIg is a sterile solution containing IgG anti-$Rh_0(D)$. It is prepared from fractionated pooled human plasma, which undergoes treatment to inactivate lipid-enveloped viruses. Preparations are available for administration by the intramuscular (IM) or intravenous (IV) route. For the sake of convenience, the intramuscular preparation is more commonly used. One standard dose of RhIg (roughly 1mL) containing 300-μg (1,500 IUI) of anti-$Rh_0(D)$ provides protection against 15mL of $Rh_0(D)$ positive red blood cells or 30mL of $Rh_0(D)$ positive whole blood. A smaller 50-μg dose is available in the United States for limited use after first-trimester pregnancy terminations and will counteract the effects of approximately 2.5 mL of $Rh_0(D)$ positive red blood cells or 5 mL of $Rh_0(D)$ positive

★ **TABLE 14-6** Indications for Rh Immune Globulin

Common pregnancy related:
  Antepartum prophylaxis (28–30 weeks)
  Postpartum when baby is Rh(D) positive
Less common pregnancy related:
  Medical interventions that increase risk of feto-maternal hemorrhage
    For example: amniocentesis, chorionic villus sampling, percutaneous umbilical blood sampling, post pharmacological or surgical treatment of ectopic pregnancy, termination of pregnancy
  Obstetrical complications that increase risk of feto-maternal hemorrhage
    For example: abdominal trauma, abruptio placentae, antepartum vaginal bleeding, placenta previa, fetal death
Transfusion related: Transfusion of Rh(D) positive red blood cell or platelet units to an Rh(D) negative patient

whole blood. An outline of the suggested indications for use of RhIg in $Rh_0(D)$ negative, unsensitized women is given in Table 14-6 ★.

Antepartum Prophylaxis

Antepartum administration of a standard 300-μg (1,500 IU) dose, given either IM or IV, of RhIg is indicated between 28 and 30 weeks of gestation in all pregnant $Rh_0(D)$ negative women who have not already made anti-$Rh_0(D)$.[23, 44] A test for weak D on the mother is not necessary.[20] If the father of the fetus is known and can be shown conclusively to be $Rh_0(D)$ negative, RhIg is not indicated. However, the RhIg is generally given anyway as a precautionary measure

because of the uncertainty of paternity and the serious consequences of not giving the RhIg for future fetuses. Since the half-life of RhIg varies from 21 to 30 days,[45] antepartum administration of RhIg will provide protection for approximately 12 weeks. Therefore, $Rh_0(D)$ negative women must receive a second dose of RhIg following delivery, provided the neonate is $Rh_0(D)$ positive.

Postpartum Prophylaxis

A minimum of at least one 300-μg (1,500 IU) dose of RhIg must be administered to all $Rh_0(D)$ negative women who deliver an $Rh_0(D)$ positive infant, provided the woman has not already made anti-$Rh_0(D)$.[20, 32] If the woman received an antepartum dose of RhIg, anti-$Rh_0(D)$ may be detected at the time of delivery. However, the amount of the passive anti-$Rh_0(D)$ given as antepartum prophylaxis does not provide sufficient protection for the postpartum period and an additional dose should be given. It is important to determine whether the presence of anti-$Rh_0(D)$ represents active or passive immunization. Typically, the standard antenatal dose of RhIg at 28 weeks' gestation will not be responsible for an anti-$Rh_0(D)$ titer greater than 4 at the time of delivery. If serologic testing results are questionable, it is advisable to administer RhIg rather than withhold it. RhIg should be administered within 72 hours of delivery, but even if administration is delayed it should still be given.

All $Rh_0(D)$ negative women who are considered candidates for RhIg should have a postpartum sample tested for excessive FMH.[20] If the degree of FMH is greater than 30mL whole blood, more than one dose of RhIg must be administered. Several screening tests are available to determine the presence of a FMH, the most common being the rosette test. Figure 14-4 ■ illustrates the rosette screening test. Note that the rosette test cannot be used if the infant is of the weak D phenotype; a different screening assay should be utilized. If the screening test is positive,

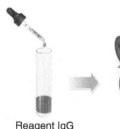 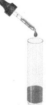 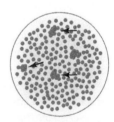

Reagent IgG anti-D is added to a suspension of maternal red blood cells and the mixture is incubated at 37°C

Fetal Rh(D) positive red blood cells that crossed into the maternal circulation will be coated with the reagent anti-D.

Maternal red blood cells are Rh(D) negative and remain uncoated.

Suspension is washed to remove any unbound anti-D reagent. Then dilute suspension of Rh(D) positive red blood cells is added and the mixture is centrifuged.

Anti-D attached to the Rh(D) positive fetal cells also attach to the reagent Rh(D) positive cells, forming a rosette with a fetal cell in the middle of a group of reagent cells.

Because the majority of the red blood cells are maternal Rh(D) negative cells, a positive reaction in the rosette test looks very similar to a mixed-field reaction when the suspension is viewed microscopically.

■ **FIGURE 14-4**   Rosette Test

The rosette test is a qualitative screen test. Most commercial kits have a sensitivity to detect a fetal maternal hemorrhage of 10–30 mL. The rosette test can only be used if the mother is $Rh_0(D)$ negative and the baby is $Rh_0(D)$ positive. False-positive results will occur if either the baby or the mother has a variant, weak D antigen.

Positive and negative control cell suspensions are run at the same time as the patient specimen(s) to ensure that the reagents are working and that the washing step was adequate.

If the rosette test is negative, a standard dose of Rh-immune globulin (RhIg) should be sufficient to prevent immunization and production of anti-$Rh_0(D)$. If the rosette test is positive, a qualitative test should be done to estimate the size of the fetal maternal bleed and subsequently the adequate dose of Rh-immune globulin (RhIg) to be given.

Not drawn to scale.

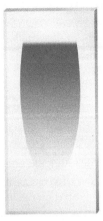

Blood film is made on a slide with maternal blood specimen. The blood film is first fixed and then incubated with a weak aid solution, such as a citrate acid buffer.

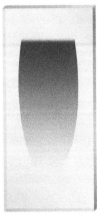

The blood film is then stained and examined microscopically.

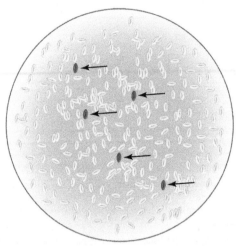

Fetal hemoglobin is resistant to acid and any fetal cells, if present, will be stained normally. Adult hemoglobin is eluted by the acid; the maternal red blood cells will appear as lightly stained "ghost" cells. The number of stained and ghost cells are counted up to a predetermined total number (such as 2,000). The count is used to estimate the percentage of fetal cells within the maternal circulation, which can then be used to calculate the volume of fetal blood in the maternal circulation.

■ FIGURE 14-5   Kleihauer-Betke Test

The Keihauer-Betke test is a quantitative test that estimates the amount of a fetal–maternal bleed. It can be done on any maternal specimen, regardless of the antigen type of the mother and baby, because it relies on the differences in adult and fetal hemoglobin.

A false-positive result will occur if the mother has abnormally high amounts of fetal hemoglobin, such as if she has sickle cell trait.

the degree of FMH should be quantitated using either flow cytometry, enzyme linked antiglobulin test, or the Klichauer-Betke (KB) acid-elution test. Figure 14-5 ■ illustrates the Kliehauer-Betke test.

Various formulas exist for calculating the required number of 300-μg (or 1,500 IU) doses of RhIg needed to cover a FMH of greater than 30 mL. A common formula using results from the KB test follows.[2] It assumes a maternal blood volume of 75 mL/kg, giving an average blood volume of 5,000 mL. The KB result is expressed as the number of fetal cells seen when counting a total of 2,000 red blood cells in a maternal peripheral blood sample. This number is then converted into the percentage of fetal cells.

(% Fetal cells)(5,000 mL or maternal volume) ÷ 30 mL

= number of doses RhIg needed [30 mL

represents the amount of fetal whole blood

covered by one dose of RhIg]

Consider this example:

If 40 fetal cells were seen while counting a total of 2,000 red blood cells on the KB test, the calculation would be:

Step 1: determine % fetal cells in a decimal format: 40/2000 = 0.02
Step 2: multiply value obtained in step 1 by 5,000 mL blood volume: (0.02) × (5,000) = 100
Step 3: divide value obtained in step 2 by 30 mL: 100/30 = 3.33 = since the number is > 0.5 it is not rounded up and is therefore 3
Step 4: add one to the value obtained in step 3: 3 + 1 = 4 doses

Note: When the decimal point is > or = .5, many institutions round up and then add one extra vial. For example, 3.6 doses would be rounded up to 4 doses and one more dose would be added to equal a total of 5 doses.

At least one additional dose may be added as a precaution, given the inherent difficulties in the performance and interpretation of the KB test. See Table 14-7 ✳ for dosages of RhIg used in several clinical conditions. Generally, no more than five doses are injected intramuscularly at one time. If a larger quantity is needed, the doses can be spaced over a 72-hour time period.

☑ CHECKPOINT 14-8

Which type(s) of HDFN can be prevented? How is this achieved?

SEROLOGICAL TESTING AND TREATMENT OF THE NEWBORN

In past years it was standard practice to collect an umbilical cord blood sample on every newborn. The degree of testing performed on the cord blood varied from institution to institution, with some facilities performing ABO, Rh, and direct antiglobulin testing on all samples and others holding the samples in the event testing was needed at a later time. It is no longer necessary to perform blood bank testing on all cord blood samples and not doing so conserves resources

✳ **TABLE 14-7** Recommended Dosage of Intramuscular Rh-Immune Globulin

Indication	Dose
Pregnancy related:	
<12 weeks gestation	50 μg (United States)*
For example: antepartum bleeding, miscarriage, medical intervention that increases risk of bleeding, obstetrical complications	
28 weeks gestation: routine prophylaxis	300 μg (standard dose in most countries)
Postpartum: if infant is Rh(D) positive or weak Rh(D) positive	300 μg minimum**
Transfusion related:	20 μg/mL of red blood cells transfused

*Repeat dose if >21 days between indications.
 Give standard 300 μg dose for same indications occurring at or later than 12 weeks gestation.
 Smaller dose size differs amongst countries (for example 120 μg dose is used in Canada).

**Additional dose(s) may be required if testing indicates a feto-maternal hemorrhage of > 30 mL
 Check manufacturer's instructions for other indications, suitability of product and dosage for intravenous administration and updates to recommendations

and money. Instead, most institutions now test the cord bloods of babies born to O mothers or other situations that could result in HDFN. Cord blood may contain a material called Wharton's jelly, which interferes with testing if adequate washing is not performed and can cause false-positive reactions. Wharton's jelly is a gelatinous substance within the umbilical cord, largely made up of mucopolysaccharides (hyaluronic acid and chondroitin sulfate). It also contains some fibroblasts, macrophages, and potentially pluripotent stem cells. The sections that follow introduce and describe the various serological testing and treatment strategies, when appropriate, for newborns.

ABO and $Rh_0(D)$ Determination

ABO and Rh typing of the newborn is usually not performed unless the mother is $Rh_0(D)$ negative. Babies born to $Rh_0(D)$ negative mothers should have their Rh type determined, including a test for weak D. Some facilities perform ABO and Rh typing on all newborns born to Group O women in an effort to identify those infants at risk for ABO HDFN. This practice has not proven to be of value and is not recommended by the American Academy of Pediatrics.[46] Obviously, if the baby will require transfusion following birth, an ABO/Rh should be performed. For the ABO, only typing of the red blood cells (forward typing) is required because any ABO antibodies in the serum are of maternal origin. Keep in mind that if the neonate received intrauterine transfusions, RBC typings may appear mixed field between the baby's true type and the transfused O $Rh_0(D)$ negative red blood cells or the newborn may type as entirely O $Rh_0(D)$ negative. If plasma products were given intrauterine, the baby's plasma may add to the confusion of trying to identify the true ABO type if tested with A and B cells (reverse type).

Direct Antiglobulin Test (DAT)

Direct antiglobulin testing (DAT) is not required on all newborns and in most institutions is not performed on a routine basis. As with ABO typing, some institutions choose to perform a DAT on all infants born to group O mothers. Often, the DAT will be negative in these infants. If ABO HDFN is strongly suspected, an eluate should be performed even if the DAT is negative. The strength of the DAT

in cases of ABO incompatibility is not indicative of the severity of the hemolytic process.

Below are important points to remember about DATs in newborns:

- If the mother has a clinically significant antibody, a DAT should be performed on the newborn's sample. If the DAT is positive, an eluate is often performed. However, one is not necessary if antibody identification studies have already been performed on the mother during admission for the delivery.[32]

- An $Rh_0(D)$ positive baby born to a mother who received RhIg during pregnancy may have a weakly positive DAT due to passive transfer of anti-$Rh_0(D)$. This passively acquired anti-$Rh_0(D)$ has not been shown to have adverse effects on the infant.[9]

- If the neonate has a positive DAT and the mother has a negative antibody screen, an antibody to a low-incidence antigen should be suspected. In such instances, testing the mother's serum/plasma against the biologic father's red blood cells can be helpful. If the mother is ABO incompatible with the father, which would cause positive reactions due to the ABO mismatch and make testing uninterpretable for a low-incidence antigen, an eluate prepared from the infant's red blood cells can be used instead.

Phototherapy

All infants should be routinely monitored for the development of jaundice. In the average full-term infant, the bilirubin level will peak at 5.0–6.0 mg/dL (5.0–6.0 μmol/L).[47] In ABO HDFN, the degree of hyperbilirubinemia is often minimal and transfusion is rarely indicated. These infants are typically treated with **phototherapy**, or light-based treatment alone. In addition, intensive phototherapy can sometimes avoid the need for exchange transfusion in infants with HDFN due to other blood group antibodies. Commonly used phototherapy units contain daylight, cool white, or blue fluorescent tubes. The most effective are those providing light in the blue-green region because bilirubin is most effectively reduced at this spectrum. Phototherapy works by converting toxic unconjugated bilirubin in the skin to a nontoxic isomer, called lumirubin, that is water-soluble and excreted in the urine.[47] The criteria for initiating phototherapy for hyperbilirubinemia vary. At the very least, it should be started well before toxic levels of bilirubin are reached in order to prevent neurologic damage to the infant. These trigger levels vary, depending on the birth weight of the infant and whether there are any other complications, such as hypoglycemia, infections, or acidosis. Premature infants are affected at lower concentrations of bilirubin than are full-term infants.

Transfusion

Transfusion of the neonate affected with HDFN depends on the degree and rate of hemolysis and the resultant increase in the bilirubin level. If the baby received intrauterine transfusions, an exchange transfusion may be unnecessary. Instead, small transfusions of red blood cells to "top off" the hemoglobin and hematocrit may be required over the course of the next 1–3 months to correct anemia due to low levels of ongoing hemolysis. Newborns are very susceptible to changes in volume and 10–15 ml of red blood cells are administered for each kilogram of the baby's body weight.

Exchange Transfusion

An **exchange transfusion** consists of replacing one or more volumes of the infant's blood with compatible red blood cells and plasma. This is done to rapidly reduce the bilirubin level in the newborn to prevent or reduce the degree of brain damage or kernicterus.[48] While HDFN is the most common indication for performing an exchange transfusion, there are other nonimmune-mediated causes of hyperbilirubinemia for which exchange transfusion may be beneficial. These include familial disorders of bilirubin conjugation including Gilbert's syndrome and Crigler-Najjar syndrome, enzymatic RBC defects including glucose-6-phosphate dehydrogenase deficiency, and infections including babesiosis.[47]

In addition to decreasing the levels of unconjugated bilirubin, an exchange transfusion will (1) remove the antibody-coated red blood cells of the infant, thereby preventing their destruction *in vivo* and the resultant anemia and increase in bilirubin; (2) remove maternal antibody that is present in the infant's circulation, preventing it from attaching to and destroying newly produced red blood cells; and (3) correct the anemia without causing volume overload. Typically, a two-blood-volume or "double-volume" exchange transfusion is performed. This will remove 85% of red blood cells and 25–45% of the bilirubin.[47] Although infrequent, newborns may require more than one exchange transfusion in order to decrease the bilirubin to nontoxic levels.

There are no set recommendations on how early an exchange transfusion should be performed. Rather, age-specific nomograms have been proposed by the American Academy of Pediatrics[49] in an effort to standardize treatment. However, infants who exhibit signs or symptoms of neurologic bilirubin toxicity or have a total bilirubin level of ≥ 25.0 mg/dL (≥ 25.0 μmol/L) should be considered for an immediate exchange transfusion.[49]

The blood used for an exchange transfusion consists of red blood cells mixed with compatible thawed FFP. The red blood cells should be ABO compatible with both the mother and infant and lack the offending antigen. In addition, they should be relatively fresh (i.e., less than 5–7 days old), leukocyte-reduced, CMV-reduced-risk, and irradiated. It is desirable to use red blood cell units lacking hemoglobin-S. Consequently, group O red blood cells are often used and reconstituted with group AB plasma. Maternal serum or plasma can be used for crossmatching; if it is not available, an eluate from the infant's red blood cells can be used.

The volume of reconstituted blood needed for an exchange transfusion is based on the baby's total blood volume. This is determined by the neonatologist as is the preferred hematocrit of the final product. Typically, a hematocrit between 40 and 50% (0.40–0.50) is requested. For a full-term baby, it may be necessary to prepare the equivalent of 2 units of reconstituted red blood cell units. Once the FFP is thawed and mixed with the red blood cells, the reconstituted product expires in 24 hours.

Exchange transfusions are usually only performed in centers with neonatal intensive care units under the guidance of experienced neonatologists. To perform an exchange transfusion, small aliquots of the infant's blood are removed and replaced with an equal volume of the reconstituted donor blood. Typically, the umbilical artery and/or umbilical vein are used for access. If there are two points of venous access, the removal of the newborn's blood and transfusion of the replacement blood can occur simultaneously, which is called **continuous exchange**. If there is access to only one

☑ CHECKPOINT 14-9

State the criteria for preparation of a blood product for an exchange transfusion.

CASE IN POINT (continued)

8. Is SC a candidate for RhIg at 28 weeks' gestation? Why or why not?

When SC arrives at the hospital for delivery, a T & S is ordered on her once more. She is still A-Rh_0(D) negative with a positive antibody screen. However, the antibody identification panel now shows both anti-C and anti-D.

9. Could the anti-Rh_0(D) be something other than active sensitization to the Rh_0(D) antigen?

Following delivery, cord blood is sent to the blood bank for ABO/Rh and DAT testing. The infant is O-Rh_0(D) positive with a positive DAT. An eluate reveals that anti-C is attached to the infant's cells.

10. What are the benefits of exchange transfusion?

In addition, a fetal cell screen (rosette test) is ordered on the mother and is positive. The blood is sent for a Kliehauer-Betke test to quantitate amount of the fetal bleed. Twenty fetal cells are seen in a total of 2,000 cells counted.

11. Given the results of the testing, how many vials of RhIg should be administered?

vessel, a small amount of blood can first be slowly removed and then replaced, which is called **discontinuous exchange**. Regardless of the method used, the exchange must take place very slowly using small volumes in order to prevent hypo- or hypervolemia in the neonate. It is, therefore, not uncommon for a two-volume exchange transfusion to require 1–2 hours to complete. In selected cases of HDFN, intravenous immune globulin (IVIG) may be given to avoid the need for exchange transfusion.[46] IVIG has also been given during pregnancy to mothers with high antibody titers or previous children with severe HDFN.

UNIQUE ASPECTS OF NEONATAL PHYSIOLOGY

There are three unique aspects of neonatal physiology pertinent to this discussion: fetal red blood cells, erythropoietin response, and immunologic status. The sections that follow provide an overview of each aspect.

Fetal Red Blood Cells

The fetal red blood cell differs in many ways from the adult red blood cell. The fetal red blood cell is larger, contains predominantly hemoglobin F (HbF; approximately 70% at term), has a shorter lifespan of 90 days, and has more lipids then adult cells. Additionally, fetal red blood cells carry a maximum oxygen load at a lower oxygen pressure of 19 mmHg compared to adult red blood cells, which carry a maximum oxygen load of 26 mmHg.[50] At birth, a full-term infant has a hemoglobin level between 14.0 and 20.0 mg/dL (140–200 g/L).[49] Since much of the increase in hemoglobin occurs during the last weeks of gestation, infants born prematurely can be expected to have lower hemoglobin levels. In addition, premature babies have a higher percentage of HbF, which may be as high as 97% in very premature children, than full-term infants. Because HbF interacts poorly with 2,3-diphosphoglycerate (2,3-DPG), the delivery of oxygen to the tissues of the premature neonate is decreased, especially if the amount of hemoglobin is also low.

Erythropoietin Response

After birth, all newborns experience a decline in the amount of circulating red blood cells, called the physiologic anemia of infancy. **Erythropoietin (EPO)** is a growth factor that stimulates the proliferation and differentiation of stem cells into red blood cell precursors. In the fetus, the majority of EPO is produced in the liver; in the adult, EPO is produced predominantly in the kidneys. The switch in production of EPO from the liver to the kidney begins during fetal life, but a complete transition may not occur until the infant is several months old. Because the liver is less responsive to tissue hypoxia and anemia than the kidneys, diminished EPO levels in the neonate are likely due to continued EPO production in the liver versus the kidneys, resulting in anemia in the newborn period.[51] In the full-term baby, hemoglobin levels gradually decrease during the first 1–2 months of age and then begin to increase. Typically, the baby tolerates this change without difficulty and no treatment is needed. Premature babies, who are already born with a lower hemoglobin

level, experience an even more dramatic decrease in hemoglobin levels following birth. This "anemia of prematurity" is thought to be mediated not only by low EPO levels and a suboptimal EPO response, but also by decreased iron stores, decreased survival of red blood cells, and high levels of HbF.[52] This may be further compounded by repeated phlebotomies for blood samples collected for testing of the sick infant.

Immunologic Status

The neonatal immune system is not fully developed at birth, such that newborns are at increased risk for a variety of infections. Both humoral and cellular immunity are functionally compromised.[2] Although the infant can produce some IgM in response to antigens, sufficient levels of IgG are not produced until about the first year of age. Most of the baby's circulating IgG is derived from the mother via placental transfer, while the baby's IgA comes from breast milk.

> ### ☑ CHECKPOINT 14-10
> Which organ is primarily responsible for erythropoietin (EPO) production during fetal development?

RED BLOOD CELL TRANSFUSIONS IN INFANTS LESS THAN 4 MONTHS OF AGE

When transfusion is required in infants, the neonate's physiology must be considered. The neonate is not a small adult and should be treated accordingly. Considerations and indications for this population in the areas of compatibility testing, red blood cell transfusion, red blood cell components, special products, transfusion administration, and recombinant human erythropoietin are addressed in the sections that follow.

Compatibility Testing

In the blood bank, the laboratorian need only test the neonate once within one hospital stay during the first 4 months of age. This testing will consist of a forward ABO and Rh type on red blood cells either from the cord or a heelstick sample. Antibody screening can be done on the serum or plasma of either the mother or the neonate. If this initial antibody screen is negative, it is not necessary to crossmatch the donor red blood cells.[20] If the antibody screen is positive due to a clinically significant antibody, compatibility testing should be performed with the neonate or mother's serum or plasma, or with an eluate prepared from the infant's red blood cells. Red blood cell units chosen for transfusion should be ABO compatible with the mother as well as with the neonate. For instance, if the neonate is group A and the mother is group O, the red blood cell units should be group O. For this reason, many institutions elect to transfuse group O red blood cells to all neonates, rather than ABO-type-specific blood. The unit must be negative for the antigen to the maternal antibody.

Indications for Red Blood Cell Transfusion

Triggers have been proposed for the transfusion of red blood cells to neonates. Unfortunately, these triggers are difficult to apply consistently because of the wide array of clinical issues that can occur in the premature newborn. Red blood cell transfusion is indicated for any baby showing signs or symptoms attributed to anemia. Red blood cell transfusions are most often given to preterm babies to replace iatrogenic blood loss, which is blood removed for clinical laboratory testing.[53] These transfusions are frequently small-volume transfusions of 10–15 mL/kg administered slowly over a period of 2–4 hours.

Red Blood Cell Components Used for Neonatal Transfusion

The optimal red blood cell product for neonatal transfusion is controversial. Fresh, defined as less than 5–7 days old, red blood cell units have traditionally been ordered by neonatologists; however, the studies of several investigators now show this is not necessary, particularly for small-volume transfusions.[53, 54] The concern over transfusing older red blood cell units has centered on the increase in extracellular potassium (K^+) with storage, the decline in 2,3-DPG with storage, and the safety of various components of additive solutions, in particular mannitol and dextrose. It is worthwhile to briefly address each of these issues because they guide clinical practice.

In donor units with an additive solution (Chapter 10), such as AS-1 or AS-3, extracellular K^+ levels increase up to 50 mEq/L by day 42 of storage.[54, 55] Although this is seemingly a very high level, the amount of bioavailable K^+ actually transfused is much smaller. For instance, 15 mL of red blood cells suspended in an additive solution will result in the infusion of approximately 0.3 mEq of K^+ to the newborn. Contrast this to an infant's normal requirement of 2–3 mEq K^+ per kg per day and one can appreciate the amount of K^+ associated with a red blood cell transfusion is very small and not associated with the development of hyperkalemia. It is, however, important to note this does not apply to larger volume transfusions or transfusions given rapidly, such as those associated with exchange transfusion, *extracorporeal membrane oxygenation (ECMO)*, or cardiopulmonary bypass circuits. Transfusion during ECMO is discussed later.

The depletion of 2,3-DPG from stored red blood cell units has been viewed as detrimental to infants. The low 2,3-DPG results in the reduced ability of hemoglobin to offload oxygen compared to fresh red blood cells. However, with small-volume transfusions, levels of 2,3-DPG increase rapidly after transfusion as long as sufficient glucose and phosphate are available.[55] On the other hand, transfusion of larger volumes of blood, such as exchange transfusion, can be associated with impaired oxygen delivery and the use of fresh red blood cell units is indicated for these situations in newborns.

As with extracellular K^+ and 2,3-DPG, the quantity and type of additive solutions present in extended storage media for red blood cells are not considered dangerous for small-volume neonatal transfusions. Studies have shown that newborns, even preterm newborns, are able to adequately metabolize or excrete the various additive components associated with small-volume transfusions up to 20 mL/kg.[49, 54, 55] However, data on the toxicities of additive solutions associated with large-volume transfusions or transfusions to extremely ill premature neonates is lacking; therefore, many institutions consider it prudent to avoid exposing these neonates to large quantities of extended storage media in red blood cell units until more is known about the effects. The use of volume-reduced red blood cell units may be indicated for critical preterm babies. Volume reduction may be as simple as storing the red blood cell product upside down and using careful manipulation to prepare the aliquot from the "settled" product to obtain red blood cells with less additive solution. Alternatively, the red blood cell product or aliquot may be centrifuged and the additive solution removed.

Therefore, based on several studies, the use of stored red blood cell units is appropriate for small-volume infant transfusions. An advantage of using stored red blood cell units up to the end of their usual expiration date is decreased donor exposure because 1 unit of red blood cells can be used for multiple small-volume transfusions over the course of several weeks. Regardless of the age of the red blood cell product used, the unit should be leukocyte-reduced, preferably by prestorage filtration. Consideration should be given to the use of irradiated, CMV-reduced-risk, and hemoglobin S–negative red blood cell units, if appropriate.

Special Products

Due to the immaturity of the neonate's immune system, it may be necessary to provide red blood cell units that are either irradiated and/or CMV-reduced-risk. Irradiated cellular blood components, including whole blood, red blood cells, platelets, and granulocytes, are indicated for any infant at risk for transfusion-associated graft versus host disease (TA-GVHD). This includes babies with congenital immunodeficiency disorders or hematologic malignancies and those receiving transfusions from blood relatives.[49] Because it may be problematic to clinically identify which infants will have an immunodeficiency disorder until they become ill, some hospitals choose to transfuse all infants less than 4 months of age with irradiated cellular blood products. While this practice may be difficult to justify based on statistical data alone, it prevents inadvertently transfusing an at-risk infant with nonirradiated blood products, resulting in serious sequelae or death.

Cytomegalovirus (CMV) infection can be a devastating disease in a fetus or newborn. Infants at risk for severe CMV infection include premature babies, those born to CMV-seronegative mothers, and those with congenital immunodeficiency disorders. However, all newborns are considered at risk for CMV infection because any protective CMV antibodies passively acquired from the mother will eventually be lost and CMV is ubiquitous among humans. Therefore, it is common practice to provide CMV-reduced-risk components to infants.[49] Because CMV is associated primarily with leukocytes, effective leukocyte reduction provides a product with minimal risk of CMV transmission. Alternatively, red blood cell units from CMV-seronegative donors may be used or the combination of blood from CMV-seronegative donors that has been leukoreduced.

☑ **CHECKPOINT 14-11**

What kinds of patients are at risk for transfusion-associated graft versus host disease (TA-GVHD)?

Transfusion Administration

The weight of the infant determines the volume of the blood transfusion. Transfusing 10–15 mL red blood cells/kg of body weight is expected to increase the hemoglobin level by approximately 2.0–3.0 g/dL (20-30 g/L).[49] The rate of transfusion depends on the clinical condition of the baby and while it should be given slowly, it should allow completion of the transfusion within 4 hours or be split into smaller volumes. All red blood cell units must be administered through a standard blood filter of 170–260 microns. Due to the small volume of red blood cells needed, this filtration step may be performed in the blood bank at the time of aliquot preparation by priming the filter first with extra blood above the amount needed for the transfusion. Small aliquots of red blood cells can be prepared by attaching one or more satellite bags using a sterile connecting device or by using a red blood cell unit with multiple integrally attached satellite bags. This allows for preparation of aliquots in a closed system so that the original expiration date of the unit can be maintained. For transfusion services without a sterile connecting device, the blood center supplying the hospital can be requested to attach additional satellite bags. Alternatively, red blood cells can be aliquoted into a syringe. If this results in an open or nonsterile system, the original unit expires 24 hours from the time the syringe is prepared. The expiration time of the syringe aliquot is dependent on the type used but will be 24 hours or less.

Recombinant Human Erythropoietin

Since a low erythropoietin (EPO) level, rather than decreased bone marrow production, is a major cause of anemia of prematurity, the use of exogenous EPO in premature infants has undergone extensive evaluation. Studies have shown that the administration of recombinant human erythropoietin (rHuEPO) decreases the need for red blood cell transfusion in some, but not all, infants.[56] To produce an adequate number of red blood cells, supplemental iron therapy is required when EPO is administered.

TRANSFUSION OF OTHER BLOOD COMPONENTS

There are instances when neonates and babies require a transfusion of a blood product other than red blood cells. The components that are worthy of discussion here are platelets, granulocytes, and components necessary to restore hemostasis.

Platelets

Platelet transfusion is indicated for thrombocytopenia or for qualitative defects in platelet function. Adults may be able to tolerate a platelet count as low as $10 \times 10^3/\mu L$ ($10 \times 10^9/L$), but newborns often cannot. This is particularly true of premature babies who are at higher risk of intraventricular hemorrhage (IVH) due to the immaturity of the brain. In general, for the neonatal population, a platelet count of $50 \times 10^3/\mu L$ ($50 \times 10^9/L$) is considered the minimum to maintain daily hemostasis.[49] However, the sick premature baby may require a platelet count as high as $100 \times 10^3/\mu L$ ($100 \times 10^9/L$) to prevent bleeding.[53] Platelets selected for transfusion should be leukocyte-reduced and ABO compatible with the baby, when possible. $Rh_0(D)$

negative infants are transfused with $Rh_0(D)$ negative platelets, again when possible. Dosage is calculated based on body weight; 5–10 mL of platelets/kg of the baby's body weight should increase the platelet count by $50–100 \times 10^3/\mu L$ ($50–100 \times 10^9/L$). An aliquot may be prepared or a single platelet unit may be dispensed. Volume reduction of platelets is generally not recommended because centrifugation has been shown to activate platelets and reduce recovery. As with red blood cell units, consideration should be made to use irradiated and/or CMV reduced-risk platelets, if appropriate.

Granulocytes

Granulocyte transfusions are very rare. However, they are utilized more frequently in the neonatal and pediatric population than in adults. Granulocyte therapy is reserved for those with severe neutropenia, an absolute neutrophil count $<500/\mu L$, ($<0.50 \times 10^9/L$) and a documented bacterial or fungal infection unresponsive to standard antimicrobial therapy for at least 24–48 hours. In addition, there must be a reasonable chance of marrow recovery. Granulocytes for newborns are collected from CMV-seronegative donors and must be irradiated prior to transfusion to prevent transfusion-associated graft versus host disease by any donor lymphocytes present. The dose of granulocytes to administer is difficult to determine, but in general the children given higher doses have a better response. For an infant, a dose of 1×10^9 to 2×10^9 PMN/kg is recommended.[49] This dose is typically repeated for five daily transfusions. Because the granulocytes should be as fresh as possible and the baby is critically ill, they are often transfused immediately after collection and before infectious disease testing can be completed. Because transfusion should occur no later than 24 hours after collection due to the short lifespan of the granulocytes, the granulocytes need to be delivered promptly. There must be close coordination between the transfusion service and the collecting facility to ensure that either the donors have been prescreened and tested or an emergency release is signed if the infectious disease testing is not yet completed. Due to the content of red blood cells in a granulocyte concentrate, it is usually necessary to perform a crossmatch. Granulocytes are administered through a standard blood filter; a leukocyte-reduction filter must never be used or the granulocytes will be lost.

TRANSFUSION TO ENHANCE HEMOSTASIS

Although newborns have lower levels of some coagulation factors at birth, transfusion of fresh frozen plasma (FFP) for newborns is generally used to prevent bleeding when multiple factors are needed, such as the vitamin K–dependent factors. Current guidelines recommend FFP transfusion primarily for bleeding due to either an acquired deficiency of coagulation factors such as DIC or a congenital factor deficiency for which no specific factor concentrates are available. FFP is not indicated for volume expansion alone. FFP should be ABO compatible with the infant. The typical dose is 10–15 mL/kg of body weight, which will result in a 15–20% increase in factor levels.[49] These small doses are typically prepared in aliquots, either in a satellite bag or a syringe.

Cryoprecipitate serves as a concentrated source of fibrinogen, factor VIII, factor XIII, and von Willebrand factor (vWF). In newborns, as in adults, it is transfused primarily for hypofibrinogenemia. Cryoprecipitate should be ABO compatible with the infant. A dose of 1–2 units/10 kg of body weight will increase the fibrinogen level by 60–100 mg/dL (1.76-2.94 μmol/L).[53] Due to the small volume (approximately 15 mL) present in a single unit of cryoprecipitate, it is usually not necessary to aliquot it into smaller volumes. A standard blood filter should be used for transfusion of both FFP and cryoprecipitate.

NEONATAL POLYCYTHEMIA

Polycythemia in an infant is defined as hematocrit of 65% (0.65) or higher.[2] There is a higher incidence of neonatal polycythemia in babies born at high altitudes, in small-for-gestational-age infants, in the recipient twin of a twin-to-twin transfusion, after delayed clamping of the umbilical cord, and in infants born to diabetic mothers. In addition, babies with cyanotic congenital heart disease may develop secondary polycythemia as a mechanism to compensate for decreased oxygen delivery to the tissues. Many infants are asymptomatic; however, in others the elevated hematocrit can result in a hyperviscosity syndrome, with respiratory distress, seizures, and renal failure. In such instances, it may be necessary to perform a therapeutic phlebotomy to reduce the red blood cell mass. In adult patients, therapeutic phlebotomy usually involves just the removal of whole blood. In contrast, neonatal patients often require replacement of the whole blood removed with saline or albumin in order to maintain an adequate blood volume.

EXTRACORPOREAL MEMBRANE OXYGENATION (ECMO)

Extracorporeal membrane oxygenation (ECMO) is a form of cardiopulmonary bypass providing artificial oxygenation to an infant with severe respiratory failure or congenital heart disease.[56, 57] The lungs of a premature baby are often not fully developed or may be otherwise compromised, resulting in inadequate delivery of oxygen to the blood and tissues. ECMO allows the infant's blood to be cycled through a mechanical pump that serves as an artificial lung. There carbon dioxide is removed and the blood is oxygenated and returned to the body, protecting the infant's lungs while they develop or heal. Figure 14-6 ▦ is a schematic of an ECMO circuit. It is unusual for an infant to be on ECMO for longer than 1–2 weeks. ECMO can be performed on adult patients, but the vast majority of procedures involve neonatal or pediatric patients.

Because ECMO involves cycling the blood through a mechanical device with systemic heparinization of the patient, it is not surprising blood components are required to support the baby. Set transfusion guidelines do not exist and standard blood orders vary by institution, often dependent upon the neonatologist and the particular ECMO

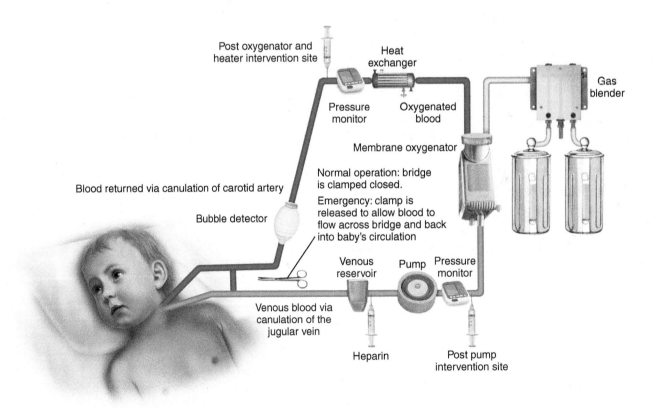

▦ FIGURE 14-6 Extracorporeal Membrane Oxygenation Circuit
This is a schematic representation of the components of an example extracorporeal membrane oxygenation (ECMO) circuit. The ECMO circuit replaces the functions of the heart via the pump and the lungs via the oxygenator. ECMO is primarily used to allow either a baby's heart and/or lungs to rest and heal when the baby is suffering from a reversible, severe cardiac or pulmonary condition. Examples of conditions where neonatal ECMO has been used include congenital diaphragmatic hernia that was not surgically repaired *in utero* and meconium aspiration.
Not drawn to scale.

circuit used. However, a common order would be 2 or 3 units of red blood cells to prime the circuit, 1 unit of FFP, and a portion of a unit of single-donor platelets. Some circuits require priming with albumin prior to the red blood cell prime. Pretransfusion testing should be performed in accordance with the institution's standard operating procedures and the red blood cell units should be fresh. Studies have shown red blood cells preserved in additive solutions such as AS1, AS3, and SAGM (not available in the United States) are safe to use on an ECMO circuit despite the high volume. Transfusion services that are concerned about additive solutions may request collection of red blood cells in CPD, CPDA1, or C2PD (not available in the United States) from their blood supplier. Nonadditive units have an increased hematocrit and viscosity compared to units with additives and FFP may be added to the unit by the transfusion service, resulting in a whole blood substitute.

Depending on birth weight, some newborns undergoing ECMO may be considered at high risk for transfusion-associated CMV infection and GVHD. Therefore, many centers choose to provide CMV-reduced-risk and irradiated cellular blood components for all babies on ECMO. During ECMO, most physicians elect to maintain the platelet count between 80 and $150 \times 10^3/\mu L$ (80-150 $\times 10^9$/L) and the hemoglobin between 10.0 and 12.0 g/dL (100–120 g/L).[47] Coagulation is often monitored by the activated clotting time (ACT) assay and point-of-care devices for this assay are available, which are sensitive to heparin. FFP and cryoprecipitate are administered on an "as-needed" basis. Close communication between the ECMO team and the transfusion service staff is vital to providing the optimal blood components in a timely manner.

Review of the Main Points

- Hemolytic disease of the fetus and newborn (HDFN) results in the shortened lifespan of the fetus' or baby's red blood cells due to maternal antibodies.
- Rh incompatibility between an $Rh_0(D)$-negative mother and an $Rh_0(D)$-positive baby used to be the most common cause of HDFN, resulting in potentially serious consequences for the second or later babies. Rh-immune globulin (RhIg) prophylaxis prevents the formation of anti-$Rh_0(D)$ in most mothers and thus prevents HDFN in their next $Rh_0(D)$-positive pregnancy.
- ABO incompatibility is now the number one cause of HDFN and is most severe in A or B babies of O mothers. It is seldom as severe as HDFN due to other blood group antibodies.
- The mother's IgG antibody can cross the placenta and cause destruction of the fetal red blood cells with increased anemia, resulting in the need for intrauterine transfusion if the anemia becomes severe enough.
- Bilirubin from red blood cell breakdown in the fetus is removed by the mother's circulation before birth, but may accumulate to dangerous levels after birth during the period before the newborn's liver becomes fully functional.
- High levels of bilirubin can be treated by phototherapy or, when very elevated, by exchange transfusion to prevent permanent brain damage and serious neurologic sequelae.

- The newborn has an immature immune system and most antibodies present are from the mother for the first 4 months of life.
- During the first 4 months of a baby's life, ABO red blood cell typing and antibody screen testing need only be done one time per hospital visit as the baby's immune system is not well developed enough to make antibodies.
- Newborns are very sensitive to volume changes and low platelet counts; therefore, laboratory collection volumes are carefully measured and titrated with the transfusion of blood products to avoid hypo- or hypervolemia.
- Many institutions transfuse fresh group O red blood cell units that are CMV-risk-reduced and irradiated to decrease the risk of CMV infections or transfusion-associated graft versus host disease (TA-GVHD) in immune-suppressed newborns.
- Erythropoietin (EPO) production in newborns is less responsive to hypoxia and is made primarily in the liver until several months after birth, rather than in the kidney as in adults. Recombinant EPO with iron supplementation may prevent or reduce the need for transfusions in some newborns.
- Newborns have different transfusion requirements, especially volume per body weight, than adults.
- Extracorporeal membrane oxygenation (ECMO) is a form of cardiopulmonary bypass providing artificial oxygenation to an infant with severe respiratory failure or congenital heart disease.

Review Questions

1. Select the conditions that are necessary for production of maternal antibody in HDFN. (Objective #1)

   A. Antibody must be IgG in class.

   B. Antibody must not cross the placenta.

   C. Mother must possess the corresponding antigen that is present on fetal red blood cells.

   D. Fetal antigen must be developed before birth.

2. Choose the class of immunoglobulin that is implicated in HDFN. (Objective #2)

   A. IgA

   B. IgM

   C. IgG

   D. IgE

3. Which of the following is *not* characteristic of HDFN due to ABO incompatibility? (Objective #3)

   A. Occurs exclusively in group O mothers

   B. Causes severe hemolysis

   C. Antibody specificity is anti-A or anti-B

   D. Can occur in the first pregnancy

4. Excessive levels of unconjugated bilirubin in the newborn cause a condition known as: (Objective #3)

   A. Hydrops fetalis

   B. Cerebral palsy

   C. Seizure

   D. Kernicterus

5. Choose the antigenic determinants that affect the severity of HDFN: (Objective #3)

   A. Late development of fetal antigen

   B. Density of fetal antigen

   C. Structure of fetal antigen

   D. Presence of tissue antigens

6. Which of the following could be a harmful consequence of the elimination of the weak D test in serological studies on maternal blood specimen? (Objective #6)

   A. Production of anti-$Rh_0(D)$ in a mother with a rare partial D phenotype

   B. Development of multiple Rh alloantibodies

   C. Administration of RhIg to an $Rh_0(D)$-positive mother

   D. Reduced potency of anti-$Rh_0(D)$ reagent

7. A low-risk method of predicting the *risk* of HDFN is: (Objective #7)

   A. Fetal blood phenotyping

   B. Amniocentesis

   C. Paternal antigen typing

   D. Cordocentesis

8. Which type of measurement is considered least invasive in monitoring the presence of anemia in HDFN? (Objective #8)

   A. Doppler

   B. Amniocentesis

   C. Percutaneous umbilical blood sampling (PUBS)

   D. Cordocentesis

9. Select *two* methods that may be used in the antepartum treatment of HDFN: (Objective #9)

   A. Amniocentesis

   B. Intrauterine transfusion

   C. Whole blood exchange transfusion

   D. Plasma exchange transfusion

10. The results of a prenatal work-up on a 32-year-old female who is 26 weeks pregnant reveal:

    Blood type A, Rh+

    Antibody screen = positive, with anti-K identified

    An intrauterine transfusion is requested for confirmed fetal anemia. What type of blood should be chosen for the transfusion? (Objective #18)

    A. Blood type A, $Rh_0(D)$ positive; Kell antigen negative

    B. Blood type A, $Rh_0(D)$ negative; Kell antigen positive

    C. Blood type O, $Rh_0(D)$; Kell antigen positive

    D. Blood type O, $Rh_0(D)$ negative; Kell antigen negative

11. Match the indications for Rh-immune globulin (RhIg) administration: (Objective #10)

    _____ $Rh_0(D)$-positive woman who is 28 weeks pregnant   A. Candidate for RhIg

    _____ $Rh_0(D)$-negative woman with ectopic pregnancy at 8 weeks   B. Not a candidate for RhIg

    _____ $Rh_0(D)$-negative woman who just gave birth to $Rh_0(D)$ positive infant

    _____ $Rh_0(D)$-positive woman with fetal demise at 18 weeks

12. When an $Rh_0(D)$-negative mother gives birth to an $Rh_0(D)$ positive infant, RhIg should be administered within _____ of delivery. (Objective #10)

    A. 24 hours

    B. 36 hours

    C. 48 hours

    D. 72 hours

13. Results of a Kleihauer-Betke test reveal 3.2% fetal cells in the maternal circulation. How many doses of RhIg should be administered if the maternal blood volume is 5,000 mL? (Objective #11)

    A. 4

    B. 5

    C. 6

    D. 7

14. A mother is blood type O, $Rh_0(D)$ negative. Her antibody screen is positive and anti-C is identified in the plasma. Cord blood results on her newborn baby boy reveal that the blood type is A, $Rh_0(D)$ positive, DAT is negative. Select the *true* statements. (Objective #10)

A. The mother is a candidate for RhIg.

B. The mother is not a candidate for RhIg.

C. The baby is suffering from HDFN due to anti-C.

D. The baby does not have HDFN.

15. Which of the following is a treatment that is typically used for a mild case of HDFN? (Objective #3)

A. Exchange transfusion

B. Cordocentesis

C. Phototherapy

D. ECMO

References

1. Venes D, ed. *Taber's Cyclopedic Medical Dictionary.* Philadelphia (PA): F.A. Davis Company; 2001.

2. Roback JD, ed. *Technical Manual,* 17th ed. Bethesda (MD): AABB Press; 2011.

3. Sgro M, Campbell D, Shah V. Incidence and causes of severe neonatal hyperbilirubinemia in Canada. *CMAJ* 2006; 175(6): 587–90.

4. Adams KM, Yan A, Steven AM, Nelson JL. The changing maternal "self" hypothesis: A mechanism for maternal tolerance of the fetus. *Placenta* 2007; 28: 378–82.

5. Dennery PH, Seidman DS, Stevenson DK. Neonatal hyperbilirubinemia. *NEJM* 2001; 344: 581–90.

6. Shapiro SM. Bilirubin toxicity in the developing nervous system. *Pediatr Neurol* 2003; 29: 410–21.

7. Klein HG, Anstee DJ. *Mollison's Blood Transfusion in Clinical Medicine,* 11th ed. Malden (MA): Blackwell Publishing; 2005.

8. Bowman J. Thirty-five years of Rh prophylaxis. *Transfusion* 2003; 43: 1661–66.

9. Hartwell EA. Use of Rh immune globulin: ASCP practice parameter. *Am J Clin Pathol* 1998; 110: 281–92.

10. Hadley, AG. Laboratory assays for predicting the severity of haemolytic disease of the fetus and newborn. *Transplant Immunology* 2002; 10: 191–98.

11. Moise KJ. Non-anti-D antibodies in red-cell alloimmunization. *Eur J Obstet Gynecol Repro Biol* 2000; 92: 750–81.

12. Vaughan JI, Manning M, Warwick RM, Letsky EA, Murray NA, Roberts IA. Inhibition of erythroid progenitor cells by anti-Kell antibodies in fetal alloimmune anemia. *N Engl J Med* 1998; 338: 798–803.

13. Novotny VMJ, Kanhai HHH, Overbeeke MAM, Schlamam-Nijp A, Harvey MS, Brand A. Misleading results in the determination of haemolytic disease of the newborn using antibody titration and ADCC in a woman with anti-Lub. *Vox Sang* 1992; 62: 49–52.

14. Skidmore I, Hadley AG. The effect of specificity on the functional activity of red cell-bound blood group antibodies. *Transfus Med* 1996; 6(supl 2): 26.

15. Simister NE. Placental transport of immunoglobulin G. *Vaccine* 2003; 21(24): 3365–69.

16. Antohe F, Radulescu, L, Gafencu A, Ghetie V, Simionescu M. Expression of functionally active FcRn and the differentiated biodirectional transport of IgG in human placental endothelial cells. *Human Immunology* 2001; 62: 93–105.

17. Hashira S, Okitsu-Negishi S, Yoshino K. Placental transfer of IgG subclasses in a Japanese population. *Pediatrics International* 2000; 42: 337–42.

18. Lambin P, Debbia M, Puillandre P, Brossard Y. IgG1 and IgG3 anti-D in maternal serum and on the RBCs of infants suffering from HDN: Relationship with the severity of the disease. *Transfusion* 2002; 42(12): 1537–46.

19. Zupanska B, Brojer E, Richards Y, Lenkiewics B, Seyfried H, Howell P. Serological and immunological characteristics of maternal anti-Rh(D) antibodies in predicting the severity of haemolytic disease of the newborn. *Vox Sang* 1989; 56: 247–53.

20. Carson TH, ed. *Standards for blood banks and transfusion services.* 27th edition. Bethesda (MD): AABB Press, 2011.

21. Judd WJ. Practice guidelines for prenatal and perinatal immunohematology, revisited. *Transfusion* 2001; 41: 1445–52.

22. Filbey D, Berseus O, Carlberg M. Occurrence of anti-D in Rh(D)-positive mothers and the outcome of the newborns. *Acta Obstet Gynecol Scand* 1996; 75: 585–87.

23. ACOG Practice Bulletin #75: management of alloimmunization. *Obstet Gynecol* 2006; 108(2): 457–64.

24. Eder AF. Update on HDFN: new information on long-standing controversies. *Immunohematology* 2006; 22(4): 188–95.

25. Avent ND, Martin PG. Kell typing by allele-specific PCR (ASP). *Br J Haemotol* 1996; 93: 728–30.

26. Lo YMD, Corbetta N, Chamberlain PF, Rai V, Sargent IL, Redman CW, Wainscoat JS. Presence of fetal DNA in maternal plasma and serum. *Lancet* 1997; 350: 485–87.

27. Lo YMD. Fetal Rh(D) genotyping from maternal plasma. *Ann Med* 1999; 31: 308–12.

28. Daniels G, Finning K, Martin P, Soothill P. Fetal blood group genotyping from DNA from maternal plasma: an important advance in the management and prevention of haemolytic disease of the fetus and newborn. *Vox Sang* 2004; 87: 225–32.

29. Nelson M, Eagle C, Langshaw M, Popp H, Kronenberg H. Genotyping fetal DNA by non-invasive means: extraction from maternal plasma. *Vox Sang* 2001; 80: 112–6.

30. Randen I, Hauge R, Kjeldsen-Kragh J, Fagerhol MK. Prenatal genotyping of *RH(D)* and *SRY* using maternal blood. *Vox Sang* 2003; 85: 300–6.

31. Arndt PA, Garratty G. A retrospective analysis of the value of monocyte monolayer assay results for predicting the clinical significance of blood group antibodies. *Transfusion* 2004; 44: 1273–81.

32. Westhoff CM (Chair, Scientific Section Coordinating Committee). *Guidelines for prenatal and perinatal immunohematology.* Bethesda (MD): AABB Press; 2005.

33. Moise KJ. Management of Rhesus alloimmunization in pregnancy. *Obstet Gynecol* 2002; 100: 600–11.

34. Oepkes D, Seaward PG, Vandenbussche F, Windrim R, Kingdom J, Beyene J, Hanhai HH, Ohlsson A, Ryan G. Doppler ultrasonography versus amniocentesis to predict fetal anemia. *N Engl J Med* 2006; 355; 2: 156–64.

35. Mari G, Andrignolo A, Abuhamad AZ, Pirhonen J, Jones DC, Ludmirsky A, Copel JA. Diagnosis of fetal anemia with Doppler ultrasound in pregnancy complicated by maternal blood group immunization. *Ultrasound Obstet Gynecol* 1995; 5: 400–5.

36. Mari G. Noninvasive diagnosis by Doppler ultrasonography of fetal anemia due to maternal red-cell alloimmunization. *N Engl J Med* 2000; 342: 9–14.

37. Szczepiorkowski ZM, Winters JL, Bandarenko N, Haewon KC, Linenberger ML, Marques MB, Sarode R, Schwartz J, Weinstein R, Shaz BH. Guidelines on the use of therapeutic apheresis in clinical practice–Evidence-based approach from the Apheresis Applications Committee of the American Society for Apheresis. *J Clinical Apheresis* 2010; 25: 83–177.

38. Fernandez-Jimenez MC, Jimenez-Marco MT, Hernandez D, Gonzalez A, Omenaca F, de la Camara C. Treatment with plasmapheresis and intravenous immunoglobulin in pregnancies complicated with anti-PP_1P^k or anti-K immunization: A report of two patients. *Vox Sang* 2001; 80: 117–20.

39. von Baeyer H. Plasmapheresis in immune hematology: review of clinical outcome data with respect to evidence-based medicine and clinical experience. *Therapeutic Apheresis and Dialysis* 2003; 7(1): 127–40.

40. Kumpel, BM. On the immunologic basis of Rh immune globulin (anti-D) prophylaxis. *Transfusion* 2006; 46: 1652–56.

41. Freda VJ, Gorman JG, Pollack W. Successful prevention of experimental Rh sensitization in man with an anti-Rh gamma2-globulin antibody preparation: A preliminary report. *Transfusion* 1964; 4: 26–32.

42. Kumpel BM, Elson CJ. Mechanism of anti-D-mediated immune suppression – a paradox awaiting resolution? *Trends Immunol* 2001; 22: 26–31.

43. Branch DR, Shabani F, Lund N, Denomme GA. Antenatal administration of Rh-immune globulin causes significant increases in the immunomodulatory cytokines transforming growth factor-β and prostaglandin E2. *Transfusion* 2006; 46: 1316–22.

44. Urbaniak SJ. The scientific basis of antenatal prophylaxis. *Br J Obstet Gynaecol* 1998; 105(suppl 18): 11–8.

45. Bichler J, Schondorfer G, Pabst G, Andresen I. Pharmacokinetics of anti-D IgG in pregnant Rh(D)-negative women. *Br J Obstet Gynaecol* 2003; 110: 39–45.

46. American Academy of Pediatrics, Subcommittee on Hyperbilirubinemia. Clinical practice guideline: Management of hyperbilirubinemia in the newborn infant 35 or more weeks of gestation. *Pediatrics* 2004; 114: 297–316.

47. Dennery PH, Seidman DS, Stevenson DK. Neonatal hyperbilirubinemia. *NEJM* 2001; 344: 581–90.

48. Smitherman H, Stark AR, Bhutani VK. Early recognition of neonatal hyperbilirubinemia and its emergent management. *Semin Fetal Neonatal Med* 2006; 11: 214–24.

49. Roseff SD, Gotschall JL eds. *Pediatric Transfusion: A Physician's Handbook*, 3rd ed. Bethesda (MD): AABB Press; 2009.

50. Crowley J, Ways P, Jones JW. Human fetal erythrocyte and plasma lipids. *Journal of Clinical Investigation* 1965; 44(6): 989–97.

51. Strauss RG. Pathogenetic mechanisms of the anaemia of prematurity. *ISBT Science Series* 2006; 1: 9–10.

52. Bain A, Blackburn S. Issues in transfusing preterm infants in the NICU. *J Perinat Neonat Nurs* 2004; 18(2): 170–82.

53. New HV. Paediatric transfusion. *Vox Sang* 2006; 90: 1–9.

54. Luban NLC. Neonatal red blood cell transfusions. *Vox Sang* 2004; 87(suppl 2): S184–S188.

55. Strauss RG. Data-driven blood banking practices for neonatal RBC transfusions. *Transfusion* 2000; 40: 1528–40.

56. Mielck F, Quintel M. Extracorporeal membrane oxygenation. *Curr Opin Crit Care* 2005; 11: 87–93.

57. Petrou S, Edwards L. Cost effectiveness analysis of neonatal extracorporeal membrane oxygenation based on four year results from the UK Collaborative ECMO Trial. *Arch Dis Child Fetal Neonatal* 2004; 89: 263–8.

58. RhoGAM Symposium. Complete proceedings of symposium held in New York, NY, April 17, 1969. Printed by Ortho Diagnostics.

Additional Resources

1. Herman JH, Manno CS. *Pediatric Transfusion Therapy.* Bethesda (MD): AABB Press; 2002.

2. Cunningham FG, Leveno KJ, Bloom SL, Hauth JC, Rouse DJ. *Williams Obstetrics*, 22nd ed. New York: McGraw-Hill Professional; 2005. pp. 1057–60, 1093–1141.

3. Behrman RE, Kliegman RM, Jenson HB (eds.) *Nelson Textbook of Pediatrics*, 16th ed. Philadelphia (PA): W.B. Saunders Company; 2000. pp. 521–5, 1456–1525.

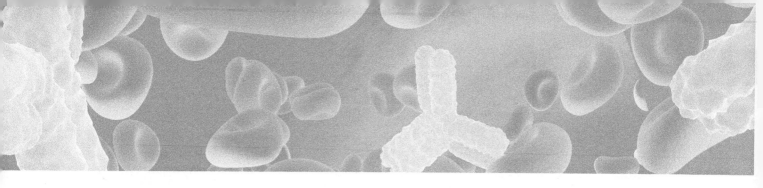

15

Autoimmune and Drug-Induced Immune Hemolytic Anemias

MARK K. FUNG AND MICHAEL RICHARD LEWIS

Chapter Objectives

Upon completion of this chapter, the student will be able to:

1. Identify and describe the laboratory tests that can be used to establish the presence of autoimmune hemolytic anemia (AIHA).
2. State the purpose and principle of the Donath-Landsteiner test.
3. Interpret direct antiglobulin test (DAT) results when assessing anemia.
4. Discuss the limitations of the DAT.
5. List the clinical findings that are associated with red blood cell hemolysis.
6. Identify and compare and contrast the clinical presentation, laboratory features, and treatment options for warm autoimmune hemolytic anemia (WAIHA), cold agglutinin syndrome (CAS), mixed autoimmune hemolytic anemia (MAIHA), paroxysmal cold hemoglobinuria (PCH), DAT-negative autoimmune hemolytic anemia, and drug-induced immune hemolytic anemia (DIIHA).
7. List common conditions that can cause secondary AIHA.
8. Describe possible mechanisms underlying drug-induced immune hemolytic anemia (DIIHA).
9. Describe two laboratory methods used to test for DIIHA.
10. Identify and describe the problems associated with antibody screen and crossmatch procedures commonly encountered when a patient has an AIHA.
11. Describe the procedures used to select blood for transfusion to patients with (AIHA).

Key Terms

Adsorption
Alloadsorption
Allogeneic adsorption
Anisopoikilocytosis
Antigen typing
Autoadsorption
Autoantibody (autoantibodies)
Autoimmune hemolytic anemia (AIHA)
Autologous adsorption

Biphasic hemolysin
Cold agglutinin(s)
Cold agglutinin disease (CAD)
Cold agglutinin syndrome (CAS)
Cold autoimmune hemolytic anemia (CAIHA)
Cyanosis
Drug-induced immune hemolytic anemia (DIIHA)

Eluate
Elution
Hapten
Hemolysis
Hemophagocytosis
Hyperhemolysis
Immune hemolysis
Immune-mediated hemolytic
  anemia

Mixed autoimmune hemolytic
  anemia (MAIHA)
Panreactive pattern
Paroxysmal cold hemoglobin-
  uria (PCH)
Transfusion trigger
Warm autoimmune hemolytic
  anemia (WAIHA)

CASE IN POINT

BH is a healthy 27-year-old male who works in a plastic factory. Three weeks ago he wasn't feeling well, so he went to see his primary care physician. The doctor ordered some bloodwork and noted that his hemoglobin and hematocrit were in the low normal range at 13.8 g/dL (138 g/L) and 42% (0.42). After testing was complete, the physician diagnosed BH with a common cold. The cold symptoms went away, but BH was still feeling extremely fatigued and short of breath. In addition, he noted that his urine was very dark. He returned to his physician's office for another visit. The doctor noted that BH had an enlarged spleen and a bit of tachycardia, so additional laboratory testing was ordered. The results showed that BH now had a hemoglobin of 6.7 g/dL (37g/L) and hematocrit of 20% (0.20). The patient was immediately admitted to the hospital where both anemia and hemolysis work-ups were performed.

What's Ahead?

There are a number of conditions when a person's immune system will make antibodies that attach and destroy corresponding antigens. If the antibodies are directed against an antigen on the red blood cell membrane, this typically results in the destruction of red blood cells, which is known as **hemolysis**, and subsequent anemia. Hemolysis due to an immune process is often referred to as **immune hemolysis**. Individuals who make antibodies against antigens on their own red blood cells (known as **autoantibodies**) with resultant hemolysis suffer from **autoimmune hemolytic anemia (AIHA)**. Some individuals experience anemia as a result of taking certain medications. This condition is called **drug-induced immune hemolytic anemia (DIIHA)**. Because both types of anemia result in destruction of red blood cells and are immune based, the general term, **immune-mediated hemolytic anemia**, is often used to describe them.

This chapter addresses the following questions:

- What laboratory tests are associated with autoimmune hemolytic anemias (AIHAs)?
- What laboratory tests are associated with drug-induced immune hemolytic anemia (DIIHA)?
- What conditions fall into the category of warm autoimmune hemolytic anemia (WAIHA)?
- What are the similarities and differences amongst the various WAIHAs?
- What are the three categories of DIIHA?
- What is the latest theory associated with DIIHA?
- What are the key issues regarding transfusion support and laboratory investigation of AIHAs and DIIHAs?

LABORATORY TESTS ASSOCIATED WITH AUTOIMMUNE HEMOLYTIC ANEMIA (AIHA)

There are a number of laboratory tests used to diagnose and monitor treatment of autoimmune hemolytic anemias (AIHAs). Each of these tests is introduced and described in the following sections.

Direct Antiglobulin Test (DAT)

The direct antiglobulin test (DAT) is the primary means for determining whether immune-mediated destruction of red blood cells is contributing to a patient's anemia (Chapter 3). A positive DAT result confirms the presence of red blood cells that are coated *in vivo* with antibodies or complement. Immune-mediated hemolytic anemia is characteristically associated with binding of IgG or IgM to red blood cells. It is difficult to demonstrate binding of IgM directly, but IgM almost always fixes complement.[1]

Method Review

The DAT can be performed by either tube or gel technique. The anti-human globulin (AHG) used may be directed against IgG alone; complement components only, specifically anti-C3d and/or anti-C3b; or polyspecific, which is a combination of anti-IgG and anticomplement.

The initial DAT is usually performed using the polyspecific reagent. A negative result with the polyspecific reagent implies, with rare exceptions, that there is no evidence of immune destruction of red blood cells and further testing is not indicated. If the initial result is positive, anti-IgG and anticomplement reagents are used to further characterize the mechanism of immune destruction.

☑ CHECKPOINT 15-1

Which reagent antisera should be used to perform an initial DAT?

Clinical Interpretation

The DAT does not distinguish between autoantibodies and alloantibodies; for this reason, the test can be useful not only in addressing the possibility of autoimmune hemolytic anemia but also in determining whether a hemolytic or serologic transfusion reaction has occurred (Chapter 12). A positive DAT result in a patient with a history of recent transfusion should be investigated as a possible transfusion reaction, even if none was reported. On occasion, clinical suspicion of autoimmune hemolytic anemia (AIHA) leads to diagnosis of a delayed hemolytic transfusion reaction. Conversely, a positive DAT result in an anemic patient who has not been recently transfused is suggestive of an AIHA.

It is important to note that a small proportion of people will have a positive DAT in the absence of anemia; thus, a positive DAT result in isolation is not sufficient to diagnose an AIHA . This low level of clinically insignificant DAT results in the general population is the reason why DAT is rarely included in routine pretransfusion testing. Using the tube method, a positive DAT occurs in approximately 1 in 7,000 to 1 in 13,000 healthy blood donors,[2, 3] and has an incidence as high as 3.5% in hospitalized patients.[4] Consistent with the higher sensitivity of the gel method, the incidence of positive DAT results among blood donors was found to be increased 10-fold with use of this method.[5]

In general, a clinically significant AIHA would be expected to have a positive DAT result, but in rare instances the DAT is negative despite an immune-mediated cause of hemolysis.

Complement Detection

A positive anticomplement DAT is generally interpreted as the presence of an IgM antibody because clinically significant destruction of red blood cells by IgM antibodies is mediated mainly through complement activation. However, IgM antibodies are not the only cause of complement-mediated red blood cell destruction. Some IgG autoantibodies that cause AIHAs specifically, warm autoimmune hemolytic anemia and paroxysmal cold hemoglobinuria (both of which are detailed later in this chapter) and some IgG alloantibodies (e.g., anti-jk[a]) can activate complement.

Complement-mediated red blood cell destruction can also occur in the absence of antibodies, as in the case of paroxysmal nocturnal hemoglobinuria, which results from acquired loss of complement regulating proteins CD55 and CD59 on the red blood cell surface. Therefore, correlation of positive anticomplement DAT results with other clinical information or laboratory results is necessary before inferring that an IgM antibody is the cause.

> ### ☑ CHECKPOINT 15-2
> List three causes of complement mediated hemolysis.

Limitations

The DAT has several technical limitations. First, the DAT should be performed on freshly drawn specimens whenever possible. False-positive results may occur after prolonged storage, particularly with cold-reactive autoantibodies, as *in vitro* binding is enhanced during cold storage of specimens. Second, a positive DAT result is dependent on sufficient numbers of antibody or complement molecules being bound to the red blood cell surface; the test may yield a negative result if the number of bound IgG molecules per cell is less than 300–500.[6] There have been instances in which detectable numbers of IgG antibodies have been eluted from the red blood cells of patients whose DAT results were negative. Third, the DAT result will be negative if complete destruction of antibody or complement-coated red blood cells has occurred, such as in an ABO-incompatible hemolytic transfusion reaction.

In addition to the technical limitations, it is also important to point out that the DAT and the autocontrol are not equivalent. The two tests serve different purposes, though positive results for each

may share the same underlying cause in a given case. While it is common for a patient with an AIHA that is IgG-mediated to have both a positive DAT and a positive autocontrol, the close correlation of the two results may not be consistent and should not be relied upon. The DAT determines whether there is *in vivo* binding of antibodies or complement to the patient's red blood cells, while the autocontrol determines whether a pattern of antibody reactivity may be due to the presence of autoantibodies binding *in vitro*.

Finally, a positive DAT must be interpreted in the context of the patient's history, symptoms, and laboratory data. Recent findings suggest that the DAT result is a prognostic indicator of AIHA occurrence after treatment for chronic lymphocytic leukemia.[7]

> ### ☑ CHECKPOINT 15-3
> Are the DAT and autocontrol tests equivalent? Why or why not?

Elution

Elution is the process of removing antibodies bound to red blood cells (Chapter 8). The supernatant liquid recovered from the elution procedure is referred to as the **eluate** and can be tested for the presence of antibodies. The antibody specificity found in the eluate can help distinguish a delayed hemolytic transfusion reaction from an AIHA. A specific pattern of antibody reactivity is expected in the former, while autoantibodies often result in a *panreactive pattern*, a concept defined later in this chapter within the discussion of warm autoimmune hemolytic anemias. Antibodies detected via elution are predominantly IgG and rarely IgM.

A DAT is usually performed before consideration is given to performing an elution, as a specimen with a negative DAT will rarely produce a positive eluate (an eluate containing demonstrable antibodies). A DAT that is positive only for complement is also unlikely to yield a positive eluate, as experience has shown that IgM antibodies do not usually remain stably bound and thus are not susceptible to recovery via elution.

> ### CASE IN POINT *(continued)*
>
> Both DAT and T & S testing was ordered on BH as part of the hemolysis work-up. The DAT was strongly positive with polyspecific AHG and with monospecific anti-IgG. The anticomplement antisera was negative when tested with BH's cells. An eluate was performed and yielded a panreactive pattern—the eluted antibody reacted with all cells tested. In addition, the patient's antibody screen is positive. The antibody identification also shows an antibody with panreactive pattern.
>
> 1. Given the DAT results, is the cause of the positive DAT more likely mediated by an IgG or IgM antibody?
> 2. The eluate is positive in this situation, which can indicate which two clinical diagnoses?
> 3. What questions need to be asked of the patient's history to determine which is the more likely diagnosis?

Adsorption

Adsorption refers to techniques that remove antibodies (frequently autoantibodies) from a plasma or serum specimen to aid in detecting any coexisting alloantibodies (Chapter 8). Adsorption is a selective process that requires careful choice of conditions during preparation. The basic principle is to use red blood cells or another substance to bind interfering antibodies, separating them from the remaining plasma. Different adsorption techniques have differing risks of unintentional removal of clinically significant alloantibodies and differing levels of success in complete removal of the autoantibody. Adsorptions can be divided into two categories: autoadsorption and alloadsorption.

Autoadsorption

The material used for **autoadsorption** (also referred to as **autologous adsorption**) is the patient's own red blood cells. Only autoantibodies should be removed because any alloantibodies should not bind to the patient's red blood cells, which lack the corresponding antigens. The autoadsorption procedure involves removing antibody (stripping them) from a sample of the patient's red blood cells and subsequently incubating the patient's plasma with their stripped red blood cells to allow more autoantibody to attach. The plasma is then separated from the recoated red blood cells (Chapter 8). The process may need to be repeated with fresh aliquots of the patient's stripped red blood cells to obtain complete removal of the autoantibody. Autoadsorptions should not be performed if the patient has been transfused in the previous 3 months.[8]

Alloadsorption

In situations when an autoadsorption cannot be used, an **alloadsorption** (also known as **allogeneic adsorption**) technique may be performed using donor or reagent red blood cells with known phenotypes (Chapter 8). Such cells will adsorb autoantibodies directed against antigens expressed by the cells and may also adsorb some alloantibodies. Ideally, the donor or reagent red blood cells should have a phenotype similar to the patient. However, this is not usually possible, so a combination of at least two and possibly three sets of donor or reagent red blood cells are frequently used. Any crossmatching with allogeneic adsorbed plasma should be performed with caution, as alloantibodies against high-incidence antigens, if present, are typically inadvertently removed.

An alternative alloadsorption technique is to use rabbit red blood cell preparations, which efficiently remove cold-reactive autoantibodies without the removal of most clinically significant alloantibodies (Chapter 8).[9, 10] However, rabbit erythrocyte stroma can remove some significant antibodies, including anti-B.[11, 12, 13] Patient plasma samples adsorbed with rabbit erythrocyte stroma should not be used for reverse ABO typing or in immediate spin crossmatches with group B or AB red blood cell units.

☑ CHECKPOINT 15-4

How is the alloadsorption technique different from the autoadsorption?

Antigen Typing

Identifying which antigens a patient's red blood cells lack (referred to as **antigen typing**) can assist in determining which clinically significant alloantibodies the patient is potentially capable of making (Chapter 8). This is of particular importance when autoantibodies are of sufficient titer or strength that their presence interferes with the ruling out or exclusion of various alloantibody specificities despite the use of adsorption techniques. Determining the patient's red blood cell antigen phenotype facilitates the transfusion of phenotype-matched red blood cells. By transfusing fully or partially matched red blood cells, the risk of developing an alloantibody is reduced, and this may allow for a less extensive evaluation for the presence of an alloantibody. Specifically, the need for performing otherwise laborious allogeneic adsorptions is reduced when fully matched red blood cells are transfused.[14]

Red blood cell phenotyping by serologic methods can only be performed on specimens from patients who have not been transfused within the last 3 months. If the patient has been recently transfused, isolation of endogenous reticulocytes can be used for serologic typing, or molecular methods can be used instead.[15]

Additionally, serologic phenotyping can be difficult in a patient with IgG autoantibodies bound to the red blood cells. The autoantibodies should not interfere with phenotyping reagents that are IgM and that use a direct agglutination technique. However, false-positive results will occur if the phenotyping requires the use of human anti-IgG for the indirect antiglobulin test, such as in Duffy and MNS phenotyping (Chapter 3). This obstacle can sometimes be overcome by stripping the autoantibodies from the patient's red blood cells prior to phenotyping, though the stripping methods are not always successful. If DAT-negative patient red blood cells cannot be produced, phenotyping of the remaining antigens can be achieved either through molecular methods[15] or through the use of mouse monoclonal IgG antibodies followed with antimouse IgG antibodies that are not reactive with human autoantibodies bound to the red blood cells.[16]

CASE IN POINT (continued)

You have obtained additional history on JH. It appears that his last transfusion was 27 years earlier when he was born prematurely and transfused in the neonatal intensive care unit. Given this information, delayed transfusion reaction has been ruled out and a diagnosis of autoimmune hemolytic anemia has been made.

The patient's hemoglobin and hematocrit has now dropped to 4.8 mg/dL (48 g/L) and 14% (0.14). The physician has asked that the blood bank put 4 units of red blood cells on hold for possible transfusion.

4. Is autologous or allogeneic adsorption recommended for this patient? Why?
5. You have performed molecular typing on the patient and know that he has the following antigenic makeup:

D+, C+, E−, c−, e+, K−, Jk^a−, Jk^b+, Fy^a−, Fy^b+, S+, s+

If time permits, it is preferred to give antigen-matched blood products. Which antigens would need to be matched for this patient?

Donath-Landsteiner Test

The Donath-Landsteiner test is an *in vitro* hemolysis assay for identifying the autoantibody that is associated with the autoimmune hemolytic anemia discussed later in this chapter known as *paroxysmal cold hemoglobinuria (PCH).*[17] This antibody, which is usually anti-P, is also known as a **biphasic hemolysin**, meaning that the IgG will bind optimally to red blood cells at cooler temperatures, such as 39.2° F (4° C), but will activate complement and cause hemolysis nearer body temperature of 98.6° F (37° C).

A patient blood specimen is collected without anticoagulant and kept at 98.6° F while the blood clots and during centrifugation. The separated serum is mixed with red blood cells in triplicate: one set of tubes is incubated at 39.2° F and then warmed to 98.6° F, another set is incubated at 39.2° F for the entire time period and the third set is incubated at 98.6° F for the entire time period. Often, a mixture of the patient's serum and fresh normal serum is tested in tandem because some patients with PCH have low levels of complement. A positive result occurs when hemolysis is detected in the set of tubes where the temperature changed from 39.2° F to 98.6° F. Anti-P specificity can be confirmed by repeating the 39.2° F/98.6° F test using p cells. Figure 15-1 ■ illustrates the preparation of a Donath-Landsteiner test and the expected results if the patient has paroxysmal cold hemoglobinuria.

☑ CHECKPOINT 15-5

What is a biphasic hemolysin?

LABORATORY TESTS ASSOCIATED WITH DRUG-INDUCED IMMUNE HEMOLYTIC ANEMIA (DIIHA)

Two methods can be used to test for DIIHA.[18] The first method uses patient serum, plasma, and/or eluate and drug-coated red blood cells and the second tests the patient's serum for antibodies that only react in the presence of the drug.

The first method detects antibodies that recognize drugs bound to red blood cells. In this method, drug-treated red blood cells are incubated with patient plasma/serum/eluate and tested for aggregation. Drug-treated cells are prepared by incubating group O red blood cells with a solution of the drug believed to be causing the anemia. The cells are washed and then the patient's plasma, serum, and/or an eluate prepared from the patient's cells is/are tested in parallel against both the drug-treated and untreated red blood cells. The test procedure involves incubating the plasma, serum, and/or eluate with the cells, observing for hemolysis or agglutination and then completing an indirect antiglobulin test (IAT) using a polyspecific antihuman globulin (AHG) reagent (Chapter 3). If hemolysis or agglutination at either test phase is observed with the treated cells only and not with the untreated cells, antibodies to the drug are likely the cause. Common drugs tested by this method are penicillin and some cephalosporins. Figure 15-2 ■ illustrates this test method.

The second method identifies antibodies that cause an *in vitro* reaction with red blood cells when the drug is present, but do not bind reliably or at all to red blood cells in the absence of the drug. In this method, a mixture containing the patient's serum and a solution of the drug is prepared. As a control another aliquot of the patient's serum is diluted to the same degree with saline. Other controls may include mixtures where normal serum replaces the patient's serum and/or where a combination of patient's serum and normal serum (as a source of complement) are tested. Group O red blood cells are added to each mixture. After incubation, the cells are observed for hemolysis or agglutination and then an indirect antiglobulin test using a polyspecific antihuman globulin reagent is performed. The drug is the likely cause of hemolysis if there is agglutination or hemolysis in the mixture containing the patient's serum and the drug and no reaction in the corresponding control(s). In certain instances, a drug metabolite is the etiologic agent and a urine sample containing the metabolite may be needed to demonstrate the association between hemolysis and the drug. Figure 15-3 ■ illustrates the test and control mixtures in this method.

SIGNS AND SYMPTOMS OF ANEMIA

Symptoms such as fatigue, tachycardia, and pallor may suggest to a clinician the diagnosis of anemia, which can be confirmed by measurement of the hemoglobin level as part of a complete blood count (CBC). Although there are many causes of anemia, laboratory findings such as an increased reticulocyte count, visible hemolysis in serum or plasma, elevated serum bilirubin level (especially indirect), depressed serum haptoglobin level, elevated serum lactate dehydrogenase (LDH) level, and the presence of schistocytes or spherocytes on peripheral blood smear review raise the possibility of accelerated red blood cell destruction. Depending on the mechanism underlying the hemolysis and resulting anemia, not all of these laboratory abnormalities may be detected.

CATEGORIES OF AUTOIMMUNE HEMOLYTIC ANEMIA (AIHA)

Autoimmune hemolytic anemia (AIHA) may be defined as an immunologically based anemia resulting in "self-destruction" of one's own red blood cells and subsequent hemolysis. As with many other conditions, AIHA has been the subject of numerous classification schemes over the years. Optimally, classification should facilitate the grouping of individual cases into distinct and clinically relevant categories for the differentiation of treatment or prognosis. At present, AIHA is classified based on two factors: the temperature at which the pathogenic antibodies react optimally and association with a recognized instigator of AIHA (Table 15-1 ✳).

Although autoantibody specificities are associated with each category of autoimmune hemolytic anemia, determining the specificity of the antibody is not necessary and is usually beyond the ability of most laboratories. Instead, the category of the autoimmune hemolytic anemia is identified by reviewing the patient's clinical history and test results to determine:

- The optimal temperature of the antibody reaction: cold, warm, or biphasic

- The presence or absence of complement activation

- The idiotype of the antibody: IgG or IgM.

The following sections introduce and describe the various types of AIHA.

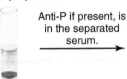
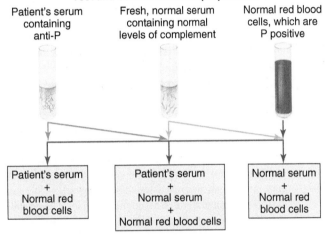

Specimen collection and preparation

Anti-P, if present, does not attach to the red blood cells because the specimen has been kept near body temperature.

Anti-P if present, is in the separated serum.

Blood specimen collected into a warmed, plain vacutainer tube. Tube placed into warm water bath immediately after collection.

After the blood has clotted, the specimen is spun in a warm centrifuge and the serum is immediately removed.

Test and control mixtures preparation

Patient's serum containing anti-P

Fresh, normal serum containing normal levels of complement

Normal red blood cells, which are P positive

Patient's serum + Normal red blood cells

Patient's serum + Normal serum + Normal red blood cells

Normal serum + Normal red blood cells

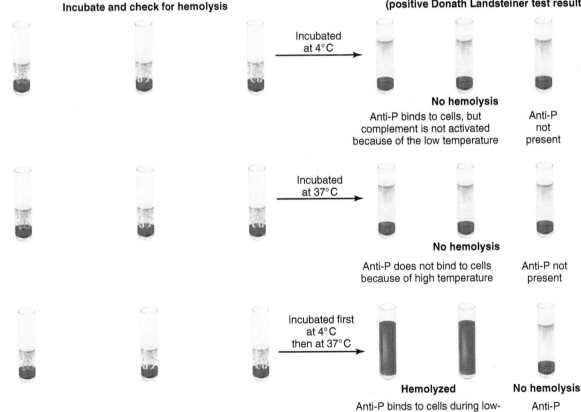

Incubate and check for hemolysis

Hemolysis pattern in a patient that has paroxysmal cold hemogobinuria (positive Donath Landsteiner test result)

Incubated at 4°C

No hemolysis

Anti-P binds to cells, but complement is not activated because of the low temperature

Anti-P not present

Incubated at 37°C

No hemolysis

Anti-P does not bind to cells because of high temperature

Anti-P not present

Incubated first at 4°C then at 37°C

Hemolyzed

Anti-P binds to cells during low-temperature incubation and then complement is activated during high-temperature incubation

No hemolysis

Anti-P not present

FIGURE 15-1 Donath-Landsteiner Test

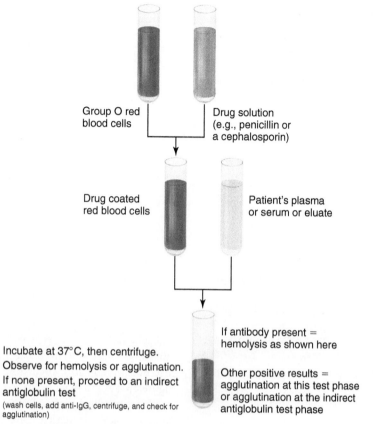

Group O red
blood cells

Drug solution
(e.g., penicillin or
a cephalosporin)

Drug coated
red blood cells

Patient's plasma
or serum or eluate

Incubate at 37°C, then centrifuge.
Observe for hemolysis or agglutination.
If none present, proceed to an indirect
antiglobulin test
(wash cells, add anti-IgG, centrifuge, and check for
agglutination)

If antibody present =
hemolysis as shown here

Other positive results =
agglutination at this test phase
or agglutination at the indirect
antiglobulin test phase

■ FIGURE 15-2   Drug-Coated Red Blood Cell Test Method

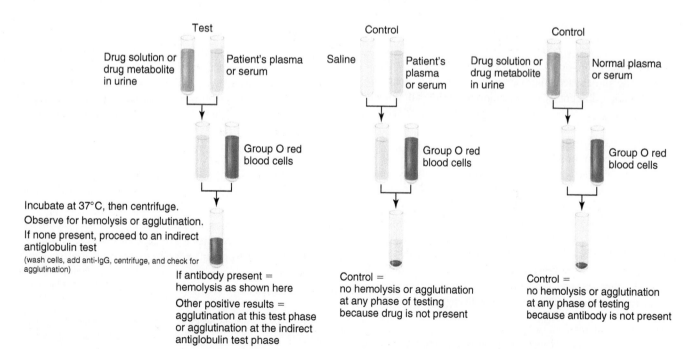

Test

Drug solution or
drug metabolite
in urine

Patient's plasma
or serum

Control

Saline

Patient's
plasma
or serum

Control

Drug solution or
drug metabolite
in urine

Normal plasma
or serum

Group O red
blood cells

Group O red
blood cells

Group O red
blood cells

Incubate at 37°C, then centrifuge.
Observe for hemolysis or agglutination.
If none present, proceed to an indirect
antiglobulin test
(wash cells, add anti-IgG, centrifuge, and check for
agglutination)

If antibody present =
hemolysis as shown here

Other positive results =
agglutination at this test phase
or agglutination at the indirect
antiglobulin test phase

Control =
no hemolysis or agglutination
at any phase of testing
because drug is not present

Control =
no hemolysis or agglutination
at any phase of testing
because antibody is not present

■ FIGURE 15-3   Addition of Drug to Test Environment Method

★ TABLE 15-1 Types of Immune-Mediated Hemolytic Anemia

Category	Incidence*	Temperature**	Associations
Warm autoimmune hemolytic anemia (WAIHA)	48–70%	98.6° F (37° C)	Lymphoproliferative disorders, autoimmune conditions, viral infections
Cold agglutinin syndrome (CAS)	16–32%	39.2–71.6° F (4–22° C) is optimal but reacts at 37° C too	*Mycoplasma pneumoniae* infection, Epstein-Barr virus infection, chronic lymphocytic leukemia, carcinomas
Mixed autoimmune hemolytic anemia (MAIHA)	<0.1–8%	Both 98.6° F (37° C) and colder	Lymphoproliferative disorders, systemic lupus erythematosus, human immunodeficiency virus infection
Paroxysmal cold hemoglobinuria (PCH)	Rare in adults; 32% in children	Biphasic	Viral infection
DAT-negative autoimmune hemolytic anemia	2–10%	98.6° F (37° C)	Lymphoproliferative disorders, autoimmune conditions, viral infections
Drug-induced immune hemolytic anemia (DIIHA)	12–18%	98.6° F (37° C)	Cephalosporin treatment, methyldopa treatment, penicillin treatment, other drug treatments

*Proportion of autoimmune hemolytic anemias (AIHAs) attributed to this category;

**Optimal temperature at which the antibody reacts; DAT, direct antiglobulin test.

☑ CHECKPOINT 15-6

How are the categories of immune-mediated hemolytic anemia identified?

Warm Autoimmune Hemolytic Anemia (WAIHA)

Warm autoimmune hemolytic anemia (WAIHA) is the most common type of autoimmune hemolytic anemia (AIHA).[18] As the name implies, primary WAIHA is mediated by autoantibodies that react optimally at 98.6° F (37° C). The antibodies are most commonly IgG, but are sometimes IgM.[19] Among the more common underlying etiologies, or causes, of secondary WAIHA are lymphoproliferative disorders and autoimmune conditions. Viral infections are another common cause and are sometimes associated with a fulminant, or severe and sudden, onset of anemia in children. The autoantibody is usually directed against a common self-antigen on the Rh proteins.

Clinical Presentation

WAIHA tends to occur most frequently in older adults. While the clinical symptoms associated with WAIHA may vary in severity, they most frequently include fatigue, dyspnea, and even angina if the hemoglobin level becomes sufficiently low. The rate of hemolysis influences the clinical picture; more rapid hemolysis may be associated with fever, dark urine, and pain in the abdomen and/or back. Physical examination often reveals splenomegaly and may also show jaundice and hepatomegaly. Lymphadenopathy may be noted in association with an underlying lymphoproliferative disorder. Venous thrombosis has been reported in cases associated with the presence of a lupus anticoagulant.[20]

Laboratory Features

Fundamental to the diagnosis of any AIHA, including WAIHA, is a decrease in hemoglobin concentration. In WAIHA the degree of anemia may be marked, with hemoglobin levels below 7 g/dl (70 g/L). Anisocytosis and macrocytosis are frequently observed and spherocytes may also be seen on review of a stained peripheral blood smear. Polychromasia is common and may be accompanied by the presence of circulating nucleated erythroid precursors. Figure 15-4 ■ is a diagrammatic representation of the features to watch for on the peripheral blood smear. While the reticulocyte count is typically increased, it may be normal or decreased because the autoantibodies may suppress erythropoeisis.[21]

Changes in numbers of leukocytes and platelets are variable; while often these counts are within the reference range, absolute neutrophilia may accompany acute hemolysis, and thrombocytosis has been reported in a minority of cases of WAIHA.[1] The combination of autoimmune hemolytic anemia and thrombocytopenia, which is called Evans syndrome, may occur in WAIHA, as may immune-mediated pancytopenia with all three cell lines decreased.[22]

The most common WAIHA testing results are those associated with a warm reactive panagglutinin (Table 15-2 ★). Typical results are of a **panreactive pattern**: positive autocontrol, positive DAT, and positive antibody screen with all reagent screen and panel cells reacting upon indirect antiglobulin test (IAT) phase testing. The eluate is usually panreactive as well.

Treatment

In addition to transfusion support as needed, first-line treatment of WAIHA includes use of corticosteroid therapy to reduce autoantibody production.[23] In steroid-refractory cases, other immunosuppressive drugs and splenectomy have been attempted. Recent publications have suggested that rituximab, which is a therapeutic monoclonal antibody directed against CD20 present on B cells, may be beneficial when there is lack of response to steroid treatment.[24, 25] Intravenous immune globulin (IVIG) therapy has been of limited benefit in this setting.[26]

☑ CHECKPOINT 15-7

What antibody class is typically implicated in warm autoimmune hemolytic anemia (WAIHA)?

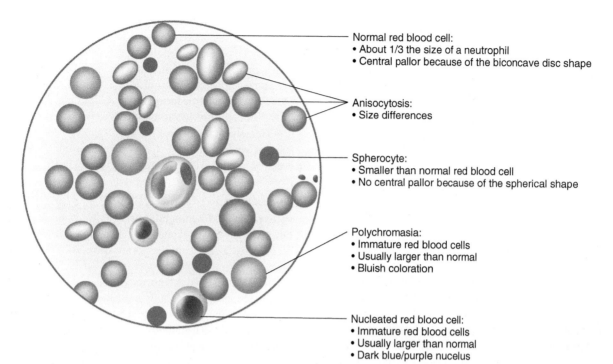

Normal red blood cell:
• About 1/3 the size of a neutrophil
• Central pallor because of the biconcave disc shape

Anisocytosis:
• Size differences

Spherocyte:
• Smaller than normal red blood cell
• No central pallor because of the spherical shape

Polychromasia:
• Immature red blood cells
• Usually larger than normal
• Bluish coloration

Nucleated red blood cell:
• Immature red blood cells
• Usually larger than normal
• Dark blue/purple nucelus

FIGURE 15-4 Peripheral Blood Smear in Warm Autoimmune Hemolytic Anemia

Cold Agglutinin Syndrome (CAS)

Cold agglutinins are primarily IgM autoantibodies with optimal reactivity at cooler temperatures and are usually not clinically significant unless there is reactivity at body temperature. Therefore, a distinction should be made between a patient who has cold agglutinins that are detectable only at room temperature or at 39.2° F (4° C) and one who has clinically significant hemolysis in association with a cold agglutinin that is weaker but still reactive at or near 98.6° F (37° C). Only the latter scenario should be referred to as **cold agglutinin syndrome (CAS)**, which is also called **cold agglutinin disease (CAD)**.

The most common underlying etiologies are infections, most notably Epstein-Barr virus infections and *Mycoplasma pneumoniae* infections. Other diseases that have been associated with cold agglutinin production include lymphoid neoplasms, such as chronic lymphocytic leukemia and carcinomas. The autoantibody is usually directed against a common self-antigen, such as the I, i, or HI carbohydrate antigens. CAS, like WAIHA, tends to be encountered more frequently in older patients than in the pediatric population.

✳ **TABLE 15-2** Transfusion Testing Results in Immune Hemolytic Anemias*

	Direct Antiglobulin Test (IgG vs. C')	Eluate Antibody Identification	Plasma Antibody Identification (Phase of reaction)	Autocontrol
Warm autoimmune hemolytic anemia (WAIHA)	Positive (IgG ≫ C')	Panreactive	Panreactive (AHG)	Positive
Cold agglutinin syndrome (CAS)	Positive (C' ≫ IgG)	Negative	Panreactive (RT/IS ≫ 98.6°F [37° C])	Positive (39.2° F [4° C] > 98.6°F [37° C])
Mixed autoimmune hemolytic anemia	Positive (IgG/C')	Panreactive	Panreactive (RT/IS, AHG)	Positive
Paroxysmal cold hemoglobinuria (PCH)	Positive (C')	Negative	Negative (Biphasic IgG hemolysin)	Negative
Delayed hemolytic transfusion reaction	Positive[1] (IgG > C')	Specific pattern	Specific pattern (AHG)	Positive[1]
Alloantibody to a high-incidence antigen	Negative[2]	Panreactive	Panreactive (AHG)	Negative[2]
Acute hemolytic transfusion reaction	Positive[1] (IgG/C')	Negative[3]	Negative[3]	Positive[1]
Drug-induced immune hemolytic anemia	Positive (IgG/C')	Negative	Negative; positive with drug	Positive

C', complement

[1] Delayed hemolytic and acute hemolytic transfusion reactions may have a negative direct antiglobulin test (DAT) and autocontrol result if all incompatible transfused red blood cells have been destroyed.

[2] DAT and autocontrol may be positive with an antibody against a high-incidence antigen if the patient was recently transfused.

[3] An acute hemolytic transfusion reaction is usually due to ABO incompatibility and antibody panel cells are always group O. However, eluate and plasma panels may be positive in cases of non-ABO acute hemolytic transfusion reactions, such as anti-Jk^a incompatibility. And in cases of ABO acute hemolytic transfusion reactions the eluate will give positive reactions if tested against group A and/or B cells.

*Adapted from reference 18.

Clinical Presentation

Symptoms of CAS are those associated with chronic, progressive hemolytic anemia, commonly fatigue and exertion-associated dyspnea. Depending on the thermal range of the antibodies that are causing the hemolysis, the symptoms may be exacerbated by exposure to cold temperatures. **Cyanosis** (defined as a bluish discoloration of the skin due to buildup of deoxygenated blood) of the extremities such as fingertips, toes, ears, and nose is associated with diminished flow in cutaneous capillaries in the cold. Progression to tissue necrosis is uncommon but can cause serious morbidity and may require amputation. Hemoglobinuria, hepatosplenomegaly, and/or jaundice may be detected in a subset of cases.

Laboratory Features

Anemia associated with cold agglutinins tends in general to be milder than that encountered in WAIHA, as do morphologic changes in the red blood cells. Spontaneous agglutination of red blood cells at room temperature may interfere with analysis by automated hematology instruments, necessitating prewarming of samples to yield accurate results for red blood cell count, mean corpuscular volume, and other indices.[27] Reticulocytes are typically increased in proportion to the degree of anemia, while leukocyte and platelet numbers are commonly within the reference ranges. Erythroid hyperplasia and a generally modest lymphocytosis are seen in bone marrow specimens.[1]

Laboratory results in cases of CAS are consistent with an IgM autoantibody (Table 15-2). There may be a discrepancy in the ABO typing due to additional positive reactions in the reverse grouping (Chapter 5). The antibody screen is positive, often with all cells, if tested at room temperature or if an immediate spin phase is included after incubation. The DAT is positive, especially with anticomplement reagents, but the eluate is usually nonreactive.

Treatment

In contrast to WAIHA, steroid therapy is of minimal benefit in most cases of CAS. Immunosuppressive therapy and rituximab have been used in more severe cases with some response reported. Avoiding exposure to cold temperatures tends to reduce symptoms and signs in milder cases.[28]

Mixed Autoimmune Hemolytic Anemia (MAIHA)

Among the least commonly encountered types of AIHAs are patients who simultaneously have two types of autoantibodies causing both WAIHA and CAS. This phenomenon is referred to as **mixed autoimmune hemolytic anemia (MAIHA)** or combined warm and the form of anemia mediated by autoantibodies that react best at room temperature or below known as **cold autoimmune hemolytic anemia (CAIHA)**. Laboratory results will demonstrate the presence of both the warm and cold reactive antibodies (Table 15-2). MAIHA is believed to be a distinct clinical entity, associated with a more severe and chronic form of AIHA. It can be idiopathic or may arise in association with a lymphoproliferative disorder, systemic lupus erythematosus, or HIV infection.[1] Treatment may lead to one form of AIHA predominating over the other.

The frequent incidental finding of cold agglutinins reactive only at 68° F (20° C) but not 98.6° F (37° C) in patients with WAIHA may lead to overdiagnosis of this entity.[1] Additionally, a recent study suggests that the incidence of this form of autoimmune hemolytic anemia may be overestimated due to confusion with cases of CAIHA with high thermal amplitudes and cases of WAIHA that are also reactive at low temperatures, mimicking a simultaneous CAIHA; if this premise holds, the true incidence of MAIHA may be much closer to 0.1% than to the previously reported 8%.[29]

Hemolysis can be severe,[30] but response to corticosteroid therapy is often dramatic.[31] A relapsing course is not uncommon, however, and rituximab has been reported to be of use in one such case.[32]

Paroxysmal Cold Hemoglobinuria (PCH)

Paroxysmal cold hemoglobinuria (PCH) is a rare AIHA historically associated with syphilis infections, but now more commonly encountered as an acute, temporary hemolytic episode in children following a viral infection. PCH is attributable to an IgG autoantibody usually directed against the P carbohydrate antigen. As previously mentioned, this antibody is also known as a biphasic hemolysin. The DAT will be positive because of the activation of complement *in vivo*, but the usual antibody detection methods will have negative results because a single incubation temperature is used (Table 15-2). The Donath-Landsteiner test, described earlier in this chapter, is an *in vitro* hemolysis assay for identifying the biphasic nature of the autoantibody that is associated with PCH.[17]

Clinical Presentation

Hemoglobinuria resulting in red-brown urine is nearly always seen and is frequently accompanied by jaundice and pallor. Fever and malaise may be present, as may abdominal pain with or without hepatosplenomegaly. Chronic PCH is a rare phenomenon.

Laboratory Features

In contrast to the mild, generally stable anemia encountered in CAS, PCH-associated anemia is frequently marked and characterized by rapid worsening during a sudden attack of symptoms known as a *paroxysm*. Peripheral blood smears typically show **anisopoikilocytosis** (red blood cells show variation in both size and shape) with polychromasia and spherocytes. A transient neutrophil-specific **hemophagocytosis** (a process that results in red blood cells found within phagocytic cells, in this case neutrophils) may be observed on the blood smears of some patients and is relatively specific for PCH.[33] Figure 15-5 ■ is a diagrammatic representation of the features to watch for on the peripheral blood smear.

Treatment

Given the acute and transient nature of most cases, treatment is typically limited to supportive care. Depending on the severity of the anemia, red blood cell transfusion may be required. Evidence supporting the use of corticosteroids or plasmapheresis is lacking. Avoidance of cold reduces hemolytic paroxysms in chronic cases.[1]

☑ CHECKPOINT 15-8

Which blood group is associated with paroxysmal cold hemoglobinuria (PCH)?

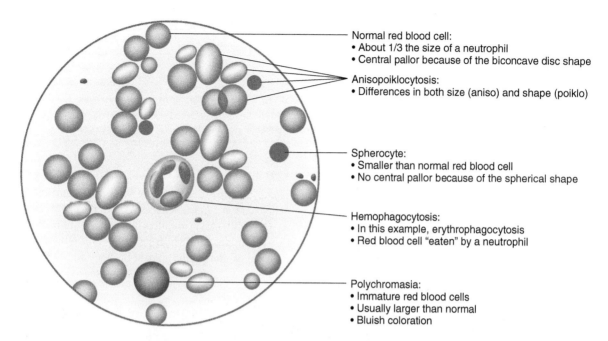

Normal red blood cell:
• About 1/3 the size of a neutrophil
• Central pallor because of the biconcave disc shape

Anisopoiklocytosis:
• Differences in both size (aniso) and shape (poiklo)

Spherocyte:
• Smaller than normal red blood cell
• No central pallor because of the spherical shape

Hemophagocytosis:
• In this example, erythrophagocytosis
• Red blood cell "eaten" by a neutrophil

Polychromasia:
• Immature red blood cells
• Usually larger than normal
• Bluish coloration

FIGURE 15-5 Peripheral Blood Smear in Paroxysmal Cold Hemoglobinuria

DAT-Negative Autoimmune Hemolytic Anemia

Although a positive DAT result is typically used to identify immune causes of hemolytic anemia, there are infrequent instances in which a hemolytic anemia may be associated with a negative DAT yet still respond to treatments for WAIHA. Reports in the literature show a frequency of DAT negativity ranging from 2 to 10% of patients with AIHA.[6]

The DAT result can be negative in instances where 50–200 IgG molecules are bound per red blood cell, which is too low to be detected by routine analysis and yet may be associated with immune destruction of red blood cells. IgG bound to red blood cells in levels too low to be detected by the DAT may be identified by other methods such as flow cytometry, various enzyme-linked methodologies, radiometric assays, solid phase, or direct polyethylene glycol (PEG).[18, 34] Many of these methods are not available in routine laboratory settings.

Testing an eluate may help identify an autoimmune cause of hemolysis even when the DAT is negative because preparation of an eluate can concentrate the antibody (Chapter 9). When there is no other identifiable cause of hemolysis, preparation of an eluate can be valuable regardless of the DAT result.[35]

Other explanations for a negative DAT when hemolysis appears to be occurring include low-affinity IgG that washes off during the testing and autoantibodies that are IgM or IgA instead of IgG. Autoantibody can also suppress antigen expression, resulting in a negative DAT, although this is usually not associated with a hemolytic anemia.[36]

DRUG-INDUCED IMMUNE HEMOLYTIC ANEMIA (DIIHA)

A hemolytic anemia with no obvious cause that starts soon after the start of a new drug regimen may be **drug-induced immune hemolytic anemia (DIIHA).** The clinical manifestations of DIIHA vary in severity. Up to 125 drugs have reasonable evidence documenting their ability to induce immune hemolytic anemia or a positive DAT.[37]

The DAT will usually be positive in DIIHA because the antibody has attached *in vivo*, but the antibody screen will usually be negative unless the drug is included in the test system (Table 15-2). As described previously, the drug can be incorporated into the test system by either coating the red blood cells with the drug prior to testing or by adding the drug or its metabolite directly into the plasma/red blood cell mixture. The detection method that will work is dependent on the drug that is causing the DIIHA.

In the past, the most common drug associated with DIIHA was methyldopa, which was a commonly prescribed antihypertensive. The second most common cause was high-dose intravenous penicillin.[38] Today, both of these drug treatments are relatively uncommon and the most common causes of DIIHA are the cephalosporins, a group of antibiotics.[39, 40] Cefotetan, which has the longest half-life of the first- and second-generation cephalosporins, is the most often implicated. Other drugs commonly associated with DIIHA currently include ceftriaxone and piperacillin.

DIIHA has been generally divided into three categories based on the results seen during laboratory testing (Table 15-3 ✳). The first category shows a pattern of reactivity identical to a warm autoantibody.[41] In the past, the second category was called the drug adsorption model because positive reactions were obtained when testing red blood cells that had been treated with the drug.[18] The third category was previously called *immune complex formation.* Positive reactivity would occur when the patient's plasma was tested against red blood cells in the presence of the suspected drug or sometimes one of the drug's metabolites.

The latest theory that explains DIIHA is called the unifying hypothesis.[18, 37] In this theory, the drug is a **hapten** that binds either strongly or weakly to the red blood cell membrane. This induces an immune response and an antibody is made to different epitopes

★ TABLE 15-3 Categories of Drug-Induced Immune Hemolytic Anemia

Laboratory Results	Index Drug	Common Drugs Today
Panreactive antibody pattern with untreated red blood cells	Methyldopa	Fludrabine (Fludara®)[41] Cladribine (Leustatin®)[41]
Negative antibody pattern with untreated red blood cells but positive results with red blood cells that were treated with the drug	Penicillin	Cephalothin
Positive antibody reactions if plasma, drug, and red blood cells are incubated together	Quinidine	Ceftriaxone

depending on the drug involved (Figure 15-6 ■). The antibody may be directed against:

- Primarily the red blood cell membrane, which will cause positive reactions with untreated red blood cells;

- Primarily the drug, which will cause positive reactions when plasma is tested against drug-treated red blood cells; or

- A combination of part of the red blood cell membrane and part of the drug, which will cause positive reactions when the antibody, red blood cell membrane, and drug are all present together in the test system.

The first line of treatment in all cases of DIIHA is to stop therapy with the implicated drug, replacing it with an alternative medication, if required.[42]

☑ CHECKPOINT 15-9

List four medications that can cause drug-induced immune hemolytic anemia (DIIHA).

TRANSFUSION SUPPORT

Depending on the mechanism of red blood cell destruction, the results of antibody screen and crossmatch testing in immune-mediated hemolytic anemia vary from negative results, which can be seen with certain types of drug-induced hemolysis, to panreactive positive results, which can be seen with warm autoantibodies. The ease of providing crossmatch-compatible red blood cells can be predicted by the antibody screen and identification testing results. Patients with panreactive results can be very challenging.

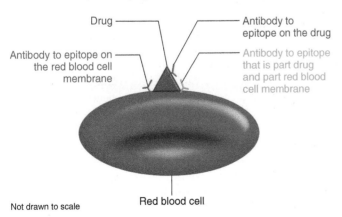

Not drawn to scale

■ FIGURE 15-6 Antibodies Believed to Cause Drug-Induced Immune Hemolytic Anemia

Compatible and Incompatible Crossmatch

There are four issues worthy of brief discussion surrounding compatible and incompatible crossmatches for patients diagnosed with AIHA or DIIHA: (1) instances in which the antibody screen is negative; (2) instances in which panreactive patterns are noted; (3) the presence of nonspecific autoantibodies; and (4) the importance of communication. A discussion of each issue follows.

Negative Antibody Screen

Obviously, crossmatch-compatible donors can be easily identified if the antibody screen is negative. However, even donor cells that are crossmatch compatible *in vitro* may not have a normal lifespan *in vivo*.

Panreactive Pattern

All donors will be crossmatch incompatible when the patient has panreactive autoantibodies. The major concern in these cases is determining if the panreactive autoantibody is masking alloantibodies, which could cause a hemolytic transfusion reaction. Obtaining an accurate history from the patient can help identify which patients are at the greatest risk. If the patient has no history of sensitizing events such as pregnancy, transfusion, or transplantation, chances are that the patient does not have a clinically significant alloantibody. If the laboratory is confident in the patient's history, they may limit the amount of additional testing performed as transfusion of ABO-compatible units carries minimal risk, even if the units appear crossmatch incompatible.

Additional testing, such as adsorptions, is likely required if the patient is transfused during this hemolytic episode or even if the patient has a history of transfusion in the past.

Nonspecific Autoantibody

In between these two extremes of test results are the patients whose plasma reacts with some but not all reagent and donor cells. Sometimes the common clinically significant red blood cell antibodies can be ruled out or excluded but sometimes one, multiple, or all of the common alloantibodies cannot be ruled out. Even when clinically significant alloantibodies are ruled out or excluded, the serologic crossmatch with donor cells may be positive. Therefore, there are many cases of AIHA where crossmatch-incompatible units are the only transfusion option.

Communication

A common practice, especially in the past, was to select for transfusion the donor units with the weakest positive crossmatch result, which would be called least incompatible. However, there is no evidence that this selection process identifies a unit that is less susceptible to hemolysis. More important is good communication between the clinical and laboratory staff members to assess the risks and benefits of crossmatch-incompatible transfusion in a particular patient's situation.[43, 44]

Laboratory Investigation

Adsorption, elution, and antigen typing are all common laboratory tests utilized in the search for red blood cell units that pose the least risk and the greatest benefit to a patient suffering from an immune hemolytic anemia (Figure 15-7 ■). However, different laboratories may use the same techniques at different times and in different ways.

For example, some laboratories will perform an elution whenever a positive DAT is discovered; others only perform an elution if the patient has been recently transfused. Some laboratories perform allogeneic adsorptions whenever an antibody screen is repeated in a patient with a warm autoantibody; others perform an initial adsorption and then repeat only if the DAT or antibody screen results

increase in strength. A third strategy is to perform an initial adsorption only, providing phenotype-matched units for all subsequent transfusions.

Crossmatch with Adsorbed Plasma

Patient plasma is often prepared via autoadsorption or alloadsorption when investigating an AIHA. The resultant adsorbed plasma is used in antibody identification procedures with the hope that alloantibodies can be identified if present or ruled out if absent (Chapter 9). There is no consensus regarding the appropriateness of using adsorbed plasma in crossmatching donor units. If alloantibodies against the common clinically significant antigens have been ruled out and a serological crossmatch with adsorbed plasma gives negative results, some may consider these results sufficient for identifying a red blood cell unit as crossmatch compatible without further qualification. Alternatively, some institutions employ the use of

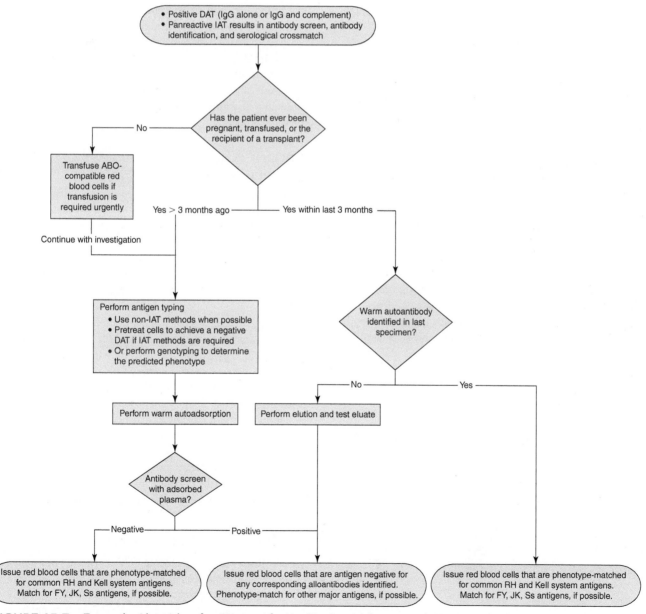

■ FIGURE 15-7   Example Algorithm for Pretransfusion Testing in Suspected Warm Autoimmune Hemolytic Anemia

electronic crossmatch criteria and issue a unit without further testing if no clinically significant alloantibodies were detected through the use of adsorption studies. Finally, some laboratories may identify the red blood cell unit as crossmatch incompatible on the issue tag, label, or voucher, with a comment that states that alloantibodies to major antigens have been excluded or ruled out. Some institutions will also include a comment that suggests that the patient be monitored continuously throughout the transfusion when issuing a red blood cell unit that appears incompatible in laboratory testing. Other laboratories may try an *in vivo* crossmatch (Chapter 8) when transfusing a red blood cell unit that appears incompatible.

Plasma Dilution

Some laboratories use diluted patient plasma in antibody identification procedures when there is not enough time to perform an adsorption. The presumption underlying this strategy is that an alloantibody would have a higher titer than an autoantibody. One method is to use a 1:5 dilution, while another recommendation is to find a dilution that causes a 1+ reaction with donor cells and use this diluted plasma to test reagent red blood cells.[38, 45]

Risk–Benefit Ratio

In general, the increased red blood cell destruction seen in patients with AIHA decreases the benefit of transfusion because the transfused cells are unlikely to have a normal lifespan. The goal of transfusion support is to provide red blood cells that hopefully will have at least a lifespan similar to the patient's own cells. The risk of hemolytic transfusion reactions may be greater than in other patients because of the interference in testing that autoantibodies cause. Autologous or allogeneic adsorptions may have reduced the sensitivity of detecting alloantibodies, either through dilution of the antibody during serial adsorptions or the adsorption of an antibody to a high-incidence antigen.

Up to 32% of patients with warm autoantibodies also have alloantibodies, and 42–77% of these alloantibodies could not be detected after adsorption studies were done.[1] Conversely, 9% of patients with alloantibodies will develop autoantibodies following transfusion.[46] Alloantibodies and autoantibodies appear to have developed simultaneously after transfusion in 34–75% of patients who have both.[46, 47] Similar to patients without autoantibodies, anti-E and anti-K are commonly found alloantibodies in patients who also have warm autoantibodies in their serum (Table 15-4 ✳).[48]

✳ **TABLE 15-4** Frequency of Alloantibodies Found in Patients with Warm Autoantibodies[47]

Alloantibody Specificity	Percentage of Patients
Anti-E	46%
Anti-K	22%
Anti-C	18%
Anti-Fy^a	15%
Anti-Jk^a	10%
Anti-c	10%
Anti-Jk^b	9.4%
Anti-S	8.4%
Anti-D	7%
Anti-e	5%

The emergence of allo- and autoantibodies together has raised the question of whether transfusion may exacerbate an AIHA. It is unknown if allogeneic red blood cells stimulate the autoimmune destructive process. **Hyperhemolysis**, which has been described in sickle cell anemia, has not been described in autoimmune hemolytic anemia.[49–54] Hyperhemolysis refers to the destruction of autologous red blood cells during a hemolytic transfusion reaction that is destroying allogeneic cells.

☑ **CHECKPOINT 15-10**

Which alloantibody is most frequently identified in patients with warm autoantibodies?

Transfusion Triggers

Like other **transfusion triggers** (conditions or changes indicating that transfusion may be indicated), the level of anemia at which a patient with autoimmune hemolytic anemia should be transfused has been debated. Given the increased risks and decreased benefits of transfusion in these patients, transfusion should be reserved for patients who have profound anemia with severe symptoms or increased risk of death due to anemia. On the other hand, transfusion should not be withheld solely because the donor units appear crossmatch incompatible.[43]

Antigen-Negative and Phenotype Matched Donors

Another controversy involves the choice of donor units when the specificity of an autoantibody is identified. The use of rare antigen-negative units, such as c-negative or e-negative when an autoanti-c or autoanti-e is identified, might be justified if the lifespan of the transfused cells will be longer than phenotype-matched cells. However, it is debatable whether the lifespan of these antigen-negative cells will be longer than that of the autologous red blood cells. Also, if the patient is homozygous for the autoantigen, exposure to the corresponding alloantigen, such as E or C, can increase the risk of alloantibody production.

One alternative is to use donor cells that are phenotypically matched with the patient. This is a commonly used strategy when the specificity of the autoantibody cannot be determined. Using phenotype-matched cells reduces the risk of a delayed hemolytic transfusion reaction due to an underlying alloantibody and also reduces the risk of alloimmunization. If phenotype-matched units are selected, allogeneic adsorptions are not necessary as the patient would already be receiving blood that is negative for any major alloantigens. However, the prolonged use of phenotype-matched blood in a patient who might or might not have alloantibodies may deplete the availability of those units for patients who do have demonstrable multiple alloantibodies.

PATIENT SUPPORT AND TREATMENT

Transfusion is a supportive therapy. The underlying cause of any case of hemolytic anemia should be identified and treated whenever possible. Successful therapy can reduce the total number of transfusions needed by increasing the lifespan of both endogenous and transfused red blood cells.

Review of the Main Points

- Hemolysis is the increased destruction of red blood cells.
- Laboratory tests often used to investigate cases of autoimmune hemolytic anemia (AIHA) include the direct antiglobulin test (DAT), antibody screen, elution, adsorption, and antigen typing.
- The DAT is usually positive in cases of immune hemolysis.
- The Donath-Landsteiner test is used to help diagnose paroxysmal cold hemoglobinuria (PCH).
- Two methods of testing for drug-induced immune hemolytic anemia (DIIHA)) include:
  - Testing patient plasma, serum, and/or eluate with red blood cells that have been treated with the suspected drug.
  - Testing the patient serum, reagent red blood cells, and suspected drug together.
- Symptoms of anemia include fatigue, tachycardia, and pallor.
- Categories of AIHA include warm autoimmune hemolytic anemia (WAIHA), cold agglutinin syndrome (CAS), mixed autoimmune hemolytic anemia (MAIHA), paroxysmal cold hemoglobinuria (PCH), and DAT-negative autoimmune hemolytic anemia.
- AIHAs are associated with various infections, cancers, and autoimmune disorders.
- Laboratory tests used to assess immune hemolytic anemia include complete blood count (CBC), serum bilirubin, serum haptoglobin, serum lactate dehydrogenase, reticulocyte count, DAT, and red blood cell antibody screen and identification.
- The most common autoimmune hemolytic anemia is WAIHA and least common is DAT-negative autoimmune hemolytic anemia.
- Common features of WAIHA include:
  - IgG autoantibody directed against a common Rh protein and reacting strongest at 98.6° F (37° C).
  - Panreactive pattern of reactivity: positive autocontrol, DAT, and indirect antiglobulin tests such as antibody screen, antibody identification panel(s), and crossmatch.
  - Usually secondary to lymphoproliferative disorders, autoimmune conditions, or viral infections.
  - Rate of hemolysis can vary and will influence the signs and symptoms experienced by the patient.
- Corticosteroid therapy may be an effective treatment in WAIHA, MAIHA, and DAT-negative autoimmune hemolytic anemia.
- Positive DAT with anticomplement is commonly seen with CAS and MAIHA.
- Common features of CAS include:
  - IgM autoantibody (usually directed against i, I, or HI antigens) that reacts best at room temperature or 39.2° F (4° C).

- DAT is positive, especially with anticomplement; antibody screen is positive especially if tested at room temperature <98.6° F (<37° C).
- Secondary to Epstein-Barr virus infection, *Mycoplasma pneumoniae* infection, chronic lymphocytic leukemia, or various carcinomas.
- Signs and symptoms of a chronic, progressive anemia.
- MAIHA is associated with laboratory test results, signs, symptoms, and treatments that reflect the contribution of both a warm-reactive IgG and a cold-reactive IgM autoantibody to the disease.
- Common features of PCH include:
  - IgG biphasic autoantibody, usually anti-P.
  - Anisopoikilocytosis and hemophagocytosis may be seen on peripheral blood smear.
  - Most common in children following a viral infection.
  - Causes an acute, temporary hemolytic episode.
- The Donath-Landsteiner test is used to help diagnose PCH.
- Laboratory indicators of hemolysis include decreased hemoglobin level, increased bilirubin level, decreased haptoglobin level, and increased lactate dehydrogenase level.
- Reasons for a negative DAT result in what otherwise looks like a WAIHA include:
  - Low levels of IgG molecules attached to each red blood cell.
  - Low-affinity IgG molecules that are released from the red blood cell during testing.
  - IgM or IgA molecules are involved rather than IgG antibodies.
- Many drugs can cause a positive DAT.
- Commonly implicated drugs in drug-induced immune hemolytic anemia (DIIHA) include various cephalosporins today and, in the past, methyldopa, penicillin, and quinidine.
- In the unified hypothesis, DIIHA may be caused by an antibody directed against:
  - Primarily an epitope on the red blood cell membrane,
  - Primarily an epitope on the drug molecule, or
  - An epitope composed partly of the red blood cell membrane and partly of the drug.
- Communication between the laboratory and clinical staff members is vital when all donor units are crossmatch incompatible, as often happens in autoimmune hemolytic anemias.
- Transfusion is only a supportive therapy; successful treatment of autoimmune hemolytic anemia relies on treating the underlying cause.

Review Questions

1. What is the basic principle of the adsorption test? (Objective #1)

   A. To remove antigens from red blood cells

   B. To separate plasma from red blood cells

   C. To remove antibodies from red blood cells

   D. To separate antibodies from plasma

2. A specimen from a male patient with suspected autoimmune hemolytic anemia (AIHA) is sent to the blood bank for testing. The patient medical history reveals that he was transfused 3 weeks ago at a different facility. The blood bank work-up reveals a positive DAT, positive antibody screen, and a panagglutinin antibody in both the plasma and eluate. Which test should the laboratorian perform next? (Objective #1)

   A. Autoadsorption

   B. Alloadsorption

   C. Antigen adsorption

   D. Reticular adsorption

3. What techniques may be used to perform antigen phenotyping on a specimen from a recently transfused patient? (Objective #1)

   A. Isolation of endogenous reticulocytes

   B. Molecular techniques

   C. Adsorption of autoantibody from patient red blood cells

   D. All of the above

4. Which laboratory procedure is used to confirm paroxysmal cold hemoglobinuria (PCH)? (Objective #2)

   A. Allogeneic adsorption

   B. Acid elution

   C. Donath-Lansteiner test

   D. Endogenous reticulocytes

5. A specimen from a 50-year-old female with a history of anemia reveals a positive DAT. The patient reports she has not been recently transfused or pregnant. The most likely explanation for the positive test is: (Objective #3)

   A. Autoimmune hemolytic anemia

   B. Hemolytic transfusion reaction

   C. Delayed serologic reaction

   D. Hemolytic disease of the newborn

6. True or false: All patients with a positive DAT are anemic. (Objective #3)

7. Which of the following circumstances can result in a false-positive DAT? (Objective #4)

   A. Low-titer IgG antibody is present

   B. Prolonged storage of specimen prior to testing

   C. Complete destruction of antibody has occurred

   D. Loss of complement-regulating protein

8. Choose all of the laboratory findings that are indicative of red blood cell hemolysis. (Objective #5)

   A. _____ Elevated reticulocyte count

   B. _____ Elevated haptoglobin

   C. _____ Elevated LDH

   D. _____ Elevated hemoglobin

   E. _____ Icteric plasma

   F. _____ Schistocytes

9. Which type of autoimmune hemolytic anemia is associated with *Mycoplasma pneumoniae*? (Objective #6)

   A. Drug-induced immune-mediated hemolytic anemia

   B. Paroxysmal cold hemoglobinuria

   C. Cold agglutinin syndrome

   D. Warm autoimmune hemolytic anemia

10. Antibody reactivity in warm autoimmune hemolytic anemia (WAIHA) is best described as: (Objective #6)

    A. Alloagglutinin

    B. Panagglutinin

    C. Low frequency

    D. Negative

11. Which type of hemolytic anemia would most likely have a nonreactive (negative) eluate? (Objective #6)

    A. Warm autoimmune hemolytic anemia

    B. Mixed autoimmune hemolytic anemia

    C. Cold agglutinin syndrome

    D. Delayed hemolytic transfusion reaction

12. Match each type of hemolytic anemia with the expected DAT results. (Objective #6)

    _____ Cold agglutinin syndrome

    _____ Mixed autoimmune hemolytic anemia

    _____ Acute hemolytic transfusion reaction

    _____ Paroxysmal cold hemoglobinuria

    _____ Warm autoimmune hemolytic anemia

    A. Positive DAT; IgG and complement

    B. Positive DAT; IgG only

    C. Positive DAT; complement only

13. A specimen from a patient with cold agglutinin syndrome is received in the hematology lab for CBC analysis. In order to obtain an accurate set of results on an automated analyzer, what step should be taken prior to testing? (Objective # 6)

A. Dilution of blood specimen with isotonic saline

B. Determination of plasma hemoglobin value

C. Removal of buffy coat

D. Prewarm the specimen to 98.6° F (37° C)

14. What is the first course of treatment for a patient with a confirmed case of drug-induced immune hemolytic anemia? (Objective #6)

A. Corticosteroids

B. Transfusion with drug-negative red blood cells

C. Alternative medication

D. Phototherapy

15. What is the most important concern when a panreactive autoantibody is identified in the blood bank laboratory? (Objective #10)

A. ABO incompatibility

B. Masking of alloantibodies

C. *In vitro* hemolysis

D. Antigen phenotyping

References

1. Petz LD, Garratty G. *Immune hemolytic anemias,* 2nd ed. Philadelphia (PA): Churchill Livingstone; 2004.

2. Win N, Islam SI, Peterkin MA, Walker ID. Positive direct antiglobulin test due to antiphospholipid antibodies in normal healthy blood donors. *Vox Sang* 1997; 72(3): 182–4.

3. Gorst DW, Rawlinson VI, Merry AH, Stratton F. Positive direct antiglobulin test in normal individuals. *Vox Sang* 1980; 38(2): 99–105.

4. Huh YO, Lichtiger B. Evaluation of a positive autologous control in pretransfusion testing. *Am J Clin Pathol* 1985; 84(5): 632–6.

5. Boulton FE. Increase of blood donations found positive in the direct antiglobulin test detected by column methods—do we need to know? *Br J Biomed Sci* 1996; 53(2): 172–3.

6. Gilliland BC. Coombs-negative immune hemolytic anemia. *Semin Hematol* 1976; 13(4): 267–75.

7. Dearden C, Wade R, Else M, Richards S, Milligan D, Hamblin T, Catovsky D; UK National Cancer Research Institute (NCRI); Haematological Oncology Clinical Studies Group; NCRI CLL Working Group. The prognostic significance of a positive direct antiglobulin test in chronic lymphocytic leukemia: A beneficial effect of the combination of fludarabine and cyclophosphamide on the incidence of hemolytic anemia. *Blood* 2008; 111(4): 1820–6.

8. Laine EP, Leger RM, Arndt PA, Calhoun L, Garratty G, Petz LD. In vitro studies of the impact of transfusion on the detection of alloantibodies after autoadsorption. *Transfusion* 2000; 40(11): 1384–7.

9. Marks MR, Reid ME, Ellisor SS. Adsorption of unwanted cold autoagglutinins by formaldehyde-treated rabbit RBCs (abstract). *Transfusion* 1980; 20(5): 629.

10. Waligora SK, Edwards JM. Use of rabbit red cells for adsorption of cold autoagglutinins. *Transfusion* 1983; 23(4): 328–30.

11. Dzik WH, Yang R, Blank J. Rabbit erythrocyte stroma treatment of serum interferes with recognition of delayed hemolytic transfusion reaction. *Transfusion* 1986; 26(3): 303–4.

12. Mechanic SA, Maurer JL, Igoe MJ, Kavitsky DM, Nance ST. Anti-Vel reactivity diminished by adsorption with rabbit RBC stroma. *Transfusion* 2002; 42(9): 1180–3.

13. Tonder O, Larsen B, Aarskog D, Haneberg B. Natural and immune antibodies to rabbit erythrocyte antigens. *Scand J Immunol* 1978; 7(3): 245–9.

14. Shirey RS, Boyd JS, Parwani AV, Tanz WS, Ness PM, King KE. Prophylactic antigen-matched donor blood for patients with warm autoantibodies: An algorithm for transfusion management. *Transfusion* 2002; 42(11): 1435–41.

15. Reid ME, Rios M, Powell VI, Charles-Pierre D, Malavade V. DNA from blood samples can be used to genotype patients who have recently received a transfusion. *Transfusion* 2000; 40(1): 48–53.

16. Lee E, Hart K, Burgess G, Halverson GR, Reid ME. Efficacy of murine monoclonal antibodies in RBC phenotyping of DAT-positive samples. *Immunohematology* 2006; 22(4): 161–5.

17. Judd WJ, Johnson ST, Storry JR. Testing for PCH using the Donath-Landsteiner test. In: Judd's *Methods in Immunohematology.* Bethesda (MD): AABB Press; 2008.

18. Roback JD, Combs MR, Grossman BJ, Hillyer CD, editors. *Technical manual,* 16th ed. Bethesda (MD): AABB Press; 2008.

19. Arndt PA, Leger RM, Garratty G. Serologic findings in autoimmune hemolytic anemia associated with immunoglobulin M warm autoantibodies. *Transfusion* 2009; 49(2): 235–42.

20. Pullarkat V, Ngo M, Iqbal S, Espina B, Liebman HA. Detection of lupus anticoagulant identifies patients with autoimmune haemolytic anaemia at increased risk for venous thromboembolism. *Br J Haematol* 2002; 118(4): 1166–9.

21. Meyer RJ, Hoffman R, Zanjani ED. Autoimmune hemolytic anemia and periodic pure red cell aplasia in systemic lupus erythematosus. *Am J Med* 1978; 65(2): 342–5.

22. Evans R, Duane R. Acquired hemolytic anemia: I. The relation of erythrocyte antibody to activity of the disease. II. The significance of thrombocytopenia and leukopenia. *Blood* 1949; 4(Nov): 1196–213.

23. King KE. Review: pharmacologic treatment of warm autoimmune hemolytic anemia. *Immunohematology* 2007; 23(3): 120–9.

24. Zecca M, Nobili B, Ramenghi U, Perrotta S, Amendola G, Rosito P, Jankovic M, Pierani P, De Stafano P, Bonora MR, Locatelli F. Rituximab for the treatment of refractory autoimmune hemolytic anemia in children. *Blood* 2003; 101(10): 3857–61.

25. Bussone G, Ribeiro E, Dechartres A, Viallard JF, Bonnotte B, Fain O, Godeau B, Michel M. Efficacy and safety of rituximab in adults' warm antibody autoimmune haemolytic anemia: Retrospective analysis of 27 cases. *Am J Hematol* 2009; 84(3): 153–7.

26. Flores G, Cunningham-Rundles C, Newland AC, Bussel JB. Efficacy of intravenous immunoglobulin in the treatment of autoimmune hemolytic anemia: results in 73 patients. *Am J Hematol* 1993; 44(4): 237–42.

27. Zandecki M, Genevieve F, Gerard J, Godon A. Spurious counts and spurious results on haematology analysers: A review. Part II: white blood cells, RBCs, haemoglobin, red cell indices and reticulocytes. *Int J Lab Hematol* 2007; 29(1): 21–41.

28. Petz LD. Cold antibody autoimmune hemolytic anemias. *Blood Rev* 2008; 22(1): 1–15.

29. Mayer B, Yurek S, Kiesewetter H, Salama A. Mixed-type autoimmune hemolytic anemia: Differential diagnosis and a critical review of reported cases. *Transfusion* 2008; 48(10): 2229–34.

30. Sokol RJ, Hewitt S, Stamps BK. Autoimmune hemolysis: Mixed warm and cold antibody type. *Acta Haematol* 1983; 69(4): 266–74.

31. Shulman IA, Branch DR, Nelson JM, Thompson JC, Saxena S, Petz LD. Autoimmune hemolytic anemia with both cold and warm autoantibodies. *JAMA* 1985; 253(12): 1746–8.

32. Morselli M, Luppi M, Potenza L, Tonelli S, Dini D, Leonardi G, Donelli A, Narni F, Torelli G. Mixed warm and cold autoimmune hemolytic anemia: Complete recovery after 2 courses of rituximab treatment. *Blood* 2002; 99(9): 3478–9.

33. Heddle NM. Acute paroxysmal cold hemoglobinuria. *Transfus Med Rev* 1989; 3(3): 219–29.

34. Lin JS, Hao TC, Lyou JY, Chen YJ, Liu HM, Tzeng CH, Chiou TJ. Clinical application of a flow cytometric direct antiglobulin test. *Transfusion* 2009; 49(7): 1335–46.

35. Gilliland BC, Baxter E, Evans RS. Red-cell antibodies in acquired hemolytic anemia with negative antiglobulin serum tests. *N Engl J Med* 1971; 285(5): 252–6.

36. Zimring JC, Hair GA, Chadwick TE, Deshpande SS, Anderson KM, Hilyer CD, Roback JD. Nonhemolytic antibody-induced loss of erythrocyte surface antigen. *Blood* 2005; 106(3): 1105–12.

37. Garratty G, Arndt PA. An update on drug-induced immune hemolytic anemia. *Immunohematology* 2007; 23(3): 105–19.

38. Petz LD, Garratty G. Acquired immune hemolytic anemias. New York: Churchill Livingstone; 1980.

39. Garratty G, Arndt PA, Leger RM. The changing spectrum of drug-induced immune hemolytic anemia over the last 25 years (abstract). *Blood* 2003; 102: 560a.

40. Garratty G. Review: Drug-induced immune hemolytic anemia—the last decade. *Immunohematology* 2004; 20(3): 138–46.

41. Garratty G, Arndt PA. Mechanisms and laboratory investigations of drug-induced immune hemolytic anemia (February 27, 2008). In: AABB Audioconferences. Bethesda (MD): AABB; 2008.

42. Packman C. Hemolytic anemia resulting from immune injury. In Lichtman M, Beutler E, Kipps T, Seligsohn U, Kaushansky K, Prchal J, eds. *Williams Hematology*, 7th ed. New York: McGraw-Hill; 2006. 729–50.

43. Ness, PM. How do I encourage clinicians to transfuse mismatched blood to patients with autoimmune hemolytic anemia in urgent situations? *Transfusion* 2006; 46(11): 1859–62.

44. Petz LD. "Least incompatible" units for transfusion in autoimmune hemolytic anemia: should we eliminate this meaningless term? A commentary for clinicians and transfusion medicine professionals. *Transfusion* 2003; 43: 1503–7.

45. Oyen R, Angeles ML. A simple screening method to evaluate the presence of alloantibodies with concomitant warm autoantibodies. *Immunohematology* 1995; 11: 85–7.

46. Ahrens N, Pruss A, Kahne A, Kiesewetter H, Salama A. Coexistence of autoantibodies and alloantibodies to RBCs due to blood transfusion. *Transfusion* 2007; 47(5): 813–6.

47. Young PP, Uzieblo A, Trulock E, Lublin DM, Goodnough LT. Autoantibody formation after alloimmunization: Are blood transfusions a risk factor for autoimmune hemolytic anemia? *Transfusion* 2004; 44(1): 67–72.

48. Garratty G, Petz LD. Approaches to selecting blood for transfusion to patients with autoimmune hemolytic anemia. *Transfusion* 2002; 42(11): 1390–2.

49. Petz LD, Calhoun L, Shulman IA, Johnson C, Herron RM. The sickle cell hemolytic transfusion reaction syndrome. *Transfusion* 1997; 37(4): 382–92.

50. King KE, Shirey RS, Lankiewicz MW, Young-Ramsaran J, Ness PM. Delayed hemolytic transfusion reactions in sickle cell disease: Simultaneous destruction of recipients' red cells. *Transfusion* 1997; 37(4): 376–81.

51. Win N, Doughty H, Telfer P, Wild BJ, Pearson TC. Hyperhemolytic transfusion reaction in sickle cell disease. *Transfusion* 2001; 41(3): 323–8.

52. Talano JA, Hillery CA, Gottschall JL, Baylerian DM, Scott JP. Delayed hemolytic transfusion reaction/hyperhemolysis syndrome in children with sickle cell disease. *Pediatrics* 2003; 111(6 Pt 1): e661–5.

53. Ballas SK, Marcolina MJ. Hyperhemolysis during the evolution of uncomplicated acute painful episodes in patients with sickle cell anemia. *Transfusion* 2006; 46(1): 105–10.

54. Petz LD. Bystander immune cytolysis. *Transfus Med Rev* 2006; 20(2): 110–40.

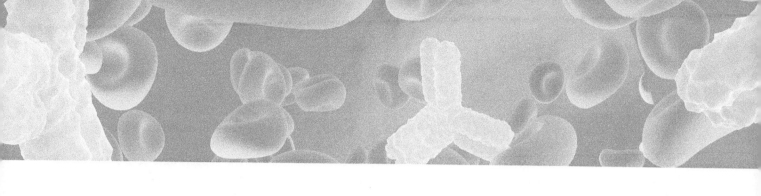

16 Platelet Refractory Patients

PAMPEE P. YOUNG AND ANDRIJ E. SVERSTIUK

Chapter Objectives

Upon completion of this chapter, the student will be able to:

1. List the risk factors for platelet refractoriness.
2. Discuss the significance of the corrected count increment (CCI) and post-transfusion platelet recovery (PPR), including threshold values, in determining refractoriness to platelet transfusion.
3. Given patient data, calculate the CCI and PPR.
4. Name the two most common causes of nonimmune- and immune-mediated platelet refractoriness.
5. Identify the medications that are associated with drug-induced thrombocytopenia.
6. Describe the conditions that cause platelet refractoriness through both immune-mediated (alloimmunization and autoimmunization) and nonimmune-mediated (sequestration, consumption, prothrombosis) mechanisms.
7. Discuss the pathophysiology, treatment and prognosis for immune- and nonimmune-mediated platelet refractoriness.
8. Discuss the factors that influence alloimmunization.
9. Identify specific antibodies that are causative agents in each of the immune-mediated platelet refractory disorders.
10. Describe the following immune-mediated thrombocytopenias including pathophysiology, testing, and treatment: idiopathic/immune thrombo-cytopenia purpura (ITP), drug induced post-transfusion purpura (PTP), neonatal alloimmune thrombocytopenia (NAIT), maternal immune thrombocytopenia.
11. Discuss the procedures for product selection for platelet refractory patients: human leukocyte antigen (HLA) antibody testing, human platelet antigen (HPA) antibody screening, HLA type and match, platelet crossmatching.
12. List the thrombocytopenic conditions that are contraindications for platelet transfusions.
13. State the percentage of total body platelets sequestered in the spleen under normal circumstances.

Key Terms

Corrected count increment
  (CCI)

Eplet(s)

Human leukocyte antigen(s)
  (HLA)

Human platelet antigen(s)
  (HPA)

Native

Panel reactive antibody (PRA)

Platelet crossmatch

Platelet refractoriness

Platelet sequestration

Post-transfusion platelet
  recovery (PPR)

Prothrombotic

CASE IN POINT

DD is a 44-year-old female who presented to the ER after being run over by a car. She had an open pelvic fracture and major injuries to her abdomen. She was actively bleeding and was brought to surgery immediately after admission for splenectomy and to fix her pelvic fracture.

   She has two biological children and underwent back surgery at the same hospital several years prior to this accident. She received a transfusion of 2 red blood cell units during her previous surgery.

What's Ahead?

Platelet transfusions are an important and often life-saving component of modern therapy. Unfortunately, many patients requiring chronic platelet transfusion support develop **platelet refractoriness**, which is an inadequate response to platelet transfusion.

   This chapter addresses the following questions:

1. How does one assess if a patient is refractory to platelet transfusion?
2. What are the common causes of platelet refractoriness?
3. What laboratory tests are used to diagnosis platelet refractoriness?
4. How are platelet units selected for transfusion to a patient who is experiencing platelet refractoriness?
5. What immune thrombocytopenias are accompanied by platelet refractoriness?
6. What thrombocytopenic conditions are relative contraindications for platelet transfusion?
7. What other treatments are used instead of or in combination with platelet transfusions in patients who may not respond to transfusion?

THROMBOCYTOPENIA AND PLATELET TRANSFUSION

Thrombocytopenia is a common complication in a number of pathologic conditions. It often occurs in hematology and oncology patients, particularly during and after chemotherapy. Severe thrombocytopenia requires regular platelet transfusion support until the patient's own bone marrow regains its functional capacity or until the cause of the incompletely compensated platelet consumption or abnormally increased platelet consumption is eliminated. Platelet transfusions may also be indicated in various platelet function disorders, when the patient's platelets are incapable of maintaining adequate hemostatic function. Often, prophylactic platelet transfusions are given based on low platelet counts, rather than on clinically evident bleeding.

   In the United States, two types of platelet products are currently available (Chapter 10). Platelet concentrates prepared from a whole blood unit are concentrated in approximately 40–70 mL of plasma and contain at least 5.5×10^{10} platelets. Four to six units of platelets prepared by this technique are considered one dose. The platelet concentrates may be pooled together or transfused separately. Apheresis platelets are harvested from one donor, are suspended in 100–500 mL of plasma, and should have a minimal platelet count of 3.0×10^{11}. This is close to the content of a pool of five to six platelet concentrates prepared from whole blood units. One transfusion of either a pooled platelet concentrate or a single apheresis product is expected to increase the platelet count in an average 150-pound (70-kilogram) person by approximately $30–50 \times 10^3/\mu L$ ($30–50 \times 10^9/L$).

   The development of platelet refractoriness should be considered when platelet transfusions fail to produce the expected platelet count increments on at least two occasions. Platelet transfusion refractoriness develops in approximately 15–20% of chronically transfused patients.[1] In the hematology and oncology populations, this incidence may be even higher,[2] probably reflecting considerably heavier donor exposure, as well as frequent significant comorbidity in this group of patients.

   Several different mechanisms may result in refractoriness to platelet transfusion. They can be separated into two large groups: nonimmune (Table 16-1 ✳) and immune (Table 16-2 ✳). Increased **platelet sequestration**, where platelets are removed from circulation and stored by the spleen and/or increased platelet consumption, are the predominant factors in nonimmune refractoriness. Immune-mediated refractoriness occurs less often, but is particularly important for transfusion medicine purposes because it includes cases requiring special handling by the transfusion service. In many cases the cause of platelet refractoriness is multifactorial and different factors may predominate at certain points in the course of the transfusion therapy. On the other hand, some patients demonstrate apparent clinical refractoriness to platelet transfusions but no plausible cause of this refractoriness can be discovered.

POST-TRANSFUSION PLATELET INCREMENT

The diagnosis of platelet refractoriness is defined by the failure to meet the expected platelet count increment and therefore depends on the accuracy of the predicted increment. In a healthy person, the majority of transfused platelets remain in the circulation, while about one-third is sequestered in the spleen. Therefore, the immediate post-transfusion platelet count increment is a function of the number of

☀ **TABLE 16-1** Nonimmune Causes of Platelet Refractoriness

Mechanism Resulting in Low Platelet Count	Clinical Condition
Sequestration	Splenomegaly
Consumption	Sepsis*
	Disseminated intravascular coagulation (DIC)
	Medications, for example:
	Amphotericin B
	Vancomycin*
	Ciprofloxacin
	Hematopoietic stem cell transplant* and potential complications including:
	Graft versus host disease (GVHD)
	Veno-occlusive disease (VOD)
	Fever
	Bleeding
Prothrombotic conditions**	Heparin-induced thrombocytopenia (HIT)
	Thrombotic thrombocytopenia purpura (TTP)
	Hemolytic uremic syndrome (HUS)

*Conditions where more than one mechanism of platelet refractoriness may be involved.

**Prothrombotic means a condition leading to the formation of blood clots.

platelets transfused, the total circulating blood volume, and the size of the spleen. In order to normalize the observed increment for these variables, several formulas have been developed.

The most popular, the **corrected count increment (CCI)**, takes into account the transfused platelet dose and the patient's blood volume, which are assumed to be proportional to the body surface area (BSA). The latter is calculated from a conventional nomogram based on body weight and height.

$$CCI = \frac{BSA\ (m^2) \times Platelet\ increment\ (per\ \mu L) \times 10^{11}}{Number\ of\ platelets\ transfused\ \times\ 10^{11}}$$

Note: This formula applies when measurement units for the BSA is m^2 and the platelet increment is per μL

For example, if a person with BSA of 1.7 m^2 is transfused with 3.5×10^{11} platelets, the pretransfusion platelet count was $10 \times 10^3/\mu L$ ($10 \times 10^9/L$) and increased to $50 \times 10^3/\mu L$ ($50 \times 10^9/L$), the CCI will be:

Step 1: Determine the platelet increment count, calculated by subtracting the pretransfusion count per μL from the posttransfusion count per μL

Pretransfusion count: $10 \times 10^3 = 10 \times 1,000 = 10,000/\mu L$

Posttransfusion count: $50 \times 10^3 = 100 \times 1,000 = 50,000/\mu L$

The 10^3 portions cancel out leaving:

50,000 (posttransfusion count) − 10,000 (pretransfusion count) = $40,000/\mu L$

Step 2: Enter the given values and that obtained in step 1 into the formula

In this case: $1.7 \times 40,000 \times 10^{11}/3.5 \times 10^{11}$

The 10^{11} portions cancel out leaving: $1.7 \times 40,000/3.5$ = 68,000/3.5 = 19,428

The calculated CCI in patients who have a spleen cannot be higher than 26,600 because that would correspond to more than 100% recovery and indicates an error in data or calculations.

☀ **TABLE 16-2** Immune-Mediated Platelet Refractoriness

Type of Immunization	Antigens or Diseases
Alloimmunization	Human leukocyte antigens (HLA) Class I (A, B, rarely C loci)
	ABO antigens
	Human platelet antigens (HPA)
	Other: CD36 deficiency type I (Nak[a])
	Post-transfusion purpura (PTP)*
	Neonatal alloimmune thrombocytopenia (NAIT)*
Autoimmunization	Immune/idiopathic thrombocytopenia purpura (ITP)*
	Drug-induced platelet antibodies*, including:
	Quinine, quinidine, amiodarone, vancomycin, gold, captopril, sulfonamides, glibenclamide, carbamazepine, ibuprofen, cimetidine, tamoxifen, ranitidine, phenytoin, piperacillin, interferon alpha, GPIIb/IIIa inhibitors, and many others

*Diseases with immune-mediated destruction of native platelets accompanied by refractoriness to allogeneic platelets.

CASE IN POINT (continued)

DD received 9 units of red blood cells during surgery. On admission, her platelet count was $388 \times 10^3/\mu L$ ($388 \times 10^9/L$). Post surgery, her platelet count fell to $89 \times 10^3/\mu L$ ($89 \times 10^9/L$). She was transfused with 2 units of plasma and one apheresis platelet unit. Immediately following platelet transfusion, her platelet count was $109 \times 10^3/\mu L$ ($109 \times 10^9/L$).

1. What is the minimum number of platelets present in one apheresis unit of platelets?
2. If DD has a BSA of 1.7 m^2 and the unit of platelets she received contained 4.0×10^{11} platelets, what is her CCI?

The alternative formula calculates the **post-transfusion platelet recovery (PPR)**, which normalizes the increment by the platelet dose, the blood volume, and optionally the spleen status. The total blood volume (TBV) is derived from body weight assuming there is 75 mL/kg blood for adult men and 65 mL/kg of blood for women. The average adult body weight of 70 kg is used in these calculations when the body weight is not specified. Some formulas take the status of the spleen into account. In these calculations, the spleen sequestration factor (F) is assumed to be 0.62 in an average person, 0.91 in an asplenic individual, and 0.23 in a patient with hypersplenism. An example of a calculation excluding and including the spleen sequestration factor follows:

EXAMPLE 1

Example 1: (excludes the spleen sequestration factor) =

$$PPR = \frac{TBV\ (mL) \times Platelet\ Increment\ (per\ \mu L) \times 10^3}{Number\ of\ Platelets\ Transfused} \times 100$$

Note: This formula applies when measurement units for the estimated total blood volume (TBV) is mL and the platelet increment is per μL

Using the information from the previous example and using the average weight of 70 kg for an average adult with a normal spleen, the PPR would be calculated as follows:

Step 1 Determine the estimated total blood volume (TBV), calculated by multiplying the assumed amount of blood for an adult male in mL/kg × the average adult weight in kg (since the patient's actual weight is not given)

75 mL/kg × 70 kg = 5250 mL

Step 2 Determine the platelet count increment calculated by subtracting the pretransfusion count per μL from the posttransfusion count per μL

Pretransfusion count: $10 \times 10^3 = 10 \times 1,000$ = 10,000 μL

Posttransfusion count: $10 \times 10^3 = 50 \times 1,000$ = 50,000 μL

The 10^3 portions cancel out leaving:

50,000 (posttransfusion count) − 10,000 (pretransfusion count) = 40,000 μL

Step 3 Enter the values obtained into the formula

To determine the numerator:

TBV × Platelet increment = 5250 × 40,000 = 210,000,000 or 2.1×10^8

Then the above result is
$\times 10^3 = 2.1 \times 10^8 \times 10^3 = 2.1 \times 10^{11}$

To determine the denominator: given = 3.5×10^{11} (number of platelets transfused)

Therefore, the calculation is:
$2.1 \times 10^{11} / 3.5 \times 10^{11}$

The 10^{11} portions cancel out leaving:
$2.1/3.5 = 0.6 \times 100 = 60\%$

EXAMPLE 2

Example 2: (includes the spleen sequestration factor) =

$$PPR = \frac{TBV\ (mL) \times Platelet\ Increment\ (per\ \mu L) \times 10^3}{Number\ of\ Platelets\ Transfused \times F(Sequestration\ factor)} \times 100$$

Note: This formula applies when measurement units for the estimated total blood volume (TBV) is mL, the platelet increment is per μL

Using the information from the previous example and using the average weight of 70 kg for an average adult with a normal spleen and the sequestration factor of 0.62 for an adult with a normal spleen, the PPR would be calculated as follows:

Step 1 Determine the estimated total blood volume (TBV), calculated by multiplying the assumed amount of blood for an adult male in mL/kg × the average adult body weight in kg

75 mL/kg × 70 kg = 5250

Step 2 Determine the platelet count increment calculated by subtracting the pretransfusion count per μL from the posttransfusion count per μL

Pretransfusion count: $10 \times 10^3 = 10 \times 1,000$ = 10,000 μL

Posttransfusion count: $50 \times 10^3 = 50 \times 1,000$ = 50,000 μL

The 10^3 portions cancel out leaving:

50,000 (posttransfusion count) − 10,000 (pretransfusion count) = 40,000 μL

Step 3 Enter the values obtained into the formula

To determine the numerator:

TBV × Platelet increment = 5250 × 40,000
= 210,000,000 or 2.1×10^8

Then the above result $\times 10^3 = 2.1 \times 10^8 \times 10^3$
$= 2.1 \times 10^{11}$

To determine the denominator: given = 3.5
$\times 10^{11}$ (number of platelets transfused)
and assumed platelet sequestration factor
for an average person with a spleen = 0.62

Number of platelets transfused × Average
sequestration factor = $3.5 \times 10^{11} \times 0.62$
$= (3.5 \times 0.62) \times 10^{11} = 2.17 \times 10^{11}$

Therefore, the calculation is:
$2.1 \times 10^{11}/2.17 \times 10^{11}$

The 10^{11} portions cancel out leaving:
$2.1/2.17 = 0.9677 \times 100 = 96.8\%$

CASE IN POINT (continued)

DD was transfused a second unit of apheresis platelets due to oozing at her surgical wounds. Her pretransfusion platelet count was $109 \times 10^3/\mu L$ ($109 \times 10^9/L$) and her post-transfusion platelet count is $129 \times 10^3/\mu L$ ($129 \times 10^9/L$). The platelet count of the unit was 3.8×10^{11}. Her spleen was removed during the earlier surgery.

3. Calculate her PPR.
4. How does the patient's splenectomy affect the post-transfusion platelet count?

CCI and PPR calculations offer considerable improvement in the accuracy and consistency of assessment of the platelet transfusion effectiveness over simply noting the post-transfusion rise in platelet numbers. However, both are based on a number of assumptions and approximations. Circulating blood volume is only estimated and may be inaccurate. CCI arguably is slightly more accurate in this respect if the BSA is calculated and not estimated. Splenic sequestration factor is not always proportional to the spleen size, even if the latter is known. The transfused platelet dose can also be subject to error. While this number for an apheresis product is available from the blood supplier, this information is not readily obtainable for platelet concentrates prepared from whole blood.

Regardless of the chosen method of transfusion response monitoring, the same method should be used consistently for an individual patient. Platelet count should be checked within 15 to 60 minutes after the transfusion, as well as 20–24 hours later, and both values should be compared with the pretransfusion baseline. An acceptable immediate increment, but significantly decreased 24-hour survival

may indicate a nonimmune cause of refractoriness. Immune-mediated platelet refractoriness shows little or no platelet increment at either 1 hour or 24 hours.

In a nonrefractory patient, the typical immediate post-transfusion CCI is at least 7,500 following a single typical adult platelet dose of either one apheresis unit or 4–6 whole blood–derived units. This corresponds to approximately 30% recovery, and should remain above 5,000, which is an approximate 20% recovery, after 24 hours. Immediate CCI below the arbitrary selected threshold of 5,000 on at least two occasions may indicate a refractory state. Figure 16-1 ■ illustrates the CCI typically occurring in nonrefractory and refractory patients following platelet transfusion. If the information necessary to calculate CCI or PPR is not available, a very rough estimate of 2,000/μL increment per 1 unit of platelet concentrate in an average patient can be used. This estimate is based on an average whole blood–derived platelet concentrate containing 7.0×10^{10} platelets and an average adult BSA of 1.76 m^2. If a patient develops a clinical transfusion reaction (Chapter 12), the CCI usually is considerably lower than expected, which does not necessarily indicate a refractory state.

☑ CHECKPOINT 16-1

Name the two formulas that can be used to determine the effectiveness of platelet transfusion.

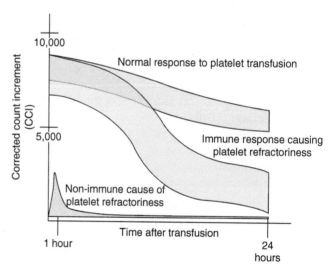

■ FIGURE 16-1 Corrected Count Increments in Nonrefractory, Immune Refractory, and Nonimmune Refractory Patients

Response in the green zone is typical of a normal response to platelet transfusion; CCI is above 7,500 at 1-hour post transfusion and CCI remains about 5,000 at 24 hours post transfusion. Response in the blue, striped zone is typical of a patient experiencing an immune response that decreases the effectiveness of platelet transfusion; the CCI soon after transfusion shows a normal response but the platelet count falls to below an expected CCI level over the next 24 hours. Response in the pink zone is typical of a patient exhibiting a nonimmune cause of platelet refractoriness; the CCI never reaches an expected value and the platelet count quickly returns to pretransfusion levels.

PLATELET SEQUESTRATION

About 30% of total body platelets are normally harbored in the spleen. Splenomegaly, therefore, often results in the increase of the sequestered fraction and lack of an adequate response to platelet transfusions. Although in many patients the size of the spleen correlates with the degree of refractoriness, this relationship is not always straightforward,[3] and some patients with massive splenomegaly still demonstrate an adequate response to transfusion.

CONSUMPTIVE PLATELET REFRACTORINESS

Markedly increased platelet consumption occurs in many conditions and can result in platelet transfusion refractoriness.

Sepsis

In bacterial or fungal sepsis the mechanism of increased platelet consumption, both **native** and transfused, is not well characterized. Native is another term to describe the patient's own platelets. Platelet consumption in sepsis is probably related to generalized vascular endothelial damage with contributions from complement activation, immune complex formation, direct effect of endotoxin, and other changes associated with infection.

Disseminated Intravascular Coagulation (DIC)

In disseminated intravascular coagulation (DIC), massive intravascular thrombin generation and decreased intrinsic anticoagulation mechanisms lead to overwhelming consumption of platelets and plasma procoagulants, anticoagulants, and fibrinolytic components. This results in simultaneous widespread microvascular thrombosis and bleeding. This condition can be triggered by a number of different factors. One cause of DIC is sepsis, which will lead to profoundly low platelet counts even with transfusion, because both sepsis and DIC increase platelet consumption.

Medications

Many medications can cause platelet refractoriness. In some cases the refractoriness is consumptive, but a number of drugs can also induce an immune refractory state. Amphotericin B, which is used to treat severe disseminated fungal infection, is a well-recognized cause of platelet refractoriness.[4] CCI decreases by 20–30% and, in addition, platelet function is affected. The mechanism of this phenomenon is not completely understood. The detrimental effect of amphotericin B on transfused platelet recovery can be reduced by scheduling transfusion and drug administration as far apart as clinically feasible.

A milder effect is seen with vancomycin and ciprofloxacin, which are commonly used antibiotics.[4] Heparin is known to induce platelet activation, and almost all patients develop a mild transient decrease in platelet counts at the beginning of the therapy, probably due to subclinical platelet consumption known as heparin-induced thrombocytopenia (HIT) type I. However, a subset of these patients develops a much more serious complication called heparin-induced thrombocytopenia type II.

Fever

Fever, even without a documented systemic infection, has often been quoted as a causative factor for platelet refractoriness.[5, 6]

Bleeding

Bleeding is traditionally listed as a cause of nonimmune platelet refractoriness. Available data, however, is confusing: only some,[7] but not all, studies[6] detected such an association. Severe hemorrhage would result in platelet consumption as the body tried to achieve hemostasis. Treatment of a severely bleeding patient would include massive volume replacement that would have a dilutional effect on platelet counts. These are probably the factors that cause some bleeding patients to appear refractory to platelet transfusion.

Bone Marrow Transplant

Bone marrow transplantation, particularly when accompanied by graft versus host disease (GVHD) is another factor that can result in apparent platelet refractoriness. Patients who develop post-transplant veno-occlusive disease invariably demonstrate consumptive thrombocytopenia.[8]

Prothrombotic Conditions

Consumptive thrombocytopenia is also one of the leading manifestations of several disorders, including heparin-induced thrombocytopenia (HIT), thrombotic thrombocytopenic purpura (TTP), and hemolytic uremic syndrome (HUS). Although some pathological immune component may be present in many cases, the mechanism of thrombocytopenia is platelet consumption rather than immune-mediated destruction. In these conditions, platelet transfusions are relatively contraindicated. These conditions are **prothrombotic**, which means that they lead to clot formation. Platelet transfusion can lead to more clot formation and can worsen the patient's symptoms. However, in rare instances, life-threatening bleeding still may occur, necessitating emergency platelet transfusions. In such circumstances, consumptive refractoriness to platelet transfusions will be evident.

Heparin-Induced Thrombocytopenia (HIT)

In heparin-induced thrombocytopenia type II (HIT), patients develop IgG antibodies against heparin-platelet factor 4 (PF4) complexes. These antibodies activate platelets, causing platelet aggregation and thrombosis. The platelet count drops and heparin must be stopped before major thrombosis develops. Despite the thrombocytopenia, HIT patients require continuous anticoagulation with anticoagulants such as low-molecular-weight heparin or nonheparin anticoagulants. Platelet counts usually stay above $15–20 \times 10^3/\mu L$ ($15–20 \times 10^9/L$) and, if bleeding develops, it is from the continuous anticoagulation rather than the thrombocytopenia. Platelet transfusions are almost never indicated in HIT and may, in fact, contribute to the development of thrombotic complications.

The causative antibodies can be detected either by a commercially available solid-phase enzyme immunoassay or by the serotonin release assay.[9] The latter, more specific functional assay detects pooled donor platelet aggregation in the presence of heparin, if the patient's sample contains antibodies against the heparin-PF4 complex. The detection is based on measuring ^{14}C-labeled serotonin released from degranulating platelets following platelet activation. Functional assays based on heparin-induced platelet aggregation measured by either conventional platelet aggregometry or flow cytometry are rarely used.

Thrombotic Thrombocytopenic Purpura (TTP)/Hemolytic Uremic Syndrome (HUS)

Patients with thrombotic thrombocytopenic purpura (TTP) present with a consumptive thrombocytopenia, as well as a microangiopathic anemia. In this disease, ultra-large multimers of von Willebrand factor accumulate in the circulation due to decreased cleavage. This leads to massive intravascular microthrombosis with resultant platelet consumption and thrombocytopenia.[10, 11] Hemolytic uremic syndrome (HUS) closely resembles TTP, but the disease is limited to the kidney vasculature. The primary event in HUS is renal endothelial damage by bacterial toxins or unopposed complement activation with resultant thrombosis.[12, 13]

All TTP and HUS patients are thrombocytopenic and occasionally very low platelet counts may be seen. Both TTP and HUS are considered relative contraindications for platelet transfusions in view of continuous intravascular platelet activation, adhesion, and aggregation. Major bleeding complications are very uncommon and platelet transfusions are very rarely indicated. When platelets are transfused, however, consumptive refractoriness to platelet transfusions may be seen.

☑ CHECKPOINT 16-2

List four causes of consumptive platelet refractoriness.

IMMUNE-MEDIATED PLATELET REFRACTORINESS

Approximately 30–40% of patients refractory to platelet transfusion demonstrate immune-mediated platelet destruction.[6, 14] In contrast to immune-mediated hemolysis, which often results in dramatic immediate clinical manifestations, immune platelet destruction is not usually evident at the time of transfusion. Platelet destruction may result in a relatively mild febrile nonhemolytic transfusion reaction or the only indication may be the absence of the expected platelet count increment.

In most cases alloantibodies are involved, but in some conditions autoantibodies cause the destruction of native platelets as well as the transfused platelets (Table 16-2). In clinical transfusion medicine practice, the most challenging cases of platelet refractoriness are related to alloimmunization to antigens expressed on the platelet membrane. These antigens can be either platelet-specific, called **human platelet antigens (HPA)**, or represent specificities shared with other cell types such as those leukocytes, platelets, and many tissue cells, known as **human leukocyte antigens (HLA)** class I (Chapter 18) and ABO group antigens (Chapter 4).

Platelet alloimmunization develops at some point in many chronically transfused hematology and oncology patients. Its prevalence has been reported to be from 15% to almost 80%, depending on inclusion criteria, platelet products used, and laboratory techniques. However, only 30–40% of alloimmunized patients demonstrate clinically relevant platelet refractoriness.

Factors Influencing Alloimmunization

There are three factors, discussed in the next sections, that influence alloimmunization: prior exposure, immune status, and antigen dose.

Prior Exposure

In contrast to naturally occurring ABO antibodies, HPA- and HLA-related alloimmunization requires prior exposure to an allogeneic antigen. Sources of exposure are previous pregnancies, transplantation, and/or multiple transfusions. The risk of alloimmunization is proportional to the number of previous exposures, so a reduction in transfusion frequency and the use of apheresis products rather than pooled platelet concentrates may decrease the incidence of platelet refractoriness.[15] This correlation, however, is lost after reaching a critical number of exposures, which is probably fewer than 20. In multiply transfused patients the alloimmunization rate becomes independent of the number of exposures.[16] Many transfusion services that utilize both pooled and apheresis platelet products reserve the latter for patients that can be expected to require continuous transfusion support.

Immune Status

An important factor that influences the development of refractoriness is the state of the patient's immune system. Immunosuppression regardless of etiology significantly reduces the incidence of alloimmunization. Increased rates of alloimmunization are seen with individuals who, for poorly understood reasons, are active antibody producers. Certain medical conditions, especially autoimmune disorders and some hemoglobinopathies, also predispose patients to alloimmunization.[17] Conversely, it has been noted that patients with acute lymphoblastic leukemia develop platelet refractoriness less often than patients with myeloid leukemia.[18] Patients with previous or concomitant alloimmunization to nonplatelet antigens—for example, red blood cell antigens—may be at higher risk for the development of antibodies against platelet antigens.[19] Some procedures, particularly those associated with extracorporeal circulation—for example, cardiopulmonary bypass and hemodialysis—are known to predispose patients to alloimmunization.[20] The exact mechanism of this phenomenon is unclear, although leukocyte activation and the release of proinflammtory cytokines have been suggested.[21]

Antigen Dose

The other factor that contributes to alloimmunization is antigen dose. HLA alloimmunization is the leading cause of immune-mediated refractoriness and leukocytes express a high density of HLA molecules. Not surprisingly, blood product leukoreduction results in at least a threefold reduction in the rate of HLA antibody formation.[22, 23] Besides a simple decrease in foreign antigen load, leukoreduction results in a significant depletion of donor antigen-presenting cells (APC). The donor APC can present donor antigens to the recipient's T cells, resulting in antigen recognition and subsequent antibody formation.

Ultraviolet-B irradiation of platelets, a technique originally developed for pathogen inactivation, has also been demonstrated in clinical trials to reduce alloimmunization rates.[23] Currently this methodology is not licensed in the United States.

Platelets express variable but a relatively high density of about 10^5 molecules per platelet for Class I HLA-A and HLA-B molecules. HLA alloimmunization is the cause of more than half of all cases of immune-mediated refractoriness. On the other hand, HLA alloantibodies can be detected in about one-third of patients who are not clinically refractory.[14] Primary immune response occurs within 3 to 4 weeks, although it can develop as early as 10 days post transfusion. In approximately 40% of cases these antibodies spontaneously vanish, sometimes within several months, even in patients on continuous transfusion support.[18] Some of these patients will never develop an anamnestic response. But in a subset of individuals, particularly multiparous women, the antibodies may persist for decades and these patients can mount an anamnestic response in 4–5 days upon subsequent antigen challenge.[22, 23]

☑ CHECKPOINT 16-3

Identify three factors that influence alloimmunization.

Alloantibody Specificities

Antibodies directed against HLAs, ABO, HPAs, and to CD36 are all of importance and brief discussions are found in the sections that follow.

Human Leukocyte Antigen (HLA) Antibodies

More than 90% of HLA antibodies are directed against *public epitopes*, which are antigens common to several different HLA molecules.[24] The cross-reactivity of HLA antibodies leads to broad platelet refractoriness during transfusion and to complications in HLA matching of platelet products.

Platelets also express HLA-C molecules, but in low density. Traditionally, HLA-C alloimmunization has been considered clinically irrelevant; however, one study found HLA-C-related alloimmunization caused platelet refractoriness in about 5% of refractory patients.[25] The density of HLA-C molecule expression on platelets is subject to considerable intraindividual variation, which may explain the controversy. The issue is complicated by the fact that the overwhelming majority of HLA-typed platelet donors are phenotyped for HLA-A and HLA-B only, and HLA-C matching, even if proven clinically useful, is problematic. Normal platelets do not carry HLA Class II molecules.

ABO Antibodies

ABH antigens are present on the platelet membrane, partially intrinsic and in part absorbed from the plasma (Chapter 4). ABO-related incompatibility, after HLA mismatch, is the second most common cause of immune platelet refractoriness and may account for 20–25% of all refractory cases.[26]

One type of ABO incompatibility occurs when the recipient's plasma has an antibody to an ABO antigen that is on the donor platelets (Table 16-3 ✳; see also Table 7-2). The clinical relevance of this type of platelet ABO mismatch correlates with the recipient's antibody titers, which in the ABO system is also called the *isoagglutinin titers*. Isoagglutinin titers vary widely among different individuals, but generally are higher in group O persons, with anti-A reactivity usually being stronger than anti-B. In many cases ABO mismatch results in a mild decrease in post-transfusion platelet increment that is clinically irrelevant. Approximately one-third of patients show a modest, statistically significant reduction in CCI, and 20% with unusually high levels of anti-A or infrequently anti-B antibodies may demonstrate clinically relevant platelet refractoriness to ABO-incompatible platelets.[27]

Another factor that affects survival of ABO-mismatched platelets, as with HLA, is the antigen dose. The ABO antigen density is relatively high on platelets, about 50,000–180,000 molecules per platelet. B antigens exhibit weaker expression than A, similar to red blood cells. Individuals of the A_2 group carry very small, often

✳ **TABLE 16-3** ABO Mismatches in Platelet Transfusion (see also Table 7-2)

Recipient Plasma Has Antibody to ABO Antigen on Transfused (Donor) Platelets		Donor Plasma Has Antibody to ABO Antigens on Recipient's Red Blood Cells and Platelets	
Recipient	Donor	Recipient	Donor
O	A, B, AB	A, B, AB	O
A	B, AB	B, AB	A
B	A, AB	A, AB	B
Platelet Transfusion Choices			
Recipient ABO	First Choice	Second Choice	Third Choice
O	O	A, B, or AB	
A	A	AB	B or O
B	B	AB	A or O
AB	AB	A or B	O

undetectable, amounts of A substance on their platelets. Approximately 7% of healthy donors are high expressers of A and/or B determinants, carrying on their platelets three to seven times more antigen than average individuals.[28] This variability in antigen expression on platelets can explain why the same patient may have an adequate response to some ABO-mismatched platelet transfusions but an inadequate response to others.

While the mechanism of platelet destruction due to recipient ABO antibodies is easy to understand, the mechanism of donor ABO antibody–related refractoriness is less obvious (Table 16-3). Some clinical observations have shown that platelet transfusions where donor antibodies are mismatched to recipient ABO antigens can result in an even worse outcome than transfusions where recipient antibodies could attach ABO antigens on the donor platelets.[26, 29] It is believed that immune complexes consisting of donor antibodies and recipient soluble A and/or B substances form. The complexes attach to the recipient's platelet immunoglobulin FcγRIIα and/or complement C1q-R receptors, resulting in platelet destruction.[30, 31]

Some data suggest that ABO-mismatched platelet transfusions may predispose recipients to a higher rate of alloimmunization for HLA or HPA.[32] Data also suggests that ABO-incompatible platelets may have lower *in vivo* hemostatic potential than ABO-identical platelets.[33] Additionally, cases of severe hemolysis attributed to ABO-incompatible platelet transfusions have been reported. Clearly, ABO-identical platelets are the preferred product and should be selected whenever possible. However, supply issues that include a short shelf life and a rising demand for platelet products mean that it is not always possible to provide ABO-identical platelet transfusions.

Human Platelet Antigen (HPA) Antibodies

Platelet refractoriness due only to HPA antibodies is much less common than cases related to HLA alloimmunization or ABO mismatch, and occurs in less than 5% of refractory patients.[34] As with HLA, the prevalence of HPA antibodies is much higher than the relevant clinical refractoriness due to these antibodies. Approximately 10–25% of HLA-alloimmunized platelet refractory patients also demonstrate HPA antibodies, but their contribution to the immune platelet destruction is unclear.[35] Conversely, most patients with HPA alloimmunization also have broadly reacting HLA antibodies. Generally, antigenicity of HPA appears to be weaker than HLA.

Currently, 24 HPAs have been described (Box 16-1).[36] The molecular basis is known for all except two, Vaᵃ and Mouᵃ. Most HPA and the corresponding antibodies were originally reported in cases of neonatal alloimmune thrombocytopenia (NAIT) or post-transfusion purpura (PTP). Only a few HPA antibodies have been implicated in platelet refractoriness: HPA-1 through -5 and -15. The most commonly identified specificities are against low-frequency antigens: HPA-1b, -2b, and -5b.[35]

CD36 Antibodies

CD36, also known as the Nakᵃ antigen, is carried on the glycoprotein IV (abbreviated as GPIV) molecule and is not included in HPA classification. Alloimmunization to CD36 is very rare in the Caucasian population. However, complete absence of CD36 occurs in 2.5% of Americans of African ethnicity, about 5% of the population

---

BOX 16-1 Human Platelet Antigens (HPAs)

ISBT Name

1a (Plᴬ¹, Zwᵃ)	8bw (Srᵃ)
1b (Plᴬ², Zwᵇ)	9bw (Maxᵃ)
2a (Koᵇ)	10bw (Laᵃ)
2b (Koᵃ, Sibᵃ)	11bw (Groᵃ)
3a (Bakᵃ, Lekᵃ)	12bw (Iyᵃ)
3b (Bakᵇ)	13bw (Sitᵃ)
4a (Yukᵇ, Penᵃ)	14bw (Oeᵃ)
4b (Yukᵃ, Penᵇ)	15a (Govᵇ)
5a (Brᵇ, Zavᵇ)	15b (Govᵃ)
5b (Brᵃ, Zavᵃ, Hcᵃ)	16bw (Duvᵃ)
6bw (Caᵃ, Tuᵃ)	Vaᵃ
7bw (Moᵃ)	Mouᵃ

International Society of Blood Transfusion (ISBT) classification (1990) revised by Platelet Nomenclature Committee (PNC) in 2003. Traditional names are given in parentheses; a "w" designation is added after the antigen name if an alloantibody against the antithetical antigen has not been reported

---

in Japan and as high as 8–11% in other Southeast Asian and sub-Saharan African populations.[37] Cases of severe CD36 antibody-related platelet refractoriness, as well as NAIT and PTP, have been reported. The transfusion support of such patients is considerably complicated due to the high prevalence of the antigen in the regular donor population; screening and recruitment of family members may be required.

CASE IN POINT (continued)

DD was returned to surgery on day 2 and day 3 of hospitalization for repair of massive abdominal injuries. On day 2, her platelet count fell to $89 \times 10^3/\mu L$ ($89 \times 10^9/L$). At that time, an additional 2 units of apheresis platelets were transfused. On day 3, her platelet count was $14 \times 10^3/\mu L$ ($14 \times 10^9/L$). She received 2 units of red blood cells and 1 unit of apheresis platelets and her post-transfusion platelet count immediately following transfusion was $11 \times 10^3/\mu L$ ($11 \times 10^9/L$).

5. Is DD's post-transfusion platelet recovery adequate? Explain.

6. List some possible reasons for poor platelet response in this patient.

7. Given the history, do you suspect the platelet destruction is immune or nonimmune mediated?

The patient was started on intravenous immune globulin (IVIG) on day 3 of hospitalization.

DIAGNOSIS AND PRODUCT SELECTION

Transfusion support of platelet refractory patients is complicated and requires coordinated efforts of the clinical team, the hospital transfusion medicine service, and the local blood supplier.

Initial Steps

When platelet refractoriness is suspected in a patient, it is important to first confirm the response to the transfusion. Measurements of platelet counts within 1 hour and at 20–24 hours post transfusion are essential because these may help both in establishing the cause of refractoriness and in selection of a rational treatment strategy. The accuracy of assessing the response will be considerably improved if CCI or PPR values are calculated.

The next important step is to obtain a complete and accurate history including relevant information on any possible condition that may result in platelet refractoriness. Sepsis, profuse bleeding, DIC, massive splenomegaly, and other factors should be considered. Medication history should also be reviewed. If a patient abruptly develops platelet refractoriness and/or worsening of thrombocytopenia concomitantly with administration of a drug known to induce platelet refractoriness, adjustments to the treatment protocol may solve the problem. Box 16-2 lists some of the more commonly prescribed medications that are known to sometimes cause thrombocytopenia.

BOX 16-2 Partial List of Medications Known to Cause Thrombocytopenia

Drug Names

Acetaminophen	Hydrochlorothiazide
Acetazolamide	Indinavir
Aminoglutethimide	Levamisole
Atorvastatin	Mesalamine
Carbamazepine	Penicillamine
Chlorothiazide	Penicillins
Chlorpromazine	Pentoxlfylline
Chlorpropamide	Phenytoin
Cimetidine	Prednisone
Diazepam	Quinidine
Diazoxide	Quinine
Diclofenace	Ranitidine
Eptifibatide	Rifampin
Famotidine	Sulfasalazine
Furosemide	Ticlopidine
Gold salts	Valproic acid
Haloperidol	Vancomycin
Heparin	

If no plausible cause of nonimmune refractoriness can be found, transfusion of ABO-identical platelets is the next step. The freshest units available should be selected, as survival of platelets in units less than 48 hours old is generally longer.[38] Adequate response to ABO-identical platelets is assessed on at least two occasions by immediate post-transfusion platelet increments. Patients in whom no clinical reason for refractoriness is evident and who subsequently do not adequately respond to ABO identical platelets should next be evaluated for immune refractoriness due to HLA- or, less likely, HPA-related alloimmunization.

HLA and HPA Antibody Screen

The next step is to screen the patient for HLA and/or HPA antibodies. Methodologies that allow for high-definition antibody identification, such as enzyme-linked immunosorbent assay (ELISA) and flow cytometry, are preferred; although the classic antibody-mediated complement–dependent lymphocytotoxicity test with antiglobulin augmentation can also be used (Chapter 18). The latter assay, while giving a good estimate of the degree of alloimmunization, which is reported as a percentage of **panel reactive antibody (PRA)**, does not allow for accurate antibody specificity identification in HLA alloimmunized patients with PRA approaching 100%.

Several ELISA and solid phase–based screening assays for HLA and HPA antibodies are commercially available.[39] While they detect the presence of both HLA and HPA antibodies, they do not discriminate between different HLA Class I antibodies. Some, however, do identify HPA antibody specificities, which is particularly advantageous in diagnosing NAIT and PTP cases. In platelet refractoriness cases a positive screening test must be followed either by a *platelet crossmatch* (described later in this chapter) or by HLA antibody identification with subsequent HLA matching. A negative screening test suggests that the patient's refractoriness is due to a nonimmune cause and that time-consuming and expensive matching tests would not be beneficial.

HLA Type and Match

When the HLA antibody screen is positive, both the antibody specificity and the HLA phenotype of the patient should be determined. High-definition antibody screening tests may have already identified the antibody or antibodies present. Hematology patients who have been assessed for a possible bone marrow transplant will likely have already been HLA typed. Intermediate- or high-resolution DNA-based techniques are preferred for HLA typing. No matter the sequence of testing, once the patient's antibody is identified and phenotype is established, the platelet unit with the closest possible HLA match is selected for transfusion, as shown in Table 16-4 ✴.

An HLA identical match is called an A match, which occurs when the donor and the recipient have the identical phenotype for all four HLA-A and -B antigens. HLA-compatible matches are called BU matches. In BU matches, one (B1U) or two (B2U) antigens in the donor phenotype are unknown, which in most cases represents homozygosity of the identified allele. HLA mismatches are called C matches when one antigen is mismatched and D matches when two or more antigens are mismatched. Table 16-4 shows contains each of these traditional designations along with its corresponding grade and potential donor-recipient phenotype matches.

✴ **TABLE 16-4** Platelet Match Grades

Grade	Traditional Designation*	Donor and Recipient Phenotype Matches
HLA identical	A	All 4 HLA-A and HLA-B antigens identical
HLA compatible	B1U	3 donor antigens identified, all present in recipient
	B2U	2 donor antigens identified, all present in recipient
HLA CREG** match	B1X	3 donor and recipient antigens identical, 1 antigen cross-reactive
	B2X	2 donor and recipient antigens identical, 2 antigens cross-reactive
Selective mismatch	N/A	No recipient antibody against donor antigens
Random crossmatch	N/A	Crossmatch compatible
Random mismatch	C	1 donor antigen not cross-reactive
	D	2 donor antigens not cross-reactive

*A description of each traditional designation is located in the corresponding text. Traditional designations may appear in older literature, especially before DNA typing methods became the routine for HLA typing (Chapter 18).

**CREG = Cross-Reacting Epitope Groups.

Availability of high-grade A or BU matches may pose a problem, even for a patient with a relatively common HLA phenotype. For example, in the Caucasian population the calculated probability of a random A match is 1:2,500, increasing nearly tenfold for all possible A and BU matches combined. Chances of finding a match for a non-Caucasian patient within the predominantly Caucasian donor pool are two to three times lower.[40] It has been shown that platelet products with grade C or D antigen mismatch perform only marginally better or no better at all than randomly selected units.[41]

In cases when a high grade–matched product is not available, alternative HLA-based strategies can be employed. Antigen avoidance, analogous to red blood cell transfusion practice, relies on the selection of products with an HLA phenotype lacking the antigens for which the patient has the corresponding antibodies. Phenotypic selection based on antibody cross-reactivity pattern takes advantage of the fact that most HLA antibodies react against so-called public epitopes, which are shared by several HLA molecules (Chapter 18). These specificities are arranged in serologically defined cross-reacting epitope groups (CREGs). If the patient's antibody is directed against an antigen from a particular CREG group, it is assumed that it may cross-react with the other antigens in this group. Therefore, the HLA phenotype of the selected platelet product should lack any of the antigens belonging to this particular CREG. On the other hand, antigens from the same CREG(s) as the patient's own phenotype are permissible, as they are unlikely to react with the patient's antibody. Attention to linked HLA specificities—for example, Bw4 and Bw6—is beneficial in some patients unresponsive to antigen-avoidance platelets; while mismatching for poorly expressed HLA-B locus antigens—for example, HLA-B44 and -B45—may be acceptable for certain donor-recipient pairs.[41, 42] The combination of these strategies is called the antibody-specificity prediction (ASP) method. A sophisticated computerized algorithm that uses ASP has been developed.[42] However, while this approach increases the availability of platelet products for refractory patients, the effectiveness of such transfusions is still inferior to high-grade HLA-matched products.

A novel technique of HLA-based selection of platelet products for refractory patients has recently been developed.[43, 44] It is based on tridimensional structural similarities of different HLA molecules defined by short, adjacent, antibody-accessible amino acid sequences called **eplets**. Eplets range from two to five amino acid residues long. In the three-dimensional structure of the HLA antigen the amino acids of the eplet are adjacent but they may not be continuous, that is, all in line if the molecule was spread out linearly rather than being twisted and folded as occurs in nature. Figure 16-2 ■ illustrates this concept. A given eplet cannot induce alloantibody production if the same sequence is present on any antigen of the recipient. A computerized algorithm for HLA matching by this methodology, called HLAMatchmaker, is available.[45] Although this approach considerably expands the number of compatible donors, it requires that a large cohort of donors be HLA typed by DNA-based intermediate or high-resolution techniques, which is expensive and not available in many areas.

Regardless of the strategy employed for HLA matching, it is important to regularly confirm a patient's antibody specificity. In some patients HLA antibodies disappear spontaneously despite continuing transfusion support,[18] whereas other patients develop new antibodies. An individual patient's response to matched platelets should be continuously followed by CCI or PPR monitoring. PRA screen and/or high-definition antibody identification panels should be repeated every 2–3 weeks or whenever patients begin to demonstrate inadequate responses, without another identified reason, to seemingly well-matched products.

☑ **CHECKPOINT 16-5**

What is the best type of HLA match for transfusion?

Platelet Crossmatch

A **platelet crossmatch** with 12–18 randomly selected, preferably ABO-identical platelet units is the alternative to HLA-based selection.[46] If all units are crossmatch compatible, immune refractoriness is assumed to be unlikely. A platelet crossmatch refers to testing where the recipient's plasma or serum is combined with donor platelets. There are several techniques that can be used for the platelet crossmatch: the platelet immunofluorescent test, which can be read either by microscopy (PIFT) or by the more sensitive flow cytometry

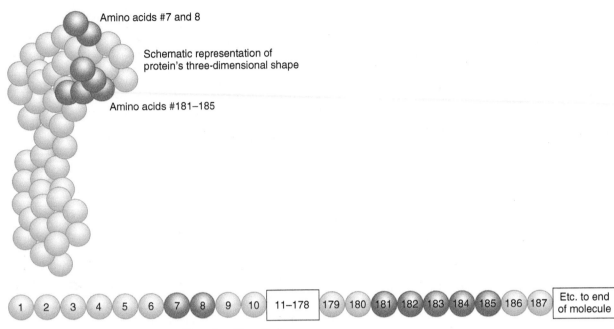

Amino acids #7 and 8

Schematic representation of protein's three-dimensional shape

Amino acids #181–185

| 1 | 2 | 3 | 4 | 5 | 6 | 7 | 8 | 9 | 10 | 11–178 | 179 | 180 | 181 | 182 | 183 | 184 | 185 | 186 | 187 | Etc. to end of molecule |

■ FIGURE 16-2   Protein Structure Showing Two Eplets

In this fictional protein molecule, amino acids 7–8 and 181–186 would be far apart if the protein molecule was a straight line of amino acids, as shown at the bottom of the diagram. When the protein molecule twists and bends into its three-dimensional shape, the two eplets are quite close together, as shown at the top of the diagram.

(FCIT); the modified antibody capture ELISA (MACE); and the solid-phase mixed red cell adherence assay (SPRCA).[39] The latter two assays are available as commercial kits.

The advantage of platelet crossmatching is the immediate availability of compatible units. Ideally, the crossmatch detects incompatibility regardless of the alloantibody specificity. Solid phase–based platelet crossmatch methodology is adaptable for high-throughput automation. An institution with a large donor collection center can utilize whole blood platelet concentrates, rather than apheresis platelets, and selected crossmatch-compatible units can be pooled.[47] The crossmatch approach is highly technique dependent. Occasionally the sensitivity of the methodology appears insufficient, and in clinical trials crossmatched platelets performed somewhat worse than high-grade HLA-matched products.[48] Also, crossmatches have to be performed fairly frequently, as the shelf life of platelet products is limited to 5 days.

Selection of the optimal strategy for a particular institution depends on multiple factors, including the patient population and available resources. It has been suggested that continuous transfusion support with high-grade HLA-matched platelets selected by a traditional HLA phenotype technique requires a platelet donor pool of optimally 6,000–10,000.[49] When a large donor pool is unavailable, platelet crossmatch is usually the preferred strategy. Platelet product selection for a refractory patient incurs considerable expense and the economic factor also has to be taken into consideration when choosing a strategy.

Finally, 20–25% of refractory patients with no obvious nonimmune cause for refractoriness do not respond even to high-grade HLA-matched platelets.[50] Crossmatching of HLA-matched units has been suggested for such patients; however, a huge pool of donors would be needed to find one or more units that would be both platelet

crossmatch compatible and high-grade HLA matched. Figure 16-3 ■ shows one algorithm for testing patients who are thought to be refractory to platelet transfusion and strategies for treating them. Again, each institution will develop their own algorithm based on patient and donor populations and the availability of test procedures and platelet products.

Patients who fail to respond to multiple well-matched platelet units may require a modification of the platelet transfusion strategy. The common strategy of maintaining a minimum platelet count level in order to prevent a bleed may have to be changed to controlling any active, clinically significant bleeds that occur. Often this can be achieved by aggressive transfusions of random, unselected platelet units, in addition to nontransfusion-based therapies.

CASE IN POINT (continued)

The transfusion service medical director was consulted regarding DD's poor platelet response. The medical director and DD's treating physician were able to rule out non-immune-mediated platelet destruction. The medical director recommended transfusing ABO-identical, crossmatch-compatible platelet products and performing an HLA/platelet antibody screen. The HLA/platelet antibody screen was sent to a reference laboratory, but in the meantime ABO-identical, crossmatch-compatible apheresis platelets were obtained.

8. DD is blood type O-positive. Why did the medical director recommend transfusing ABO-identical, group O platelets to the patient?

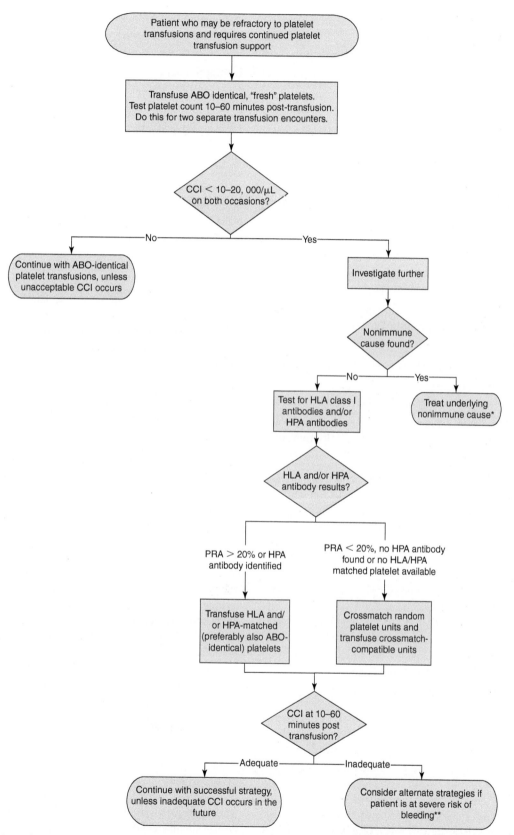

■ FIGURE 16-3 Algorithm of Treatment for Platelet Refractory Patients CCI (Corrected Count Increment)

Facility-specific algorithms should be developed that take into account the patient and donor populations in the area and the testing methods available to the laboratory. This figure is only one example of many acceptable algorithms.

*Nonimmune causes include disseminated intravascular coagulation (DIC), sepsis, medications, fever, bleeding, and splenomegaly.

**Alternative strategies include massive platelet transfusion; slow, continuous platelet infusion; antifibrinolytic agents; activated Factor VII; or prothrombin complex concentrates.

✓ CHECKPOINT 16-6

List three techniques that can be used to perform a platelet crossmatch.

IMMUNE-MEDIATED THROMBOCYTOPENIAS

Immune-mediated thrombocytopenia is a symptom in several clinical conditions. Platelet transfusions are rarely indicated for these patients because the transfused platelets are usually destroyed by the same disease process that is destroying the patient's own platelets.

Immune/Idiopathic Thrombocytopenia Purpura (ITP)

Immune thrombocytopenic purpura (ITP), also known as Werlhof's disease, is a relatively common disorder. Autoimmune platelet destruction can occur secondary to other conditions:

- Autoimmune diseases, for example, systemic lupus erythematosus and antiphospholipid antibody syndrome.
- Neoplastic disorders, particularly lymphoproliferative disorders.
- Viral infections such as HIV, where the pathogenesis of the thrombocytopenia is multifactorial, and only partially results from autoimmune destruction.

When ITP develops without an identifiable underlying disease, it is called idiopathic thrombocytopenic purpura instead of immune, but retains the same abbreviation (ITP). Autoantibodies in ITP are usually directed against the glycoprotein (GP) complexes GPIIb/IIIa and/or GPIb/IX, while many patients with chronic ITP develop antibodies that react broadly against multiple platelet antigens. Antibody detection and identification is generally not done because conventional laboratory tests for platelet antibodies lack sufficient specificity to be clinically useful in most cases of acute ITP. More elaborate tests based on radioactive, enzyme-linked or fluorescent-based detection of specific platelet glycoprotein antibodies have been recently introduced. They include modifications of monoclonal antibody immobilization of platelet antigen (MAIPA) capture assay, radioactive immunobead assay, and several flow cytometry–based assays employing microbeads loaded with platelet GP molecules. While some of these newer tests have good specificity, they are not used to diagnose ITP because of their lack of standardization, technical difficulties, limited availability, and relatively low sensitivity, especially in chronic ITP cases. At present, ITP remains a clinical diagnosis of exclusion.[39]

Fortunately, severe bleeding complications are rare in acute ITP and platelet transfusions are almost never indicated. However, patients with chronic ITP can develop severe bleeding complications that may require platelet transfusions, often in combination with high-dose intravenous immunoglobulin (IVIG). The effect of such transfusions is only transient. Considering the broad, often panreactive specificity of platelet antibodies in patients with ITP, platelet product selection is not feasible, and random pooled concentrates or random apheresis products are used.

Drug-Induced Thrombocytopenia

Drug-induced thrombocytopenia related to quinine was first described in 1865.[51] The condition is also known as cocktail or tonic water purpura, as cases of thrombocytopenia have been linked to ingestion of these beverages, which have a small amount of quinine. Quinine remains the most common compound implicated in drug-induced immune thrombocytopenia.

A number of other drugs have been linked to thrombocytopenia, but only some are associated with immune destruction of platelets (Box 16-2). Heparin-induced thrombocytopenia (HIT) is the most common drug-induced thrombocytopenia. Although the condition is antibody mediated, the thrombocytopenia in HIT is primarily a result of platelet consumption rather than immune destruction.

In a typical case of drug-induced thrombocytopenia, the patient's platelet count drops 1–2 weeks after the beginning of treatment.[52] Occasionally, however, this period may be as long as several months or as short as several hours, as in cases of repeat or intermittent drug exposure. Sometimes the drug exposure is not obvious; for example, a street drug such as heroin containing another substance as an adulterant or quinine in beverages or herbal preparations. Severe thrombocytopenia, defined as a platelet count below $10 \times 10^3/\mu L$ ($10 \times 10^9/L$), usually lasts for several days after the discontinuation of the offending medication, depending on the half-life of the drug or metabolite causing the immune destruction. However, gold-associated thrombocytopenia may last for months, resembling chronic ITP. The mechanism causing the prolonged thrombocytopenia associated with gold salt preparation treatments is unclear.

Another cause of drug-induced thrombocytopenia is related to platelet integrin GPIIb/IIIa inhibitors used as antiplatelet medications in cardiothoracic and vascular surgery. Currently approved agents in this group of drugs include abciximab, tirofiban, and eptifibatide. Naturally occurring antibodies that cross-react with these drugs have been implicated as the cause of the thrombocytopenia. Abciximab (ReoPro®) can cause thrombocytopenia in 24 hours or less and occasionally within 30 minutes.

Diagnosis of drug-induced thrombocytopenia requires a high degree of clinical alertness. If a patient's platelet count drops abruptly for no apparent reason or the patient ceases to respond to well-matched products, a careful review of medication history and comparison with a list of drugs implicated in drug-induced thrombocytopenia may provide the answer.[53] Laboratory confirmation of the diagnosis, however, is technically difficult.[39] Some assays developed for platelet antibody screening can be adapted for drug-dependent antibody testing. There is, however, no single assay that works best for all drugs and ideally several different tests are performed simultaneously.

During the period of profound thrombocytopenia, patients are at high risk for life-threatening hemorrhage and platelet transfusions, usually with concomitant administration of IVIG, are indicated in bleeding patients. However, as long as the antibody and the implicated drug are present in circulation, the response to transfusions as measured by platelet count increment will be modest and transient.

CASE IN POINT (continued)

On day 5 of hospitalization an artery that was damaged by DD's broken pelvic bone was disrupted and began to bleed. She was returned to surgery to repair the bleed and began to ooze once more. She was given 11 ABO-identical, crossmatch-compatible apheresis platelets, but her post-transfusion platelet count never rose above $4 \times 10^3/\mu L$ ($4 \times 10^9/L$). Her HLA/platelet antibody screen result was positive and the reference laboratory identified anti-HPA-5b (Br^a) in DD's plasma. DD was diagnosed with post-transfusion purpura.

9. What factors influence immune-mediated platelet destruction?

On day 6 of hospitalization (3 days after beginning treatment with IVIG), DD's platelet counts began going up. Further transfusions and surgeries were not necessary.

☑ CHECKPOINT 16-7

Which type of drug-induced thrombocytopenia is the most common?

Post-Transfusion Purpura (PTP)

Post-transfusion purpura (PTP) is a rare but potentially serious complication of transfusions. Its incidence is estimated at 1:100,000 transfusions, which is probably an underestimate due to misdiagnosis.[54] It is associated most often with red blood cell transfusions. In PTP an acute thrombocytopenia occurs due to an alloimmune mechanism. In more than 95% of cases the patient is a multiparous woman alloimmunized during her previous pregnancies. Male patients suffering from PTP have often been alloimmunized by previous multiple transfusions. The most common antigenic target is HPA-1a in patients homozygous for HPA-1b. Significantly less often HPA-1b, -2b, -3a, -3b, -4a, -5b, and -CD36 (Nak^a) antibodies are involved. Sometimes patients are alloimmunized against several platelet antigens. An association between HLA-DR52a phenotype and HPA-1a alloimmunization has been noted.

The pathogenesis of PTP is not completely understood. The presence of a recipient's alloantibodies explains the destruction of transfused, allogeneic platelets that have the corresponding antigen. Even in red blood cell concentrates there are a small number of platelets that can trigger an anamnestic response of the platelet antibody or antibodies. However, the mechanism of brisk destruction of the patient's own platelets, which lack the corresponding antigen, remains obscure. Several explanations of this enigmatic phenomenon have been proposed and include antigen–antibody complex formation, shedding of antigen from destroyed allogeneic platelets with absorption onto native platelets, or cross-reacting antibodies.[55]

Clinically PTP presents as acute thrombocytopenia that develops 5–10 days after the implicated transfusion, which may have been complicated by a febrile nonhemolytic transfusion reaction. The severity of thrombocytopenia varies, but platelet counts commonly decrease to less than $10 \times 10^3/\mu L$ ($10 \times 10^9/L$). If untreated, the thrombocytopenia usually resolves in 2–3 weeks, but protracted cases have been reported. Severe bleeding complications are not uncommon, leading to a 5–10% mortality rate. High-dose IVIG and/or therapeutic plasma exchange are used for treatment.[56] Rare patients with delayed response to treatment and severe bleeding may benefit from massive transfusions of antigen-negative platelets. Obviously, platelet count increment will be modest at best, but clinical hemostasis can be achieved. Availability of antigen-negative platelets may pose a problem, and recruiting and antigen typing of family members may be considered. Red blood cell transfusions preferably should be postponed until recovery, but in urgent situations washed red blood cell components may be used.[55]

☑ CHECKPOINT 16-8

What blood product is most frequently implicated in post-transfusion purpura?

Neonatal Alloimmune Thrombocytopenia (NAIT)

Neonatal alloimmune thrombocytopenia (NAIT) develops in fetuses when maternal platelet IgG antibodies directed against a fetal platelet antigen cross the placenta (Box 16-1). This situation is analogous to hemolytic disease of the fetus and newborn (Chapter 14). The most commonly involved target platelet antigen is HPA-1a, formerly known as Pl^{A1}. About 98% of Caucasians express at least one copy of the HPA-1a antigen, while 2% are homozygous for HPA-1b (PL^{A2}). NAIT occurs in approximately 0.4–2 per 1,000 live births and about 75–80% of cases are caused by anti-HPA-1a. This observed frequency of NAIT due to anti-HPA-1a is much lower than would be expected from calculations based on the antigen frequency. There is a strong association between HPA-1a alloimmunization and HLA-DR52a (DRB3*0101 allele) and DQ2 (DQB1*0201 allele) expression. Apparently, these HLA Class II molecules are required for HPA-1a polypeptide presentation and immune response in antigen-negative individuals. In fact, individuals who do not express either HLA-DR52a or -DQ2 are at very low risk of developing anti-HPA-1a.

HPA-5b is the second most often encountered specificity, followed by HPA-15a or -15b. Anti-HPA-5b is implicated in approximately 15% of NAIT cases in people of European ethnicity. Cases involving anti-HPA-4b and anti-Nak^a (CD36 deletion) are more prevalent in people of Asian ethnicity. Only a few reports of NAIT due to immunization against other platelet antigens have been published. Approximately 5% of affected mothers demonstrate multiple or broadly reactive platelet antibodies. Many pregnant women develop HLA antibodies; however, their role in NAIT is questionable. Similarly, a role for ABO antibodies in NAIT remains unproven.

In contrast to hemolytic disease of the fetus and newborn (HDFN), about 30% of NAIT cases develop in children of first-time mothers. NAIT can affect the fetus as early as 17 weeks of gestation, but most hemorrhagic complications develop after 20 weeks' gestation. NAIT can result in intrauterine fetal demise or severely debilitating congenital defects.[57, 58] Half of all central nervous system bleeding due to NAIT occurs *in utero*. Affected neonates typically present with isolated thrombocytopenia at birth or within the first several hours of life. Hemorrhagic manifestations vary widely from a few petechiae to intracranial hemorrhaging, seen in about 20% of cases. This severe bleeding is usually in cases with platelet counts below $10 \times 10^3/\mu L$ ($10 \times 10^9/L$). Platelet destruction is more severe with antibodies directed against highly expressed antigens such as the GPIIb/IIIa complex. Thrombocytopenia usually lasts 1–3 weeks, but protracted cases have been reported. The reported fetal mortality is 10–15% and is mostly due to central nervous system bleeding. Subsequent pregnancies tend to be complicated by NAIT of the same or increased severity, which emphasizes the importance of accurate diagnosis during the first occurrence.

Diagnosis of NAIT depends on a high degree of clinical suspicion.[58] An isolated thrombocytopenia in a newborn with no apparent nonimmune cause should be treated as NAIT unless proven otherwise. The laboratory confirmation requires demonstration of an HPA antibody in the mother, who is negative for the corresponding antigen. The work-up should start with the incompatibility most prevalent in the patient's particular ethnic population. If possible, the most sensitive technique available, such as the MAIPA assay, should be employed,[39] as some antibodies, such as anti-HPA-5a and -5b, are often undetectable in immunofluorescent tests with relatively low sensitivity.

The correlation between maternal antibody titer and the severity of NAIT remains controversial. Recent data suggests that antibody levels may have predictive value for NAIT, particularly if a sufficiently sensitive and standardized laboratory technique is used.[59] It has been suggested that the IgG subclass may also play a role, with IgG_3 being associated with more severe thrombocytopenia.[60] In about one-quarter of clinically apparent NAIT cases, no platelet antibodies can be demonstrated by conventional screening tests. Occasionally, however, antibodies may become detectable 3–6 months postpartum.

If no HPA antibodies can be identified in the maternal sample, a crossmatch of maternal serum against paternal platelets, if the latter are available, can be performed.[39] In cases of ABO incompatibility, which may produce a false-positive result, the allogeneic absorption of maternal anti-A and/or -B agglutinins using washed red blood cells can be attempted. If the mother has concomitant HLA antibodies, which also can result in false-positive platelet antibody tests, treatment of paternal or reagent panel platelets with chloroquin may be helpful. This reagent removes as much as 75% of class I HLA molecules from the platelet membrane, rendering them nonreactive with HLA antibodies, thus allowing better detection of platelet antibodies.

Regardless of whether maternal antibodies are demonstrable or not, maternal typing for an implicated HPA(s) is essential. However, serological phenotyping, for antigens other than HPA-1,

is complicated by the lack of typing sera and lack of reagent standardization.[61] Presently, monoclonal antibody is available for HPA-1a phenotyping only. Fortunately, genotyping for HPA is fairly simple because almost all HPA alleles are determined by single-nucleotide polymorphisms (SNP). DNA-based genotyping techniques can be used for *in utero* diagnosis of NAIT; they require only a small volume of sample and they can be performed on a variety of specimens including amniotic fluid.

Another important aspect of the NAIT laboratory work-up is determining the zygosity of the father. As mentioned earlier, subsequent pregnancies carry a very high risk of NAIT recurrence. Paternal homozygosity is an indication for invasive fetal platelet count monitoring and, if the fetus is affected, aggressive fetal platelet transfusion support. On the other hand, fetuses of fathers who are heterozygous will have a 50% chance of being homozygous for the maternal antigen and thus not at risk of NAIT. For HPA-1 incompatibility, about 25% of fathers are heterozygous and half of their children may be affected by the maternal antibody.

Treatment of NAIT includes intrauterine and/or postnatal platelet transfusions, often concurrent with IVIG.[58] Maternal administration of high-dose IVIG during pregnancy can also be of benefit in decreasing the strength of the mother's platelet antibody. In some large collection centers a pool of antigen-negative donors is maintained. In the United States, this is usually limited to HPA-1a only. When antigen-negative allogeneic platelets are not available, washed maternal platelets can be used for transfusion. Washing, however, causes significant platelet loss and can result in considerable deterioration of platelet function. When neither allogeneic antigen-negative nor maternal platelet products are available, massive transfusion of antigen-mismatched volume-reduced platelets may prevent bleeding complications.[62] Irradiation of the transfused platelets for GVHD prevention is mandatory, particularly if maternal platelets are transfused. In prenatal management, the transfusion support continues until the gestational age when the least traumatic delivery, typically Caesarian section, is safe and feasible.

☑ CHECKPOINT 16-9

What antibody is most frequently identified in neonatal alloimmune thrombocytopenia?

Maternal Immune Thrombocytopenia Purpura

Neonatal immune thrombocytopenia can also develop in mothers with ITP.[63] Maternal IgG platelet autoantibodies cross the placenta and destroy fetal platelets. In contrast to NAIT, the mother presents with significant thrombocytopenia, while fetal/neonatal impairment is usually mild. The incidence of ITP mothers giving birth to affected babies is relatively low. A rarely occurring complication of such babies is the development of intracranial hemorrhage. The treatment of choice in affected newborns is IVIG, and unlike NAIT, platelet transfusions are almost never indicated.

Review of the Main Points

- Platelet transfusion refractoriness is a common condition.
- The diagnosis of platelet refractoriness depends on accurate assessment of platelet transfusion effectiveness.
- The most common causes of platelet transfusion refractoriness are nonimmune sequestration and consumption.
- Recurrent antigen exposure may result in alloimmunization and immune-mediated platelet transfusion refractoriness.
- The most common cause of immune refractoriness is human leukocyte antigen (HLA) alloimmunization.
- Selection of platelets for refractory patients can be done either by HLA matching or crossmatching.
- ABO incompatibility and human platelet antigen (HPA) alloimmunization are infrequent causes of refractoriness.
- A number of disorders share similarities with platelet refractoriness and if transfusion occurs, poor platelet count increments are common:

- Heparin-induced thrombocytopenia (HIT) and other drug-related thrombocytopenias
- Thrombocytic thrombocytopenia purpura (TTP) and hemolytic uremic syndrome (HUS)
- Immune thrombocytopenia purpura and idiopathic thrombocytopenia purpura (ITP)
- Post-transfusion purpura (PTP)
- Neonatal alloimmune thrombocytopenia (NAIT) and maternal immune ITP affecting the neonate
- Platelet transfusion is a relative contraindication in HIT, TTP, HUS, and ITP. Transfusions are only considered if life-threatening bleeds occur.
- Platelet transfusions are rarely required in PTP.
- Platelet transfusions, in the postnatal period and sometimes *in utero*, are often required to treat NAIT.

Review Questions

1. A patient is considered to be responsive to platelet therapy if the immediate post-transfusion corrected count increment (CCI) is at least: (Objective #2)

   A. 5,000

   B. 7,500

   C. 10,000

   D. 12,000

2. GC was transfused with 1 unit of apheresis platelets. The immediate post-transfusion corrected count increment (CCI) was within the normal range; however, decreased platelet survival was noted 24 hours post-transfusion. What could be a possible explanation for this finding? (Objective #2)

   A. ITP

   B. HLA antibody

   C. PTP

   D. DIC

3. Use the following information to calculate the CCI for a 50-year-old female patient: (Objective #3)

   BSA = $1.7m^2$

   # of platelets transfused = 4.0×10^{11}

   Pretransfusion platelet count = $5.0 \times 10^3/\mu L$ ($5.0 \times 10^9/L$)

   Post-transfusion platelet count at
   60 minutes = $45.0 \times 10^3/\mu L$ ($45.0 \times 10^9/L$)

   A. 2,125

   B. 12,500

   C. 17,000

   D. 19,125

4. The corrected count increment (CCI) calculation is based on which of the following assumptions? Select all that apply. (Objective #2)

   A. Accurate report of circulating blood volume

   B. Splenic sequestration is in proportion to spleen size

   C. Accurate report of the number of platelets transfused

   D. Initial calculation is performed within 5 minutes of transfusion

5. Select *two* medications that are known to cause thrombocytopenia after administration to the patient: (Objective #5)

   A. Acetaminophen

   B. Heparin

   C. Keflex

   D. Digoxin

6. Select the condition that causes platelet refractoriness through the mechanism of platelet consumption: (Objective #6)

   A. NAIT

   B. PTP

   C. HPA

   D. DIC

7. Treatments for neonatal alloimmune thrombocytopenia (NAIT) typically include all of the following except: (Objective #10)

   A. Intrauterine platelet transfusion

   B. Whole blood exchange transfusion

   C. Postnatal platelet transfusion

   D. IVIG

8. Under normal circumstances, what percentage of total body platelets is sequestered in the spleen? (Objective #13)

   A. 10%

   B. 15%

   C. 30%

   D. 45%

9. Which of the following is not a clinical finding in heparin-induced thrombocytopenia type II? (Objective #7)

   A. Decreased platelet count

   B. IgG antibody production

   C. Abnormal bleeding

   D. Complement activation

10. Alloantibody specificity in immune-mediated platelet refractoriness may include all of the following except: (Objective #6)

    A. GPB

    B. ABO

    C. HPA

    D. HLA

11. The severity of ABO antibody-related platelet refractoriness is highly dependent on which two factors? (Objective #8)

    A. Antibody titer

    B. GP receptor

    C. Antigen dose

    D. Avidity

12. Which condition is known to cause nonimmune platelet refractoriness? (Objective #6)

    A. ITP

    B. DIC

    C. NAIT

    D. PTP

13. Which procedure can be used as an alternative to finding HLA-matched platelets for a refractory patient? (Objective #11)

    A. Platelet crossmatch

    B. Antibody identification

    C. Molecular phenotyping

    D. Cytotoxicity

14. Idiopathic thrombocytopenia purpura (ITP) can occur as a secondary condition to which of the following diseases? (Objective #10)

    A. Bernard-Soulier

    B. Hemophilia A

    C. Systemic lupus erythematosus

    D. bacterial infection

15. Post-transfusion purpura (PTP) occurs most often in: (Objective #10)

    A. Newborns

    B. Multiparous patients

    C. Males less than age 50

    D. Elderly patients

References

1. Rebulla P. A min-review on platelet refractoriness. Haematologica 2005; 90(2): 247–53.
2. Slichter SJ, Davis K, Enright H, Braine H, Gernsheimer T, et al. Factors affecting posttransfusion platelet increments, platelet refractoriness, and platelet transfusion intervals in thrombocytopenic patients. Blood 2005; 105(10): 4106–14.
3. Hussein MA, Lee EJ, Schiffer CA. Platelet transfusions administered to patients with splenomegaly. Transfusion 1990; 30(6): 508–10.
4. Bock M, Muggenthaler KH, Schmidt U, Heim MU. Influence of antibiotics on posttransfusion platelet increment. Transfusion 1996; 36(11–12): 952–4.

5. Doughty HA, Murphy MF, Metcalfe P, Rohatiner AZ, Lister TA, Waters AH. Relative importance of immune and non-immune causes of platelet refractoriness. *Vox Sang* 1994; 66(3): 200–5.

6. McFarland JG, Anderson AJ, Slichter SJ. Factors influencing the transfusion response to HLA-selected apheresis donor platelets in patients refractory to random platelet concentrates. *Br J Haematol* 1989; 73(3): 380–6.

7. Friedberg RC, Donnelly SF, Boyd JC, Gray LS, Mintz PD. Clinical and blood bank factors in the management of platelet refractoriness and alloimmunization. *Blood* 1993; 81(12): 3428–34.

8. Carreras E, Granena A, Rozman C. Hepatic veno-occlusive disease after bone marrow transplant. *Blood Rev* 1993 Mar; 7(1): 43–51.

9. Warkentin TE, Sheppard JA. Testing for heparin-induced thrombocytopenia antibodies. *Transfus Med Rev* 2006; 20(4): 259–72.

10. Bowen DJ, Collins PW. Insights into von Willebrand factor proteolysis: clinical implications. *Br J Haematol* 2006; 133(5): 457–67.

11. Mannucci PM. Thrombotic thromboytopenic purpura: another example of immunomediated thrombosis. *Pathophysiol Haemost Thromb* 2006; 35(1–2): 89–97.

12. Karch H, Friedrich AW, Gerber A, Zimmerhackl LB, Schmidt MA, et al. New aspects in the pathogenesis of enteropathic hemolytic uremic syndrome.*Semin Thromb Hemost* 2006; 32(2): 105–12.

13. Zimmerhackl LB, Besbas N, Jungraithmayr T, van de Kar N, Karch H, et al.; European Study Group for Haemolytic Uraemic Syndromes and Related Disorders. Epidemiology, clinical presentation, and pathophysiology of atypical and recurrent hemolytic uremic syndrome. *Semin Thromb Hemost* 2006; 32(2): 113–20.

14. Sintnicolaas K, van Marwijk Kooij M, van Prooijen HC, van Dijk BA, van Putten WL, et al. Leukocyte depletion of random single-donor platelet transfusions does not prevent secondary human leukocyte antigen-alloimmunization and refractoriness: A randomized prospective study. *Blood* 1995; 85(3): 824–8.

15. Gmur J, von Felten A, Osterwalder B, Honegger H, Hormann A, et al. Delayed alloimmunization using random single donor platelet transfusions: A prospective study in thrombocytopenic patients with acute leukemia. *Blood* 1983; 62(2): 473–9.

16. Dutcher JP, Schiffer CA, Aisner J, Wiernik PH. Alloimmunization following platelet transfusion: The absence of a dose-response relationship. *Blood* 1981; 57(3): 395–8.

17. Friedman DF, Lukas MB, Jawad A, Larson PJ, Ohene-Frempong K, et al. Alloimmunization to platelets in heavily transfused patients with sickle cell disease. *Blood* 1996; 88(8): 3216–22.

18. Lee EJ, Schiffer CA. Serial measurement of lymphocytotoxic antibody and response to nonmatched platelet transfusions in alloimmunized patients. *Blood* 1987; 70(6): 1727–9.

19. Buetens O, Shirey RS, Goble-Lee M, Houp J, Zachary A, et al. Prevalence of HLA antibodies in transfused patients with and without red cell antibodies. *Transfusion* 2006; 46(5): 754–6.

20. McKenna DH Jr, Eastlund T, Segall M, Noreen HJ, Park S. HLA alloimmunization in patients requiring ventricular assist device support. *J Heart Lung Transplant* 2002; 21(11): 1218–24.

21. Lante W, Franke A, Weinhold C, Markewitz A. Immunoglobulin levels and lymphocyte subsets following cardiac operations: Further evidence for a T-helper cell shifting. *Thorac Cardiovasc Surg* 2005; 53(1): 16–22.

22. Seftel MD, Growe GH, Petraszko T, Benny WB, Le A, et al. Universal prestorage leukoreduction in Canada decreases platelet alloimmunization and refractoriness. *Blood* 2004; 103(1): 333–9.

23. Leukocyte reduction and ultraviolet B irradiation of platelets to prevent alloimmunization and refractoriness to platelet transfusions. The Trial to Reduce Alloimmunization to Platelets Study Group. *N Engl J Med* 1997; 337(26): 1861–9.

24. Rodey GE, Neylan JF, Whelchel JD, Revels KW, Bray RA. Epitope specificity of HLA class I alloantibodies. I. Frequency analysis of antibodies to private versus public specificities in potential transplant recipients. *Hum Immunol* 1994; 39(4): 272–80.

25. Saito S, Ota S, Seshimo H, Yamazaki Y, Nomura S, et al. Platelet transfusion refractoriness caused by a mismatch in HLA-C antigens. *Transfusion* 2002; 42(3): 302–8.

26. Heal JM, Rowe JM, Blumberg N. ABO and platelet transfusion revisited. *Ann Hematol* 1993; 66(6): 309–14.

27. Brand A, Sintnicolaas K, Claas FH, Eernisse JG. ABH antibodies causing platelet transfusion refractoriness. *Transfusion* 1986; 26(5): 463–6.

28. Ogasawara K, Ueki J, Takenaka M, Furihata K. Study on the expression of ABH antigens on platelets. *Blood* 1993; 82(3): 993–9.

29. Heal JM, Rowe JM, McMican A, Masel D, Finke C, Blumberg N. The role of ABO matching in platelet transfusion. *Eur J Haematol* 1993; 50(2): 110–7.

30. Heal JM, Masel D, Rowe JM, Blumberg N. Circulating immune complexes involving the ABO system after platelet transfusion. *Br J Haematol* 1993; 85: 566–72.

31. Heal JM, Masel D, Blumberg N. Interaction of platelet fc and complement receptors with circulating immune complexes involving the ABO system. *Vox Sang* 1996; 71(4): 205–11.

32. Carr R, Hutton JL, Jenkins JA, Lucas GF, Amphlett NW. Transfusion of ABO-mismatched platelets leads to early platelet refractoriness. *Br J Haematol* 1990; 75(3): 408–13.

33. Heal JM, Blumberg N. Optimizing platelet transfusion therapy. *Blood Rev* 2004; 18(3): 149–65.

34. Sanz C, Freire C, Alcorta I, Ordinas A, Pereira A. Platelet-specific antibodies in HLA-immunized patients receiving chronic platelet support. *Transfusion* 2001; 41(6): 762–5.

35. Schnaidt M, Northoff H, Wernet D. Frequency and specificity of platelet-specific alloantibodies in HLA-immunized haematologic-oncologic patients. *Transfus Med* 1996 Jun; 6(2): 111–4.

36. IPD—The Immuno Polymorphism Database [Internet]. Hinxton (United Kingdom): European Molecular Biology Laboratory—European Bioinformatics Institute. c2009—[cited 2009 Aug 07]. Available from: http://www.ebi.ac.uk/ipd/hpa/.

37. Curtis BR, Aster RH. Incidence of the Nak(a)-negative platelet phenotype in African Americans is similar to that of Asians. *Transfusion* 1996; 36(4): 331–4.

38. Slichter SJ. Algorithm for managing the platelet refractory patient. *J Clin Apher* 1997; 12(1): 4–9.

39. McFarland JG. Detection and identification of platelet antibodies in clinical disorders. *Transfus Apher Sci* 2003; 28(3): 297–305.

40. McFarland JG. Matched apheresis platelets. In: McLeod BC, Price TH, Weinstein RA, eds. *Apheresis: principles and practice*, 2nd ed. Bethesda (MD): AABB Press; 2003. pp. 210–5.

41. Duquesnoy RJ, Filip DJ, Rodey GE, Rimm AA, Aster RH. Successful transfusion of platelets "mismatched" for HLA antigens to alloimmunized thrombocytopenic patients. *Am J Hematol* 1977; 2(3): 219–26.

42. Petz LD, Garratty G, Calhoun L, Clark BD, Terasaki PI, et al. Selecting donors of platelets for refractory patients on the basis of HLA antibody specificity. *Transfusion* 2000; 40(12): 1446–56.

43. Duquesnoy RJ. A structurally based approach to determine HLA compatibility at the humoral immune level. *Hum Immunol* 2006; 67(11): 847–62.

44. Nambiar A, Duquesnoy RJ, Adams S, Zhao Y, Oblitas J, et al. HLAMatchmaker-driven analysis of responses to HLA-typed platelet transfusions in alloimmunized thrombocytopenic patients. *Blood* 2006; 107(4): 1680–7.

45. HLAMatchmaker [Internet]. Pittsburgh: HLAMatchmaker; c2009 [cited 2009 Aug 7]. Available from: http://www.hlamatchmaker.net/.

46. von dem Borne AE, Ouwehand WH, Kuijpers RW. Theoretic and practical aspects of platelet crossmatching. *Transfus Med Rev* 1990; 4(4): 265–78.

47. Rebulla P, Morelati F, Revelli N, Villa MA, Paccapelo C, et al. Outcomes of an automated procedure for the selection of effective platelets for patients refractory to random donors based on cross-matching locally available platelet products. *Br J Haematol* 2004; 125(1): 83–9.

48. Moroff G, Garratty G, Heal JM, MacPherson BR, Stroncek D, et al. Selection of platelets for refractory patients by HLA matching and prospective cross-matching. *Transfusion* 1992; 32(7): 633–40.

49. Rodey GE. *HLA beyond tears*, 2nd ed. Atlanta: De Novo, 2000. pp. 235.

50. Kickler T. Pretransfusion testing for platelet transfusions. *Transfusion* 2000; 40(12): 1425–6.

51. Vipan WH. Quinine as a cause of purpura. *Lancet* 1865; ii: 37.

52. Vandendries ER, Drews RE. Drug-associated disease: hematologic dysfunction. *Crit Care Clin* 2006; 22(2): 347–55, viii.

53. Platelets on the Web [Internet]. Oklahoma City: Platelets on the Web; c2007 [updated 2009 Mar 2; cited 2009 Aug 7]. Drug-Induced Thrombocytopenia; Available from: http://www.ouhsc.edu/platelets/ditp.html.

54. Shtalrid M, Shvidel L, Vorst E, Weinmann EE, Berrebi A, Sigler E. Post-transfusion purpura: a challenging diagnosis. *Isr Med Assoc J* 2006; 8(10): 672–4.

55. Klein HG, Anstee D. *Mollison's blood transfusion in clinical medicine*, 11th ed. Malden (MA): Blackwell: 2005. pp. 676–79.

56. Gonzalez CE, Pengetze YM. Post-transfusion purpura. *Curr Hematol Rep* 2005; 4(2): 154–9.

57. Rothenberger S. Neonatal alloimmune thrombocytopenia. *Ther Apher* 2002; 6(1): 32–5.

58. Berkowitz RL, Bussel JB, McFarland JG. Alloimmune thrombocytopenia: State of the art 2006. *Am J Obstet Gynecol* 2006 Oct; 195(4): 907–13.

59. Killie MK, Husebekk A, Kaplan C, Taaning E, Skogen B. Maternal human platelet antigen-1a antibody level correlates with the platelet count in the newborns: a retrospective study. *Transfusion* 2007; 47(1): 55–8.

60. Mawas F, Wiener E, Williamson LM, Rodeck CH. Immunoglobulin G subclasses of anti-human platelet antigen 1a in maternal sera: relation to the severity of neonatal alloimmune thrombocytopenia. *Eur J Haematol* 1997; 59(5): 287–92.

61. Metcalfe P. Platelet antigens and antibody detection. *Vox Sang* 2004; 87 Suppl 1: 82–6.

62. Kiefel V, Bassler D, Kroll H, Paes B, Giers G, et al. Antigen-positive platelet transfusion in neonatal alloimmune thrombocytopenia (NAIT). *Blood* 2006; 107(9): 3761–3.

63. Webert KE, Mittal R, Sigouin C, Heddle NM, Kelton JG. A retrospective 11-year analysis of obstetric patients with idiopathic thrombocytopenic purpura. *Blood* 2003; 102(13): 4306–11.

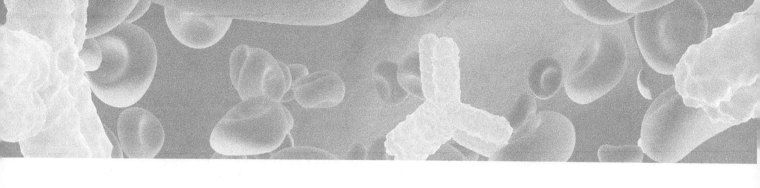

17 Transfusion Support of Selected Patient Populations

JOSHUA J. FIELD

Chapter Objectives

Upon completion of this chapter, the student will be able to:

1. Discuss the etiology and symptoms associated with hemophilia A and B.
2. Identify the severity levels of hemophilia.
3. List the indications for treating hemophiliacs with factor replacement therapy.
4. Describe how to calculate an appropriate factor replacement dose schedule for patients with hemophilia A or B.
5. List the requirements for transfusion of red blood cells in individuals with sickle cell disease.
6. List the most common complications of transfusion in individuals with sickle cell disease.
7. Describe strategies to reduce the common complications of transfusion in individuals with sickle cell disease.
8. Summarize the specialized blood products used in hematopoietic progenitor cell transplant.
9. Describe the plasma exchange procedure and indications for its use.
10. Discuss how the antibody class affects the plasma exchange schedule.
11. State the most common reason for anemia and treatment of chronic kidney disease.
12. Discuss compatibility in organ transplantation.
13. Describe the complications of liver disease including the strategies for correction of coagulopathy.
14. Discuss the risk factors, pathophysiology, and prevention of transfusion-associated CMV and transfusion-associated graft versus host disease (TA-GVHD).

Key Terms

Erythropoietin
Hemophilia A
Hemophilia B
Hyperhemolysis
Inhibitor(s)
Passenger lymphocyte
  syndrome

Sickle cell disease (SCD)
Therapeutic apheresis
Transfusion-associated
  graft versus host disease
  (TA-GVHD)
Tumor lysis syndrome

What's Ahead?

Clinicians encounter a variety of disease processes that require transfusion therapy and they depend on the transfusion medicine service for guidance in the management of these complex problems.

This chapter addresses the following questions:

- What are the common transfusion therapies used in patients with coagulation-factor deficiencies, hemoglobinopathies, renal failure, and kidney failure?
- How is transfusion therapy used to improve clinical outcomes in patients receiving transplants?
- What are the different types of therapeutic apheresis and what are the indications for their use?

CASE IN POINT

AC is a 17-year-old female with severe sickle cell disease. She has been receiving regular blood transfusions for years to treat anemia and prevent complications. She is group O Rh$_0$(D) positive and has a history of multiple alloantibodies and several febrile, nonhemolytic transfusion reactions.

HEMOPHILIA A AND B

There are three aspects associated with these disorders worthy of discussion here: cause and symptoms, therapy, and inhibitors.

Cause and Symptoms

Hemophilia A and **hemophilia B** are inherited bleeding disorders due to deficiencies in coagulation Factors VIII and IX, respectively. They are X-linked disorders; males are almost exclusively affected. Hemophilia A occurs in 1 in 10,000 males, while hemophilia B is much less common.[1] They are the most common forms of hemophilia, although less prevalent than von Willebrand's disease, which occurs in 1 in 100 persons and is the most common inherited bleeding disorder.

The severity of hemophilia correlates with the factor activity level: mild, 5–20%; moderate, 1–5%; severe, <1%.[2] Severe hemophiliacs suffer from recurrent bleeds in their joints and, over time, develop pain and immobility, leading to disability. Additionally, spontaneous intracranial (brain) and gastrointestinal (gut) hemorrhages as well as bleeding in other sites can occur. Spontaneous bleeding rarely occurs in patients with mild or moderate hemophilia and, consequently, their management differs from the severe type.

Therapy

Replacement of Factor VIII or Factor IX is the cornerstone of management in patients with severe hemophilia. It can be administered prior to a medical procedure, in response to a bleed, or as long-term prophylaxis to prevent bleeding episodes. Table 17-1 ✻ outlines typical treatment goals in patients with severe hemophilia A who are bleeding or scheduled for surgery. Factor VIII has a half-life of 12 hours and, generally, 1 IU/kg of Factor VIII will increase factor activity by 2%. Thus, to achieve a Factor VIII activity of 100%, assuming an endogenous patient activity of 0%, a dose of 50 IU/kg would be

needed and, typically, the patient would then be maintained with a dose of 25 IU/kg every 12 hours.

The half-life of Factor IX is 24 hours and 1 IU/kg of replacement factor should result in a 1% increment of factor IX activity. Therefore, a 100% increase in Factor IX requires a dose of 100 IU/kg of replacement factor with additional maintenance doses of 50 IU/kg every 24 hours.

☑ CHECKPOINT 17-1

What is the effect on factor activity of a 1 IU/kg dose of Factor VIII or Factor IX?

Prophylactic therapy in severe hemophilia aims to maintain a factor activity of 1–4% to prevent bleeding and the consequent long-term sequelae of recurrent bleeds, such as joint damage, muscle damage, and neurologic conditions. The premise of prophylactic therapy

✻ **TABLE 17-1** Factor VIII Activity Treatment Goal

Procedure or Site of Bleeding	Goal—FVIII Activity*	Duration (Days)*
Surgery	~100%	7–10
Bleeding		
Central nervous system	~100%	7–10
Gastrointestinal	50–70%	5–7
Hemarthrosis (into joints)	~50%	1–2
Oral mucosa	~30%	Resolution
Hematuria	~30%	Resolution

*Percent activity and duration can be tailored to the patient's bleeding episode.

is to attain factor activities similar to people with moderate hemophilia, who generally have mild disease. Studies of pediatric hemophilia A patients have demonstrated that beginning treatment with Factor VIII by the age of 1–2 preserves joint function. Typical regimens are 20–40 IU/kg of factor concentrate. Hemophilia A patients receive Factor VIII three times per week and hemophilia B patients receive biweekly doses of factor IX.[3]

Both recombinant and plasma-derived preparations are available for Factor VIII and Factor IX. Recombinant products are produced without human plasma (Chapter 10), thereby eliminating the risk of infectious disease transmission. Conversely, plasma-derived factor replacements are prepared from large pools of up to 20,000 donors and carry a risk of infection transmission despite viral testing, filtration, and heat or solvent/detergent treatment.[2] Disadvantages of recombinant factor therapy include the increased cost of treatment.

Inhibitors

Whether recombinant or plasma-derived products are used for treatment, there is no difference in the number of patients who form **inhibitors**, which are antibodies to human Factor VIII or IX. Approximately 30% of patients with severe hemophilia A will form an inhibitor, while fewer than 5% of patients with hemophilia B will form an inhibitor.[4] Low-titer inhibitors of less than 10 Bethesda units may be overcome by higher doses of factor replacement; however, this treatment is ineffective in the case of high-titer inhibitors.[5] Patients who are bleeding and have a high-titer inhibitor may be treated with activated Factor VII (FVIIa), which is a recombinant product that activates Factor X, which in turn activates thrombin, bypassing the need for Factors VIII or IX. Unfortunately, FVIIa has a half-life of 2 hours and, therefore, it is not practical to use as long-term prophylactic therapy.[4] The primary method to eradicate an inhibitor is immune tolerance, which exposes the patient to high doses of factor replacement with or without an immune suppressant; this approach is effective in 85% of cases.[2]

SICKLE CELL DISEASE

In order to fully examine the transfusion support of individuals suffering from *sickle cell disease*, this discussion covers the important topics of cause and symptoms, transfusion, product requirements, alloimmunization, and iron overload

Cause and Symptoms

Sickle cell disease (SCD) is the most common inherited disease in people with African ethnicity.[6] SCD is caused by a single amino acid substitution from valine to glutamic acid (Val → Glu) in the sixth position on the β-hemoglobin chain, resulting in the production of hemoglobin S (HbS). Individuals who inherit this mutation from each parent are diagnosed with SCD, while a single mutation causes sickle cell trait, which is generally a benign condition. In patients with SCD, the insoluble HbS polymerizes and causes a deformation of the red blood cell membrane, resulting in red blood cells with a sickle or crescent appearance on a blood smear, as illustrated in Figure 17-1 ■.

The red blood cells of patients with SCD occlude blood vessels and hemolyze more easily, causing tissue ischemia (lack of blood flow), organ damage, and pain. The predominant clinical characteristics of

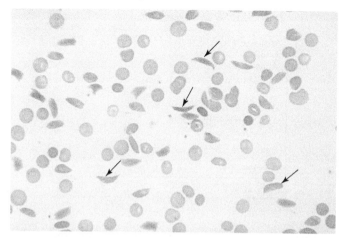

■ FIGURE 17-1 Sickle Cells on a Stained Blood Smear

A stained blood smear showing typical red blood cell deformities associated with sickle cell anemia. Some of the classic sickle-shaped red blood cells for which the condition is named are highlighted with arrows.

Source: Southern Illinois University/Getty Images.

SCD are pain crises and hemolytic anemia. Other common manifestations include stroke, pulmonary hypertension (high blood pressure in the lungs), avascular necrosis of bones (deterioration of bone due to lack of blood flow), acute chest syndrome, infections, priapism (abnormal, persistent erection of the penis), and ankle ulcers.

☑ CHECKPOINT 17-2

What is the genetic difference between sickle cell disease and sickle cell trait?

Transfusion

Indications for transfusing red blood cells to patients with SCD are twofold: to increase hemoglobin and thereby increase oxygen-carrying capacity and to dilute red blood cells containing HbS with healthy donor red blood cells. There is no accepted hemoglobin value that should trigger a red blood cell transfusion in an anemic SCD patient. SCD patients, like others with chronic anemia, tolerate the anemia well and therefore the decision to transfuse is often based on the patient's other symptoms. Additionally, several clinical conditions in SCD require dilution of HbS by red blood cell transfusion to ameliorate or prevent symptoms. Table 17-2 ✱ lists common indications for transfusion in sickle cell disease as well as the associated treatment goals.

In SCD, red blood cells can be transfused in a simple transfusion or as part of a red blood cell exchange. In a red blood cell exchange, the transfusion of donor cells is paired with the removal of patient cells. The patient cells can be removed by phlebotomy, in which case the procedure is called a *manual exchange*; or using a pheresis machine, as illustrated in Figure 17-2 ■, in which case the procedure is called *erythrocytapheresis*. Simple transfusions will increase the patient's hemoglobin and cause a small dilution of the sickle cells. Conversely,

✴ **TABLE 17-2** Transfusion Indications in Sickle Cell Disease

Indication	Goal	Delivery
Anemia	↑O_2 carrying capacity	Episodic
Aplastic crisis	↑O_2 carrying capacity	Episodic
Stroke	RBC dilution*	Emergent + chronic
Acute chest syndrome	RBC dilution*	Emergent ± chronic
Priapism	RBC dilution*	Episodic
Splenic/hepatic sequestration	RBC dilution*	Episodic
Preoperative	RBC dilution*	Preoperative

*RBC dilution = HbS <30%

exchange transfusions have the capacity to rapidly lower the percentage of sickle cells while increasing the hemoglobin to a targeted value and leaving the patient without excess volume. Exchange transfusion is the preferred method of transfusion for life-threatening complications of sickle cell disease such as acute chest syndrome or stroke. For these indications, the target HbS level is typically less than 30%.

Strokes are a devastating complication of SCD. The risk of stroke in the pediatric population is about 1% per year. By age 20, 11% of patients with SCD will have an overt stroke.[7] Measurements of blood velocity through the internal carotid or middle cerebral artery can identify patients who have a higher risk of stroke. Stroke risk increases to 10% per year for patients with elevated velocities.[8, 9] Individuals with a history of stroke or those who are found to be at high risk to develop a stroke benefit from chronic transfusion therapy. In high-risk patients, preventative transfusion therapy reduces the risk of stroke by 92% and for patients with a history of stroke, the risk of recurrence is reduced from 70% to 13%.[7, 9] Because chronic transfusion therapy is complicated by iron overload, exchange transfusions are preferred. The goal of transfusion therapy is to maintain an HbS of less than 30% for at least the first 2 years following a stroke, which typically requires a procedure every 4–6 weeks. While the optimal duration of transfusion is unknown, at least one study demonstrated that discontinuation of transfusions after a minimum of 30 months resulted in a reversion to high-velocity measurements on Doppler studies and a recurrence of strokes.[10]

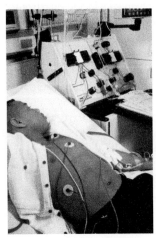

▦ **FIGURE 17-2** Automated Red Blood Cell Exchange Transfusion
Source: Spencer Grant/Science Source.

Patients with SCD have a high rate of morbidity and mortality in the perioperative period. In one series, the complication rate for SCD patients undergoing total hip arthroplasty was 67%.[11] Preoperative transfusions diminish the risk of perioperative complications.[12] The National Preoperative Transfusion in Sickle Cell Disease Group study compared an aggressive preoperative transfusion strategy where HbS was reduced to less than 30% to a less aggressive approach where simple transfusions were used to increase a patient's hemoglobin to 100 g/L (10 g/dL). They found the two strategies to be equally efficacious.[13] Consequently, patients with SCD are routinely transfused to a hemoglobin level of 100 g/L (10 g/dL) preoperatively. Minor procedures without anesthesia do not require a preoperative transfusion.

Product Requirements

Leukoreduced red blood cell units are generally indicated for patients with SCD. Leukoreduction reduces the incidence of febrile nonhemolytic transfusion reactions.[14] If bone marrow transplant is a consideration, the patient should receive anti-CMV-negative cellular blood products as well. HbS may be present in donor red blood cell units because individuals with sickle cell trait are allowed to donate. About 40% of the hemoglobin in these products is hemoglobin S, which may impact the efficacy of a transfusion to a patient with SCD. Many institutions consequently stipulate that SCD patients, especially children, should receive donor red blood cell units that have been tested and found negative for HbS.

Alloimmunization

Alloimmunization is a serious problem in SCD. Approximately one-third of patients with SCD have alloantibodies and the rate of alloantibody formation is 3%/unit.[15, 16] Alloantibodies may cause a delayed hemolytic transfusion reaction if they are not detected during pretransfusion testing. Even when detected, alloimmunization causes problems as it can be difficult to find compatible blood if the patient develops multiple antibodies or an antibody to a high-incidence antigen.

In North America, most blood donors are of European ethnicity, but SCD is prevalent in patients of African ethnicity. This ethnic mismatch causes a high degree of antigen mismatches, which contributes to the prevalence of alloimmunization in transfused SCD patients.[17]

Transfusion therapy with units antigen-matched for C, E, and K reduces the rate of alloantibody formation from 3%/unit to 0.5%/unit and decreases delayed hemolytic reactions by 90%.[18]

CASE IN POINT *(continued)*

AC is due for her laboratory work, which is assessed on a regular basis. Her physician receives the following results:

AC's results:

Reference range:

- Hemoglobin = 10.8 g/dL (108 g/L)
- Hemoglobin A = 23.8% (0.238)
- Hemoglobin A2 = 3.4% (0.034)
- Hemoglobin F = 5.6% (0.056)
- Hemoglobin S = 67.2% (0.672)
- Relative reticulocyte count = 8.0% (0.080)

- 11.5–16.0 g/dL (115–160 g/L)
- >96.0% (>0.960)
- 1.8–3.5% (0.018–0.035)
- <2.0% (<0.020)
- 0.0% (0.000)
- 0.6–2.7% (0.006–0.027)

The laboratorian working on AC's crossmatch that the physician ordered at the same time sees the following in the transfusion history file:

- Previously typed as O Rh₀(D) positive
- Known antibodies: anti-I, anti-V, Anti-Fyᵃ, Anti-Jkᵇ, Anti-Jsᵃ, Anti-K.
- Transfuse Fyᵃ negative, Goᵃ negative, Jkᵇ negative, Jsᵃ negative, K negative, C negative, E negative red blood cell units

1. Which laboratory result suggests that transfusion is indicated?
2. Why is the laboratory providing C-negative, E-negative red blood cell units if AC does not have anti-C or anti-E?
3. What other requirements for red blood cell transfusion are likely to be considered for AC?

Hyperhemolysis, which is a delayed hemolytic transfusion reaction where both donor and recipient red blood cells are destroyed resulting in profound anemia, occurs most often in multiply transfused patients such as those with sickle cell disease (Chapter 12). Reducing the rate of alloimmunization also reduces the risk of hyperhemolysis. The provision of donor red blood cells phenotypically matched for C, E, and K has become the accepted transfusion standard for patients with SCD.

Iron Overload

Transfusion related iron overload is common in patients with SCD who receive regular transfusions (Chapter 12). Iron overload in SCD is treated with chelators that bind to iron. The resulting complex is excreted in the urine, stool, or both. Deferoxamine was the first commonly used iron chelator. It was administered by subcutaneous or intravenous infusion 10–12 hours per day 5 days per week.[19] In 2005, an oral iron chelator, deferasirox, was approved by the U.S. Food and Drug Administration for the treatment of transfusion-related iron overload. Deferasirox is well tolerated, taken once per day, and equally efficacious to deferoxamine.

HEMATOPOIETIC PROGENITOR CELL TRANSPLANT

Many hematological malignancies, including acute leukemia, chronic leukemia, lymphoma, and multiple myeloma, are treated with a hematopoietic progenitor cell (HPC) transplant (Chapter 11). HPC transplants can be autologous or allogenic and use cells collected from the bone marrow or peripheral circulation. Allogenic transplants may also use cells collected from cord samples. Both autologous and allogenic HPC transplant patients require red blood cell and platelet transfusion support until engraftment occurs, which typically takes about 14 days.

Transfusion Triggers

The hemoglobin value at which patients derive the most benefit from transfusion therapy is controversial. In general, for patients who are not at risk of cardiac ischemia (lack of blood flow to the heart), a transfusion threshold of 8 g/dL (80 g/L) is used, while a hemoglobin value of 10 g/dL (100 g/L) may prevent increased mortality in the subgroup of patients at risk for cardiac ischemia.[20]

Two randomized, controlled trials have evaluated prophylactic platelet transfusions in patients with acute leukemia receiving chemotherapy.[21, 22] Each trial required randomized patients to receive prophylactic platelet transfusions at $10 \times 10^3/\mu L$ or $20 \times 10^3/\mu L$ ($10 \times 10^9/L$ or $20 \times 10^9/L$) and neither study found a significant difference in bleeding episodes between the groups. Based on this data, a transfusion threshold of $10 \times 10^3/\mu L$ ($10 \times 10^9/L$) is appropriate for hospitalized patients receiving chemotherapy or a HPC transplant.

ABO-Incompatible Transplant

Allogeneic HPC transplants are matched for human leukocyte antigen (HLA) compatibility between the donor and the recipient (Chapter 18). On the other hand, ABO compatibility is not critical to the success of an HPC transplant and therefore ABO-incompatible transplants are performed. Patients receiving non-ABO identical HPC transplants will switch their ABO group over time. Choosing the correct ABO group for either red blood cell or plasma product transfusion is based on the type of ABO incompatibility—either major or minor—and the stage in the transplant process—pretransplantation, post-transplantation but pre-engraftment, or postengraftment (Chapter 4).

Cytomegalovirus Risk

Cytomegalovirus (CMV) is a major cause of morbidity and mortality in patients who undergo an allogeneic HPC transplant. CMV reactivation is primarily associated with allogeneic HPC transplants; the risk of CMV reactivation following an autologous transplant is very low.[23] Common manifestations of CMV disease include pneumonia, hepatitis, and gastroenteritis.[24]

> ### ☑ CHECKPOINT 17-3
>
> What are two common manifestations of cytomegalovirus (CMV) infection in immunocompromised people?

Transfusion transmission of CMV is prevented through the use of serologically tested anti-CMV-negative or leukoreduced cellular blood products. Current or potential HPC transplant recipients who are CMV negative should receive CMV-reduced-risk red blood cell and platelet products. A large prospective study performed in patients with acute myelogenous leukemia did not demonstrate a significant difference in the rate of CMV infection between patients who received anti-CMV-negative blood products and those who were treated with leukoreduced products. However, more patients treated with leukoreduced blood products developed CMV-related disease manifestations.[25] Although the practice is controversial, based on this data, many physicians request anti-CMV-negative products for their patients who have had or may have a HPC transplant.

> ### CASE IN POINT (continued)
>
> AC is scheduled to receive a HPC transplant using cells harvested from cord blood as treatment for her sickle cell disease. In preparation, her physician orders a serological test for antibodies to the cytomegalovirus (CMV) and determines she is negative. AC is transplanted with cord blood from two donors. One of the donors is O Rh$_0$(D) positive, which is the same blood type as AC, and the other donor is A Rh$_0$(D) positive.
>
> 4. Once AC is identified as a potential HPC transplant recipient, what type of red blood cell and platelet units should she receive?
> 5. What blood type of red blood cell or plasma products should AC receive in the timeframe soon after her HPC transplant? (*Hint:* See Chapter 4 for further details.)

Transfusion-Associated Graft versus Host Disease

Transfusion-associated graft versus host disease (TA-GVHD) is a devastating complication of transfusion therapy that is almost universally fatal. TA-GVHD occurs when transfused T lymphocytes engraft in the bone marrow of immunosuppressed patients, such as HPC transplant recipients. The resulting clinical symptoms include bone marrow failure, rash, and liver dysfunction.

TA-GVHD cannot be prevented through leukoreduction, but instead requires the irradiation of cellular blood products (Chapter 10).[26] All cellular blood components should be irradiated before transfusion from the time the conditioning chemotherapy or radiation begins and should continue until the patient's lymphocyte count stabilizes above $1 \times 10^3/\mu L$ ($1 \times 10^9/L$) or graft versus host disease prophylaxis is discontinued, which is commonly 1 year after transplantation. Some patients require irradiated blood products for longer times after their transplantation.

> ### ☑ CHECKPOINT 17-4
>
> What are two symptoms of transfusion-associated graft versus host disease (TA-GVHD)?

Platelet Refractoriness

HPC transplant recipients are at risk for developing platelet refractoriness because of the large number of platelet transfusions that they typically receive. Leukoreduction of red blood cell and platelet products reduces the incidence of platelet refractoriness, which is an inadequate response to platelet transfusion (Chapter 16). HLA antigens are present on both white blood cells and platelets (Chapter 18). Leukoreduction reduces the number of white blood cells with foreign HLA antigens that the patient is exposed to and therefore decreases the risk that the patient will form antibodies to the foreign HLA antigens. Patients with platelet refractoriness and antibodies to HLA antigens should receive HLA-matched platelet units.

Granulocyte Transfusion

Overwhelming infection can occur when patients have low neutrophil counts following chemotherapy or HPC transplant. The transfusion of donor granulocytes to a recipient with neutropenia of less than $0.50 \times 10^3/\mu l$ ($0.50 \times 10^9/L$) and an infection may be a helpful adjunct to antibiotics (Chapter 11). Patients with fungal infections show improvement after granulocyte transfusion more often than patients with bacterial infections.[27, 28, 29]

SOLID ORGAN TRANSPLANT

Transfusion practices in solid organ transplantation differ significantly from HPC transplantation. Unlike HPC transplants, donor organs are usually ABO-compatible and with the exception of kidney transplants, HLA matching is often not necessary. In general, leukoreduced blood products are administered to solid organ transplant recipients to diminish HLA alloimmunization; however, irradiation of blood products is unnecessary. To date, there have been only a few case reports of TA-GVHD in the setting of solid organ transplant and this limited data does not support the routine practice of irradiating blood products.[30] CMV reactivation occurs following transplantation and, thus, CMV-reduced-risk products should be used.[30]

ABO Incompatible

The ABO barrier is rarely crossed in solid organ transplantation, as hyperacute rejection of the donor organ can result. ABO-mismatched solid organ transplants are most common in kidney transplants, where HLA matching is critical to prevent organ rejection. When the decision is made to transplant an ABO-incompatible graft, measures must be taken to prevent hyperacute rejection.[31]

Patients who will be receiving an ABO-incompatible kidney transplant undergo treatment aimed at decreasing hemagglutinin titers, which is the test result that estimates the amount of ABO antibodies in the patient's plasma. Plasmapheresis can be used in combination with immune-suppression drugs and sometimes splenectomy.[32] The goal is a hemagglutinin titer of less than 16 prior to transplantation. Kidneys from A_2 donors, who express less A antigen than A_1 individuals, are rejected less often than kidneys from A_1 donors when transplanted into a group O or B individual.[33, 34]

In contrast to kidney transplantation, hyperacute rejection is rare in ABO-incompatible liver transplants.[30] ABO-compatible transplants are still the standard of care as graft survival is better in ABO compatible rather than ABO-incompatible transplants.[35] Nevertheless, ABO-incompatible livers are transplanted in some cases due to the scarcity of donors and the urgent need of the recipient. As in kidney transplant, plasmapheresis, immune suppression, and utilization of A_2 donors have successfully prevented rejection of ABO-incompatible liver allografts.[31]

Minor ABO incompatibilities—for example, a group O organ transplanted to a group A, B, or AB patient—can result in red blood cell hemolysis. On average, hemolysis occurs 7–14 days following transplant and is usually not severe.[30] Hemagglutinin-producing lymphocytes in the transplanted organ are responsible for this phenomenon, which is called **passenger lymphocyte syndrome**. Passenger lymphocyte syndrome is a self-limited process that subsides with donor lymphocyte death. Patients can be supported through the hemolysis with transfusion of red blood cells that lack the corresponding ABO antigen. Additional treatment options include plasma exchange, immune suppression, and splenectomy.[36]

Human Leukocyte Antigen (HLA) Alloantibodies

Preexisting HLA antibodies may cause acute or chronic rejection of a transplanted organ. Consequently, HLA-sensitized patients are identified prior to transplant and the antibody titer is reduced in the peri-transplant period to prevent rejection. Plasma exchange and immune suppression in combination are the most commonly used methods to decrease the HLA antibody titer. In many regimens, one plasma exchange procedure is performed prior to the transplant with an additional four procedures performed postoperatively. Despite these aggressive measures, HLA sensitization is still a risk for mortality.[37]

LIVER DISEASE

One of the common consequences of liver disease is bleeding. The liver is responsible for the production, activation, and modification of many proteins involved in blood clotting. The liver stores vitamin K, which is necessary for the activation of coagulation Factors II, VII, IX, and X. Other complications of liver disease that contribute to bleeding include abnormalities of fibrinogen, which affects the formation of fibrin clots, and low platelet counts due to enlargement of the spleen. Hepatic dysfunction can also cause dilated blood vessels in the esophagus and stomach, which can lead to massive bleeding when combined with poor coagulation.

The mainstay of treatment in a bleeding patient with liver disease is correction of the coagulopathy and platelet count. Fresh frozen plasma (FFP) raises coagulation factor levels. The typical dose of FFP is 15–30 ml/kg; generally, a unit of FFP will produce a 7% increase in coagulation factors. Of the coagulation factors, Factor VII has the shortest half-life of 4–7 hours and, consequently, FFP is administered about every 6 hours. Vitamin K should also be given along with FFP. In a vitamin K–deficient patient, administration of vitamin K can correct the coagulopathy within 24 hours. Additionally, to achieve hemostasis in a patient with liver dysfunction, a platelet count of greater than $100 \times 10^3/\mu L$ ($100 \times 10^9/L$) is the therapeutic target. Platelet transfusions may be required to achieve this target and stop or prevent bleeding. Activated Factor VII (FVIIa) may be given to a bleeding patient who has not responded to or cannot receive FFP, for example, a patient at risk for volume overload.[38] Adequate fibrinogen levels are required for FVIIa to be effective. Therefore, in bleeding patients receiving FVIIa, it is recommended that fibrinogen levels be monitored and cryoprecipitate be transfused, if required.

☑ CHECKPOINT 17-5

What vitamin is a co-factor in the activation of several coagulation factors?

KIDNEY DISEASE

While anemia is a common complication of kidney disease, transfusion therapy is not the mainstay of treatment. In the setting of kidney disease, anemia is typically the result of decreased **erythropoietin** production. Erythropoietin is a glycoprotein, synthesized in the kidneys, that stimulates red blood cell precursors in the bone marrow to differentiate into mature red blood cells.

In patients with kidney dysfunction, anemia is associated with left ventricular hypertrophy (thickening), heart failure, and myocardial events. Correction of anemia has been demonstrated to benefit quality-of-life measures, decrease left ventricular hypertrophy, and prevent the progression of kidney disease.[39] Thus, therapy to improve anemia is vital to the management of patients with kidney dysfunction.

Clinicians must thoroughly investigate other causes of anemia—for example, vitamin deficiencies, hemolysis, or malignancy—prior to attributing anemia solely to low erythropoietin levels. Although the most appropriate target hemoglobin and hematocrit in patients

✳ **TABLE 17-3** Common Indications for Therapeutic Plasma Exchange

Indication	Antibody Class	Replacement Fluid	Schedule*
Thrombotic thrombocytopenic purpura	IgG	Plasma or plasma cryoprecipitate reduced	Daily
Waldenström's macroglobulinemia	IgM	Albumin ± plasma	Daily
Myasthenia gravis	IgG	Albumin ± plasma	QOD
Guillain-Barré syndrome	IgG	Albumin ± plasma	QOD
Goodpasture's syndrome	IgG	Albumin ± plasma	Daily
Prior to solid organ transplant	IgG	Albumin ± plasma	QOD

*Schedule may be adjusted based on clinical setting; QOD, every other day.

with end-stage renal disease is not well defined, consensus guidelines have recommended a goal hematocrit of 33–36% (0.33–0.36).[40] To achieve this goal, erythropoietin is administered subcutaneously or intravenously with variable dosing schedules. Typically, patients on hemodialysis receive erythropoietin three times per week unless the pegylated formulation, called darbepoetin, is used. Darbepoetin requires less frequent weekly or every-other-week dosing. In patients with renal insufficiency not severe enough to require hemodialysis, erythropoietin is given weekly, while darbepoetin is administered every 2–3 weeks.[39] To achieve the best response from erythropoietin, adequate iron stores are necessary. Consensus guidelines recommend a serum ferritin ≥200 ng/mL (≥450 pmol/L) and a transferrin saturation ≥20%.[41] As oral iron is poorly absorbed in patients with chronic renal disease, iron is usually given intravenously.

☑ CHECKPOINT 17-6

What does erythropoietin do?

THERAPEUTIC APHERESIS

Therapeutic apheresis involves the removal of a whole blood component, such as plasma, red blood cells, platelets, or white blood cells. Most commonly, blood is removed from the patient through a central venous catheter or peripheral vein and travels through an extracorporeal circuit to a centrifuge where the blood components are separated. The desired fraction is removed by the machine and the remainder of the blood is returned to the patient. Throughout this process the blood must be anticoagulated with either citrate or less commonly, heparin. Citrate is the most frequently used anticoagulant as it causes little or no systemic anticoagulation. However, calcium must be administered to the patient during the procedure because citrate binds calcium and causes hypocalcemia.

Plasma Exchange

In plasma exchange, which is also called plasmapheresis, plasma is removed from the patient and replaced with albumin, donor plasma, or both. With the removal of plasma and replacement with albumin, a coagulopathy may develop as blood clotting factors are removed. If plasma exchange is performed every other day or less frequently,

donor plasma is usually not required to maintain normal coagulation and prevent bleeding. Alternatively, daily plasma exchange with albumin replacement will eventually deplete the blood clotting factors, necessitating at least partial replacement with plasma, for example, 50/50 albumin/plasma or last liter of plasma.

Plasma exchange is performed for many indications, usually to remove a disease-provoking antibody. Table 17-3 ✳ lists common indications for plasma exchange therapy. The efficacy of plasma exchange is dependent upon the type of antibody targeted, IgG or IgM. IgG is about 55% extravascular and, thus, it requires approximately five procedures with 1.5 blood volumes processed per procedure to remove 90% of IgG antibodies. In contrast, IgM is predominantly intravascular and in two to three procedures about 90% of the antibody is removed. Schedules of plasma exchange vary depending on the underlying disease process and the offending antibody involved.

Thrombotic thrombocytopenic purpura (TTP) is a common indication for plasma exchange and may require specific replacement therapy. The mechanism of TTP involves an IgG antibody directed against an enzyme, ADAMTS13. Without ADAMTS13, large multimers of von Willebrand factor (vWF) accumulate and cause red blood cell hemolysis, thrombocytopenia, and organ damage. Plasma exchange is effective because the procedure removes the IgG antibody and the donor plasma used as replacement fluid provides ADAMTS13. However, vWF is present in FFP and may exacerbate TTP. When patients with TTP have not responded to several plasma exchange procedures, clinicians may request plasma cryoprecipitate reduced, which contains ADAMTS13 but lacks vWF.

☑ CHECKPOINT 17-7

Is there more IgG in the intravascular or extravascular space?

Red Blood Cell Exchange

Red blood cell exchange procedures are used to treat patients with sickle cell disease who are experiencing an acute crisis such as a stroke or acute chest syndrome. Red blood cell exchange rapidly reduces the amount of sickle cells in circulation, replacing them with donor red blood cells.

Cellular Reduction

White blood cells, red blood cells, or platelets may be removed by apheresis. The typical indication for white blood cell apheresis is hyperviscosity in acute leukemia, which can cause mental status changes, dizziness, vision changes, shortness of breath, or bleeding. The extremely large number of blasts and/or other immature white blood cells in the circulation causes these symptoms and prompt removal of the cells via leukoreduction can prevent clinical deterioration. Although there is variation, the goal for leukoreduction is often a blast count of less than $50 \times 10^3/\mu L$ ($50 \times 10^9/L$) for symptomatic improvement.

Clinicians may choose to perform white blood cell apheresis in an asymptomatic patient with acute leukemia prior to the initiation of chemotherapy. Chemotherapy causes the breakdown of a large number of cells in a short time period. The breakdown products can cause kidney dysfunction and electrolyte changes, which is called **tumor lysis syndrome**. Reducing the number of leukemia cells before chemotherapy can prevent these complications.

Less commonly, red blood cells or platelets may be removed in patients with elevated blood counts due to a myeloproliferative disorder in the setting of blood clots or bleeding.

☑ **CHECKPOINT 17-8**

What causes tumor lysis syndrome?

Review of the Main Points

- Hemophilia A is an X-linked inherited disease that causes low levels of Factor VIII.
- Hemophilia B is an X-linked inherited disease that causes low levels of Factor IX.
- Hemophilia is categorized as mild if factor levels are 5–20% of normal, moderate if factor levels are 1–5%, and severe if factor levels are <1%.
- Factor VIII and Factor IX concentrates are used to treat hemophilia.
- Factor VIII has a half-life of 12 hours and 1 IU/kg will raise the factor activity by 2%.
- Factor IX has a half-life of 24 hours and 1 IU/kg will raise the factor activity by 1%.
- Hemophilia patients may develop inhibitors, which are antibodies to Factor VIII or IX.
- Sickle cell disease (SCD) is an inherited disease that results in abnormal hemoglobin, called hemoglobin S (HbS).
- Red blood cells with HbS have an abnormal shape that causes them to block blood vessels, leading to various complications.
- Red blood cell transfusion in sickle cell disease increases oxygen-carrying capacity and dilutes abnormal sickle cells with healthy donor red blood cells.
- Patients with sickle cell disease are treated with simple red blood cell transfusions or exchange transfusions in three situations: prophylactically to reduce the risk of stroke, emergently when the patient experiences a life-threatening complication, and preoperatively to decrease postoperative complications.
- Donor red blood cells transfused to patients with sickle cell disease are usually leukoreduced, HbS negative, and phenotype-matched for C, E, and K antigens.
- Iron overload is a complication of frequent transfusion.
- Exchange transfusion or treatment with iron chelators can reduce the risk of iron overload.

- Hematopoietic progenitor cell (HPC) transplant patients require red blood cell and platelet transfusion support until engraftment occurs.
- Donor platelet and red blood cell units for hematopoietic progenitor cell transplant patients should be leukoreduced and irradiated.
- Cytomegalovirus (CMV)-reduced-risk units may be required for hematopoietic progenitor cell transplant patients if the patient is seronegative for cytomegalovirus.
- Granulocyte transfusions are used as an adjunct therapy in severely neutropenic patients who have an infection that is not responding to antimicrobial therapy.
- Bleeding in patients with liver failure is usually treated with transfusions of fresh frozen plasma (FFP) and platelets.
- Activated Factor VII (FVIIa) may be used in patients with massive hemorrhage who do not respond to plasma transfusion.
- Anemia in kidney disease is caused by decreased levels of erythropoietin and patients are treated with erythropoietin once other causes of anemia are ruled out.
- Therapeutic apheresis is the removal of a blood component with the return of the other blood components.
- Plasma exchange is often used to remove an antibody that is causing disease.
- IgG is 55% extravascular and requires more plasma exchange procedures to reduce the amount of antibody compared to IgM, which is mostly intravascular.
- Replacement fluids used in plasma exchange include fresh frozen plasma, albumin, or a combination of both.
- Plasma cryoprecipitate reduced may be requested as replacement fluid for patients undergoing plasma exchange to treat thrombotic thrombocytopenic purpura (TTP).
- Apheresis to remove white blood cells may be used to treat hyperviscosity syndrome or prevent tumor lysis syndrome in leukemia patients.

Review Questions

1. How are hemophilia A and hemophilia B similar? Select all that apply. (Objective #1)

   A. Genetic disorder

   B. Pattern of inheritance is autosomal

   C. Occur mainly in males

   D. Deficient protein is Factor VIII

2. A mild case of hemophilia A correlates with a _____ Factor VIII activity level. (Objective #2)

   A. <1%

   B. 1–5%

   C. 5–20%

   D. 30–50%

3. What is the half-life of Factor VIII? (Objective #3)

   A. 2 hours

   B. 12 hours

   C. 24 hours

   D. 48 hours

4. Disease manifestations in patients with sickle cell disease include: (Objective #6)

   A. Organ damage

   B. Bone necrosis

   C. Stroke

   D. Pulmonary hypertension

5. A physician orders an exchange transfusion for a patient with sickle cell disease. What are the anticipated benefits of this type of transfusion? (Objective #7)

   A. Decreased hemoglobin level

   B. Decreased percentage of sickle cells

   C. Increased blood volume

   D. Increased blood viscosity

6. Blood transfusion requirements for a patient with sickle cell disease typically include: (Objective #5)

   A. HbS negative

   B. Leukoreduced

   C. CMV positive

   D. Irradiated

7. Which of the following techniques reduces the risk of hyper-hemolysis in sickle cell anemia patients? (Objective #7)

   A. Irradiation

   B. Leukoreduction

   C. Phenotype-matched RBCs

   D. Iron chelation

8. Allogeneic hematopoietic progenitor cell (HPC) transplants require donor and recipient to be: (Objective #8)

   A. ABO identical

   B. ABO compatible

   C. HLA compatible

   D. None of the above

9. How is transfusion-transmitted CMV prevented? (Objective #14)

   A. Serologically tested CMV-negative product

   B. Leukoreduction of RBC product

   C. Irradiation of RBC product

   D. Deferral of CMV-positive donors

10. Transfusion-associated graft versus host disease (TA-GVHD) is preventable with which of the following methods? (Objective #14)

    A. Leukoreduction

    B. Irradiation

    C. Washing

    D. High-speed centrifugation

11. Red blood cell hemolysis that occurs approximately 7–14 days after transplant of an organ with minor ABO incompatibility is termed: (Objective #12)

    A. Lymphocytotoxicity

    B. Hyperacute rejection

    C. Passenger lymphocyte syndrome

    D. HLA sensitization

12. Complications of liver disease include: (Objective #13)

    A. Abnormal bleeding

    B. Depletion of vitamin K–dependent factors

    C. Decreased fibrinogen

    D. Low platelet count

13. Which coagulation factor has the shortest half life? (Objective #13)

   A. Factor II

   B. Factor V

   C. Factor VII

   D. Factor IX

14. The process that is used to remove circulating antibody that is causing disease is called: (Objective #9)

   A. Dialysis

   B. Plasmapheresis

   C. Hemodilution

   D. Irradiation

15. Select the diseases in which plasma exchange therapy is often indicated as a course of treatment. (Objective #9)

   A. Glanzmann's thrombasthemia

   B. Goodpasture's syndrome

   C. von Willebrand's disease

   D. Myasthenia gravis

References

1. Jacquemin MG, Saint-Remy JM. Factor VIII alloantibodies in hemophilia. *Curr Opin Hematol* 2004; 11: 146–50.

2. Bolton-Maggs PH, Pasi KJ. Haemophilias A and B. *Lancet* 2003; 361: 1801–9.

3. Carcao MD, Aledort L. Prophylactic factor replacement in hemophilia. *Blood Rev* 2004; 18: 101–13.

4. Young G. New approaches in the management of inhibitor patients. *Acta Haematol* 2006; 115: 172–9.

5. Freedman J, Garvey MB. Immunoadsorption of factor VIII inhibitors. *Curr Opin Hematol* 2004; 11: 327–33.

6. Knight J, Murphy TM, Browning I. The lung in sickle cell disease. *Pediatr Pulmonol* 1999; 28: 205–16.

7. Switzer JA, Hess DC, Nichols FT, Adams RJ. Pathophysiology and treatment of stroke in sickle-cell disease: Present and future. *Lancet Neurol* 2006; 5: 501–12.

8. Adams R, McKie V, Nichols F, Carl E, Zhang DL, McKie K, Figueroa R, Litaker M, Thompson W, Hess D. The use of transcranial ultrasonography to predict stroke in sickle cell disease. *N Engl J Med* 1992; 326: 605–10.

9. Pegelow CH, Adams RJ, McKie V, Abboud M, Berman B, Miller ST, Olivieri N, Vichinsky E, Wang W, Brambilla D. Risk of recurrent stroke in patients with sickle cell disease treated with erythrocyte transfusions. *J Pediatr* 1995; 126: 896–9.

10. Adams RJ, Brambilla D; Optimizing Primary Stroke Prevention in Sickle Cell Anemia (STOP2) Trial Investigators. Discontinuing prophylactic transfusions used to prevent stroke in sickle cell disease. *N Engl J Med* 2005; 353: 2769–78.

11. Vichinsky EP, Neumayr LD, Haberkern C, Earles AN, Eckman J, Koshy M, Black DM. The perioperative complication rate of orthopedic surgery in sickle cell disease: Report of the national sickle cell surgery study group. *Am J Hematol* 1999; 62: 129–38.

12. Koshy M, Weiner SJ, Miller ST, Sleeper LA, Vichinsky E, Brown AE, Khakoo Y, Kinnery TR; The Cooperative Study of Sickle Cell Disease. Surgery and anesthesia in sickle cell disease. *Blood* 1995; 86: 3676–84.

13. Vichinsky EP, Haberkern CM, Neumayr L, Earles AN, Black D, Koshy M, Pegelow C, Abboud M, Ohene-Frempong K, Iyer RV; The Preoperative Transfusion in Sickle Cell Disease Study Group. A comparison of conservative and aggressive transfusion regimens in the perioperative management of sickle cell disease. *N Engl J Med* 1995; 333: 206–13.

14. The Trial to Reduce Alloimmunization to Platelets Study Group. Leukocyte reduction and ultraviolet B irradiation of platelets to prevent alloimmunization and refractoriness to platelet transfusions. *N Engl J Med* 1997; 337: 1861–9.

15. Coles SM, Klein HG, Holland PV. Alloimmunization in two multitransfused patient populations. *Transfusion* 1981; 21: 462–6.

16. Cox JV, Steane E, Cunningham G, Frenkel EP. Risk of alloimmunization and delayed hemolytic transfusion reactions in patients with sickle cell disease. *Arch Intern Med* 1988; 148: 2485–9.

17. Vichinsky EP, Earles A, Johnson RA, Hoag MS, Williams A, Lubin B. Alloimmunization in sickle cell anemia and transfusion of racially unmatched blood. *N Engl J Med* 1990; 322: 1617–21.

18. Vichinsky EP, Luban NL, Wright E, Oliveri N, Driscoll C, Pegelow CH, Adams RJ; Stroke Prevention Trial in Sickle Cell Anemia. Prospective RBC phenotype matching in a stroke-prevention trial in sickle cell anemia: A multicenter transfusion trial. *Transfusion* 2001; 41: 1086–92.

19. Cohen AR, Martin MB. Iron chelation therapy in sickle cell disease. *Semin Hematol* 2001; 38: 69–72.

20. Wu WC, Rathore SS, Wang Y, Radford MJ, Krumhoz HM. Blood transfusion in elderly patients with acute myocardial infarction. *N Engl J Med* 2001; 345: 1230–6.

21. Rebulla P, Finazzi G, Marangoni F, Awisati G, Gugliotta L, Tognoni G, Barbui T, Mandelli F, Sirchia G; Gruppo Italiano Malattie Ematologiche Maligne dell'Adulto. The threshold for prophylactic platelet transfusions in adults with acute myeloid leukemia. *N Engl J Med* 1997; 337: 1870–5.

22. Wandt H, Frank M, Ehninger G, Schneider C, Brack N, Daoud A, Fackler-Schwalbe I, Fischer J, Gäckle R, Geer T, Harms P, Löffler B, Ohl S, Otremba B, Raab M, Schönrock-Nabulsi P, Strobel G, Winter R, Link H. Safety and cost effectiveness of a $10 \times 10(9)$/L trigger for prophylactic platelet transfusions compared with the traditional $20 \times 10(9)$/L trigger: A prospective comparative trial in 105 patients with acute myeloid leukemia. *Blood* 1998; 91: 3601–6.

23. Holmberg LA, Boeckh M, Hooper H, Leisenring W, Rowley S, Heimfeld S, Press O, Maloney DG, McSweeney P, Corey L, Maziarz RT, Appelbaum FR, Bensinger W. Increased incidence of cytomegalovirus disease after autologous CD 34-selected peripheral blood stem cell transplantation. *Blood* 1999; 94: 4029–35.

24. Hebart H, Einsele H. Clinical aspects of CMV infection after stem cell transplantation. *Hum Immunol* 2004; 65: 432–6.

25. Bowden RA, Slichter SJ, Sayers M, Sayers M, Weisdorf D, Cays M, Schoch G, Manaji M, Haake R, Welk K, Fisher L, McCullough J, Miller W. A comparison of filtered leukocyte-reduced and cytomegalovirus (CMV) seronegative blood products for the prevention of transfusion-associated CMV infection after marrow transplant. *Blood* 1995; 86: 3598–603.

26. Williamson LM, Warwick RM. Transfusion-associated graft-versus-host disease and its prevention. *Blood Rev* 1995; 9: 251–61.

27. Lee JJ, Song HC, Chung IJ, Bom HS, Cho D, Kim HJ. Clinical efficacy and prediction of response to granulocyte transfusion therapy for patients with neutropenia-related infections. *Haematologica* 2004; 89: 632–3.

28. Hester JP, Dignani MC, Anaissie EJ, Kantarjian HM, O'Brien S, Freireich EJ. Collection and transfusion of granulocyte concentrates from donors primed with granulocyte stimulating factor and response of myelosuppressed patients with established infection. *J Clin Apher* 1995; 10: 188–93.

29. Price TH, Bowden RA, Boeckh M, Bux J, Nelson K, Liles WC, Dale DC. Phase I/II trial of neutrophil transfusions from donors stimulated with G-CSF and

dexamethasone for treatment of patients with infections in hematopoietic stem cell transplantation. *Blood* 2000; 95: 3302–9.

30. Triulzi DJ. Specialized transfusion support for solid organ transplantation. *Curr Opin Hematol* 2002; 9: 527–32.

31. Rydberg L. ABO-incompatibility in solid organ transplantation. *Transfus Med* 2001; 11: 325–42.

32. Tanabe K, Takahashi K, Sonda K, Tokumoto T, Ishikawa N, Kawai T, Fuchinoue S, Oshima T, Yagisawa T, Nakazawa H, Goya N, Koga S, Kawaguchi H, Ito K, Toma H, Agishi T, Ota K. Long-term results of ABO-incompatible living kidney transplantation: A single-center experience. *Transplantation* 1998; 65: 224–8.

33. Bryan CF, Winklhofer FT, Murillo D, Ross G, Nelson PW, Shield CF 3rd, Warady BA. Improving access to kidney transplantation without decreasing graft survival: long-term outcomes of blood group A2/A2B deceased donor kidneys in B recipients. *Transplantation* 2005; 80: 75–80.

34. Nelson PW, Helling TS, Shield CF, Beck M, Bryan CF. Current experience with renal transplantation across the ABO barrier. *Am J Surg* 1992; 164: 541–4; discussion 544–5.

35. Farges O, Kalil AN, Samuel D, Saliba F, Arulnaden JL, Debat P, Bismuth A, Castaing D, Bismuth H. The use of ABO-incompatible grafts in liver transplantation: A life-saving procedure in highly selected patients. *Transplantation* 1995; 59: 1124–33.

36. Sokol RJ, Stamps R, Booker DJ, Scott FM, Laidlaw ST, Vandenberghe EA, Barker HF. Posttransplant immune-mediated hemolysis. *Transfusion* 2002; 42: 198–204.

37. Jacobs JP, Quintessenza JA, Boucek RJ, Morell VO, Botero LM, Badhwar V, van Gelder HM, Asante-Korang A, McCormack J, Daicoff GR. Pediatric cardiac transplantation in children with high panel reactive antibody. *Ann Thorac Surg* 2004; 78: 1703–9.

38. Goodnough LT, Lublin DM, Zhang L, Despotis G, Eby C. Transfusion medicine service policies for recombinant factor VIIa administration. *Transfusion* 2004; 44: 1325–31.

39. Fishbane S. Anemia treatment in chronic renal insufficiency. *Semin Nephrol* 2002; 22: 474–8.

40. Eschbach JW. Current concepts of anemia management in chronic renal failure: Impact of NFK-DOQI. *Semin Nephrol* 2000; 20: 320–9.

41. Kausz AT, Obrador GT, Pereira BJ. Anemia management in patients with chronic renal insufficiency. *Am J Kidney Dis* 2000;36:S39–51.

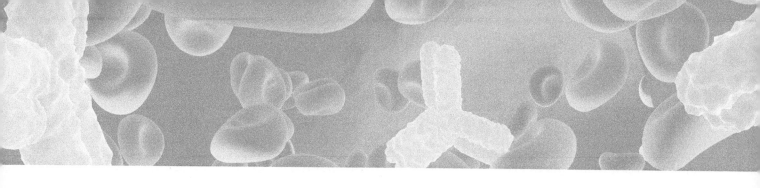

18 Human Histocompatibility

BRIAN F. DUFFY, RALPH J. GRAFF, AND BEVERLY HOOVER

Chapter Objectives

Upon completion of this chapter, the student will be able to:

1. Describe the anamnestic response and its role in adaptive immunity.
2. Identify the two classes of human leukocyte antigens (HLAs) and describe the role of each in the immune response.
3. Describe the biochemistry of the class I and class II molecules.
4. Describe the biochemistry and action of the peptide-binding domains.
5. Describe the genetics of and designations associated with the major histocompatibility complex (MHC).
6. Interpret the HLA nomenclature of serologically defined specificities and sequence-defined alleles.
7. Discuss cross-reactivity of HLA antibodies and the designation of cross-reactive groups (CREGs).
8. Interpret family study data of HLA typings.
9. Identify and describe the techniques used in and the interpretation and reporting of results associated with HLA antigen typing, crossmatching, and antibody screening.
10. Discuss the complications that can occur post-transplant (i.e., graft rejection), including the methods through which they can be monitored.
11. Describe the common pretransplant testing protocols for hematopoietic progenitor cell (HPC), kidney, and other solid organ transplants.

Key Terms

α helix (helices)
β-pleated sheet
Haplotype
Histocompatibility
Human leukocyte antigen(s) (HLA[s])
Major histocompatibility complex (MHC)
Panel reactive antibody (PRA) level
Polygenic
Polymorphic

CASE IN POINT

HT is a 72-year-old male with a diagnosis of acute myelogenous leukemia (AML) and thrombocytopenia. He is currently seen in the outpatient transfusion clinic every other week for bloodwork and has standing orders for transfusion of two apheresis platelets if his platelet count drops below $10 \times 10^3/\mu L$ ($10 \times 10^9/L$) and 2 units of red blood cells if his hemoglobin falls below 7.0 g/dL (70 g/L).

What's Ahead?

Histocompatibility (the ability of tissues to exist together) testing refers to the analyses performed to increase the chance of transplanted tissue survival. Transfusion is actually a transplant of blood cells. Transfusion and transplantation medicine are therefore related and share parallel histories. The two fields of study are separate because histocompatibility relies on **human leukocyte antigens (HLAs)** (antigens on the surface of most nucleated cells including white blood cells, platelets, and many tissue cells) matches whereas routine transfusion compatibility relies on red blood cell antigen matches. The term *histocompatibility* is also called *HLA* in the same way that transfusion medicine may be referred to as blood bank or immunohematology. HLA typing is performed when a transplant may occur and also when platelet matching is required (Chapter 16) or when investigating some types of transfusion reactions (Chapter 12). This chapter addresses the following questions:

- What biochemistry mechanisms are associated with the HLA system?
- How do genetics participate in the development of the HLA system?
- What nomenclature is associated with the HLA system?
- What techniques have been developed to determine histocompatibility between organ and hematopoietic progenitor cell (HPC) donors and recipients?

HISTORICAL BACKGROUND

The history of histocompatibility began in 1901 and continues today with ongoing research and development.[1, 2, 3, 4] In 1901, Loeb noted that cancer cells transferred between genetically identical mice would grow, but cancer cells transferred between unrelated mice would not grow. Many of the early advances in the understanding of histocompatibility were fortunate discoveries made by researchers who were studying other questions at the time. Discoveries were often initially made in laboratory mice with other researchers concurrently or soon after correlating the results to humans. Figure 18-1 ■ illustrates the major events in the early history of the scientific discovery of human leukocyte antigens (HLA).

Over the last 50 years, transplantation has evolved from an experimental procedure to an important and life-saving therapy. Figure 18-2 ■ highlights some of the key events in the history of transplantation science. As of 2007, 752,481 kidney; 21,867 kidney–pancreas; 7,195 pancreas; 696 pancreatic islet; 81,969 heart; 4,090 heart–lung; 25,456 lung; 171,288 liver; 774 intestine; and 176,501 hematopoietic progenitor cell–bone marrow–stem cell allogeneic transplants have been performed worldwide.[5] This achievement constitutes a classic example of multidisciplinary collaboration: the recognition of the phenomenon of rejection by biologists, the appreciation by geneticists that the targets of rejection were inherited, the elucidation of the mechanism of rejection by immunologists, and the adaptation of this knowledge to the histocompatibility laboratory by laboratorians and to the bedside by clinicians. Figure 18-3 ■ outlines some of the major developments in laboratory testing used to predict histocompatibility.

☑ CHECKPOINT 18-1

The development of transplant science from research to a clinical treatment is a classic example of _____.

HUMAN LEUKOCYTE ANTIGENS (HLAs) AND THE IMMUNE SYSTEM

The immune response can be divided into innate and adaptive systems (Chapter 1). Only the adaptive system is involved in allograft rejection. The adaptive system displays an anamnestic, or memory, response, which is a rapid increase in antibody production when a previously encountered antigen is reintroduced. HLA molecules, including both class I and class II, are critical components of the adaptive immune response.

☑ CHECKPOINT 18-2

Which system of the immune response is responsible for transplant rejection?

The adaptive immune system consists of antigen-presenting cells, such as macrophages, dendritic cells, and B lymphocytes, and antigen-recognition cells, most notably T lymphocytes but also B lymphocytes. Foreign proteins found outside the antigen-presenting cell are bound to a corresponding receptor, then internalized, broken down into fragments, complexed with HLA class II molecules, and displayed on

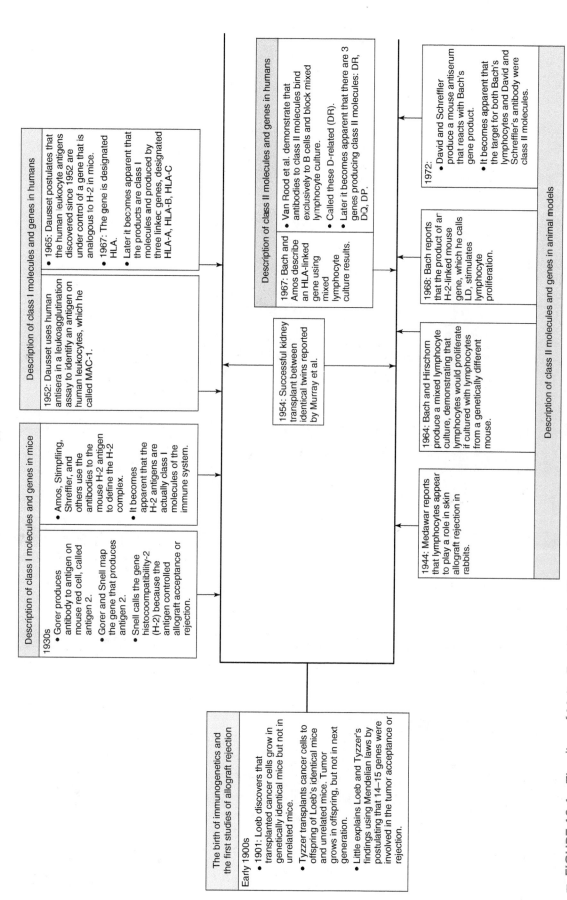

FIGURE 18-1 Timeline of Major Events in the History of HLA Description

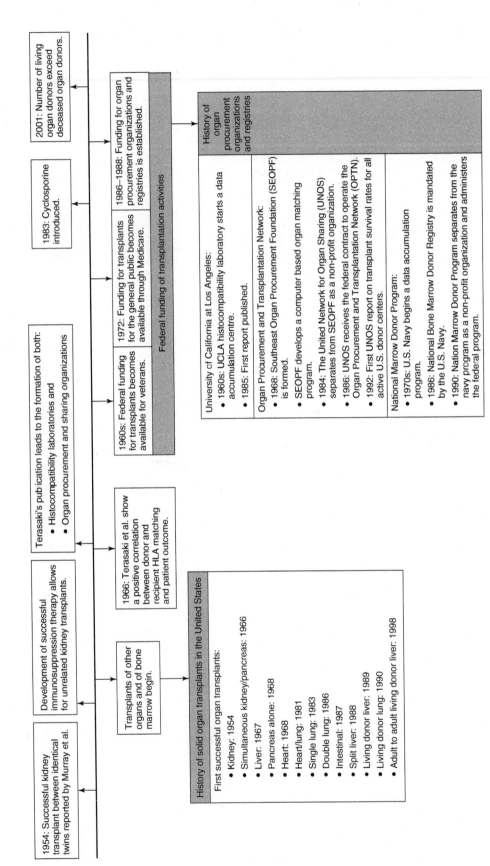

■ FIGURE 18-2 Timeline of Major Events in the History of Transplantation

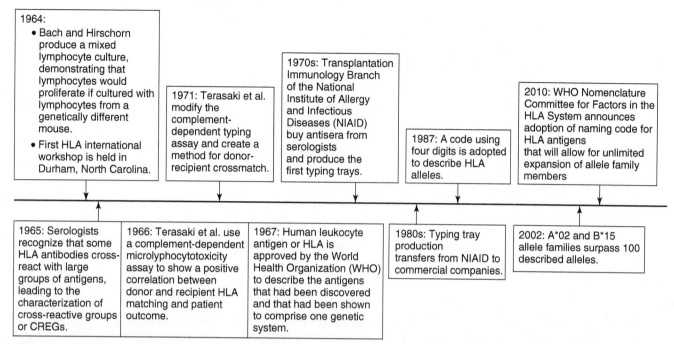

1964:
- Bach and Hirschorn produce a mixed lymphocyte culture, demonstrating that lymphocytes would proliferate if cultured with lymphocytes from a genetically different mouse.
- First HLA international workshop is held in Durham, North Carolina.

1971: Terasaki et al. modify the complement-dependent typing assay and create a method for donor-recipient crossmatch.

1970s: Transplantation Immunology Branch of the National Institute of Allergy and Infectious Diseases (NIAID) buy antisera from serologists and produce the first typing trays.

1987: A code using four digits is adopted to describe HLA alleles.

2010: WHO Nomenclature Committee for Factors in the HLA System announces adoption of naming code for HLA antigens that will allow for unlimited expansion of allele family members

1965: Serologists recognize that some HLA antibodies cross-react with large groups of antigens, leading to the characterization of cross-reactive groups or CREGs.

1966: Terasaki et al. use a complement-dependent microlyphocytotoxicity assay to show a positive correlation between donor and recipient HLA matching and patient outcome.

1967: Human leukocyte antigen or HLA is approved by the World Health Organization (WHO) to describe the antigens that had been discovered and that had been shown to comprise one genetic system.

1980s: Typing tray production transfers from NIAID to commercial companies.

2002: A*02 and B*15 allele families surpass 100 described alleles.

FIGURE 18-3   Timeline of Major Events in the History of Histocompatibility Testing

the cell surface. A common example would be a bacterium that was engulfed by a macrophage, as illustrated in Figure 18-4 ▪. Nonself proteins formed inside the antigen-presenting cell are complexed with HLA class I molecules and displayed on the cell surface. A common example would be an altered self-protein formed by a cancerous cell, as illustrated in Figure 18-5 ▪.

Antigen-presenting cells displaying foreign proteins activate antigen-recognition cells. Antigen-recognition cells produce both the cell-mediated and antibody-mediated immune responses designed to destroy cells displaying foreign protein(s). This is the basis of organ rejection. Cells that display nonself class I and class II molecules, such as cells of a non-HLA-identical transplanted organ, will initiate the cellular and humoral immune responses.

Class I and II molecules are part of the **major histocompatibility complex (MHC)** (a complex containing multiple genes located on chromosome 6 that are found in all mammals and that code for major targets of rejection). The genetic aspects associated with HLAs are described later in this chapter.

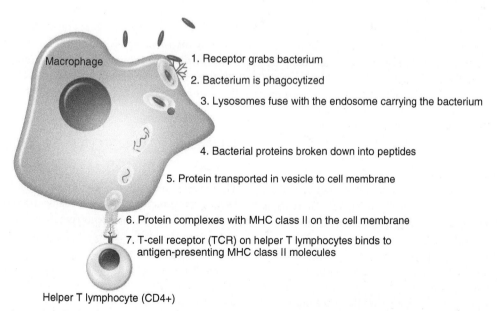

Macrophage

1. Receptor grabs bacterium
2. Bacterium is phagocytized
3. Lysosomes fuse with the endosome carrying the bacterium
4. Bacterial proteins broken down into peptides
5. Protein transported in vesicle to cell membrane
6. Protein complexes with MHC class II on the cell membrane
7. T-cell receptor (TCR) on helper T lymphocytes binds to antigen-presenting MHC class II molecules

Helper T lymphocyte (CD4+)

FIGURE 18-4   Immune Response to a Bacteria and Role of MHC Class II Molecules

HLA class II molecules are part of the immune response to foreign proteins found outside the antigen-presenting cell, in this example bacterial proteins.

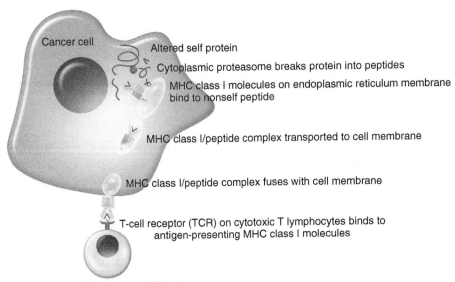

Cancer cell
Altered self protein
Cytoplasmic proteasome breaks protein into peptides
MHC class I molecules on endoplasmic reticulum membrane bind to nonself peptide
MHC class I/peptide complex transported to cell membrane
MHC class I/peptide complex fuses with cell membrane
T-cell receptor (TCR) on cytotoxic T lymphocytes binds to antigen-presenting MHC class I molecules
Cytotoxic T lymphocyte (CD8+)

■ **FIGURE 18-5**   Immune Response to a Cancer Cell and Role of MHC Class I Molecules

HLA class I molecules are part of the immune response to foreign proteins found inside an antigen-presenting cell. Examples include altered self proteins found in cancerous cells or viral proteins found within infected cells.

HUMAN LEUKOCYTE ANTIGEN (HLA) BIOCHEMISTRY

HLA molecules are constructed to bind peptides. The HLA class I molecule consists of a 45 kDa α glycoprotein heavy chain that is anchored to the plasma membrane and a noncovalently associated 12 kDa β-2 microglobulin light chain. No variation has been described in the light chain. The heavy chain consists of α1, α2, and α3 extracellular domains, a transmembrane anchor, and a cytoplasmic tail. The α1 and α2 domains are extremely *polymorphic*, a concept described later, the α3 domain less so. Together, the α1 and α2 domains form two α **helices** (protein chains coiled into right-handed coils) on a **β-pleated sheet** (an almost fully extended and folded protein chain whose folds are fixed with lateral hydrogen bonds) platform. The α helices create a groove, or peptide-binding cleft, that can accommodate a variety of peptides less than 13 amino acids in length. One end of the groove binds the carboxyl end of the peptide; the other end binds the amino end. Pockets along the course of the groove bind particular anchor amino acids, giving specificity to the binding. Class I molecules are found on almost all cells.

HLA class I and class II molecules share a similar structure, as illustrated in Figure 18-6 ■. The HLA class II molecule is a heterodimer composed of a 34 kDa α glycoprotein chain and a 29 kDa β glycoprotein chain. Each chain consists of two extracellular domains, a transmembrane domain anchor, and a cytoplasmic tail. The α1 and β1 domains create a groove similar to the α1 and α2 domains of the class I molecule. Polymorphism is less than that of the class I domains. Also the class II α1 domain is less polymorphic than the class II β1 domain. The class II peptide-binding cleft is open at both ends, allowing the binding of peptides greater than 13 amino acids. Binding does not involve the carboxyl or amino ends of the peptide. Class II molecules are found primarily on antigen-presenting cells, which includes lymphocytes, macrophages, and dendritic cells.

GENETICS REVIEW

Information is transmitted from one generation to the next via deoxyribonucleic acid (DNA). DNA is arranged into double helical chains that form chromosomes. Each human has a total of 46 chromosomes and receives one set of 23 chromosomes from each parent (Chapter 2). If the specific genes on each corresponding chromosome are the same, the alleles are called *homozygous*. If the genes are different, the person is called *heterozygous* for that allele. The term *genotype* refers to the genes present in general or at a particular location in an individual. The term *phenotype* refers to the products of those genes.

HUMAN LEUKOCYTE ANTIGEN (HLA) GENETICS

The genes of the MHC are inherited together from each parent as a **haplotype** (group of alleles on the same chromosome that are transmitted together). Neither genotyping with DNA-based techniques nor phenotyping with serologic techniques can identify which genes were inherited on the same chromosome. Separation of alleles into haplotypes requires family studies (Chapter 2). Similar to most blood group system genes, the genes of the MHC are expressed in a codominant fashion (Chapter 2).

In humans, the MHC is called the HLA system. The approximately 4 million nucleotides that code for the HLA system are located on the short arm of chromosome 6. The HLA system genes are

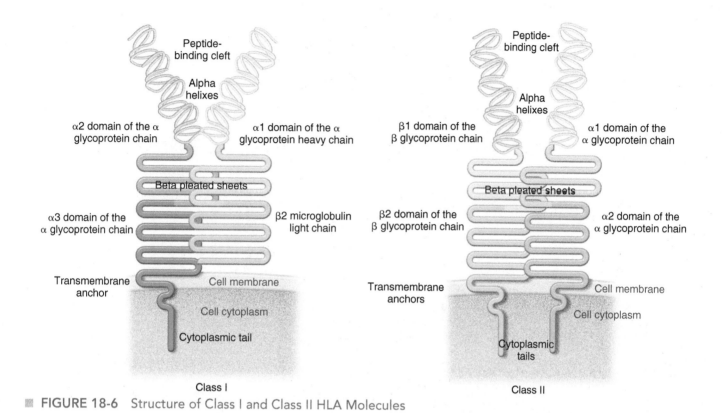

FIGURE 18-6   Structure of Class I and Class II HLA Molecules

divided into three regions, as illustrated in Figure 18-7 ■.[6] The class I region, which contains the genes that produce the class I molecules, is located closest to the telomere. The class II region, which contains the genes that produce the class II molecules, is located closest to the centromere. The class III region, which contains genes that produce some of the complement components, is located between the class I and II regions. These regions also contain genes with other functions.

☑ **CHECKPOINT 18-4**

HLA genes are on which chromosome?

The class I region contains 10 genes designated HLA and five genes designated MIC. The classic HLA molecules HLA-A, HLA-B, and HLA-C are coded by their corresponding class I region genes: *HLA-A, HLA-B,* and *HLA-C.* (It is important to point out here that the proper format used when referring to genes in written documents is *italics.*) The products of *HLA-E* and *HLA-G* are inhibitory ligands for natural killer cell receptors. The function of the *HLA-F* product is not known. *HLA-H, HLA-J, HLA-K,* and *HLA-L* are pseudogenes, which produce no protein or a nonfunctional protein. The products of *MIC-A* and *MIC-B* are HLA-like molecules that are expressed without β-2 microglobulin and function as activating ligands for natural killer cell receptors. *MIC-C, MIC-D,* and *MIC-E* are pseudogenes. All human populations carry the six expressed HLA genes, although deletions of pseudogenes have been described.

The class II region is divided into DP, DO/DM, DQ, and DR subregions. The products of the class II region genes combine to form four class II molecules: one HLA-DP, one HLA-DQ, and two HLA-DR.

The DP subregion contains *DPA1* and *DPB1* genes, whose products combine to make a DP molecule, and *DPA2* and *DPB2* pseudogenes. The DO/DM subregion contains *DOA, DOB, DMA,* and *DMB* genes. Their products combine to make DO and DM molecules. The DQ subregion contains two *DQA* and three *DQB* genes. Only two genes, *DQA1* and *DQB1,* produce products that combine to make a DQ molecule; the rest are pseudogenes.

The DR subregion is more complicated (Figure 18-8 ■). One *DRA* gene and nine *DRB* genes (four *DRB* genes and five pseudogenes, as noted below) exist in the human population, but individual HLA systems do not contain every *DRB* gene. Five different arrangements have been described.[6] All five possess the *DRA* gene, *DRB1* gene, and *DRB9* pseudogene plus one of the following:

- No additional genes
- *DRB6* pseudogene
- *DRB3* gene and *DRB2* pseudogene
- *DRB5* gene and *DRB6* pseudogene
- *DRB4* gene, *DRB7* pseudogene, and *DRB8* pseudogene

In summary, each HLA system can produce six or seven antigenic products: one each of HLA-A, HLA-B, HLA-C, HLA-DP, and HLA-DQ and one or two HLA-DR.

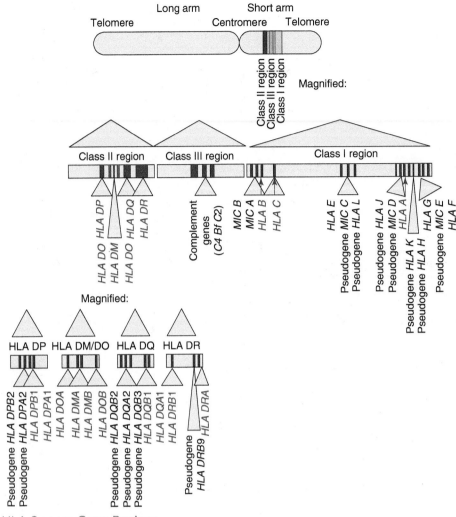

FIGURE 18-7 HLA System Gene Regions

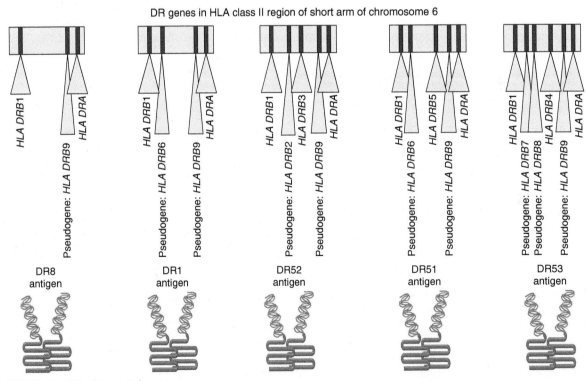

FIGURE 18-8 DR Gene Subregion

POLYMORPHISM AND POLYGENISM

Sometimes a mutation that disrupts the function of a gene puts the individual with the mutation at a survival disadvantage. Such genes are usually not **polymorphic** (the presence of multiple alleles of a given gene in a species). Generally, HLA gene mutations do not hinder the function of their products, and they may create a selective advantage to the species. As a result, the HLA genes are among the most polymorphic in the human genome. Tables 18-1 ✶ and 18-2 ✶ enumerate alleles and resulting antigens described as of 2012 in the HLA class I and class II gene regions, respectively.[7]

The HLA system is also very **polygenic** (multiple genes expressed in an individual that produce similar products); each individual expresses up to a maximum of 14 antigen-presenting HLA molecules. Although each molecule is able to bind many different peptides, the HLA molecules of a given individual may not be able to bind every peptide. Therefore, the individual may be susceptible to a particular pathogen because his or her HLA could not bind the peptides produced by that pathogen.

On the other hand, because the HLA system genes are very polymorphic, the human species possesses an immense variety of HLA molecules with the ability to respond to almost every peptide and protect the species against almost every disease. The magnitude of polygenism is protective to the individual, whereas polymorphism is protective to the species.

✶ **TABLE 18-1** HLA Class I Genes, Alleles, and Antigens

Genes	Alleles[#]	Antigens[#]
A	2,013	28
B	2,605	62
C	1,551	10
E	11	
F	22	
G	16	

[#]Numbers change over time as new alleles are discovered.

✶ **TABLE 18-2** HLA Class II Antigens, Genes, and Alleles

Antigens[#]	Genes	Alleles[#]
6	DPA1	34
	DPB1	155
9	DQA1	47
	DQB1	176
24	DRA	7
	DRB	1,260
	DMA	7
	DMB	13
	DOA	12
	DOB	13

[#]Numbers change over time as new alleles are discovered.

NOMENCLATURE OF THE HUMAN LEUKOCYTE ANTIGEN (HLA) SYSTEM

There are two systems associated with the nomenclature of the HLA system. The first system involves incorporation of the antibodies that bind HLA specificities. The second system is based on sequence-defined alleles. A description of each system follows.

Serologically Defined Specificities

Many HLA specificities have been identified by the antibodies that will bind to them. Theoretically, an individual can make antibodies against any allogeneic HLA molecule that differs from his or her own by at least one amino acid. Of the multiple thousands of amino acid differences that exist between HLA alleles, antibodies against only 88 variations of class I and 65 variations of class II have been identified.

History

The early descriptions of HLA specificities came from laboratories working individually, each developing its own nomenclature. As these laboratories came together at workshops, the need for a standard nomenclature became apparent. The compromise designation HLA was chosen,[3] and the reported specificities were given temporary designations HLA-w1, -w2, -w3, -w4, -w5, -w6, -w7, and -w8. The *w* signified workshop. When an antigen was confirmed by antibody reactivity in a sufficient number of laboratories, the *w* was dropped.

Class I

HLA-A and HLA-B antigens were the first HLA gene products described. Thus, the first eight specificities were designated HLA-A1, HLA-A2, HLA-A3, HLA-Bw4, HLA-B5, HLA-Bw6, HLA-B7, and HLA-B8. As additional HLA-A and HLA-B antigens were identified, they were given sequential HLA-A or HLA-B numbers. When new antisera defined a third locus, it was named HLA-C and its antigens were designated with sequential HLA-Cw numbers. To differentiate the HLA-C antigens from complement components, serologic HLA-C nomenclature has never dropped the *w* designation. Table 18-3 ✶ lists the HLA class I antigens recognized as of 2012.[7, 8]

> ### ☑ CHECKPOINT 18-5
> Why was the letter *w* kept in the HLA-C serologic names?

Class II

Identification of the class II antigens followed identification of the class I antigens. Class II specificities that were first identified in tissue culture with the mixed lymphocyte reaction (MLR) were named with HLA-Dw sequential numbers. As antisera were obtained and characterized, it was appreciated that two independently segregating groups of antigens existed. The molecules and the genes producing them were named HLA-DR and HLA-DQ. Then MLR reactivity identified a third gene and its product, which were called HLA-DP. Subsequently, anti-DP antibodies have been identified.

✳ **TABLE 18-3** HLA Class I Antigens

HLA-A	HLA-B		HLA-C
A1	B5	B51(5)	Cw1
A2	B7	B5102	Cw2
A203	B703	B5103	Cw3
A210	B8	B52(5)	Cw4
A3	B12	B53	Cw5
A9	B13	B54(22)	Cw6
A10	B14	B55(22)	Cw7
A11	B15	B56(22)	Cw8
A19	B16	B57(17)	Cw9(w3)
A23(9)	B17	B58(17)	Cw10(w3)
A24(9)	B18	B59	
A2403	B21	B60(40)	
A25(10)	B22	B61(40)	
A26(10)	B27	B62(15)	
A28	B2708	B63(15)	
A29(19)	B35	B64(14)	
A30(19)	B37	B65(14)	
A31(19)	B38(16)	B67	
A32(19)	B39(16)	B70	
A33(19)	B3901	B71(70)	
A34(10)	B3902	B72(70)	
A36	B40	B73	
A43	B4005	B75(15)	
A66(10)	B41	B76(15)	
A68(28)	B42	B77(15)	
A69(28)	B44(12)	B78	
A74(19)	B45(12)	B81	
A80	B46	B82	
	B47		
	B48	Bw4	
	B49(21)	Bw6	
	B50(21)		

The numbers in parentheses are the parent antigens of the splits, which are explained later in the section on cross-reactions.

✳ **TABLE 18-4** HLA Class II Antigens

HLA-D	HLA-DP	HLA-DQ	HLA-DR
Dw1	DPw1	DQ1	DR1
Dw2	DPw2	DQ2	DR103
Dw3	DPw3	DQ3	DR2
Dw4	DPw4	DQ4	DR3
Dw5	DPw5	DQ5(1)	DR4
Dw6	DPw6	DQ6(1)	DR5
Dw7		DQ7(3)	DR6
Dw8		DQ8(3)	DR7
Dw9		DQ9(3)	DR8
Dw10			DR9
Dw11(w7)			DR10
Dw12			DR11(5)
Dw13			DR12(5)
Dw14			DR13(6)
Dw15			DR14(6)
Dw16			DR1403
Dw17(w7)			DR1404
Dw18(w6)			DR15(2)
Dw19(w6)			DR16(2)
Dw20			DR17(3)
Dw21			DR18(3)
Dw22			
Dw23			DR51
Dw24			DR52
Dw25			DR53
Dw26			

The numbers in parentheses are the parent antigens of the splits, which are explained below in the section on cross-reactions.

The *w* is incorporated into the names of specificities that were originally identified by MLR. This includes the HLA-DP antigens, as well as the broad HLA-Dw specificities, which are now known to reflect a recipient's combined immune response to HLA-DP, HLA-DQ, and HLA-DR antigens. Table 18-4 ✳ lists the HLA class II antigens recognized as of 2012.[7, 8]

Cross-Reactions

As more antibodies were discovered and serologic techniques improved, it was recognized that some antibodies thought to be specific for a single antigen were actually specific for an epitope found on two or more antigens. When this occurred the original antigen designation would be appended to the new designations in parentheses. For example, there is one antibody that reacts with HLA-A9, but antibodies were also discovered that react with two different subsets, or splits, of HLA-A9. These splits

are designated HLA-A23 and HLA-A24, which can be written as HLA-A23(9) and HLA-A24(9) to identify both the specific antigens and their shared epitope. Family studies showing independent segregation of the antigens and then later genetic analysis confirmed this phenomenon that was originally identified serologically.

Conversely, some individually identified antigens share common protein sequences. Antibodies specific to the shared epitopes will cross-react with several antigens, which are grouped into cross-reactive groups (CREGs). For example, the class I antigens were divided into seven CREGs, as listed in Table 18-5 ✳.[7, 8, 9]

When a particular sequence of proteins, as defined by a cross-reacting antibody, appears in a large number of antigens, even those in different groups of HLA antigens, it is sometimes called a *public epitope*. For example, as listed in Table 18-6 ✳, anti-HLA-Bw4 and anti-HLA-Bw6 were found to react with most HLA-B antigens and anti-HLA-Bw4 reacts with some HLA-A antigens as well.[7, 8] This is the third instance in the HLA nomenclature where the *w* that originally designated workshop was kept, in this case to identify that Bw4 and Bw6 are not distinct HLA molecules, but are actually epitopes that are shared by many HLA.

✷ **TABLE 18-5** HLA Class 1 Cross-Reactive Groups (CREGs)

Cross-Reactive Group (CREG)	Associated Individual Epitopes
1C	A1, 3, 9, 11, 23(9), 24(9), 29, 30, 31, 36, 80
2C	A2, 9, 23(9), 24(9), 28, 68(28), 69(28), B17, 57(17), 58(17)
5C	B5, 15, 17, 18, 21, 35, 46, 51(5), 52(5), 53, 62(15), 63(15), 70, 71(70), 72(70), 73, 75(15), 76(15), 77(15), 78
7C	B7, 8, 13, 22, 27, 40, 41, 42, 47, 48, 54(22), 55(22), 56(22), 59, 60(40), 61(40), 67, 81, 82
8C	B8, 14, 16, 18, 38(16), 39(16), 59, 64(14), 65(14), 67
12C	B12, 13, 21, 37, 40, 41, 44(12), 45(12), 47, 49(21), 50(21), 60(40), 61(40)

✷ **TABLE 18-6** HLA Class 1 Public Epitopes

Public Epitope	Associated Private Epitopes
4C (Bw4)	A9, 23(9), 24(9), 2403, 25(10), 32(19), B5, 5102, 5103, 13, 17, 27, 37, 38(16), 44(12), 47, 49(21), 51(5), 52(5), 53, 57(17), 58(17), 59, 63(15), 77(15)
6C (Bw6)	B7, 703, 8, 14, 18, 22, 2708, 35, 39(16), 3901, 3902, 40, 4005, 41, 42 45(12), 46, 48, 50(21), 54(22), 55(22), 56(22), 60(40), 61(40), 62(15), 64(14), 65(14), 67, 70, 71(70), 72(70), 73, 75(15), 76(15), 78, 81, 82

☑ **CHECKPOINT 18-6**

What is the definition of a public epitope?

Sequence-Defined Alleles

As HLA antigens were confirmed genetically by identifying the corresponding gene, the *w*, if present, would be dropped from the name. Then in 2010, a new system for naming HLA alleles was introduced.[7] The new nomenclature uses a series of number sets separated by colons to name specific gene sequences. An asterisk is placed following the HLA locus designation to indicate that the specificity is an allele defined by DNA.

History

This naming convention was adopted in April 2010. The prior naming system was similar in that number pairs described the various alleles in the same manner, but the pairs were not separated by colons. Before 1989, the letter *w* would be kept in the allele name when it was described serologically but had not been confirmed by gene sequencing. After 1989, gene sequencing became a requirement for identification of a new allele, so the *w* was dropped from allele names except in the case of HLA-C where it was kept to differentiate the genes from complement genes. By 2002, however, more than 100 alleles had been described in several allele families. This resulted in difficulties in using a system based on pairs of numbers. For example, the 99th allele of the A*02 family was called A*0299, but the 100th allele of the A*02 family was called A*9201. Similarly, the 100th allele of the B*15 family was called B*9501.

Class I

In the 2010 naming convention, the first set of numbers is called the allele family and often describes the serologic specificity with which the allele was associated. The second set of numbers is assigned in order of the allele's discovery. In this set, the nucleotide difference must result in an amino acid sequence difference in the resulting protein antigen.

The third set of numbers differentiates silent mutations, where the nucleotide sequence is different but the resulting amino acid sequence is the same. This can occur because more than one nucleotide triplet can produce the same amino acid (Chapter 2). If the mutation prevents the production of a product, which is called a null mutation, an *N* is appended to the allele name in place of this third set of numbers.

The fourth set of numbers differentiates alleles that have different DNA sequences in the noncoding, or intron, areas of the gene or in the untranslated end pieces of DNA. Both of these types of nucleotide substitutions do not affect the amino acid sequence of the resulting protein. However, mutations within the introns may affect the production of the antigen. A nucleotide substitution that results in low production of antigen is designated with an *L*. Box 18-1 illustrates the naming convention for HLA class I alleles.

☑ **CHECKPOINT 18-7**

In the 2010 naming convention for HLA genes, which set of numbers is used to identify a silent mutation?

BOX 18-1 Examples of HLA Class I Allele Names

HLA-A Naming Convention Examples
A*01:01:01:01
A*01*03
A*01:11N
A*24:02:01:02L
A*74:02

Five of the 965 identified alleles as of January 2010.

BOX 18-2   Examples of HLA Class II Allele Names

Example alleles of DRA, DRB, DQA, DQB, DPA, DPB Genes
DRA*01:01
DRA*01:02:02
DRB1*01:01:01
DRB1*16:15
DRB2*01:01
DRB9*01:01
DQA1*01:01:01
DQA1*04:03N
DQA1*06:02
DQB1*05:01:01
DQB1*06:39
DPA1*01:03:01
DPA1*04:01
DPB1*01:01:01
DPB1*99:01

some of the alleles in the string contain different nucleotides in the exons coding for these domains, the string is reported as the allele with the lowest possible number followed by a capital *P*. Table 18-7 ✶ gives an example of reporting an ambiguous string.[7, 8] The peptide-binding domains are coded by exons 2 and 3 for class I molecules and exon 2 for class II molecules.

CASE IN POINT (continued)

After several months of regular transfusions, HT seems to be coming into the clinic more frequently for bleeding and bruising. He is now being seen twice per week and receives two apheresis platelets at each visit. Yet, despite the high number of transfusions, his platelet count seems to always be less than $4.0 \times 10^3/\mu L$ ($4.0 \times 10^9/L$). The physician requests a platelet antibody test and HLA typing of the patient.

1. Your laboratory does not perform HLA typing. The reference laboratory that you use offers separate tests to determine HLA class I and HLA class II antigens. Which will you order and why?

Class II

The same principles apply to class II allele names. However, a single gene controls the polymorphic areas of class I molecules (α glycoprotein heavy chain; Figure 18-6) but two molecules and therefore two genes control the polymorphic areas of class II molecules (α glycoprotein chain and β glycoprotein chain; Figure 18-6). Hence class I alleles are either A, B, or C; but class II alleles are DPA1, DPB1, DQA1, DQB1, DRA1, or DRB1. HLA-DR alleles may also include DRB3, DRB4, or DRB5 (Figure 18-8). Box 18-2 illustrates the naming convention for HLA class II alleles.

Ambiguous Strings

Not all testing methods will identify an HLA allele down to the level of every nucleotide present in the gene. Rather, the test may narrow the possible identity of the gene to one of several related genes, which all result in the same or similar peptide-binding domains. The list of possible alleles is called an *ambiguous string*.

If all the possible alleles have the same nucleotide sequence in the exons coding for the peptide-binding domains, the string is reported as the possible allele with the lowest number followed by a capital *G*. If the amino acids in the peptide-binding domains are the same but

LABORATORY TEST METHODOLOGIES

Histocompatibility laboratories employ various techniques to type for HLA, screen for HLA antibodies, crossmatch donor and recipient samples, and monitor recipient status post transplant.

HLA class I molecules are widely distributed in the body and are present on platelets and almost all nucleated cells. HLA class II molecules are expressed on only a few cell types, including B lymphocytes. Blood specimens, which are easy to obtain, are used for most routine HLA tests. The following sections describe a range of laboratory test methodologies that, depending on the test setting, have been or currently are being used to perform histocompatibility testing.

Complement-Dependent Microlymphocytotoxicity Typing

In complement-dependent microlymphocytotoxicity typing, abbreviated as CDC (complement-dependent cytotoxicity for the purposes of the remainder of this chapter), T lymphocytes are used to type for HLA-A, HLA-B, and HLA-C antigens, and B lymphocytes are used for HLA-DR and HLA-DQ typing. Lymphocytes are separated from other blood cells by differential centrifugation or by magnetic

✶ **TABLE 18-7** Example of Ambiguous Allele Typing String

	String	Report
Same nucleotides in exons[+]	02:03:01/02:253/02:264/02:370	A*02:03:01G
Same amino acid sequence[§]	A*02:03:01/A*02:03:02/A*02:03:03/A*02:03:04/A*02:253/A*02:264/A*02:370	A*02:03P

[+]Exons coding for protein binding domains; [§]In protein-binding domains.

beads. Magnetic beads can also enrich a lymphocyte preparation for T or B cells.

☑ CHECKPOINT 18-8

Which type of cell is used for HLA class II antigen typing?

The CDC methodology consists of incubating T or B lymphocytes with a panel of well-characterized HLA antisera. First, lymphocytes are added to a commercial microtiter tray, where each well contains one microliter of antiserum. After incubation at room temperature, unbound antibodies are removed by washing. Rabbit

serum containing complement is added to the cells and the mixture is incubated at room temperature. Rabbit complement will react with antibodies bound to the lymphocyte surface, resulting in cell membrane injury and lysis. Cell lysis is assayed using a vital stain and visualized by phase-contrast microscopy. If the lymphocyte sample is positive for the HLA corresponding to the antiserum in the well, the cells in that well will have taken up the dye. The dyed, dead cells will appear large and nonrefractile, or dull and dark, because the cell is not refracting the light. The unstained, live, antigen-negative cells by comparison will look small and refractile, or shiny. Fluorescently labeled dyes and a fluorescent microscope can be used in a manner similar to the vital stains to differentiate live and dead cells. The main steps in the CDC method are illustrated in Figure 18-9.

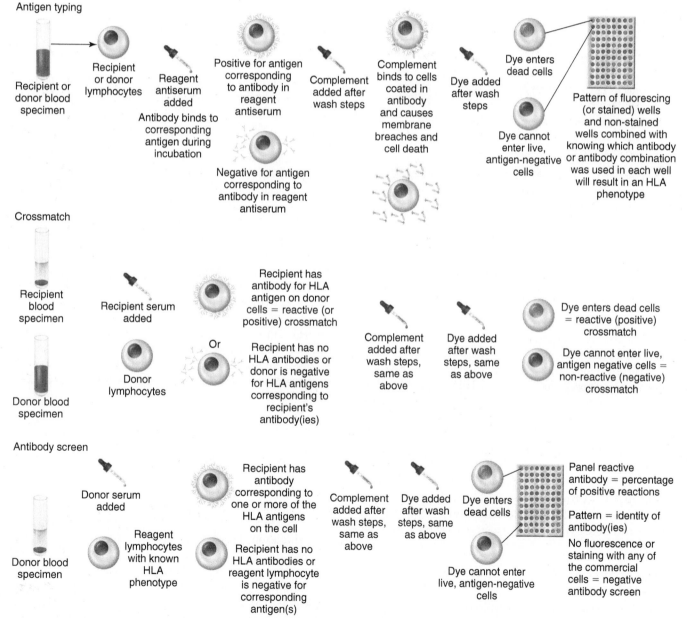

FIGURE 18-9 Complement-Dependent Microlymphocytotoxicity

Not drawn to scale.
Only the major steps in the procedure and a representative few cells/ antibodies are illustrated.
When used for antibody screen or identification purposes, 30–60 commercial cells are used, either singly or more often in different combinations.

Commercial HLA typing trays have 60 or 72 wells, each containing a different antiserum. The reaction pattern is analyzed to determine the HLA alleles. If only one allele is identified at a locus, the other is called a *blank*. A blank may occur if the person is homozygous for the identified allele or if the person has an allele for which there was no antiserum on the panel. For example, a panel may result in the phenotype A3, --; B7, B44; DR1, DR13. This would be read as A3, blank. The person may be A3, A3 or A3, unknown allele.

CASE IN POINT (continued)

While you are waiting for HT's HLA typing results to arrive from the reference laboratory, the physician reviews HT's medical records and discovers historical HLA typing results from another laboratory that at the time used a microlymphocytotoxicity testing method. HT's historical HLA typing results were A2, --; B08, B52; Cw02, Cw03.

2. Given the test methodology, why does the patient only have one A locus allele listed?
3. What is the term to describe this?
4. Your blood center currently has three apheresis platelets in inventory that have had HLA typing performed and seem to be partial matches.

   Platelet 1 = A*29, A*31; B*27, B*62; Cw*02, Cw*03

   Platelet 2 = A*02, A*03; B*08, B*52; Cw*02, Cw*03

   Platelet 3 = A*02, B*08, B52; Cw*02, Cw*03

   In what order would you transfuse these platelets?

DNA Typing

Polymerase chain reaction (PCR) methods are used to type DNA for HLA alleles and are today the most common methods used for HLA typing. These methods have largely replaced complement-dependent microlymphocytotoxicity in a number of HLA laboratory settings. DNA typing methods bypass the need for antigen expression on living cells, reduce the required specimen volume, and can often resolve blanks and ambiguities that would occur with cytotoxic methods. PCR uses repeated cycles of denaturation, primer annealing, and extension by DNA polymerase to result in an exponential increase in the HLA allele flanked by the primers. Three PCR-based variations in HLA DNA typing are described in the following sections: reverse sequence-specific oligonucleotide (SSO) probe hybridization, sequence-specific primer (SSP) typing, and sequence-based typing (SBT).

Sequence-Specific Oligonucleotide (SSO) Probe Hybridization

The reverse sequence-specific oligonucleotide (SSO) probe hybridization method begins with amplification of the target DNA, in this case the DNA at the HLA gene sites. The target DNA is amplified by using primers that are consensus sequence for the DNA sequence beside the target HLA gene DNA on the 3' end. When the PCR occurs the primer hybridizes with the single-stranded patient DNA and the polymerase continues to read the patient DNA in the 5' to 3' direction, resulting in the target DNA being produced. The primers are biotinylated on their 5' end. Biotin is a small molecule that can be attached to protein or nucleic acids. Biotin binds to streptavidin and avidin; therefore, it is often used in biochemical procedures to separate out a protein or nucleic acid of interest.

The amplified DNA sample is added to sequence-specific probe DNA, also called oligonucleotide probes because the probes are less than 20 nucleotides long. The probe is often immobilized; in the past nylon membranes were used; more recently beads are commonly used. Beads allow for multiplex testing, such as Luminex®, where multiple amplifications and detections occur simultaneously. The amplified sample DNA will bind only to exactly matched sequences of the oligonucleotide probe. Binding is detected after addition of strepavidin to the biotin–primer–probe complex and subsequent visualization with substrate, such as phycoerythrin. The beads can also have different fluorescent markers incorporated to identify them. Flow cytometry is used to determine which beads are reactive and software analyzes the results and reports the HLA type. Figure 18-10 ■ illustrates the main steps in SSO typing.

Sequence-Specific Primer (SSP) Typing

Sequence-specific primer (SSP) typing employs primer pairs that are specific for unique sequences within an exon. If the sample tested exactly matches both primers, amplification continues and a double-stranded DNA fragment will be produced. Visualization occurs after the DNA fragment is loaded onto an agarose gel and exposed to an electric current. Ethidium bromide in the gel inserts between the DNA bases and fluoresces under ultraviolet light. Each well also includes a primer pair specific for a target sequence present in all patients, such as human growth hormone, to serve as a positive control. Patterns of HLA-specific fragments are compared to known HLA sequences to determine an HLA genotype.

SSP can be low resolution (*A*01*, *A*02*) or high resolution (*A*01:01*, *A*02:01*). Low-resolution SSP can be used for stat typing because it can be completed in a relatively short period of time. High-resolution SSP can sometimes be used to resolve ambiguities in SSO typing.

Sequence-Based Typing (SBT)

Both SSO and SSP evaluate known polymorphisms in variable regions, but assume that constant regions are conserved. Sequence-based typing (SBT), which is typically a high-resolution method, determines the nucleotide sequence of the entire exon, including the regions that are usually constant. SBT uses two rounds of PCR. In the initial PCR, consensus primers amplify a specific exon. The second cycle of PCR uses cycle sequencing, resulting in DNA fragments of different sizes, each tagged with a fluorescent-labeled nucleotide. An automated sequencer identifies the fragments based on size and fluorescent terminal nucleotide. The sequence of the fluorescent nucleotides represents the sequence of the HLA exon amplified in the first PCR. The sequence along the length of the entire exon is compared to known HLA sequences to determine a genotype.

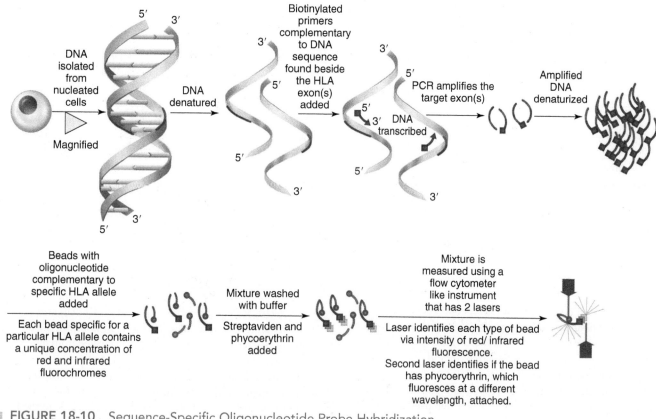

FIGURE 18-10 Sequence-Specific Oligonucleotide Probe Hybridization

Purple line `\`, DNA at HLA gene locus (target)

Blue line `\`, DNA sequence next to target DNA sequence

Dark blue square ■, biotin
Medium blue shape ◢, steptaviden
Light blue shape ◹, phycoerythrin
Not drawn to scale.
One example of multiple variations illustrated.
Exons amplified are 2 and 3 for HLA class I alleles and exon 2 for HLA class II alleles.
Hundreds of beads can be added to a single mixture of amplified DNA.
Each bead may be coated with a single allele sequence or a combination of several allele sequences.

Donor–Recipient Crossmatch

Scientists are attempting to develop assays with the ability to detect activation of the immune response cells *in vitro*. In the meantime, histocompatibility laboratories rely on the presence of donor-specific antibodies in recipient serum to indicate sensitization to donor antigens. Antibodies to donor antigens, if present, may be detected by crossmatching the recipient serum with donor lymphocytes. Three methods for conducting such testing follow.

Complement-Dependent Microlymphocytotoxicity

The complement-dependent microlymphocytotoxity (designated as CDC in this chapter) crossmatch is analogous to the CDC method used for HLA typing, except that in a crossmatch the recipient's serum is used rather than reagent antisera. Donor lymphocytes are incubated with the recipient's serum. The washing, addition of complement, and staining steps are all the same as in the CDC antigen typing method. If antibody is present in the recipient's serum, the donor lymphocytes will be lysed. The addition of an antihuman globulin (AHG) reagent

prior to complement increases the test's sensitivity and can result in the detection of some low-level class I antibodies. AHG increases the binding efficiency of complement, allowing antibodies that normally cannot fix complement to lyse cells.

Flow Cytometry

Despite the increase in sensitivity achieved by adding AHG to the CDC crossmatch, it still sometimes fails to predict antibody-mediated rejection. Crossmatch by flow cytometry, which is more sensitive than CDC, was introduced in the early 1980s.[10]

In the flow crossmatch, unseparated donor lymphocytes are incubated with patient serum. Unbound antibody is washed away after the incubation period. Goat antihuman IgG labeled with fluorescein isothiocyanate (FITC), which fluoresces green, binds to the antibodies on the donor lymphocytes. An antibody to CD3, labeled with peridinin chlorophyll protein (PerCP), which will fluoresce orange, is used to identify T lymphocytes. B lymphocytes are labeled with an antibody to CD19 that has been complexed with phycoerythrin (PE), which will fluoresce red. The lymphocytes are suspended in isotonic media and passed single file in front of a laser. Detectors determine the proportion of cells exhibiting the various combinations of fluorescence, green and orange or green and red. The resulting semiquantitative measure of the recipient's serum reactivity is compared to reactivity of antibody-negative serum to determine the immune status of the recipient specific to the donor.

Differentiation of HLA and Non-HLA Antibodies

A positive crossmatch indicates the presence of a recipient antibody that is reactive with any antigen on the donor cells. Although such reactivity is usually directed against HLA class I or class II molecules, it might be reactive with other lymphocyte membrane antigens or with a foreign antigen that the lymphocyte had processed and that is now presented by the HLA molecules on the lymphocyte's surface. The antibody may be an alloantibody or an autoantibody. Crossmatching alone also does not differentiate whether the antibody is IgG or IgM. Techniques are available to partially characterize antibodies.

HLA antibodies can be distinguished from non-HLA antibodies using solubilized HLA molecules adhered to a solid matrix. The antigen may be bound to microtiter plate wells, such as in enzyme-linked immunoassay (ELISA), or microbeads, such as in flow cytometry. Platelets can be used to remove antibodies to class I antigens, leaving only antibodies to class II antigens in the adsorbed serum.

A crossmatch using autologous lymphocytes can indicate if autoantibody is present. Autoantibody may be removed from recipient serum by adsorption using autologous tissue. The adsorbed serum can then be tested for alloantibodies.

As in red blood cell antibody identification (Chapter 8), treating the recipient serum with dithiothreitol (DTT) will destroy IgM antibodies, thus allowing differentiation between IgG and IgM. Antibodies to HLA are generally IgG.

Antibody Screen

HLA antibody screening identifies all HLA antibodies in the recipient serum in contrast to a crossmatch, which detects only donor-specific antibody. Early antibody screening techniques used panels of lymphocytes with known HLA specificities as targets. Because each cell possessed multiple HLA and non-HLA antigens, the HLA targets could be inferred only indirectly and non-HLA reactivity could not be excluded.

The use of solubilized HLA molecules adhered to a solid matrix or microparticle has resulted in more accurate identification of HLA antibodies. Single-antigen targets have been of particular value. The improvement in identifying HLA antibodies in sensitized patients has led some investigators to suggest that antibody screening may now predict crossmatch results with sufficient accuracy to replace the crossmatch.[11]

However, this assertion is controversial and other authors point out the limitations of the solid phase antibody screen.[12] Donor information concerning HLA-DP and DQA1 generally is not available, though anti-DP and anti-DQA1 are detected in some recipients. The antibodies expressed by a sensitized potential recipient can change with time or if the patient experiences another sensitizing event, thus previous antibody screens may not reflect the recipient's antibody status at the time of transplant. In addition, the significance of antibodies that react with the modified antigens on solid-state targets but not with antigens on living cells, or vice versa, is not clearly understood.

Complement-Dependent Microlymphocytotoxicity

The CDC antibody screen is similar to HLA typing or crossmatching using the CDC methodology. In the antibody screen, recipient serum acts as the unknown and is tested against a panel of previously HLA-typed lymphocytes. As with the CDC crossmatch, AHG can be added to increase the sensitivity. Commercial panels typically represent 30 or 60 donors. Most positive antibody screens are multispecific, having more than one antibody reacting, making the analysis even more complex. Computer software is used to help define antibody specificities. Antibody screen results in HLA are often expressed as a percentage of the cells that reacted, called a **panel reactive antibody (PRA) level**.

Solid-Phase Assays

The interest in transplanting across the HLA barrier spurred research in techniques to determine if a donor antibody is truly HLA specific. CDC screens detect antibodies bound to intact cells that express numerous antigens in addition to HLA. In contrast, solid-phase assays use HLA class I or class II molecules purified from human cell cultures. The culture lines usually used include Epstein-Barr virus–transformed human B lymphocytes or transfected HLA-deficient human lymphoid cells. The purified antigens are used in ELISA and flow cytometry assays to detect antibodies specific to the HLA system.

In ELISA testing, the recipient serum is added to plastic trays where the wells are coated with HLA class I or class II molecules. After incubation, the unbound antibodies are washed away. Alkaline phosphatase labeled with goat antihuman IgG is added as the conjugate and a second incubation occurs. The plate is washed again and p-nitrophenyl phosphate substrate is added. If the antibody is present, this will result in a sandwich of HLA antibody–goat antihuman IgG conjugate–p-nitrophenyl phosphate substrate all bound to the antigen, which in turn is fixed to the plate well. The alkaline phosphatase will react with the p-nitrophenyl phosphate, resulting in a color change that can be read by a spectrophotometer.

In flow cytometry HLA antibody screening, the recipient serum is incubated with microbeads coated with class I or class II molecules. Each bead can be coated with a single HLA antigen or with a combination of HLA antigens, depending on the assay and the level of differentiation desired. The beads with class II molecules attached are also coated with a PE label. After incubation, unbound antibody is washed away and FITC-labeled antihuman IgG is added. The beads are transferred from the microtiter tray wells where the reactions have occurred into plastic tubes, which are loaded onto the flow cytometer. The flow cytometer will pass the beads single file in front of a laser and will measure the fluorescence. Beads coated with a class I molecule or molecules to which the recipient has a corresponding antibody will demonstrate FITC fluorescence. Beads with a class II molecule or molecules will display both PE and FITC fluorescence if the recipient has a corresponding antibody. The fluorescence of the recipient serum is compared to that of a serum known to be negative for HLA antibody to determine if the antibody is present. The pattern of positivity is analyzed to assign HLA specificity and PRA level.

Figure 18-11 ■ illustrates the main steps in an antibody screen using antigen-coated beads counted by flow cytometry.

Multiplex procedures, such as Luminex® technology, are based on simultaneous laser analysis of multicolored beads, similar to the technique illustrated in Figure 18-9. The beads used may be coated with a single antigen or may be coated with a combination of antigens. Each type of bead is identified by varying concentrations of usually two fluorochromes incorporated into the bead. Recipient serum is incubated with a mixture of the beads. Unbound antibody is removed by washing and PE-conjugated goat antihuman IgG is added. The beads are analyzed by two lasers. One excites the PE, causing antibody-coated beads to fluoresce. The second excites the internal dye of the fluorescing beads, identifying which color bead and therefore which antigen has reacted with the antibody. If beads with multiple antigens are used, then the combination of which beads reacted and which did not can often identify the antibody present. For example, software assigns PRA level and HLA antibody specificity.[13]

Post-Transplant Immunological Monitoring

Graft rejection can occur at any time post transplant in either solid organ or hematopoietic progenitor cell (HPC) transplants. HPC transplant recipients are also at risk for graft versus host disease (GVHD), where the immunocompetent transplanted cells attack the recipient's cells. To prevent both graft rejection and GVHD, immunosuppressive drugs are a permanent therapy even in HLA-matched recipients. Antirejection drug therapy carries its own risks, including infection, cancer, and drug toxicity. The goal of post-transplant monitoring is regulation of drug dosage to minimize toxic side effects and recognition of graft rejection or GVHD as early as possible.

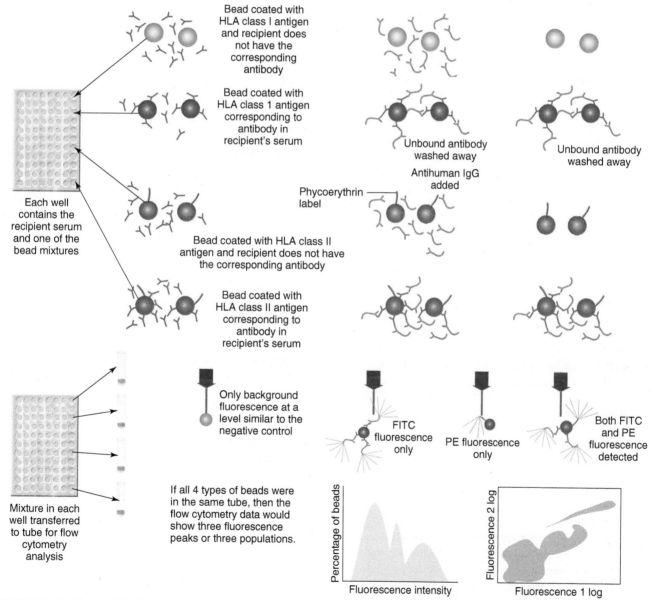

FIGURE 18-11 Solid-Phase HLA Antibody Screen Using Beads and Flow Cytometry

Not drawn to scale.

Only the major steps in the procedure and a representative few beads/ antibodies are illustrated.

Standard post-transplant monitoring techniques involve detecting injury to the graft or the host by the immune system, but adjusting immunosuppressive therapy before injury occurs would be ideal. Therefore, researchers are developing assays that identify immune activation even before injury has occurred. Although the long-term clinical outcomes of post-transplant immunological monitoring are unknown, technology to provide noninvasive meaningful indicators of allograft rejection and infection are on the verge of routine clinical practice. Assays developed to date include the detection of signal transduction,[14] DNA synthesis, gene activation,[15, 16] cytokine production,[17, 18] or antibody production.

Signal Transduction

The ImmunKnow® assay detects levels of adenosine triphosphate (ATP) in CD4-positive T lymphocytes. ATP is a nucleotide that provides energy for signal transduction, which is the process of a cell activating a series of biochemical pathways in response to a stimulus. For example, T-lymphocyte activation after interaction with an antigen-presenting cell that is presenting a foreign antigen.

Whole blood from the recipient is incubated with phytohemagglutinin (PHA), which will stimulate immunocompetent CD4-positive T lymphocytes. CD4-positive cells are selected with monoclonal anti-CD4-coated magnetic beads. The CD4 cells are lysed and ATP is released. The ATP emits light when luciferin, which is a luminescent reagent, is added. The light emission is measured with a luminometer and is proportional to the amount of ATP released. A baseline of ATP level in unstimulated T lymphocytes is determined by parallel testing of the recipient's blood without the addition of PHA. Ranges of ATP concentration predict underimmunosuppression that can lead to rejection or overimmunosuppression that can lead to infection.[14]

DNA Synthesis

DNA synthesis can be measured with mixed lymphocyte culture (MLC), which is also called mixed lymphocyte reaction (MLR). In the MLC, lymphocytes from two different people are mixed and cultured together. If there are differences in the class II molecules, the lymphocytes will activate and proliferate, increasing the level of DNA synthesis. Radioactive thymidine is added to the culture and the uptake is proportional to the amount of cell proliferation. Historically, the MLC was used to type for class II antigens, but for this purpose it has been replaced by DNA typing techniques.

Gene Activation

Microarray technology can screen many genes at once, determining which are currently active and which are not. Multicenter trials have correlated gene expression with acute rejection, chronic rejection, organ dysfunction, and well-functioning transplants.

Samples tested by microarray technology include peripheral blood lymphocytes and biopsies. Active genes produce messenger RNA (Chapter 2). The first step in the analysis is reverse transcription, which produces complementary DNA from the messenger RNA, if present.

PCR is used to increase the number of copies of complimentary DNA to a detectable level. The amount of messenger RNA produced as measured by the number of copies of complimentary DNA formed is proportional to the amount of protein expressed by the gene. If the gene is active, it is producing more protein than when it is inactive. Microarray technology uses fluorescently labeled DNA probes attached to a solid glass matrix. Each DNA probe represents a specific gene or a functional group of genes. The amplified patient DNA is added and "reacts" with the probes, causing them to fluoresce. One color indicates an upregulation of a gene and a second color indicates downregulation. Computer analysis determines which groups of genes are expressed.

Cytokine Production

Cytokines are molecules produced and secreted by activated cells. Specific cytokines are produced during an immune response, such as graft rejection. An increase in serum or biopsy cytokines may predict acute or chronic rejection. The enzyme-linked immunosorbent spot (ELISPOT) assay[17] is used to detect cytokine-producing cells. In this assay ELISA is used to measure specific cytokine levels, including interleukins, tumor necrosis factors, transforming growth factors, interferons, and colony-stimulating factors.

Antibody Detection

Antibody detection is often considered as the most common/most important post-transfusion monitoring technique performed in the HLA laboratory. CDC and solid-phase assays can be used to detect the post-transplant development of HLA antibodies. Detected antibodies are compared to the donor's HLA type to determine donor-specific antibody. If donor cells are available, HLA crossmatch techniques can also be performed to detect donor-specific antibody. In addition, a modification of the solid-phase antibody screen that uses recipient serum and solubilized donor HLA molecules bound to ELISA trays or beads has been developed.[19]

CASE IN POINT *(continued)*

HT has now been approved for a HPC transplant to treat his AML. His three siblings that are potential donors were HLA-typed. The results of HT and his siblings' typing results obtained using a DNA-based method show the following:

HT (recipient): A*02, 24; B*18, 44, C*05,*07; DRB1*04, 13; DQB1*03, 06

Sister: A*01, 02; B*08, 44, C*05, 07; DRB1*04, 03; DQB1*02, 03

Brother 1: A*02, 24; B*18, 40, C*03,*07; DRB1*01, 13; DQB1*05, 06

Brother 2: A*02, 24; B*18, 44, C*05,*07; DRB1*04, 13; DQB1*03, 06

5. Are any of the siblings potential matches?
6. Monitoring for GVHD is very important following a HPC transplant. What is GVHD?
7. After HT's HPC transplant, his CBC counts steadily rise each day. This is an indication of what?

✳ **TABLE 18-8** Current Status of Testing in Various Types of Transplants*

Transplant Type	Pretransplant Testing on Recipient	Matching of Recipient and Donor	Post-Transplant Monitoring
Hematopoietic progenitor cells	• No antibody screen performed if transplant is HLA identical. • Antibody screen occasionally performed if transplant is HLA nonidentical.	10 alleles are identified in the donor and recipient by high-resolution genetic testing: HLA-A, HLA-B, HLA-C, HLA-DR, HLA-DQ.	• Complete blood counts are used to assess engraftment. • Tests that evaluate organ function are used to assess graft versus host disease.
Kidney	Periodic antibody screens for HLA antibodies.	• 8 alleles are identified in the donor and recipient by serologic antigen typing or low-resolution genetic testing: HLA-A, HLA-B, HLA-C, HLA-DR. • Crossmatch between recipient plasma and donor lymphocytes.	• Urinary output. • Serum creatinine level. • C4D staining and histological analysis of kidney biopsy.
Other solid organs	Varies among transplant type and transplant program.	Limited use in most other organ transplants. Avoided in liver transplants.	Varies.

*General guidelines; specific protocols may vary among different transplant centers.

Transplant-Specific Testing Protocols

Table 18-8 ✳ lists the status of testing in various types of transplants. Protocols change over time.

Hematopoietic Progenitor Cell Transplants

Hematopoietic progenitor cell (HPC) transplants, also called *bone marrow transplants*, are frequently used to treat genetic and acquired dysfunction of the bone marrow and also malignant disease. Table 18-9 ✳ lists the most common indications for HPC transplants in 2009.[20] As with solid organ transplants, HPC transplants carry a risk of transplant rejection. However, unlike solid organ transplants, there is also the risk of GVHD.

GVHD plays a major role in HPC recipient morbidity and mortality. The risk of GVHD increases with the degree of HLA mismatch, therefore the majority of HPC grafts are HLA identical. Whether the donor is related or unrelated, attempts are made to match the donor and recipient at 10 alleles (two alleles each at HLA-A, -B, -C, -DRB1 and -DQ loci) using high-resolution DNA

typing techniques. Figure 18-12 ▪ illustrates HLA typing results of a prospective recipient and his related potential donors.

> ☑ **CHECKPOINT 18-10**
>
> How many HLA alleles are matched between donor and recipient in a hematopoietic progenitor cell transplant?

HLA crossmatch and antibody screen are not usually performed in HPC transplants because the transplant is usually HLA identical. In the rare cases when transplant of HLA nonidentical cells are considered, crossmatching and/or antibody testing may be requested.

Post-transplant monitoring of HPC transplants must consider both rejection and GVHD. The appearance of a full spectrum of red and white blood cells, measured by complete blood count (CBC) and bone marrow analysis, indicates engraftment. A subsequent

✳ **TABLE 18-9** Indications for Hematopoietic Progenitor Cell Transplant*

Allogeneic	Autologous
• Acute myelogenous leukemia (AML) • Acute lymphocytic leukemia (ALL) • Myelodysplastic and myeloproliferative syndromes • Nonmalignant diseases** • Non-Hodgkin's lymphoma • Other leukemias • Aplastic anemia • Chronic myelogenous leukemia (CML)	Multiple myeloma Non-Hodgkin's lymphoma Hodgkin's disease Other cancers Acute myelogenous leukemia (AML)

*In order from most common to least common overall. The most common indications are different for adult and child recipients.

**Hereditary immune system disorders (e.g., severe combined immunodeficiency, Wiskott-Aldrich syndrome), hemoglobinopathies (e.g., beta thalassemia major, sickle cell disease), hereditary metabolic disorders (e.g., Hurler's syndrome, adrenoleukodystrophy, metachromatic leukodystrophy).

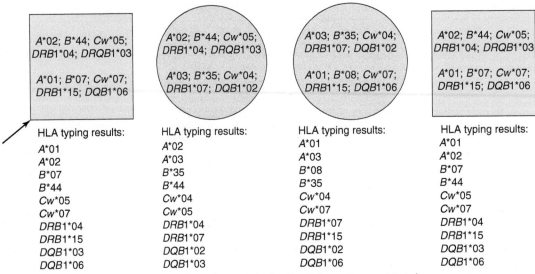

FIGURE 18-12   Comparing HLA Typing Results to Find a Recipient Donor Match

The prospective recipient is marked with an arrow and has three siblings, who are antigen-typed. Low-resolution results are shown for simplicity. The haplotypes of all four people can be inferred from the laboratory results and are included. Both of the patient's sisters are partial matches, having inherited one haplotype in common with the affected brother but having inherited a different second haplotype. The brother of the patient is a complete match, having inherited the same two haplotypes from their parents.

decline in the number of these cells indicates rejection. Because most donor–recipient pairs are HLA identical, HLA typing is of no value in quantifying donor and recipient cells. PCR characterization of variable-number tandem repeats (VNTR) (Chapter 19) is used to determine percentages of donor and recipient cells.[21] Although immunological techniques to predict GVHD are being sought, none have been considered reliable enough for clinical application. GVHD is diagnosed by evaluating organ function and morphology.

Success of HPC transplants varies depending on the aggressiveness of the primary disease, especially in the case of malignancies.

Kidney Transplants

Mismatching is better tolerated in solid organ transplants than in HPC transplants. Acceptable outcomes are achieved with mismatches in kidney transplants, but HLA matching is associated with better outcomes.

Potential recipients awaiting kidney transplantation undergo periodic HLA antibody screening. The frequency and technique used vary among transplant centers. In most centers, antibodies specific for a donor's HLA are a contraindication to transplantation. The antibody screen results also have prognostic value; recipients with high PRA levels have worse outcomes post transplant than those with negative antibody screens.[2]

Once a potential kidney donor is found, antigen matching, which is based on the donor and recipient's HLA types and the recipient's antibody screen, and crossmatching are both performed. Potential kidney donor and recipient pairs are typed for six or eight antigens (HLA-A, -B, and –DR and in some programs HLA-C), most often using a low-resolution DNA typing technique. HLA identical transplants from living sibling donors have a better success rate than lesser-matched living donor transplants, which in turn have a better

success rate than transplants from deceased donors. The number of antigen mismatches correlates with recipient mortality, especially as time progresses past the first year.

☑ CHECKPOINT 18-11

Which HLA alleles are usually typed for when matching a donor and recipient for a kidney transplant?

The United Network for Organ Sharing (UNOS) uses a point system to allocate organs from deceased donors to recipients who are likely to gain the most benefit. The point system is updated constantly based on the latest research data. For kidney transplants both ABO and HLA match are considered, along with a host of other criteria.

HLA crossmatch is generally performed prior to kidney transplantation. A negative pretransplant crossmatch has been considered a requirement in the past.[4] More recent UNOS data indicates that a negative crossmatch is not an absolute necessity.[22] Under some circumstances transplantation may occur in spite of a positive crossmatch, for example, if the risk associated with a positive crossmatch is smaller than the risk of staying on dialysis. The crossmatch must be performed using a technique that is more sensitive than the original CDC. If a serologic assay is used, the sensitivity of the CDC must be increased, for example, by adding AHG. Increasingly, flow cytometry crossmatch has become the method of choice.

Classic post-transplant monitoring includes tests that evaluate kidney function and morphology. Staining for CD4, which is a fragment of complement, identifies antibody-mediated damage to the kidney.[23] All of these tests indicate that the transplanted kidney has already been damaged.

Immunologic monitoring has not yet become a routine part of post-transplant monitoring protocols, but is performed upon request.[24] Various immunologic monitoring techniques have been used in kidney transplantation. For example, distinct microarray images for both biopsies and peripheral blood lymphocytes in cases of acute rejection, chronic rejection, acute dysfunction without rejection, and well-functioning kidney transplants have been characterized.[15]

Other Solid Organ Transplants

Preoperative HLA matching and crossmatching may be of value in other transplants. However, it is not performed often because of the limited deceased donor pool, relative unavailability of living donors, and critical timing to reduce cold ischemia effects in organs from deceased donors.

Transplant protocols vary among centers. Some transplant facilities may perform testing, including crossmatch, after the solid organ transplant surgery is completed. In PRA-negative recipients, a virtual crossmatch based on recipient antibody identity and donor corresponding antigen type may be used instead of a serological crossmatch. Pretransplant antibody status of the recipient is often determined because it can help in evaluating the significance of positive post-transplant antibody screens. Microarray technology has been used to distinguish biopsy-defined rejection from quiescence, or no rejection, in heart transplant recipients.[16]

NONTRANSPLANT-SPECIFIC TESTING PROTOCOLS

HLA typing is used for nontransplant purposes such as:

- Platelet matching for patients who are refractory (Chapter 16)
- Investigation of febrile and TRALI reactions (Chapter 12)
- Diagnosis of certain autoimmune diseases that show correlations with specific HLA types
- Paternity testing (Chapter 19)
- Forensic investigations

Review of the Main Points

- The primary use of HLA typing is to match potential transplant donors and recipients; however, the value of partial matching is a subject of debate.
- Human leukocyte antigen (HLA) class I and class II molecules are critical components in the adaptive immune system.
- Class I molecules consist of a transmembrane α glycoprotein heavy chain and a β-2 microglobulin light chain.
- The peptide-binding cleft of class I molecules is formed by the α1 and α2 domains.
- Class II molecules consist of two transmembrane chains: α and β.
- The peptide-binding cleft of class II molecules is formed by the α1 and β1 domains.
- The genes producing HLA are part of the major histocompatibility complex (MHC).
- MHC genes are inherited as haplotypes.
- In humans, MHC genes are located on chromosome 6.
- The HLA-A, HLA-B, and HLA-C genes are located in the class I region of the HLA system.
- The products of the genes located in the class II region of the HLA system combine to form four molecules: two HLA-DR, one HLA-DQ, and one HLA-DP.
- The HLA system is polymorphic, which means that there are multiple alleles for each HLA gene in humans, and polygenic, which means that there are multiple but similar gene products produced in any one individual.

- HLA type is usually reported based on DNA typing. A new allele naming convention was adopted as of 2010. The allele name starts with the allele (A, B, C, DRA, DRB, DQA, DQB, DPA, or DPB), followed by an asterisk, then two numbers that represent the allele family, which correlates to the serological specificity. If the DNA is sequenced to a higher resolution, up to three more pairs of numbers separated by colons may follow. The next number pair is assigned in chronological order of the allele's discovery, the third number pair differentiates silent mutations, and the last number pair differentiates alleles with DNA differences in areas of the gene that do not affect the amino acid sequence of the translated protein.
- Some antibodies used in serologic antigen-typing methods can cross-react with more than one HLA, resulting in cross-reactive groups (CREGs).
- HLA typing is performed using serologic techniques such as complement-based microlymphocytotoxicity (CDC) or DNA-based techniques such as reverse single-stranded oligonucleotide (SSO) probe hybridization, sequence-specific primer (SSP) typing, and sequence-based typing (SBT).
- HLA crossmatches are performed using CDC methodology or flow cytometry.
- Techniques that have been used to perform HLA antibody screens include complement-based microlymphocytotoxicity (CDC) methodology or solid-phase techniques such as enzyme-linked immunoassay (ELISA), flow cytometry, and Luminex®-based assays.

- Antibody screen results can be reported as percent of panel cells reacting, which is called a panel reactive antibody (PRA) level.
- Post-transplant monitoring traditionally uses tests that detect injury to the graft or host.
- Increasingly, immunologic monitoring is being added to post-transplant testing to detect immune system activation before graft or host injury occurs.
- Immunologic monitoring includes tests to detect signal transduction, DNA synthesis, gene activation, cytokine production, or antibody production.
- The importance of matching in terms of HLA testing varies with different types of transplants.
- Donors and recipients for hematopoietic progenitor cell (HPC) transplants are matched at 10 alleles using high-resolution DNA-typing techniques.
- Pretransplant HLA antibody screens are done periodically on the serum of patients awaiting kidney transplantation.
- Donors and recipients for kidney transplant are matched at six or eight alleles using serologic or low-resolution DNA-typing techniques. A crossmatch is also performed pretransplant.
- HLA typing is used mainly to match potential transplant donors and recipients.
- Other uses for HLA typing include platelet matching, investigation of transfusion reactions, diagnosis of certain autoimmune diseases, paternity testing, and forensic investigation.

Review Questions

1. Which term accurately describes the rapid increase in antibody production that occurs when a previously encountered antigen is reintroduced? (Objective #1)

   A. Transfusion

   B. Anamnestic

   C. Innate

   D. Foreign

2. Select the antigen-presenting cells that are involved in adaptive immunity: (Objective #1)

   A. Macrophages

   B. Dendritic cells

   C. T lymphocytes

   D. Neutrophils

3. What types of molecules make up the major histocompatibility complex (MHC)? (Objective #2)

   A. HLA class I

   B. HLA class II

   C. HLA class III

   D. HLA class IV

4. The HLA domain with the highest degree of polymorphism is: (Objective #3)

   A. HLA class I

   B. HLA class IIα1

   C. HLA class IIβ1

   D. HLA class III

5. Choose the appropriate designation for class II region molecules. (Objective #5)

   A. HLA-A, HLA-B, HLA-C

   B. HLA-DP, HLA-DQ, HLA-DR

   C. HLA-F, HLA-G

   D. MIC-C, MIC-D, MIC-E

6. How many HLA genes are typically expressed in humans? (Objective #5)

   A. 3

   B. 4

   C. 5

   D. 6

7. HLA antibodies that are specific for an epitope found on two or more antigens are designated as: (Objective #7)

   A. Polymorphic

   B. Polygenic

   C. Cross-reactive

   D. Mutagenic

8. Assign the correct order of the number sets in accordance with the 2010 HLA gene-naming convention criteria. (Objective #7)

   _____ Silent mutation

   _____ Allele family

   _____ Noncoding, intron areas

   _____ Order of allele discovery

9. When only one HLA allele is identified at a particular locus in a commercial HLA-typing procedure, the other allele is designated as: (Objective #9)

   A. Amorph

   B. Silent

   C. Blank

   D. Mutagene

10. Which of the following is *not* a DNA-typing method for HLA antigen identification? (Objective #9)

    A. Sequence-specific oligonucleotide

    B. Microlymphocytotoxicity

    C. Sequence-specific primer

    D. Sequence-based typing

11. Select the HLA typing method that determines the nucleotide sequence of an entire exon, including the regions that are usually constant: (Objective #9)

    A. Sequence-based typing

    B. Sequence-specific primer

    C. Microlymphotoxicity

    D. Sequence-specific oligonucleotide

12. What is the interpretation of a microlymphocytotoxicity crossmatching test if lysis of donor lymphocyte occurs at the end of the procedure? (Objective #9)

    A. HLA antibody is present.

    B. HLA antibody is not present.

    C. The test is invalid.

    D. None of the above.

13. Which substance, when produced post transplant, is a predictor of acute or chronic rejection? (Objective #10)

    A. HLA antigen

    B. RBC antibody

    C. Cytokine

    D. Albumin

14. Which of the following consequences can occur as a result of an HLA mismatch in a human progenitor cell (HPC) transplant? (Objective #10)

    A. GVHD

    B. Wiskott-Aldrich syndrome

    C. CMV

    D. HTLV

15. A positive HLA antibody screen test result is typically reported as: (Objective #9)

    A. Panagglutinin

    B. Incompatible

    C. Titration level

    D. Percentage of cells reactive

References

1. Snell G, Stimpfling J. Genetics of tissue transplantation. In: Green E, ed. *Biology of the Laboratory Mouse*. New York: McGraw Hill; 1966; 457–92.

2. Hahn AB, Rodey GE, eds. *ASHI: The First 25 Years*. New York: American Society for Histocompatibility and Immunogenetics; 1999.

3. Terasaki PI, ed. *History of HLA: Ten Recollections*. Los Angeles: UCLA Tissue Typing Laboratory; 1990.

4. Terasaki PI, ed. *History of Transplantation: Thirty-Five Recollections*. Los Angeles: UCLA Tissue Typing Laboratory; 1991.

5. Cecka MJ, Terasaki PI. Worldwide Transplant Center Directory, Kidney Pancreas Transplant. In: Cecka MJ, Terasaki PI, eds. *Clinical Transplants, 2007*. Los Angeles: UCLA Immunogenetics Center; 2008. pp. 397–555.

6. Marsh GE, Parham P, Barber LD. *The HLA FactsBook*. San Diego (CA): Academic Press; 2000.

7. Robinson J, Mistry K, McWilliam H, Lopez R, Parham P, Marsh SGE. The IMGT/HLA database. *Nucleic Acids Research* 2011; 39(suppl 1): D1171-6HLA in Informatics Group in HLA antigens [Internet]. London: Anthony Nolan Research Institute. [updated 2011 Dec 05; cited 2012 Sept 20]. Available from: http://hla.alleles.org

8. Marsh SGE, Albert ED, Bodmer WF, Bontrop RE, Dupont B, Erlich HA, Fernández-Vina M, Geraghty DE, Holdsworth R, Hurley DK, Lau M, Lee KW, Mach B, Mayr WR, Maiers M, Müller CR, Parham P, Petersdorf EW, Sasazuki T, Strominger JL, Svejgaard A, Terasaki PI, Tiercy JM, Trowsdale J. Nomenclature for factors of the HLA system, 2010. *Tissue Antigens* 2010; 75: 291–455 in HLA Informatics Group. Nomenclature for factors of the HLA system [Internet]. London: Anthony Nolan Research Institute. [updated 2012 Aug 02; cited 2012 Sept 20]. Available from: http://hla.alleles.org

9. Wade JA, Hurley CK, Takemoto SK, Thompson J, Davies SM, Fuller TC, Rodey G, Conter DL, Noreen H, Haagenson M, Kan F, Klein J, Eapen M, Spellman S, Kollman C. HLA mismatching within or outside of cross-reactive groups (CREGs) is associated with similar outcomes after unrelated hematopoietic stem cell transplantation. *Blood* 2007; 109(9): 6064–70.

10. Garovoy MR, Rheischmidt, Bigos M, Perkins H, Colombe BN, Salvatierra O. Flow cytometry analysis: a high technology crossmatch technique facilitating transplantation. *Transplant Proc* 1983; 15: 1939–44.

11. Kerman RH, Susskind B, Ruth J, Katz S, van Buren CT, Kahan BD. Can an immunologically, nonreactive potential allograft recipient undergo

transplantation without a donor-specific crossmatch? *Transplantation* 1998; 66(12): 1833–4.

12. Kerman R, Lappin J, Kahan B, Katz S, McKissick E, Hosek K, Acorda N, Wooley N, Hoover A, Miller K, Rodriguez L, Moore B, Melcher P, Biedermann B, Van Buren C. The crossmatch test may still be the most clinically relevant histocompatibility test performed. *Clin Transpl* 2007: 227–9.

13. Vaidya S, Partlow D, Susskind B, Noor M, Barnes T, Gugliuzza K. Prediction of crossmatch outcome of highly sensitized patients by single and/or multiple antigen bead luminex assay. *Transplantation* 2006: 82(11): 1524–8.

14. Kowalski RJ, Post DR, Mannon RB, Sebastian A, Wright HI, Sigle G, Burdick J, Elmagd KA, Zeevi A, Lopez-Cepero M, Daller JA, Gritsch HA, Reed EF, Jonsson J, Hawkins D, Britz JA. Assessing relative risks of infection and rejection: A meta-analysis using an immune function assay. *Transplantation* 2006; 15; 82(5): 663–8.

15. Flechner SM, Kurian SM, Head SR, Sharp SM, Whisenant TC, Zhang J, Chismar JD, Horath S, Mondala T, Gilmartin T, Cook DJ, Kay SA, Walker JR, Salomon DR. Kidney transplant rejection and tissue injury by gene profiling of biopsies and peripheral blood lymphocytes. *Am J Transplant* 2004; 4(9): 1475–89.

16. Deng MC, Eisen HJ, Mehra MR. Methodological challenges of genomic research—The CARGO study. *Am J Transplant* 2006; 6(5 Pt 1): 1086–7.

17. Miyahira Y, Murata K, Rodriguez D, Rodriguez JR, Esteban M, Rodrigues MM, Zavala F. Quantification of antigen specific CD8+ T cells using an ELISPOT assay. *J Immunol Methods* 1995; 181(1): 45–54.

18. Pelzl S, Opelz G, Wiesel M, Schnülle P, Schönemann C, Süsal C. Soluble CD30 as a predictor of kidney graft outcome. *Transplantation* 2002; 73(1): 3–6.

19. Book BK, Agarwal A, Milgrom AB, Bearden CM, Sidner RA, Higgins NG, Pescovitz MD. New crossmatch technique eliminates interference by humanized and chimeric monoclonal antibodies. *Transplant Proc* 2005; 37(2): 640–642.

20. Pasquini MC, Wang Z. Current use and outcome of hematopoietic stem cell transplantation: CIBMTR Summary Slides, 2011. Reference center [Internet]. Minnesota (USA): Center for international blood and marrow transplant research. [updated 2010 Nov 01; cited 2012 Oct 05]. Available from: http://www.cibmtr.org

21. Leclair B, Fregeau CJ, Aye MT, Fourney RM. DNA typing for bone marrow engraftment follow-up after allogeneic transplant: a comparative study of current technologies. *Bone Marrow Transplant* 1995; 16: 43–55.

22. Salvalaggio PR, Graff RJ, Pinsky B, Schnitzler MA, Takemoto SK, Burroughs TE, Santos LS, Lentine KL. Crossmatch testing in kidney transplantation: patterns of practice and associations with rejection and graft survival. *Saudi J Kidney Dis Transpl* 2009; 20(4): 577–89.

23. Worthington JE, McEwen A, McWilliams LJ, Picton ML, Martin S. Association between C4D staining in renal transplantation biopsies, production of donor-specific HLA antibodies and graft outcome. *Transplantation* 2007; 83(4): 398–403.

24. Norin AJ, Glenn K, Bow L, Pancoska C, Eckels D. Review of post-transplant immune monitoring survey. *ASHI Quarterly* 2006; 30: 110–2.

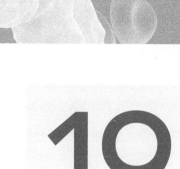

19

Methods in Parentage Testing

ROBERT W. ALLEN

Chapter Objectives

Upon completion of this chapter, the student will be able to:

1. State the role of the blood bank in early parentage testing.
2. Discuss the process of using blood groups for exclusion in early parentage testing.
3. List the blood groups that were used for early parentage testing.
4. Identify two legislative acts that assisted with disputed parentage in the early 1900s.
5. Discuss the role of human leukocyte antigen (HLA) testing and its importance in calculating both exclusion and probability of paternity.
6. Describe the molecular methods that have been developed for DNA profiling.
7. State the advantages of using DNA profiling in parentage testing.
8. Describe the short tandem repeat (STR) procedure that is used to identify genetic markers.
9. Define the likelihood ratio (parentage index).
10. Distinguish the H0 and H1 counterhypotheses with respect to how they are used to estimate probability of an alleged parent.
11. Describe the principles of the probability of parentage and the probability of exclusion.
13. Name the formula that is used to predict the frequency of homozygous and heterozygous phenotypes in the population.
14. Discuss the Bayes' theorem, including its application in parentage testing.

Key Terms

Conditional probability
Discriminatory power
Likelihood ratio (LR)
Parentage index
Parentage testing

Paternity testing
Posterior probability
Prior probability
Probability of exclusion (PEx)

CASE IN POINT

TN is a 23-year-old woman with a 6-month-old baby. The baby has two possible fathers due to circumstances that took place at the time the baby was conceived. TN has asked both alleged fathers to participate in paternity (parentage) testing to determine the identity of the biological father.

What's Ahead?

The purpose of this chapter is to introduce the reader to the fascinating topic of **parentage testing**, which is testing on the mother, child, and alleged father to determine the probability that the alleged father is the biological parent of the tested child, by addressing the following questions:

- What historical occurrence contributed to the eventual development of parentage testing?
- What is the significance of red blood cell antigens, legislation, human leukocyte antigens, standards, and accreditation in the field of parentage testing?
- What two technological advances have had a dramatic impact on the field of parentage testing?
- What are the key aspects in the production, interpretation, and analysis of STR-DNA profile testing?

INTRODUCTION TO PARENTAGE TESTING

There are five aspects, described in the following sections, associated with parentage testing, that in combination provide a framework of this important field of immunohematology: early history, red blood cell antigens, legislation, human leukocyte antigens, and standards and accreditation.

Early History

The first documented case of disputed parentage can be found in the Old Testament in I Kings, Chapter 3, verses 16–27 in the story of King Solomon. Two women in a household gave birth to children at about the same time and one child died. The mother of the child who died switched her dead child for the living child while its mother slept and then claimed the living child as her own. While judging this case, Solomon ordered the living child to be cleaved in half and each mother to be given one half of the child. The true mother, hearing the King's ruling, begged the King to rule the thieving mother to be the child's true parent, thereby sparing the child's life. Solomon accepted the woman's plea but ruled she was the child's true mother and ordered the thief to be put to death.

Parentage testing has changed significantly since the 10th century B.C. Judges do not order children to be halved or alleged parents to be punished. Moreover, decisions regarding the true parentage of a child incorporate the results of genetic marker testing considered within the framework of Mendel's laws in deciding who is and who is not the true (biological) parent of a child.

Red Blood Cell Antigens

The field of parentage testing began in the 1950s and 1960s with the analysis of red blood cell antigens. The most common type of parentage testing designed to determine the biological father of a child is referred to as **paternity testing**. Red blood cell antigens were chosen as paternity markers based on whether their inheritance patterns were well characterized, there were readily available serological reagents, and whether the testing could be routinely performed in blood banks. Testing during this period was principally done for clients in the private sector when paternity was in dispute and an enlightened judge was aware of the value of genetic testing to help resolve the issue. However, because of the rather weak discriminatory power associated with red blood cell antigens of the ABO, MN, and Rh systems, paternity tests could only realistically exclude a man who was falsely accused in about half of the cases. In addition, for a man who could not be excluded, the chance he was not the father and just coincidentally had the same blood type as the child was high. Thus blood typing had as its goal the exclusion of an alleged father, who was falsely accused, but occasionally at this time, the test results were ignored and the decision regarding paternity was made on other grounds. Such was the case in the high-profile paternity suit brought by Joan Barry against Charlie Chaplin in 1943. ABO blood grouping excluded Charlie Chaplin as the father of the child. However, the California courts did not recognize blood-typing results in matters of disputed parentage at that time and accordingly, ordered him to pay child support in spite of the blood test results.[1]

☑ CHECKPOINT 19-1

What paternity markers were used for parentage testing as early as the 1950s?

Legislation

The use of genetic testing in disputed parentage became more widespread during the 1960s, along with the dramatic rise in children born out of wedlock during this 10-year period.[2] In the United States, the Aid to Families with Dependent Children (AFDC) legislation (passed in the 1930s) was originally intended to provide widows from the recent world war with additional income to support their dependent children.[3] However, the dramatic rise in the 1970s of single-parent families taxed the AFDC funding with additional, unanticipated demand. This social and funding crisis led to the enactment of the Child Support Enforcement Act by the U.S. Congress in 1974, with the goal of reducing welfare costs by collecting from delinquent parents and included funding for genetic testing in disputed paternity cases as necessary.[3]

Human Leukocyte Antigens

Paralleling these social and legislative developments surrounding disputed parentage was the discovery of the human leukocyte antigen (HLA) system (Chapter 18) and the development of reagents for routine typing using peripheral blood. For the first time, it was possible to exclude a high proportion of falsely accused men (~98%) and even to calculate the probability of paternity for men who could not be excluded. As the use of parentage testing by child-support agencies increased, standardization of sample collection, testing procedures, and result interpretation became more important. The need for standardization was formally recognized by several organizations including the American Medical Association (AMA), American Bar Association (ABA), and American Association of Blood Banks (AABB). In 1978, the AABB formed the Committee on Parentage Testing charged with developing an accreditation program. A survey of known parentage testing laboratories in 1978 revealed a total annual case volume of approximately 11,000 cases processed by 259 laboratories.[4] By 2004, the number of cases of disputed parentage testing had increased to over 390,928 being processed by only 38 laboratories.[5]

☑ CHECKPOINT 19-2

How did the process of parentage testing become standardized?

CASE IN POINT (continued)

There are several laboratories in the state that TN could use for the parentage testing.

1. What type of assurance that standards are being followed can TN look for when choosing a parentage testing laboratory?
2. Name one set of standards that are likely used by the testing laboratories?
3. How often are these standards revised?

Standards and Accreditation

In 1982, a meeting of experts in the field was jointly sponsored by the AMA, the ABA, and the AABB with a grant from the Department of Health and Human Services. The overall goal of this meeting, known as the Arlie conference due to the meeting site, was to standardize the calculations used in parentage testing and the interpretation and communication of the results. To that end, a monograph was published containing the meeting contents as well as casework examples and the consensus opinion from the experts for the correct method of calculating exclusion and inclusion probabilities in paternity cases.[6]

Recommendations for standardization were published in 1983 by the Parentage Testing Committee of the AABB.[4] A year later, many of the recommendations became mandatory standards for laboratories seeking accreditation. Since 1984, the Standards for Parentage Testing Laboratories, published by the AABB, have been updated on a 2-year cycle. More recent editions have been named the Standards for Relationship Testing Laboratories.

CASE IN POINT (continued)

TN chooses a testing laboratory and notifies the alleged fathers. She obtains specimen collection kits for herself and her baby.

4. What type of sample is likely to be collected from TN, her baby, and the alleged fathers?
5. What is the primary methodology the laboratory is likely to use in testing the samples?

TECHNICAL CONSIDERATIONS

Two technological advances have occurred that have had a dramatic impact on the field of parentage testing. The first was HLA testing, which was principally responsible for the evolution of the statistical calculations associated with testing. Previously the exclusion of parentage was the primary focus, but now, with the mathematical emphasis, the probability of paternity could be calculated.

The second major advance came in the mid-1980s with the discovery of hypervariable DNA polymorphisms that could be revealed using restriction fragment-length polymorphism (RFLP) mapping or polymerase chain reaction (PCR) amplification, using tiny amounts of DNA to generate millions of copies. RFLP analysis refers to the digesting of a DNA sample by restriction enzymes into fragments that are different lengths in different individuals depending on the location of the specific short sequence of DNA digested by the enzymes. The RFLP analysis has largely been replaced by other methodologies, but was the first widely used DNA technique in parentage testing.

Variable-number tandem repeat (VNTR) loci was the next major advance in DNA testing and makes use of the repeating of specific sequences at specific locations in the genome. The number of repeats of each of these sequences differs between individuals and exhibits levels of polymorphism comparable to the HLA system. One advantage over HLA testing is that the type of acceptable samples is broader. No longer is freshly procured blood with viable cells an absolute must for testing as required for HLA typing. Every nucleated cell in the body contains DNA and the DNA contained within each cell is reasonably stable, allowing blood stains, tissue samples, and even buccal (cheek) swabs to be used as a source of material for testing. Figure 19-1 ■ illustrates two simple examples of a VNTR analysis. Short tandem repeat (STR) loci, which became the next focus for DNA-based parentage testing, are repeated sequences from 2 to 16 base pairs that are typically in the noncoding intron region of genes. Several thousand STRs are known in the human genome.

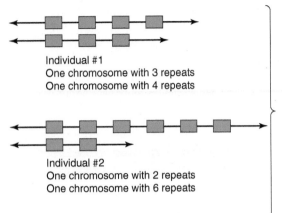

1. Digest DNA with restriction enzyme cutting outside the VNTR, or, amplify using primers that bind outside VNTR.

2. Electrophorese DNA fragments using size separation medium (e.g., agarose or acrylamide gels).

3. Visualize specific VNTR alleles. Size is proportional to the number of repeats.

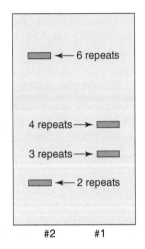

■ FIGURE 19-1   Variable-Number Tandem Repeat (VNTR) Analysis

This is a simplified schematic of polymorphisms at a single VNTR locus in two heterozygous individuals (#1 and #2). The three main steps in the analysis are digestion with restriction enzymes (or alternately amplification with primers), separation of the fragments (or amplified VNTR loci), and visualization of the alleles. Each fragment size is proportional to the number of repeats within the VNTR tandem array.

In 1992, DNA-typing procedures were incorporated into parentage testing standards.[7] Later that year the first laboratories were accredited for this technology. RFLP analysis for DNA typing was the first technology covered by parentage testing accreditation standards.[7] Soon after standards were developed to cover analysis of STR loci amplified using PCR.[4] STR typing avoids some of the issues seen with other techniques such as allele designation, population frequencies, use of toxic chemicals, and sample requirements without sacrificing discriminatory power. In 1995, approximately equal numbers of laboratories used RFLP and STR typing for parentage testing[8] and by 2002, 90% of laboratories reported using STR typing as their principal technology.[9]

☑ CHECKPOINT 19-3

What is a short tandem repeat (STR)?

STR-DNA Profiles

Since STR typing is considered the primary methodology for parentage testing, an in-depth discussion of STR-DNA profiles follow. The aspects associated with this testing are presented in two broad categories: (1) production and interpretation and (2) analysis.

Production and Interpretation

Once DNA has been extracted and quantified, the production of an STR profile is rather straightforward. Multiplex kits are available from several suppliers that contain all the components needed to produce a highly discriminatory DNA profile from about a nanogram of input DNA. Primers included with such kits are often chemically linked to fluorescent dyes. STR products amplified from a template are separated by electrophoresis and then visualized through fluorescence, which eliminates the need for radioactivity that was used in early methods.

Early during the evolution of STR technology, different laboratories used various different loci for testing.[10] Standardization within the identity testing community occurred primarily because the U.S. Federal Bureau of Investigation (FBI) took a lead in defining 13 STR systems that it called the *core loci*.[11] These 13 core loci, which represent an extremely powerful collection of genetic markers for use in identification, have become the standard test battery for most crime laboratories and for many parentage testing laboratories as well.

The inherent **discriminatory power** associated with a genetic marker reflects its ability to discriminate two samples coming from different sources. This capability is proportional to both the number of alleles exhibited by that marker in the population as well as the degree to which those alleles are evenly distributed in terms of their frequency. Thus, a genetic marker with two alleles, one of which exhibits a population frequency of 80%, will not be as effective or as powerful as another marker with two alleles, each with a 50% frequency in the population. This logic extends to markers with numerous alleles as well. The 13 core loci exhibit an average random-match probability of about 1 in a trillion.[12] Table 19-1 ✶ lists the individual STR loci that are in widespread use for identity testing, including those that comprise the 13 core systems. In addition, the random-match probabilities and exclusion probabilities are shown for each locus and for the multiplex kit as a whole.

Once STR loci have been amplified, electrophoresis is used to separate alleles by size. The size, combined with the color of light emitted by a fluorescent amplicon when irradiated by laser light, allows for identification of the STR allele. Currently, two electrophoretic platforms are used among identity testing laboratories: polyacrylamide gel electrophoresis and capillary electrophoresis. Each platform has advantages and disadvantages, but both use lasers to excite the fluorescent dyes incorporated into STR alleles and a charge-coupled device (CCD) camera to capture their fluorescent emissions. In addition, some platforms perform allele detection in real-time fashion; the laser is fixed and continuously illuminates a detection area in the

✶ TABLE 19-1 Commonly Used Short Tandem Repeat Loci

Locus*	Chromosome	Discriminatory Power**	
		Probability of Identity***	Probability of Exclusion****
CSF1PO	5	0.119	0.475
D2S1338	2	0.033	0.636
D3S1358	3	0.111	0.557
D5S818	5	0.119	0.518
D7S820	7	0.078	0.560
D8S1179	8	0.083	0.615
D13S317	13	0.081	0.470
D16S539	16	0.087	0.553
D18S51	18	0.035	0.647
D19S433	19	0.056	0.543
D21S11	21	0.051	0.608
FGA	4	0.033	0.644
THO1	11	0.105	0.581
TPOX	2	0.151	0.482
VWA	12	0.079	0.604
Cumulative values		$\sim 2 \times 10^{-18}$	>99.99%

*The 13 core loci are shown in **bold** type.

**Numbers shown represent averages across the major population groups: European, African, Hispanic, and Native American. The 15 STR loci shown are all co-amplified along with the amelogenin locus when using the AmpFISTR Identifiler® multiplex DNA typing kit (Applied Biosystems, Foster City, CA).

***The chance two samples selected at random from the population would exhibit the same phenotype.

****The chance of excluding a randomly selected individual as the parent of a child, when the known parent is also tested.

slab gel or capillary. Fluorescent data is collected as STR products move past. Other systems scan the entire gel or capillary after the electrophoresis is complete. In either case, the ultimate product is a DNA profile consisting of alleles portrayed to an analyst either as a banding pattern or as a histogram, as seen in Figure 19-2 ■.

Identification of alleles in the profile is accomplished by comparison of unknown alleles against a reference ladder of several known, common allelic variants for each STR locus, which are supplied with the multiplex kits. Thus, the size and fluorescent emission of an unknown allele will generally match to within 0.25–0.5 base pairs of an allele in the reference ladder whose identity is known. Computer software on the genetic analyzers determines the size of the unknown STR using the internal size standards co-electrophoresed with each sample in conjunction with size-estimation algorithms.[13] Other software applications estimate the size in number of base pairs of DNA fragments labeled with fluorescent dyes, as shown in Figure 19-3 ■.[14] Another software program then imports the size estimates for unknowns, matches them against known allele sizes, and displays the STR allele in a profile as the number of tandem repeats it contains, as shown in Figure 19-4 ■, p. 364.[15]

☑ CHECKPOINT 19-4

What are the 13 core loci?

Analysis

One of the most commonly encountered scenarios in parentage testing involves a trio of individuals: the child, a known parent of the child, and an alleged parent. Generally, the parent in question is the father (paternity) and the testing will be initiated by the mother, the state, or both to compel the father to help provide for the child.

CASE IN POINT (continued)

The laboratory receives the specimens from TN, her baby, and the two alleged fathers. The specimens are tested and the results analyzed.

6. What are two statistical terms that can be used to report parentage testing results?
7. What prior probability is the laboratory likely to use in analyzing the results in this case and why?
8. Prior probability is part of what statistical logic?

Likelihood Ratio

The scenario introduced in the previous section is the easiest type to analyze statistically because the collection of genetic markers from each member of the trio are known and can be compared directly. Mendel's laws of genetics require one-half of the alleles in the child's

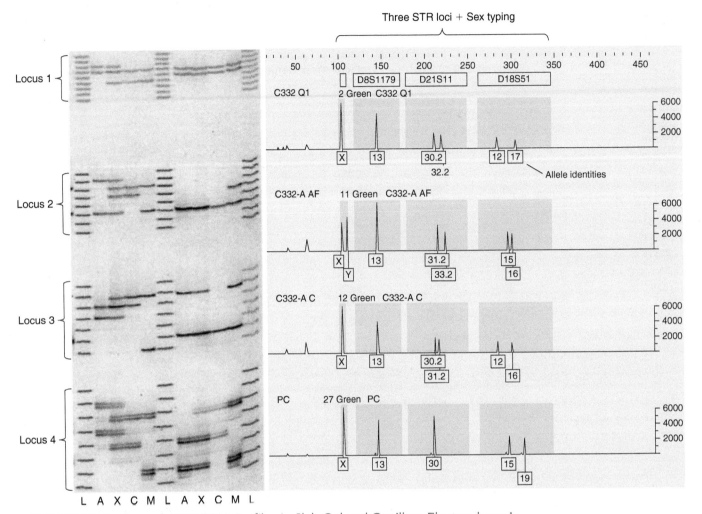

FIGURE 19-2 Example STR-DNA Profiles in Slab Gel and Capillary Electrophoresis

Left panel shows a slab gel electrophoresis. In three positions within the gel, allelic ladders for the four loci shown are added to aid in the manual identification of the alleles in each of the samples in two parentage tests.

    L, lane containing allelic ladder for each locus.
    A, 4 locus profile for the alleged father.
    X, mixed profiles for the alleged father and the child.
    C, 4 locus profile for the child.
    M, 4 locus profile for the mother.

Right panel shows a capillary electrophoresis. Capillary electrophoresis was used in conjunction with automated software to facilitate allele identification for three STR loci labeled with the same green fluorescent dye. Sex-typing products are labeled X and Y and alleles for the three loci are labeled in the boxes under each peak in the electropherogram.

sample to be traceable to each parent, since the child receives half their genes from the mom and half from the dad. Thus, one allele in the child's profile for a given marker must match a marker from the known parent, while the other allele in the child's profile is compared directly with the markers in the alleged parent's DNA. Having one person designated as a "known parent" enables certain assumptions to be used to formulate two hypotheses that will be used to evaluate the possibility that the alleged parent is indeed the parent of the child. This comparison between the child's alleles with the alleged parent's alleles is expressed as a **likelihood ratio (LR)**, which indicates to the court or other interested persons how strongly the evidence either supports or contradicts the hypothesis that the alleged parent is the

true parent of the child. The LR is typically referred to as the **parentage index**. However, the term *likelihood ratio* will be used predominantly here since it applies to the various relatedness scenarios possible. Phrases like *paternity index*, *maternity index*, and *sibling index* are all just more specific terms that describe the nature of the relationship of the likelihood ratio being calculated in each situation.

Consider the STR test results for four genetic loci shown in Table 19-2 ✶, p. 365.

The sharing of one or more alleles between each member of the trio is easily confirmed by looking at the table. Overall, one can see the alleged parent shares at least one allele from each marker with the child and, more importantly, the allele shared is one of the possible

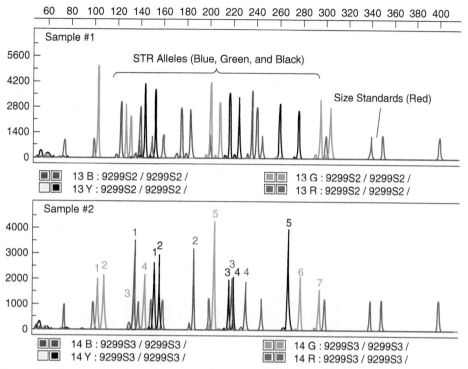

■ FIGURE 19-3   Example Electropherograms of Fluorescently Labeled STR-DNA

Fluorescently labeled short tandem repeat (STR-DNA) alleles were separated by capillary electrophoresis. Shown is the fluorescent data captured by the charge-coupled device camera during electrophoresis of STR alleles produced from two samples of chromosomal DNA. Included with each sample is a collection of size standards shown in red, upon which size estimates for each unknown PCR product are made by the GeneScan® software. The unknown PCR products found in the samples appear as green, blue, and black peaks. The top x-axis shows the base-pair lengths of the product peaks. The y-axis shows the peak heights of the products in relative fluorescent units (rfu).

obligate alleles (i.e., the allele not from the known parent, which therefore must be from the unknown parent) for each locus. For example, at the D3S1358 locus, the known parent shares allele 18 with the child. Based on our assumption that the known parent is a true parent, allele 18 was inherited from the known parent, which defines allele 15 as the one inherited from the parent whose identity we wish to establish. The alleged parent happens to have an allele 15 in his or her profile and therefore is included among the pool of possible parents in the population who also have allele 15 in their profiles.

In assigning weight to the match for allele 15 between alleged parent and child, two hypotheses are compared and represented numerically in the LR. One hypothesis, called H0, estimates the likelihood or probability of the alleged parent–child–known parent trio, if the alleged parent is the true parent of the child; in other words, the chance of producing a child who looks like this child at the D3S1358 locus through a mating of the alleged parent and the known parent. H0 is determined by this formula: the chance of the known parent passing on the allele to the child X the chance of the alleged parent passing on the allele to the child. In this case, since the known parent is heterozygous, the chance of passing an 18 to a child is 50% or 0.5. Likewise, since the alleged parent is heterozygous, the chance of passing a 15 to a child is also 0.5. Therefore,

$$H0 = (0.50)(0.50) = 0.25$$

Thus, a mating between the alleged parent and the known parent will produce a 15, 18 child 25% of the time.

The counterhypothesis, called H1, predicts the likelihood of the results in the alleged parent–child–known parent trio if the alleged parent is not the true parent of the child. The calculation for determining H1 incorporates the allele population frequency and consists of the probability of the known parent passing on the allele to the child X the probability of a an untested, unknown individual in the population passing on the allele to the child. In other words, the probability of producing a child who looks genetically like this child through a mating of the known parent with an unknown, untested individual in the population, who is random, is of the same ethnic background as the alleged parent, and is unrelated to the known parent. This individual must have allele 15 and therefore his or her existence and probability of transmitting allele 15 to the child is defined by the population frequency of allele 15. If allele 15 has a frequency of 0.246 or is present in 24.6% of randomly selected individuals, then

$$H1 = (0.50)(0.246) = 0.123$$

This means that a mating between the known parent and a random individual will produce a child like the one whose parentage is in question 12.3% of the time.

The likelihood ratio for the D3S1358 test result thus becomes a mathematical comparison of the probabilities of the two hypotheses: H0 and H1. In this case,

$$H0 = (0.50) \times (0.50) = 0.25 \text{ (each parent has a 50\%}$$
probability of passing the allele on to the child)

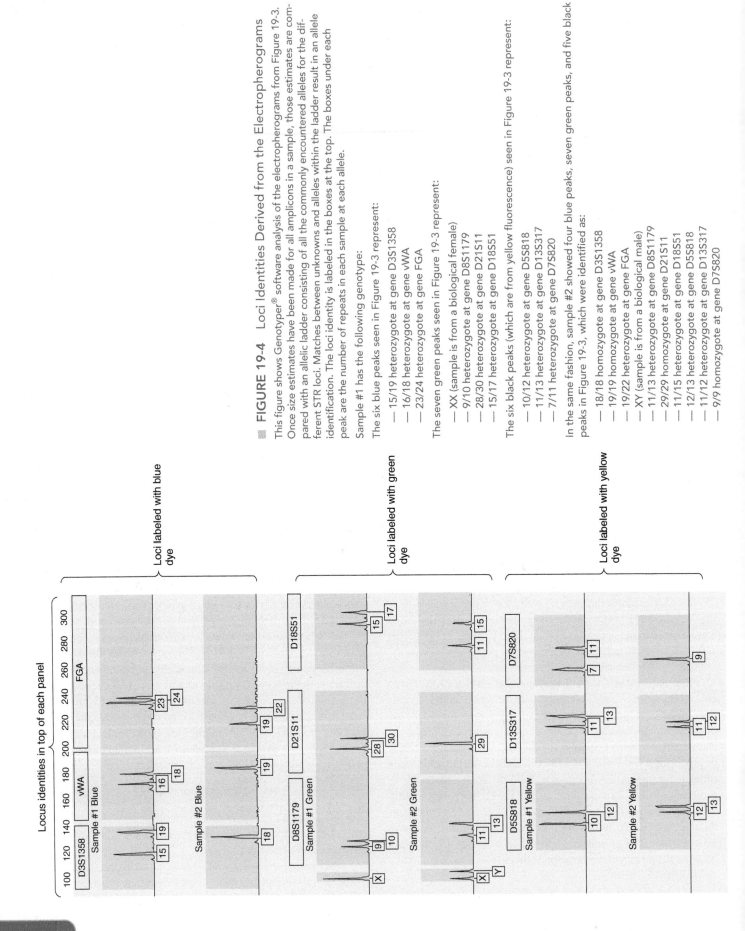

Locus identities in top of each panel

Loci labeled with blue dye

Loci labeled with green dye

Loci labeled with yellow dye

■ **FIGURE 19-4** Loci Identities Derived from the Electropherograms

This figure shows Genotyper® software analysis of the electropherograms from Figure 19-3. Once size estimates have been made for all amplicons in a sample, those estimates are compared with an allelic ladder consisting of all the commonly encountered alleles for the different STR loci. Matches between unknowns and alleles within the ladder result in an allele identification. The loci identity is labeled in the boxes at the top. The boxes under each peak are the number of repeats in each sample at each allele.

Sample #1 has the following genotype:

The six blue peaks seen in Figure 19-3 represent:

— 15/19 heterozygote at gene D3S1358
— 16/18 heterozygote at gene vWA
— 23/24 heterozygote at gene FGA

The seven green peaks seen in Figure 19-3 represent:

— XX (sample is from a biological female)
— 9/10 heterozygote at gene D8S1179
— 28/30 heterozygote at gene D21S11
— 15/17 heterozygote at gene D18S51

The six black peaks (which are from yellow fluorescence) seen in Figure 19-3 represent:

— 10/12 heterozygote at gene D5S818
— 11/13 heterozygote at gene D13S317
— 7/11 heterozygote at gene D7S820

In the same fashion, sample #2 showed four blue peaks, seven green peaks, and five black peaks in Figure 19-3, which were identified as:

— 18/18 homozygote at gene D3S1358
— 19/19 homozygote at gene vWA
— 19/22 heterozygote at gene FGA
— XY (sample is from a biological male)
— 11/13 heterozygote at gene D8S1179
— 29/29 homozygote at gene D21S11
— 11/15 heterozygote at gene D18S51
— 12/13 heterozygote at gene D5S818
— 11/12 heterozygote at gene D13S317
— 9/9 homozygote at gene D7S820

✳ **TABLE 19-2** Example of STR Testing Results

Marker Locus	Alleged Parent	Child	Known Parent
D3S1358	15, 17	15, 18	18, 19
D21S11	28	28, 32.2	31.2, 32.2
FGA	18, 20	19, 20	19, 20
D8S1179	9, 11	11, 13	13

$H1 = (0.50) \times (0.246) = 0.123$ (there is a 12.3% probability of an untested individual in the population passing on the allele)

Therefore,

$$LR = H0/H1 = 0.25/0.123 = 2.03$$

Given the test result of 2.03 obtained from data regarding the D3S1358 locus, the results are a little over twice as likely that the alleged parent is the true parent of the child versus a random person who is unrelated to the alleged parent and of the same ethnic group. Stated a different way, the probability of producing a 15, 18 child from a mating of the alleged parent with the known parent is favored by a factor of about twofold over the probability of producing the child from a mating of the known parent with a randomly selected individual.

Next, consider the test results for the D21S11 locus. In this case, the known parent shares allele 32.2 with the child, defining allele 28 as the obligate allele for the unknown parent (the second required parental allele). The two hypotheses being compared for the D21S11 locus are identical to those expressed above, but the probability of the alleged parent passing allele 28 is different because he or she is homozygous. Therefore, the chance of passing allele 28 to the child is increased to 1.0; the alleged parent can only pass allele 28 to his or her offspring (due to homozygosity it is the only one available to transmit). If the population frequency of allele 28 is 0.166, the LR calculation thus becomes:

$$LR = H0/H1 = (0.50)(1.0)/(0.50)(0.166) = 6.02$$

Note that the denominator of the equation does not change just because the alleged parent's transmission of allele 28 has increased twofold. The random parent is still represented in the equation by the frequency of the obligate allele in the population. The LR increases by a factor of two for the tested homozygous alleged parent versus one who is heterozygous, reflecting the alleged parent's twofold increased probability of passing the obligate allele.

Consider the results for the FGA locus, which introduces another layer of complexity to the analysis. The known parent and the child are genotypically identical. Because of the identical phenotypes present in both individuals, we don't know which allele, 19 or 20, was passed to the child by the known parent. This ambiguity must be considered in the LR calculation, producing a compound equation consisting of two parts representing the two possible mating scenarios that could produce the child in question. First, if the known parent (KP) transmits allele 20 to the child, which occurs with a 50% frequency, allele 19 becomes the obligate allele. The alleged parent (AP) does not harbor allele 19 in their profile and so the chance he or she will transmit 19 is 0. This of course would be evidence of nonparentage. Second, if the known parent transmits allele 19 to the

child, which occurs with a frequency of 50%, allele 20 becomes the obligate allele. The alleged parent has allele 20 and transmits it with a frequency of 50%. The hypotheses H0 and H1 are the same as before, but their mathematical expression must consider both possible conception schemes. Therefore, assuming allele 19 has a population frequency of 0.056 and allele 20 a frequency of 0.145:

$$H0 = (0.50_{KP\ transmits\ 20})(0_{AP\ transmits\ 19}) + (0.50_{KP\ transmits\ 19})$$
$$(0.50_{AP\ transmits\ 20}) = 0.25$$

and

$$H1 = (0.50_{KP\ transmits\ 20})(0.056_{Random\ 19}) + (0.50_{KP\ transmits\ 19})$$
$$(0.145_{Random\ 20}) = 0.028 + 0.073$$

H1 reflects the possibilities of the known parent mating with random individuals who possess either allele 19 or allele 20. Ultimately, the likelihood ratio takes the form:

$$LR = 0.25/(0.028 + 0.073) = 2.48$$

The reduction in the LR reflects not knowing which allele is inherited by the child from the known parent.

If the alleged parent in this case were also genotypically identical to the child (i.e., 19, 20), he or she could transmit either allele to the child. The mathematical expression of this possibility would be considered in the formula:

$$LR = [(0.50)(0.50) + (0.50)(0.50)]/[(0.50)(0.056)$$
$$+ (0.50)(0.145)] = 0.50/0.1005 = 4.98$$

The LR increases twofold simply because the alleged parent can transmit either potential obligate allele to the child.

Finally, consider the results for the D8S1179 locus. At this locus, the known parent is homozygous for allele 13, making allele 11, which has a population frequency of 0.059, the obligate allele. The alleged parent has that allele and will transmit it 50% of the time. The LR becomes:

$$LR = (1.0)(0.50)/(1.0)(0.059) = 8.48$$

Now that we have calculated the individual likelihood ratios for each genetic locus, we can combine all the data because we are ultimately evaluating whether or not the alleged parent is capable of producing a single sperm or egg capable of transmitting all of the necessary genetic markers to the child. Because each STR locus used is independently inherited, each LR can be multiplied by every other LR to arrive at a combined value. The goal is to achieve a level of certainty regarding parentage that is convincing. Accreditation standards mandate a combined LR of at least 100 as the threshold of certainty that must be achieved, except in special circumstances.[16] In our example, the combined LR (2.03 × 6.02 × 2.49 × 8.48) exceeds the minimum, the cumulative value being over 250.

☑ CHECKPOINT 19-5

What is the significance of the likelihood ratio when it is used in parentage testing?

Probability of Exclusion

Another way to evaluate the test results is the **probability of exclusion (PEx)** for a locus or combination of loci. The PEx provides the analyst with information regarding the discriminatory power of a given test or group of tests. The PEx indicates the proportion of the population who would have been excluded from parentage because they lacked the obligate allele(s). Stated another way, the PEx is the probability the alleged parent would be excluded if they were falsely accused. Our previous discussion was of inclusion, now we shift to exclusion.

To calculate PEx, we must first calculate the proportion of the population who would not be excluded. This depends on the population frequency of the obligate allele(s) identified in the child. The rarer an obligate allele is found in the population, the less chance it will be present among members of the random population. Using the D3S1358 locus example, the obligate allele is 15, which has a population frequency of 0.246. To calculate the proportion of the population harboring allele 15, who could be potential parents of the child, we use the Hardy-Weinberg equation (Chapter 8) to estimate homozygous (p) and heterozygous (q) phenotypes containing allele 15:

$$p^2 + 2pq = (0.246)^2 + 2[(0.246)(1 - 0.246)]$$
$$= (0.061) + (0.371) = 0.432$$

The part of the Hardy-Weinberg equation predicting the frequency of people who are homozygous for allele 15 is 0.246^2. The part of the equation predicting who are heterozygous is $2(0.246)(1 - 0.246)$. The part of the equation that represents the combined frequency of all other alleles except allele 15 at the D3S1358 locus is $1 - 0.246$.

From the equation above we can deduce that 43.2% of the population would be expected to have allele 15 and therefore be included as a possible parent of the child based on an allele frequency of 24.6% and the genotype predictions of the Hardy-Weinberg equation. In an extension of this logic, 100% of people minus those who would not have allele 15 in their profile would be excluded as the parent of this child. In this case the PEx equals 56.8% ($100 - 43.2$), indicating that 56.8% of the population would be expected to be excluded if tested. Of special note is the fact that the PEx value is calculated ignoring the genotype or DNA profile of the alleged parent. The only information needed to calculate PEx is the identity of the obligate gene in the child, deduced by comparing the profiles of the child and the known parent.

☑ CHECKPOINT 19-6

What is the name of the formula that is used to predict the frequency of homozygous and heterozygous phenotypes?

Bayesian Logic

Familiarization with the statistics used in parentage testing requires a discussion of Bayesian statistical logic. In its most simplistic form, Bayes' theorem allows a level of certainty for a given belief or hypothesis, such as relatedness, to be modified either positively or negatively by incorporating new information pertinent to the hypothesis. Three terms are incorporated into the Bayesian formula: **prior probability**, **conditional probability**, and **posterior probability**. When trying to establish relatedness, the level of certainty of a relationship before the genetic testing is performed is the prior probability. The prior probability may include such things as evidence that the alleged and known parent were living together or acknowledged publicly they had a sexual relationship during the period of conception.

Following genetic testing, which represents the conditional probability, the level of certainty of relatedness will be modified downward or upward. Combining the results of prior and conditional probabilities (as reflected by the LR) results in the posterior probability reflect the revised level of certainty regarding the relationship.

The calculation leading to the posterior probability involves creating a ratio comparing the evidence favoring parentage with the probability both for and against parentage. Assume for our discussion that the alleged father convinces a judge that he was not in contact with the mother during the period of conception. The judge could assign a prior probability of 10%, meaning there is a low probability the alleged parent is the true parent of the child based on nongenetic information. If the genetic testing does not exclude the alleged parent and moreover produces a combined LR of 100 (or more), the initial 10% level of certainty will be modified upward. The posterior probability calculation would take the following form:

$$W_{10} = [(0.10_{Prior\ for})(100_{LR})]/[(0.10_{Prior\ for})(100_{LR})$$
$$+ (0.90_{Prior\ against})] = 10/10.9 = 0.917\ or\ 91.7\%$$

The term W_{10} refers to the posterior probability calculated using a prior probability of 10%. A probability of 91.7% reflects the upgraded level of conviction that the alleged parent is the true parent of the child. Typically, however, a report would simply state "the probability of parentage (assuming a 10% prior chance) is 91.7%." Stated in this way, the conclusion appears as fact rather than opinion. It is important to continually remember that the 91.7% value is simply a different way to reveal how committed the laboratory is to their opinion favoring parentage based on the test results considered with other, nongenetic evidence either for or against parentage. The interpretation of parentage testing results is opinion, as evidenced by the fact it is impossible to produce a probability of parentage equal to 100% for an alleged parent, no matter how much inclusionary genetic testing is performed.

Look at what happens to the posterior probability if the judge, knowing the alleged and known parents were together on an island during the period of conception, assigns a prior probability of 90%:

$$W_{90} = (0.90)(100)/[(0.90)(100) + (0.10)] = 90/90.1$$
$$= 0.9989\ or\ 99.89\%$$

Clearly, a much higher level of certainty regarding the parentage of the child is produced under a 90% prior probability for the same LR of 100, but the posterior probability is still less than 100%.

Most relatedness testing laboratories assign a prior probability of 50% unless instructed by the court to do otherwise. The reason for choosing 50% relates primarily to the neutrality of the laboratory. A prior probability of 50% ensures that the posterior probability that appears on the report is based only on the genetic test results and not on any nongenetic information. Using a prior probability of 50% means that nongenetic evidence is given equal weight in supporting

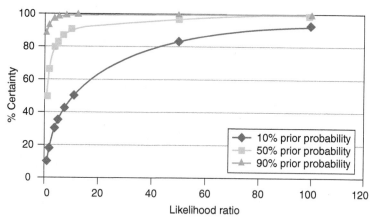

FIGURE 19-5   Posterior Probability versus Likelihood Ratio at Different Prior Probabilities

The relationship between the likelihood ratio (LR) and the probability of parentage are shown for three different prior probabilities (10%, 50%, and 90%). Notice how lower prior probability values require additional testing to achieve the same final posterior probability compared to the use of higher prior probability values.

or rejecting a claim of parentage. To achieve a 99% probability of parentage using a prior probability of 10%, we will almost always have to perform more testing to increase the LR than if we use prior probabilities of 50% or 90%. The relationship between prior probability and LR is shown in Figure 19-5 ▦. It is important to note that Bayes' theorem can be used to attach probability to virtually any likelihood ratio produced in any situation. The only requirement is that a prior probability be assigned to the calculation.

Review of the Main Points

- Early parentage testing was based on exclusion of parentage based on red blood cell antigen testing, particularly using the ABO, MN, and Rh systems.
- The human leukocyte antigen (HLA) system began to be utilized in the 1970s to determine parentage and has much stronger discriminatory power than the red blood cell antigens.
- The HLA system was high-powered enough to allow calculation of the probability of paternity (or maternity or other first-degree relationship) for the people who could not be excluded.
- The discovery of hypervariable DNA polymorphisms led to paternity testing using DNA profiles instead of HLA typing.

- Methodologies could accurately test DNA from a wide variety of samples, including aged samples and very small-volume samples.
- Initially restriction fragment-length polymorphism (RFLP) analysis was used.
- Single tandem repeat (STR) loci are commonly used in the analysis of DNA and calculation of likelihood ratios of being related or the probability of exclusion.
- The probability of parentage approaches, but never quite reaches, 100%. The higher the prior probability, the closer the posterior probability can get to 100%.

Review Questions

1. The practice of using blood groups for parentage testing in the 1950s was based on which principle? (Objective #2)

   A. Inclusion

   B. Exclusion

   C. Confirmation

   D. Probability

2. Select the advantages to using DNA typing instead of HLA typing for parentage testing. (Objective #7)

   A. DNA is more stable.

   B. Old blood specimen can be used.

   C. Many specimen types are acceptable.

   D. Testing can be performed at any temperature.

3. How many short tandem repeat (STR) loci exist in the human genome? (Objective #8)

   A. Less than 100

   B. Between 100 and 500

   C. Between 500 and 1,000

   D. More than 1,000

4. What technology was the first to be used for DNA profiling? (Objective #6)

   A. RFLP

   B. PCR

   C. STR

   D. VNTR

5. How are alleles separated by size after STR loci have been amplified? (Objective #8)

   A. Centrifugation

   B. Capillary action

   C. Electrophoresis

   D. Fluorescence

6. After STR alleles have been separated by size, which process is needed for specific identification? (Objective #6)

   A. Radioactivity

   B. Fluorescence

   C. Electrophoresis

   D. Centrifugation

7. In parentage testing, which hypothesis estimates the likelihood or probability that the alleged parent is the true parent of the child? (Objective #10)

   A. H0

   B. H1

   C. H2

   D. H3

8. How is the probability of exclusion used in parentage testing? (Objective #11)

   A. It estimates the probability that an alleged parent is the true parent of the child.

   B. It estimates the population that possesses an obligate allele.

   C. It estimates the population that lacks an obligate allele.

   D. It estimates the population frequency of the obligate allele.

9. The statistical logic that allows a level of certainty for a hypothesis to be modified by incorporating new information is referred to as: (Objective #14)

   A. Likelihood ratio

   B. Parentage

   C. Discriminatory power

   D. Bayes' theorem

10. True or False: In parentage testing, it is possible to achieve a 100% probability that an alleged parent is the true parent of a child. (Objective #11)

References

1. Fade to Black Comedy Magazine. Who was Charlie Chaplin and why did the FBI investigate him? [Internet]. [cited 18 March 2009] Available from: http://www.fadetoblack.com/foi/charliechaplin/bio2.html

2. Krause HD. Concerns of the legal profession. In: Walker RH, ed. *Inclusion probabilities in parentage testing*. Bethesda (MD): American Association of Blood Banks; 1983. pp. 13–20.

3. Schutzman F. Interests of the Office of Child Support Enforcement, U.S. Department of Health and Human Services. In: Walker RH, ed. *Inclusion probabilities in parentage testing*. Bethesda (MD): American Association of Blood Banks; 1983. pp. 7–12.

4. Allen RW. Parentage testing in the United States: The role of the American Association of Blood Banks. *Profiles in DNA* 2; 1998: 7–8.

5. AABB Relationship Testing Program Unit. Annual report summary for testing in 2004 [Internet]. Bethesda (MD): AABB; 2012. [cited 2012 October 11]. Available from http://www.aabb.org/sa/facilities/Documents/rtannrpt04.pdf

6. Walker RH, ed. *Inclusion probabilities in parentage testing*. Bethesda (MD): American Association of Blood Banks, 1983.

7. American Association of Blood Banks. *Standards for parentage testing laboratories*, 2nd ed. Bethesda (MD): American Association of Blood Banks; 1992.

8. AABB Parentage Testing Standards Committee. Annual report summary for testing in 1995 and 1996. American Association of Blood Banks, Bethesda (MD): American Association of Blood Banks; 1997.

9. AABB Relationship Testing Program Unit. Annual report summary for testing in 2002 [Internet]. Bethesda (MD): AABB; 2012. [cited 2012 October 11]. Available from http://www.aabb.org/sa/facilities/Documents/ptannrpt02.pdf

10. Hammond HA, Jin L, Zhong Y, Caskey CT, Chakraborty R. Evaluation of 13 short tandem repeat loci for use in personal identification applications. *Am J Hum Genet*. 1994; 55(1): 175–89.

11. Budowle B, Moretti TR, Niezgoda SJ, Brown BL. CODIS and PCR based short tandem repeat loci: Law enforcement tools. In: *Proceedings of the second European symposium on human identification*. Innsbruck, Austria: Promega Corporation; 1998. pp. 73–88.

12. Chakraborty R, Stivers DN, Su B, Zhong Y, Budowle B. The utility of short tandem repeat loci beyond human identification: implications for development of new DNA typing systems. *Electrophoresis* 1999; 20(8): 1682–96.

13. Elder JK, Southern EM. Measurement of DNA length by gel electrophoresis II: comparison of methods for relating mobility to fragment length. *Anal Biochem* 1983; 128(1): 227–31.

14. Applied Biosystems Inc. GeneScan product bulletin for the ABI Prism 310 and 377 genetic analyzers. Foster City (CA); Applied Biosystems Inc.; 2000.

15. Applied Biosystems Inc. ABI Prism Genotyper software product bulletin using AmpFlster for the 310 and 377 genetic analyzers. Foster, City (CA); Applied Biosystems Inc.; 2001.

16. AABB. *Standards for relationship testing laboratories*, 6th ed. Bethesda (MD): AABB Press; 2003.

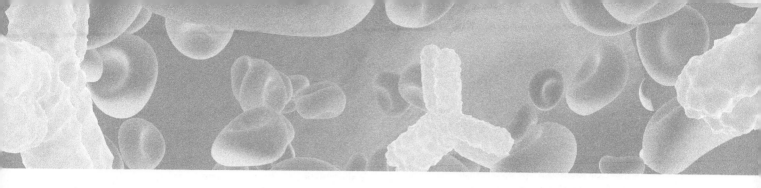

20 Transfusion Safety and Regulatory Issues

KAREN NIELSON AND LISA DENESIUK

Chapter Objectives

Upon completion of this chapter, the student will be able to:

1. Detail major historical events, with their significance, that resulted in regulation of the blood industry.
2. Identify the federal regulations that currently apply to the blood industry in the United States.
3. Identify when a facility requires or does not require licensure or registration with the Food and Drug Administration (FDA).
4. Describe the inspection processes of the FDA and common voluntary accreditation agencies.
5. State examples of and actions available to the FDA when responding to a reported violation.
6. Briefly describe the Clinical Laboratory Improvement Amendments (CLIA).
7. Compare and contrast the United States and European regulations regarding the manufacture and use of medical devices and blood products.
8. Summarize the responsibilities of laboratory professionals related to certification and licensure.
9. State three benefits of seeking voluntary accreditation for blood banks and transfusion services.
10. Discuss the responsibility of the International Organization for Standardization (ISO) as it relates to clinical laboratory services.

Key Terms

Biologic(s)
Certification
Drug(s)
Hemovigilance

Licensure
Medical device(s)
Nonconformance
Variance

CASE IN POINT

LD applied to be a volunteer American Association of Blood Banks (AABB) assessor. Her application was successful and she attended the assessor training session at last year's AABB meeting. Four months later she completed an assessment as a trainee. The assessment was of a small, single-site transfusion service and the assessment team consisted of LD and the lead assessor. LD has just received an invitation to participate on another AABB assessment team, which would be her first assignment as an official AABB assessor.

a minimum level of safety, the blood industry is highly regulated in developed countries.

Some regulations are mandated by law; others are voluntary standards defined by professional organizations. In addition to federal regulations, blood banks and transfusion services may have to comply with state or other regionally defined requirements.

This chapter addresses the following questions:

- What historical events contributed to the development of regulation of the blood industry?
- In the United States, what agencies enforce mandatory and voluntary requirements?
- What are some key features of the regulation requirements in Europe and Canada?
- What regulations outline requirements for blood banks and transfusion services operating in the United States?

What's Ahead?

While it is impossible to achieve zero risk with blood products and pharmaceuticals, blood transfusions have become increasingly safe with advances in testing, production, and storage. To ensure

HISTORY OF REGULATION OF DRUGS[1]

The foundation for the sciences of bacteriology, virology, and immunology, including acceptance of germ theory, was developed by scientists between 1800 and 1900. By the end of the 19th century, the first vaccines and antitoxins were developed and began to be widely used.

By 1885, laws had been enacted in several European countries to control the licensing, inspection, and labeling of products and to authorize inspection of manufacturing facilities.[1] However, in the United States at this time, individual states bore the primary responsibility for regulation of foods and **drugs**. Drugs are defined as chemicals used to treat, cure, prevent, or diagnose disease. Regulatory control was markedly inconsistent from state to state.

Unfortunately, it took a series of major catastrophes, including disease outbreaks, to spur increased regulatory oversight of drugs and therapeutic agents in general, and the blood industry specifically. This trend of public outcry over a tragedy followed by strengthened regulation began with the 1901 diphtheria outbreak and continued into the 1960s. Figure 20-1 ■ illustrates the concurrent development of regulation and regulatory agencies with widely publicized food and drug scandals.[1, 2]

Fortunately, regulation and quality management systems (Chapter 21) have evolved to a point where the blood industry now attempts to proactively diminish threats to the safety of the blood supply. Additionally, current regulation and systems allow the industry to respond quickly to emerging hazards, as illustrated by the reaction to more recent outbreaks such as the spread of the West Nile virus in North America that began in 1999.

Landmark Legislation

The Biologics Control Act of 1902, which was also known as the Virus-Toxin Law, was the first American legislation to deal with **biologics**, which are substances that are used to treat illness and that are isolated from a naturally occurring source. The Biologics Control Act

required that biologics be manufactured in a manner that ensured the safety, purity, and potency of the product.[1]

The Federal Food and Drugs Act enacted in 1906 was the first broad food and drug act in the United States. The new act did not require a list of ingredients on the product label, but it did require that the ingredient list be accurate if a list was provided.[1]

The Federal Food and Drugs Act of 1906 had no provisions to block the sale of dangerous drugs. The modern era of pharmaceutical law was born with the passage of the Federal Food, Drug and Cosmetic Act in 1938. This latest law further defined the government's authority to ensure that a drug was proven safe before marketing, and required that drugs be labeled with adequate directions for safe use. It set limits for certain poisonous substances and formally authorized factory inspections. It established the notion that a scientific approach would be the standard; no longer could commercial or anecdotal evidence form the basis for marketing a drug.[1]

In 1944, laws relating to public health were revised and consolidated in the Public Health Service Act. The earlier 1902 Biologics Control Act was incorporated in Section 351 of the new Act.[1] An important change was that now both biological products and the facilities producing them would need licenses.

In 1962, in response to the thalidomide tragedy in Europe, the Kefauver-Harris drug amendments were passed. These amendments required that manufacturers provide substantial evidence that drugs were effective for the intended use.[1] They further required good manufacturing practices and inspection of commercial manufacturers every 2 years. In addition, manufacturers, including blood banks, had to register annually.

☑ CHECKPOINT 20-1

What was the first law in the United States that addressed biologics?

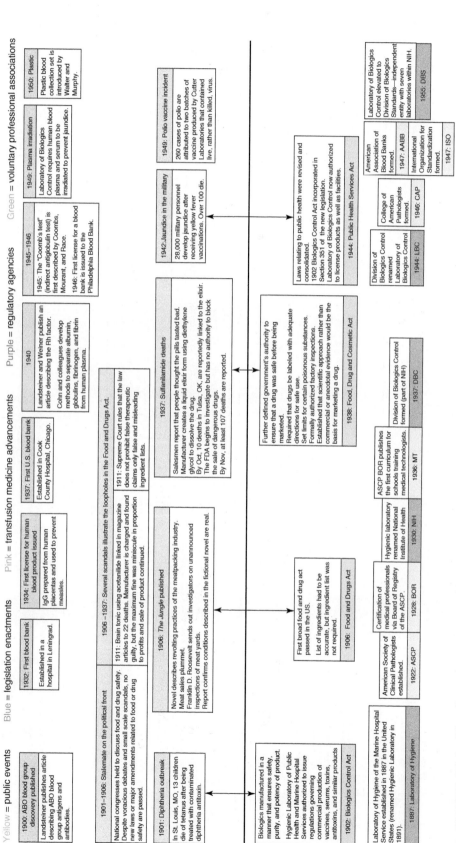

Yellow = public events   Blue = legislation enactments   Pink = transfusion medicine advancements   Purple = regulatory agencies   Green = voluntary professional associations

1900: ABO blood group discovery published

Landsteiner publishes article describing ABO blood group antigens and antibodies.

1901–1906: Stalemate on the political front

National congresses held to discuss food and drug safety. Despite voracious debates and small scale scandals, no new laws or major amendments related to food or drug safety are passed.

1901: Diphtheria outbreak

In St. Louis, MO, 13 children die of tetanus after being treated with contaminated diphtheria antitoxin.

Biologics manufactured in a manner that ensures safety, purity, and potency of product.

Hygienic Laboratory of Public Health and Marine Hospital Services authorized to issue regulations governing commercial production of vaccines, serums, toxins, antitoxins, and similar products

1902: Biologics Control Act

Laboratory of Hygiene of the Marine Hospital Service established in 1887 in the United States (renamed Hygienic Laboratory in 1891).

1887: Laboratory of Hygiene

1906: The Jungle published

Novel describes revolting practices of the meatpacking industry. Meat sales plummet. Franklin D. Roosevelt sends out investigators on unannounced inspections of meat yards. Report confirms conditions described in the fictional novel are real.

First broad food and drug act passed in the US.
List of ingredients had to be accurate, but ingredient list was not required.

1906: Food and Drugs Act

American Society of Clinical Pathologists established.

1922: ASCP

Certification of medical professionals via Board of Registry of the ASCP.

1928: BOR

Hygienic laboratory renamed National Institute of Health

1930: NIH

ASCP BOR publishes the first curriculum for schools training medical technologists.

1936: MT

1906 –1937: Several scandals illustrate the loopholes in the Food and Drugs Act.

1911: Brain tonic using acetanilide linked in magazine articles to 22 deaths. Manufacturer is charged and found guilty, but the maximum fine was miniscule in proportion to profits and sale of product continued.

1911: Supreme Court rules that the law does not prohibit false therapeutic claims only false and misleading ingredient lists.

1937: Sulfanilamide deaths

Salesmen report that people thought the pills tasted bad. Manufacturer creates a liquid elixir form using diethylene glycol to dissolve the drug.
By Oct, 10 deaths in Tulsa, OK, are reportedly linked to the elixir. The FDA begins to investigate but has no authority to block the sale of dangerous drugs.
By Nov, at least 107 deaths are reported.

Further defined government's authority to ensure that a drug was safe before being marketed.
Required that drugs be labeled with adequate directions for safe use.
Set limits for certain poisonous substances.
Formally authorized factory inspections.
Established that scientific approach rather than commercial or anecdotal evidence would be the basis for marketing a drug.

1938: Food, Drug and Cosmetic Act

Division of Biologics Control formed (part of NIH)

1937: DBC

1932: First blood bank

Established in a hospital in Leningrad.

1934: First license for human blood product issued

IgG prepared from human placentas and used to prevent measles.

1937: First U.S. blood bank

Established in Cook County Hospital, Chicago.

1940

Landsteiner and Weiner publish an article describing the Rh factor.

Cohn and colleagues develop methods to separate albumin, globulins, fibrinogen, and fibrin from human plasma.

1942: Jaundice in the military

28,000 military personnel develop jaundice after receiving yellow fever vaccinations. Over 100 die.

Laws relating to public health were revised and consolidated.
1902 Biologics Control Act incorporated in Section 351 of the new legislation. Laboratory of Biologics Control now authorized to license products as well as facilities.

1944: Public Health Services Act

Division of Biologics Control renamed Laboratory of Biologics Control

1944: LBC

College of American Pathologists formed.

1946: CAP

1945–1946: The "Coomb's test" (indirect antiglobulin test) is first described by Coombs, Mourant, and Race.

1946: First license for a blood bank is issued to the Philadelphia Blood Bank.

1949: Plasma irradiation

Laboratory of Biologics Control requires human blood plasma and serum to be irradiated to prevent jaundice.

1949: Polio vaccine incident

260 cases of polio are attributed to two batches of vaccine produced by Cutter Laboratories that contained live, rather than killed, virus.

American Association of Blood Banks formed.

1947: AABB

International Organization for Standardization formed.

1947: ISO

1950: Plastic

Plastic blood collection is introduced by Walter and Murphy.

Laboratory of Biologics Control elevated to Division of Biologics Standards—independent entity with seven laboratories within NIH.

1955: DBS

■ FIGURE 20-1   Timeline of Major Events in Regulation of Blood and Blood Products in the United States

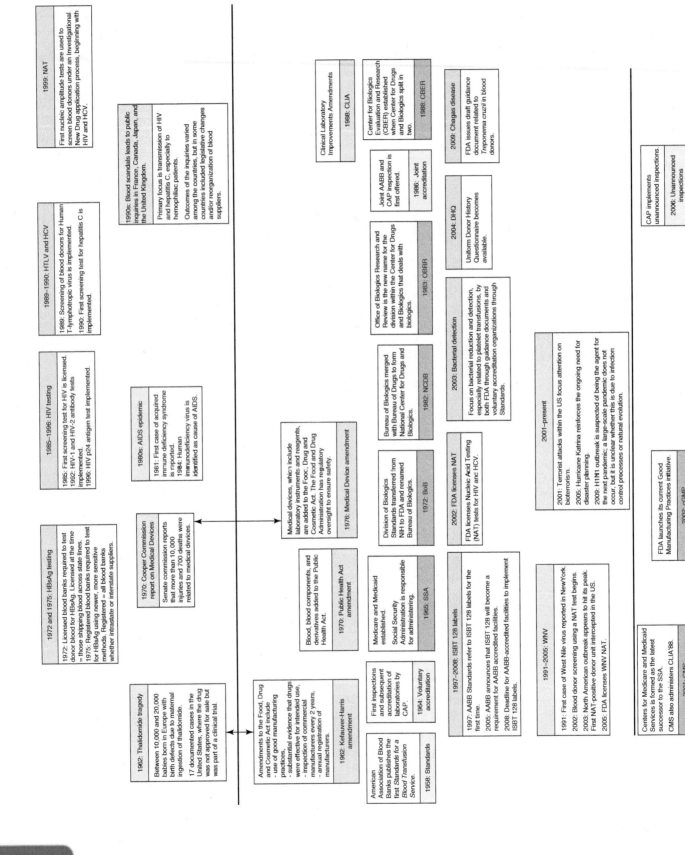

■ FIGURE 20-1 (continued)

Evolution of Regulatory Agencies

The Biologics Control Act of 1902 authorized the Hygienic Laboratory of the Public Health and Marine Hospital Services to issue regulations that governed all aspects of commercial production of vaccines, serums, toxins, antitoxins, and similar products, which eventually included human blood and products made from human blood.

The Bureau of Chemistry administered the Food and Drugs Act of 1905 and was charged with prohibiting the interstate transport of unlawful food and drugs.

The Hygienic Laboratory was renamed the National Institute of Health (NIH) in 1930. The Division of Biologic Control was established within the NIH during World War II with the mandate to supervise the safe production of plasma used to treat the war-wounded. In 1944, the Division of Biologic Control was renamed the Laboratory of Biologics Control, which administered licenses under the provisions of the Public Health Services Act of 1944.

In 1955, following an incident involving live polio virus in a vaccine that was supposed to be produced with killed virus, the Laboratory of Biologics Control was elevated to the Division of Biologics Standards within the NIH. It was an independent entity with seven laboratories.

In 1972, the Division of Biologics Standards was moved from the NIH to the Food and Drug Administration (FDA) and renamed the Bureau of Biologics. Through the 1980s there was a series of reorganizations within the FDA. In 1988, one of these reorganizations led to the creation of the Center for Biologics Evaluation and Research (CBER), which is the regulatory agency licensing blood banks today.

☑ CHECKPOINT 20-2

Which agency licenses blood banks in the United States?

Medical Laboratory Legislation

Medical laboratories within the United States must comply with the Clinical Laboratory Improvement Amendments (CLIA) of 1988. The CLIA applies to any laboratory performing testing on specimens from humans with the intent of providing information that will be used to assess health or diagnose, prevent, or treat disease.[3] Both blood banks and transfusion services fall under the authority of the CLIA.

The CLIA is currently administered by the Centers for Medicare and Medicaid Services (CMS). The CMS was formed in 2001 and traces its history back to the Social Security Administration, which was the first agency to coordinate Medicare and Medicaid services when they were established in 1965.

☑ CHECKPOINT 20-3

What facilities must comply with the Clinical Laboratory Improvement Amendments?

Historic Events in Blood Regulation

In 1934, the NIH issued the first license for a product produced from human blood. This immunoglobulin preparation was an extract made from human placentas and was used to prevent measles.

The first license for a blood bank was issued to the Philadelphia Blood Bank in 1946. Only blood banks operating in interstate commerce (shipping blood across state lines) were required to be licensed at this time.[1]

In 1949, the Laboratory of Biologics Control required that human blood plasma and serum be irradiated to prevent jaundice.

In 1970, as a result of a mislabeling scandal, the terms "blood, blood components, and derivatives" were inserted into the 1944 Public Health Services Act.

Around 1970, methods for detection of the hepatitis B virus were developed and on July 1, 1972, licensed blood banks engaged in interstate commerce were required to test for hepatitis. This requirement did not include blood banks operating only within individual states. More sensitive tests for hepatitis continued to be developed, and by December 1975, all registered blood banks, which included those operating only within state borders, were required to test for hepatitis using these more sensitive methods.

When the Bureau of Biologics was created in 1972, the agency reviewed the safety, effectiveness, and labeling of all previously licensed biologics. Regulatory activity for blood and blood products increased dramatically.

In 1976, *medical devices*, which include instruments and reagents, were added to the Food and Drug Act. While the definition of medical devices may vary somewhat among countries and legislation, generally speaking, the legal definition of a **medical device** is health or medical instruments used in the treatment, mitigation, diagnosis, or prevention of a disease.

The first case of acquired immunodeficiency syndrome (AIDS) was reported in 1981 and the human immunodeficiency virus (HIV) was identified in 1984. Early in the epidemic, it was apparent that the causative agent of AIDS could be transmitted via transfusion. The first test used to screen blood donors for HIV was licensed in 1985 and was followed by increasingly more sensitive test methods. In countries outside the United States, notably France, Canada, and Japan, the tragedy of transfusion-transmitted HIV and hepatitis C, especially within the hemophiliac community, resulted in public inquiries.

While good manufacturing practices had been enshrined in the legislation since the 1962 Kefauver-Harris drug amendments, current good manufacturing practices (cGMPs) became a focus for blood banks when the FDA launched a cGMPs project in 2002.

Regulations are periodically updated via amendments; so it is that the Food, Drug and Cosmetic Act of 1938 and the Public Health Services Act of 1944 still provide the framework for regulation of the blood industry in the United States.

CLIA, originally passed in 1988, were amendments to the Public Health Services Act. All of these acts and their current amendments are captured within the current legislation framework: the United States Code and the Code of Federal Regulations.

☑ CHECKPOINT 20-4

When was the first HIV screen for blood donors approved by the FDA?

CURRENT LEGISLATIVE FRAMEWORK

Today in the United States, when laws are enacted, they are published in the United States Code. The United States Code is divided by subject into 50 parts called *titles*. The government agency responsible for each new law writes proposed rules to enforce the law. These proposed rules are published daily in the *Federal Register*. After a comment period, final rules along with background, interpretive information, and comments are published in the *Federal Register*. All rules are gathered annually and published under the appropriate title in the Code of Federal Regulations (CFR).

Rules for blood products are found in CFR Title 21, parts 210, 211, 600–680. Rules for human cells, tissues, and cellular and tissue-based products are found in parts 1270–1271. The regulations require adherence to current good manufacturing practices (cGMPs), describe the specific requirements for different products, and describe licensing and registration requirements. Rules related to CLIA are in CFR Title 42, part 493.

☑ CHECKPOINT 20-5

What does CFR mean?

In addition to the CFR, the FDA issues guidance documents that provide additional information and current thinking about regulatory topics. Although these guidance documents are not mandatory, they do set a standard of care and are usually followed by the industry.

FOOD AND DRUG ADMINISTRATION (FDA)

Blood establishments are classified in one of three general categories for the purpose of regulation by the Food and Drug Administration (FDA),[4] as outlined in Table 20-1 ✱.

All licensed and/or registered blood collection and processing facilities are subject to inspection by the FDA. Transfusion services that perform only minimal manufacturing of blood products (e.g., thawing plasma and pooling products) and that are certified for reimbursement by CMS are not usually inspected by the FDA. The FDA accepts CMS approval, according to the terms of a memorandum of understanding with CMS. However, the FDA still has the authority to inspect if warranted.

CASE IN POINT *(continued)*

The facility identified in the assessment notice is a large blood bank and the accreditation team will consist of six members. LD recognizes the name of the blood bank and upon further investigation discovers that this facility is an alternate blood supplier that the transfusion service she works in uses when their primary blood supplier is unable to meet a request.

1. What is the most correct course of action for LD to take and why?
   (a) Accept the invitation to participate on the assessment team because the transfusion service that she works in only rarely deals with this blood supplier.
   (b) Decline the invitation and cite conflict of interest as the reason because LD is sometimes a customer of the facility being assessed.
   (c) Accept the invitation because as a junior member on a large team, LD won't have much authority to identify deficiencies anyhow.
   (d) Decline the invitation because she works in a transfusion service and the facility is a blood bank.

Licensure and Registration

Facilities must register annually with the FDA, via form FDA 2830, if they collect, manufacture, prepare, or process blood products. Facilities that want to ship products across state lines must apply for *licensure* (later discussed in State and Local Regulations) using the Biologics License Application (BLA; Form 356h). The licensure application applies to both the facility and to the product(s). Most forms can be filled out electronically using the FDA website.

Inspection

New facilities are inspected within 1 year by a team from the CBER and Office of Regulatory Affairs (ORA). Subsequent inspections occur at least every 2 years, depending on the compliance history of the facility. The ORA publishes guidelines for inspectors, licensed facilities, and registered facilities.

✱ **TABLE 20-1** FDA Categories for Blood Establishments

Requirement	Description	Example
Licensure and registration	Establishments collecting and producing blood products that engage in interstate commerce	Large blood product suppliers and plasma product producers
Registration only	Establishments collecting and producing blood products but acting solely within state borders	Hospital-affiliated blood banks that collect and process blood from donors
Exempt from registration and licensure	Transfusion services performing only minimal manufacturing activities and who are certified by Centers for Medicare and Medicaid Services (CMS)	Hospital transfusion services that do not collect donor blood but receive blood products from a blood supplier

☑ **CHECKPOINT 20-6**

What is the routine inspection cycle for FDA-licensed facilities?

Routine inspections include evaluation of the five layers of blood safety, which are listed in Figure 20-2 ■. Investigators will examine the operational systems that contribute to these layers of safety, including standard operating procedures (SOPs), personnel and training records, equipment validation, calibration and maintenance records, quality-assurance activities, quality-control records, and all related documents.

A full inspection of all systems are designated as Level I inspections. If a facility has a favorable inspection profile, subsequent inspections may be abbreviated Level II inspections that focus on three systems. If the investigator determines that objectionable practices or violations of regulations have occurred, they will document these observations in writing on Form 483 that is then presented to the facility. The investigator is required to document management's intention to correct those deficiencies. Most facilities also respond in writing to the FDA, with documentation of corrective actions that address the deficiencies noted on Form 483.

Violations

The FDA can respond to reported violations in several ways. They may take no action at all if the violation has been addressed and is considered to have posed a small degree of danger to the public.

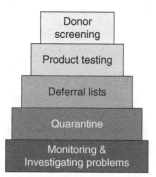

■ **FIGURE 20-2** United States Food and Drug Administration (FDA) Inspection

The FDA blood-safety system focuses on the safety of blood transfusion recipients by ensuring the quality of blood components produced by blood establishments.

- Donor screening includes questions that identify factors that may impact the suitability of the donor's blood for transfusion.
- Product testing includes tests for infectious diseases that are mandated by the FDA.
- Deferral lists ensure that a donor whose blood is unsafe for transfusion will not be able to donate in the future.
- Blood and blood components are quarantined until all infectious disease testing is completed and reviewed.
- Blood establishments must monitor their processes and investigate and correct any manufacturing problems. All product deviations are reported to the FDA.

✱ **TABLE 20-2** FDA Categories for Enforcement Actions

Requirement	Example(s)
Advisory	Warning letter
Recall	Voluntary recall initiated by manufacturer FDA-requested recall FDA-mandated recall
Administrative	License suspension License revocation Orders of retention, recall, destruction, and cessation of manufacturing related to human cell, tissue, and cellular and tissue-based products
Judicial	Seizure of product Court injunctions Civil litigation seeking monetary penalties Criminal prosecution

Alternately, they may choose to issue a warning letter, which allows the facility to remedy the violation. Or in cases where the risk to public safety is great, where a facility has repeated violations, or where a facility has not corrected reported violations, the FDA can and often will take more severe action. The FDA divides enforcement actions into advisory, administrative, judicial, and recall actions. Table 20-2 ✱ lists examples of FDA enforcement actions in each category.[5]

Biological Product Deviation Reports

Manufacturers of blood components and plasma products are required to report all instances of errors or accidents that could potentially affect the safety, potency, or purity of a distributed product. Postdonation information is the most frequent biological product deviation reported.[6] Table 20-3 ✱ lists the categories of biological product deviation codes for blood products.[7]

The same form and online system are used to report biological deviations related to human tissue, cellular, and tissue-based products (HCT/P). The rules around HCT/P reporting concentrate on the potential to transmit communicable disease.

☑ **CHECKPOINT 20-7**

When must a blood component manufacturer report a biological product deviation?

Medical Devices

Medical device regulations are mainly enforced by the Center for Devices and Radiological Health. However, because of the CBER's jurisdiction over the blood industry, the CBER also regulates some medical devices that are used in the manufacture of biologics. Medical devices include software and reagents as well as testing and therapeutic instruments.

Medical devices are sorted into three classes; Class I poses the least risk and Class III, which includes new devices that are unlike anything else on the market, poses the most potential risk.[8] Many instruments and reagents used in blood banks and transfusion

✳ **TABLE 20-3** Biological Product Deviation Code Categories for Blood Products

Requirement	Examples
Donor suitability	Postdonor information, such as changes to answers on screening questions and/or diagnosis of infectious disease. Errors occurring during donor screening.
Blood collection	Outdated or incorrect donor collection set used. Collection time exceeded.
Component preparation	Components not prepared in appropriate timeframe or at appropriate temperature. Platelet product made from a donor who took medication that affects platelet function.
Laboratory testing	Problems that occurred with transfusion testing such as ABO/Rh and antibody screen or infectious disease testing such as HIV and hepatitis screening.
Labeling	Label missing required information. Incorrect information on label.
Quality control and distribution	Failure to quarantine unit. Shipping did not meet time or temperature requirements. Product that did not meet special requirements was used (e.g., irradiated, washed, phenotype specific, negative for hemoglobin S).
Miscellaneous	Units involved in a lookback.

services fall into Class II. New Class II products can often apply for 510(k) clearance. In a 510(k) clearance the manufacturer must show substantial equivalency between the new device and a previously approved similar device.[9] Table 20-4 ✳ lists some transfusion-related examples of medical devices.

☑ **CHECKPOINT 20-8**

What is a 510(k) clearance?

Manufacturers and users must report any fatalities or serious adverse events that are related to or suspected to be related to the use of medical devices to the FDA using Form 3500A.

Fatality Reporting

Blood product manufacturers, blood banks, and transfusion services must report all deaths that are related to blood donation or blood transfusion to the CBER. The death must be reported as soon as possible, usually by telephone or e-mail, and must be followed up with a written report within 7 days.

✳ **TABLE 20-4** Regulated Medical Device Examples in Transfusion

Requirement	Example
Class I	Copper sulfate solutions for hemoglobin screening Heat sealers
Class II	Blood bank computer software systems Donor blood collection sets
Class III	Reagents for diagnostic tests for HIV, HCV, HBV
Biologics License Application	Reagents for donor screening tests for HIV, HCV, HBV

Human Tissue, Cellular, and Tissue-Based Products

The FDA enforces the regulations around human tissue and cellular products, but not solid organs. Solid organ transplants are monitored by the Health Resources Services Administration. The FDA focuses on three areas of regulation of tissue and cellular products[10]: minimizing the risk of communicable disease transmission; establishing good manufacturing processes that will reduce risk of contamination; and requiring that higher-risk products demonstrate safety and efficacy. The FDA regulations focus on facilities that collect or manipulate tissues and cells, not on facilities that only receive, store, and administer tissue products.

CENTERS FOR MEDICARE AND MEDICAID SERVICES (CMS)

The Clinical Laboratory Improvement Ammendment (CLIA) is enforced by the Centers for Medicare and Medicaid Services (CMS). All laboratories testing specimens from humans, except those performing only research, must be certified under the CLIA. This includes both blood banks, which are testing samples from donors, and transfusion services, which are testing samples from potential transfusion recipients.

Laboratories are inspected every 2 years under CLIA. Inspections may be conducted by a state health department using CMS requirements, by a CMS-approved accreditation agency, or by a licensure program in states that are CMS exempt. As of 2010, there are two CMS-exempt states, Washington and New York, and there are six approved accreditation agencies,[11] which are listed in Figure 20-3 ▪.

The CLIA divides laboratory tests based on their complexity, which is assessed using a scoring system.[3] Tests are classified as waived, moderate complexity, or high complexity. Waived tests are easily performed with minimal technical training. Generally, over-the-counter tests and some point-of-collection (also known as point-of-care) tests are classified as waived. Laboratories or physician offices that only perform waived tests may apply for a certificate of waiver

Inspection Meets CLIA Regulations

1. AABB (formerly the American Association of Blood Banks)
2. American Osteopathic Association (AOA)
3. American Society for Histocompatibility and Immunogenetics (ASHI)
4. College of American Pathologists (CAP)
5. COLA (formerly the Commission of Office Laboratory Accreditation)
6. Joint Commission (formerly the Joint Commission on Accreditation of Healthcare Organizations or JCAHO)

■ **FIGURE 20-3** Accreditation Agencies Approved by the Centers for Medicare and Medicaid

and do not need to undergo inspection. Most laboratory tests performed in blood banks and transfusion services are nonwaived tests.

CLIA regulations cover facilities, quality system, and personnel requirements. The CLIA has specific rules around proficiency testing for nonwaived tests. For some tests, the regulations set out a minimum number of challenges and minimum pass rates. The CMS also approves proficiency testing programs and providers.

☑ **CHECKPOINT 20-9**

What agencies conduct CLIA inspections?

INTERNATIONAL PERSPECTIVE

Similar regulations and regulatory agencies govern medical devices, blood suppliers, and blood and tissue products in other developed countries. And even in developing countries, there are many examples of the implementation of quality management systems (Chapter 21) in the blood system and/or regulation of the blood industry.

Manufacturers and suppliers working in one or more countries within the European Union (EU) must comply with EU rules. Generally speaking, the EU agrees upon and then publishes directives that lay out the minimum requirements on a subject. The EU does not enforce the directive; the member countries adopt the EU directive and establish enforcement processes through their own national laws.[12] The national laws may be more stringent than the EU directive but must at least meet the EU directive as a minimum requirement.

The European Commission administers the EU directives related to medical devices.[12] Manufacturers of medical devices must register the device with the European Commission and show compliance with the minimum standards. The device will receive a designation known as a *CE mark* that signifies that the product meets the applicable European Commission directives. This mark is assigned once the manufacturer has successfully completed the conformity assessment.[12] A key difference between the European and American regulatory systems for medical devices is that the responsibility for ensuring that the applicable minimum standards for safety and efficiency have been met lie with the manufacturer in the European

model rather than with a government agency in the American model. Conformity assessments are usually conducted by notified bodies, which are independent companies that are monitored and audited by the EU's member states. Once a device has a CE mark it can be marketed freely within all the EU's member states.[12] One of the four pillars of the EU is freedom of movement of goods. EU member states can only restrict movement of legally manufactured goods from other member states if there is a risk to health or safety of consumers or to the environment.

The European regulation of blood and blood products is outlined in four directives[13] as of 2011. The directives outline common goals for quality and safety. The directives touch on many of the same topics as the applicable American laws, such as quality systems, donor eligibility, blood collection, processing, testing, storage, distribution, and **hemovigilance**, which is the reporting of adverse events in blood donors and recipients. As with other EU directives, the member states enforce the provisions by aligning their national laws with the directive. Blood establishments must be licensed by a competent authority, which generally means some arm of the government or other regulatory agency. Licensed establishments must be inspected at least once every 2 years.[14] The regulation of blood products was mandated at the EU level rather than a national government level to allow the member states to have confidence in the safety of blood products if they have to import the products from another member state during a shortage or crisis.

In Canada, Health Canada plays a similar role to the FDA in the United States. Health Canada regulates medical devices and pharmaceutical drugs.[15] Health Canada also regulates blood suppliers and manufacturers.[16] Canada, similar to the United Kingdom, has a national blood supply with only two blood suppliers, Canadian Blood Services and Héma-Québec. The Canadian Standards Association has published national Standards for Blood and Blood Components[17] called CAN/CSA-Z902. The standards applicable to blood suppliers, both the two national suppliers and any hospital transfusion service processing blood, are enforced by licensure and inspection procedures administered by Health Canada. Unlike in the United States, hospitals do not generally run blood banks in Canada. Instead, hospitals usually fall under Health Canada's mandate for regulating blood if they operate an autologous donation program or if they further process blood products received from the blood supplier. Enforcement of the standards applicable to transfusion services is more complicated because the standards are national but health care falls under provincial (equivalent to state) jurisdiction. Mandatory accreditation programs for laboratories exist in some provinces but not in others. And in some, but not all, provinces the accreditation program has adopted CAN/CSA-Z902 or the Canadian Society for Transfusion Medicine's (CSTM) Standards for Hospital Transfusion Services as the standard against which accredited laboratories will be assessed. The CSTM Standards are aligned with CAN/CSA-Z902 but focus and expand on transfusion services.[18]

STATE AND LOCAL REGULATIONS

Laboratories must also comply with all applicable state and local regulations. In some cases, the state or local regulation may be more stringent or more detailed, and therefore would supersede the federal regulation.

Laboratories, as employers, must also comply with applicable occupational health and safety regulations, which may be at the federal, state, or local level. And as health care providers and employers, laboratories and laboratory professionals must be aware of and follow the federal and state privacy laws that apply to their practices. Two federal privacy laws that routinely affect laboratory operations in the United States are the Health Insurance Portability and Accountability Act of 1996 (HIPAA) and the Health Information Technology for Economic and Reinvestment Act of 2009 (HITECH).

Most states or regions also have mandatory reporting of notifiable infections to a public health agency. Notifiable infections are ones that have public health implications. The public health agency will contact the person identified as carrying the infection to ensure that he or she is receiving proper treatment and/or counseling and to identify contacts to whom the person may have transmitted the infection. Some of the diseases often on notifiable disease lists that blood donors are screened for are syphilis, hepatitis B, hepatitis C, human immunodeficiency virus, and West Nile virus. Blood banks performing infectious disease testing on donors must report positive results as mandated by their state or local regulations.

☑ CHECKPOINT 20-10

What are two infections that are commonly on a notifiable list?

Certification and Licensure of Professionals

States also set out the requirements for licensure of medical professionals. Requirements for certification or licensure of medical laboratory professionals vary among states. Certification and licensure are very similar terms and are often used interchangeably. In general, professional **certification** is usually issued by a professional society to indicate that a person has met a set of qualifications and is therefore qualified to perform a particular job. Often certification follows writing and passing some type of examination(s). While some certifications require periodic renewal, others are valid for the life of the person or product. Professional **licensure** often refers to a similar assessment of qualifications but one that is mandated by law. Therefore, licenses are often issued by a government department or a regulatory body designated by law to administer licensure on the government's behalf. Most licenses require periodic renewal but some are issued only once.

As of 2011, certification for clinical laboratory scientists is offered by the following organizations in the United States: American Medical Technologists (AMT), American Association of Bioanalysts (AAB),[19] and the Board of Certification of the American Society of Clinical Pathologists (ASCP).[20] These professional societies also offer certification for a variety of other clinical laboratory personnel. Additionally, some subspecialties within the clinical laboratory field may have certifying agencies specific to the specialty. Certification in the United States and in other countries usually occurs at a national level and involves successful completion of an applicable accredited training program followed by passing an examination administered by the certifying agency and maintaining that certification through continuing education.

Licensure often occurs at the state level or in other countries the state equivalent, and may include successfully completing a state-specific examination, either instead of or in addition to the applicable national certification. Licensure may also include annual requirements designed to assess that the professional is keeping current in their knowledge. Examples of activities that are used by various licensure agencies around the world are listed in Figure 20-4 ■.

VOLUNTARY ACCREDITATION

Blood banks or transfusion services may also choose to seek voluntary accreditation. Some of the agencies that offer voluntary accreditation are also CMS-approved inspection agencies. If the laboratory is using the inspection to meet their CLIA obligations, then the accreditation is mandatory. However, some laboratories may meet their CLIA

Requirements vary amongst licensing agencies[1]

Minimum number of hours of employment in the profession

Minimum number of continuing education hours

Completion of a continuing education program

Completion of a learning plan or professional portfolio

Completion of written or oral examinations

Practice visits[2]

[1] Requirements often encompass either one activity or a combination of activities. For example, in 2011, California requires clinical laboratory scientists to provide proof of 24 hours of continuing education from an approved provider in a 2-year cycle to maintain licensure. Whereas, in 2011, the Canadian province of Alberta requires both a minimum of 900 hours of work in the field in the last 4 years and submission for approval and then completion of an annual learning plan, which often contains participation in continuing education.

[2] Practice visits, where an independent observer watches the professional perform their job and then reports any deficiencies or the lack of deficiencies back to the licensing body, are common practice within some professions, such as dentistry, but are relatively uncommon for laboratory professionals. However, practice visits may be used to investigate professionals who have not successfully complied with ongoing licensure requirements or when a complaint has been lodged involving the professional. Practice visits may rarely be a regular part of annual licensure renewal. For example, the Canadian province of Ontario requires the regulatory College to conduct practice visits each year on a predetermined number of randomly selected registered laboratory professionals.

■ **FIGURE 20-4** Examples of Annual Activities for Maintaining Licensure

obligations by a different route and still choose to be inspected by a voluntary accreditation agency. Additionally, these agencies may offer accreditation to laboratories outside the United States, which are not subject to CLIA.

CASE IN POINT (continued)

LD declines the invitation to assess the blood bank facility. A month later she receives another invitation. The facility being assessed is a large transfusion service operating in two hospitals within the same city located in another state, but within driving distance of LD's home. The transfusion service holds voluntary accreditation with both AABB and CAP and has requested a combined assessment. The assessment is estimated to take 2 days, one for each hospital site. The other laboratory departments will be undergoing their CAP assessment on the same days; the entire assessment team consists of 10 members, with two designated to observe transfusion-related activities. LD accepts the invitation and receives her preassessment package.

2. After reviewing the information forwarded to her, what is LD's best choice for her next action?

   (a) Take the CAP online training for assessors as indicated in her preassessment package because she has never done a CAP inspection before.

   (b) Contact the other team member who will be observing transfusion-related activities because she has never met this person.

   (c) Talk to her coworkers about what she may be able to learn from seeing another transfusion service.

   (d) Wait to get more instructions from the AABB office.

LD attends a regional educational event and is seated at lunch next to someone who works at the facility she will be assessing.

3. Are any of the following acceptable actions? Why or why not?

   (a) LD could announce that she is excited to be visiting the person's place of employment next month.

   (b) LD could tell just the person next to her that she is part of the assessment team but not what day the team will be arriving.

   (c) LD could ask the person for the best routes to take if driving between her hometown and the city where the person lives.

   (d) LD could ask the person if the transfusion service is ready for their upcoming assessment.

Some of the reasons for seeking a voluntary accreditation include those listed in Table 20-5 ✱. Generally speaking, voluntary accreditation agencies use a peer-review assessment process. This

means that people working in the field perform the assessment. Most voluntary accreditation agencies align their assessment tools to ensure regulatory compliance but also to promote excellence beyond the minimum requirements outlined by regulation.

The two most common voluntary accreditations that apply to medical laboratories, including blood banks and transfusion services, are AABB and College of American Pathologists (CAP). Both are also CMS-approved agencies and both assess medical laboratories outside the United States. A voluntary accreditation for plasma product producers is the International Quality Plasma Program certification from the Plasma Protein Therapeutics Association.

☑ CHECKPOINT 20-11

Name one voluntary laboratory accreditation program in the United States.

American Association of Blood Banks

AABB, which was formerly known as the American Association of Blood Banks, was formed in 1947. AABB publishes various standards, including Standards for Blood Banks and Transfusion Services. The first AABB Standards were published in 1958 and currently are updated every 18 months. AABB-accredited facilities are assessed to the current, applicable AABB Standard using a peer-review process.[21]

AABB assessors must initially complete a training course and participate in an assessment as a trainee and then to remain an assessor they must complete a minimum number of assessments annually and ongoing continuing education on a 2-year cycle. Renewal assessment visits are unannounced if occurring within the United States or Canada and occur every 2 years.[21] Unannounced assessments mean that the facility knows that the assessment will occur within a particular timeframe, usually a 6-month window, but not what day the assessment team will arrive. Additional assessments may occur if a complaint is lodged against the facility or there is concern about the facility's performance, such as significant problems identified during the regular assessment, failures in proficiency testing, or failure to address identified nonconformances. A **nonconformance** occurs when a facility is not meeting an applicable standard. Initial assessments and reassessments are announced.

During the assessment visit, the assessor(s) will evaluate the facility's operations and quality management system. Assessors use a tool that lists applicable requirements with sample questions or means for assessing. Findings are communicated to the facility throughout the assessment and a summary of both nonconformances and commendable practices identified during the assessment are presented to the facility's management during a summary session. A written summary report outlining any nonconformances is left with the facility's management. The facility has 30 days in which to provide an action plan that addresses each reported nonconformance to the AABB.[22] There are also processes for a facility to challenge the validity of a nonconformance citing.

If an assessor notices a nonconformance that potentially poses a significant danger to donors, recipients, or staff members, the assessor should immediately notify the facility personnel and AABB. The facility is required to take immediate action to correct the nonconformance.

✴ TABLE 20-5 Potential Benefits of Voluntary Accreditation

Benefit	Achieved by
Educational opportunities	Peer-review process allows interaction with other experts in the same field.
Patient and donor care improvements	Reduction in errors due to adoption of strong quality management systems to meet voluntary accreditation standards.
Confidence that facility is ready for regulatory assessment(s)	Voluntary accreditation standards are usually aligned with and often more stringent than regulatory requirements. Therefore, preparation for a voluntary accreditation will often ensure that a facility is compliant with regulations.
Control costs	Reduction in errors should result in less rework, which saves costs.
Recognition	Some voluntary accreditations (e.g., *International Organization for Standardization (ISO)* certification (described later in the chapter), are widely recognized by external customers and/or reimbursement agencies).

Sometimes accredited facilities have a valid reason for not being able to meet a particular standard. If this occurs the facility can apply for a **variance**. A variance is an alternate way to meet the intent of a particular standard without actually meeting the letter of the standard. This commonly occurs with facilities that are outside the United States when the standard relates to compliance with American regulation; AABB Standards comply with both CLIA and applicable CFR.

 CASE IN POINT *(continued)*

LD joins the assessment team the night before the scheduled assessment. The team arrives at the larger of the two hospitals the next morning. LD and the rest of the team members sign the hospital's confidentiality agreement, meet the medical director and chief laboratorians, take a brief tour of the laboratory, and complete a quick introductory meeting. LD and the other assessor assigned to transfusion services divide up the checklist, review some procedures and quality control charts, then head off to the laboratory to observe the staff members at work. LD notes that one of the laboratory's procedures and the staff members' actions do not appear to conform to a Standard that came into effect about 6 months ago. She tells the transfusion service supervisor of her finding. The supervisor replies that at a conference she attended the audience was told that having a plan to implement the Standard was sufficient and shows LD a procedure validation plan with a timeline to start and complete the validation within the next year.

4. Place the following actions in the best sequence.

   (a) At the coffee break, ask the other team member who is assessing the transfusion service if she has questions for AABB.

   (b) Call the AABB head office and ask for clarification.

   (c) Discuss the controversial finding with the lead assessor.

   (d) Tell the supervisor what will be written on the nonconformance and/or recommendation summary reports.

LD obtains clarification from AABB and lets the lead assessor and the transfusion service supervisor know what AABB head office has advised her to do. The lead assessor has asked all the assessors to return to the conference room 45 minutes before the scheduled summation meeting. One of the items that LD has noted as a nonconformance is that five of the transfusion service procedures have cover sheets with the last entry being a former medical director's signature just over 18 months ago. The facility's quality manual states that the medical director will document approval of an annual review by signing a cover sheet for each procedure. When each of the assessor outlines the nonconformances he or she has found, the team discovers that there are a handful of procedures in each of the laboratory departments that are missing evidence of annual review as per the facility's policy.

5. What is the best way for the team to write this nonconformance on the report and why?

   (a) Each assessor writes a nonconformance for each procedure where he or she has seen evidence of the missing review because each incident is a nonconformance.

   (b) Each assessor writes a single nonconformance covering procedure annual review on each department checklist because the departments have different supervisors.

   (c) The assessor who reviewed the items on the quality system checklist writes a single nonconformance using a couple of examples from different departments because multiple occurrences indicate that the root cause may be a flaw in the system or process.

   (d) No one writes a nonconformance on the procedure review policy because the number of procedures missing a signature was less than 10% of the total.

Facilities that are both AABB- and CAP-accredited can request a joint assessment, where the same assessor(s) uses one visit to complete an assessment and submit paperwork to both organizations. Joint assessments can only be done for regular renewal assessments, not for initial or reassessments. Additionally, the anniversary dates for renewal must be sufficiently close to allow an unannounced assessment to meet both organizations' timelines.

College of American Pathologists

The College of American Pathologists (CAP) was founded in 1946 and issued the first CAP accreditation certificates in 1964. CAP-accredited facilities undergo an on-site inspection every second year and complete a self-inspection during the intervening year. Checklists are used to complete both the external and self-inspections. The on-site inspections by an external team are unannounced. CAP volunteer inspectors are employees of a CAP-accredited facility and complete an online learning course about inspections. Inspection teams may also include a professional inspector employed by CAP.

The inspection visit follows a similar process to an AABB assessment. There is usually an introductory meeting followed by a tour of the laboratory, then the inspectors evaluate the facility's performance by reviewing written documents and records, watching staff members work, and asking questions. The inspection team uses standardized forms to prepare a written summary that includes a list of the identified deficiencies and presents their findings at a summation meeting with the facility's management. CAP checklist items are identified as either phase I or phase II. Laboratories must respond in writing to CAP within 30 days of the inspection and must address all identified deficiencies. For phase I deficiencies that have not been noted on previous inspections, the laboratory must outline the corrective action(s) taken. If a particular phase I deficiency has reoccurred, CAP is likely to request additional information or documentation. For phase II deficiencies, the laboratory must submit its corrective action plan with supporting documentation; for example, new or revised policies or procedures, communication to customers or staff members, or records that support that the deficiency has been corrected.

INTERNATIONAL ORGANIZATION FOR STANDARDIZATION (ISO)

The International Organization for Standardization (ISO) was formed in 1947. ISO was chosen at the founding meeting as the organization's shorthand name to be used in all languages. ISO was allegedly derived from the Greek word *isos*, which means equal.[23] However, one of the participants at the founding meeting reports that *isos* was never discussed at the meeting.[24] ISO is a nongovernmental organization that develops technical standards that are adopted widely throughout the world. ISO has published more than 18,000 standards in various fields.

Medical laboratories first became aware of ISO with the publication of ISO 9000 in 1988. ISO 9000 was originally based on a British Standards Institution document that outlined components of a quality management system (Chapter 21). Currently, in 2011, there is a series of ISO 9000 standards with ISO 9000 outlining the fundamentals of a quality system and ISO 9001 listing the minimum requirements. ISO 9000 and 9001 have been widely adopted by companies in different business sectors, including health care.

ISO standards are drafted by technical committees composed of subject-matter experts from around the world. Before a standard is published, there is a review phase where the draft is available to the public and sent to ISO member bodies. Both members of the public and ISO member bodies can comment on the draft. This allows for experts outside ISO member bodies, but within the particular field, to be heard. Once a standard has been approved and published, it undergoes a first review 3 years later and then is reviewed at least every 5 years.[25] The reviews are conducted by ISO member bodies.

ISO does not assess companies for compliance with standards. Most commonly, companies wish to achieve certification to a particular standard to show their customers. Certifications are issued by organizations that are independent of ISO and of the company being assessed. ISO does not monitor or register these certifying agencies but does publish standards that outline how proper assessment for compliance with ISO standards should occur.

ISO 15189, which are standards specific for clinical laboratories, was first published in 2003 and updated in 2007. In North America in

CASE IN POINT (continued)

LD and the team complete the assessment the next day. While observing a transfusion at the second hospital, LD observes the nursing staff using a checklist that is printed on the red blood cell unit tag generated by the laboratory information system. LD thinks that a similar checklist would be very helpful for the nursing staff in the hospital where she works.

6. Are the following statements true or false?

   (a) LD can tell the transfusion safety officer she works with about the checklist because the assessment was voluntary not mandatory for the transfusion service she visited.

   (b) LD can take a copy of the tag checklist home with her because both AABB and CAP are peer-review assessments.

   (c) LD can ask the transfusion medicine supervisor if she can share the checklist with her staff members at home because one of the goals of voluntary assessments is education and sharing of best practices.

   (d) LD has no alternative but to forget that she ever saw the checklist because everything related to an assessment is confidential.

   (e) LD can compliment the transfusion supervisor on the utility of the nursing checklist and ask if the facility would be willing to share the checklist with AABB if LD recommends that it be recognized as a commendable practice.

2011, the three organizations most recognized for accrediting to ISO 15189 standards are the College of American Pathologists (CAP), the Ontario Laboratory Accreditation (OLA) program, and the American Association of Laboratory Accreditation (A2LA). ISO 15189 contains both management and technical requirements.[26,27] The requirements correlate with ISO 9001, which outlines quality management systems and ISO/IEC 17025, which outlines standards for testing and calibration laboratories, and include the addition of technical requirements specific to the clinical laboratory. Table 20-6 ✳ gives an overview of the 23 requirements set out in ISO 15189-2007.

> ☑ **CHECKPOINT 20-12**
>
> What ISO standard was specifically written for clinical laboratory operations?

✳ **TABLE 20-6** ISO 15189-2007 Requirements

Category	Title	Example
Management requirements 4.1–4.15	Organization and management	Define responsibilities of personnel
	Quality management system	Quality policy statement and quality manual
	Document control	Revision and approval of procedures
	Review of contracts	If laboratory provides services based on contract(s), contracts are reviewed
	Examination by referral laboratories	Evaluation and selection of laboratories to which specimens will be referred
	External services and supplies	Evaluation and selection of external suppliers
	Advisory services	Meetings between laboratory professionals and clinical staff who use the laboratory
	Resolution of complaints	Analysis of complaints for patterns
	Corrective action	Root cause analysis (Chapter 21)
	Identification and control of nonconformances	Policy for release of results when a nonconformance is identified
	Preventive action	Risk analysis
	Continual improvement	Action plan for improvement
	Quality and technical records	Record retention
	Internal audits	Personnel will not audit their own processes
	Management review	List of items that require management review
Technical requirements 5.1–5.8	Personnel	Continuing education
	Accommodation and environmental conditions	Physical barriers to prevent cross-contamination, where applicable
	Laboratory equipment	Reagent storage
	Pre-examination procedures	Phlebotomy procedures
	Examination procedures	Establishment of reference ranges
	Assuring quality of examination procedures	Quality control systems
	Postexamination procedures	Specimen storage and retention
	Reporting of results	Report format
Annexes A–C	Correlation with ISO 9001:2000 and ISO/IEC 17025:2005	
	Recommendations for protection of laboratory information systems (LIS)	
	Ethics in laboratory medicine	

Review of the Main Points

- The first law in the United States that dealt with biologics was the Biologics Control Act of 1902.
- The first law in the United States that dealt broadly with food and drugs was the Federal Food and Drugs Act of 1906.
- The Clinical Laboratory Improvement Amendments (CLIA), which provide regulations for laboratories testing human specimens for health, wellness, and disease assessment, were originally enacted in 1988.
- Currently blood banks and transfusion services in the United States are governed by the Food, Drug and Cosmetic Act of 1938 and the Public Health Services Act of 1944.
- Rules for blood products are found in CFR Title 21, parts 210, 211, 600–680.
- Rules for human tissues and related products are found in CFR Title 21, parts 1270–1271.
- Rules related to the Clinical Laboratory Improvement Amendments are found in CFR Title 42, part 493.
- The U.S. Food and Drug Administration (FDA) requires both licensure and registration for establishments that collect donor blood, produce blood products, and engage in interstate commerce.
- Blood banks that collect and process donor blood into blood products but do not routinely ship products across state lines are required to register with the FDA.
- FDA inspections occur within 1 year of a new facility beginning operations and at least every 2 years thereafter. Inspections are performed by FDA staff inspectors.
- The FDA may take advisory, recall, administrative, or judicial actions to respond to an identified violation.
- Biological product deviation reports outline errors or accidents that occurred that might affect the safety, potency, or purity of a distributed blood product.

- Fatalities related to blood donation or blood transfusion must be reported to the Center for Biologics Evaluation and Research (CBER).
- The CLIA requires that clinical laboratories be inspected every 2 years.
- American Association of Blood Banks (AABB) inspections occur every 2 years, are unannounced, and are conducted by trained, volunteer assessors, AABB staff inspectors, or a combination.
- College of American Pathologists' (CAP) inspections occur every 2 years, are unannounced, and are conducted by volunteer assessors from other CAP-accredited facilities, CAP staff inspectors, or a combination.
- Medical devices, which include laboratory automation, information systems, and reagents, must be approved by the FDA.
- Examples of state regulations that affect blood banks and transfusion services include occupational health and safety legislation, privacy laws, professional certification or licensure; and state regulations related to blood suppliers or clinical laboratories.
- Professional certification usually refers to obtaining initial training and proving entry-level knowledge, often by passing a national examination.
- Professional licensure usually refers to an assessment of qualifications that is required by law.
- Professional certification and licensure can be one-time events or can require periodic renewal.
- International Organization for Standardization (ISO) 15189, which are international standards specific to clinical laboratories, were first published in 2003 and contain 23 requirements.

Review Questions

1. The Federal Food, Drug and Cosmetic Act of 1938 defined governmental authority over which aspects of the pharmaceutical industry? (Objective #1)

   A. Drug safety

   B. Drug labeling

   C. Limits for poisonous substances

   D. Factory inspections

2. The Kefauver-Harris drug amendments of 1962 required _____ registration of blood banks. (Objective #1)

   A. Monthly

   B. Quarterly

   C. Annual

   D. Biannual

3. What year did the National Institutes of Health (NIH) issue the first license for a product produced from human blood? (Objective #1)

   A. 1930

   B. 1934

   C. 1949

   D. 1972

4. Which infectious disease was required to be tested for in all donated blood as of 1970? (Objective #1)

   A. Hepatitis B

   B. Hepatitis C

   C. HIV

   D. WNV

5. The guidelines that are used for manufacturing and pro-cessing quality products in the blood bank are called: (Objective #2)

   A. CFR

   B. FDA

   C. cGMPs

   D. CLIA

6. Select the FDA requirement for each type of blood bank facility. (Objective #3)

   _____ Small community hospital with a blood bank that receives donor blood from an outside supplier

   _____ Blood donor center that collects and processes donor blood

   _____ Trauma center hospital with blood bank donor room services for autologous and directed donors

   A. Licensure and registration

   B. Registration only

   C. Exempt from registration and licensure

7. The inspection of an FDA-licensed blood bank facility includes the evaluation of which of the following aspects of service? (Objective #4)

   A. Standard operating procedures (SOPs)

   B. Blood safety practices

   C. Equipment validation

   D. Shift scheduling

8. Choose the appropriate FDA category for enforcement based on the action taken. (Objective #5)

   _____ A license to practice is suspended

   _____ A warning letter is issued

   _____ A facility is prosecuted for engaging in llegal practices

   _____ Voluntary recall of product by the manufacturer

   A. Advisory

   B. Recall

   C. Administrative

   D. Judicial

9. An example of a reportable incident during the manufac-ture and processing of blood components is: (Objective #5)

   A. Donor blood is discarded due to self-exclusion of the donor.

   B. Blood unit is quarantined pending transmissible dis-ease test results.

   C. Donor reports a diagnosis of hepatitis B 2 weeks after his last donation.

   D. Blood typing of donor unit is repeated due to weak isoagglutinins.

10. The most frequent biological product deviation category that is reported by blood bank facilities is: (Objective #5)

    A. Donor suitability

    B. Component preparation

    C. Laboratory testing

    D. Labeling

11. According to CLIA regulations, how frequently must a cer-tified blood bank laboratory be inspected? (Objective #6)

    A. Semi-annually

    B. Annually

    C. Every 2 years

    D. Every 5 years

12. How does the responsibility for minimum safety and effi-ciency of medical devices differ between the European and the American regulatory system? (Objective #7)

    A. In the United States, responsibility lies with the government.

    B. In the European system, responsibility lies with inde-pendent companies.

    C. In the European system, responsibility lies with the manufacturer.

    D. In both systems, responsibility lies with the consumer.

13. Which of the following criteria are required for certifica-tion of medical laboratory professionals? (Objective #8)

    A. Completion of an accredited training program

    B. Mandated by law

    C. Continuing education

    D. Passing an examination

14. Select the benefits of seeking voluntary accreditation for blood banks. (Objective #9)

    A. Interaction with experts in the field

    B. Error reduction

    C. Cost savings

    D. Patient-care improvements

15. Which of the following is not a primary responsibility of the International Organization for Standardization (ISO)? (Objective #10)

    A. Develop technical standards

    B. Perform compliance checks of technical standards

    C. Outline assessment protocols for compliance with technical standards

    D. Periodic review of published technical standards

References

1. U.S. Food and Drug Administration [Internet]. Science and the regulation of biological products; From a rich history to a challenging future. Rockville (MD): FDA [cited 15 July 2010]. Available from: http://www.fda.gov/downloads/AboutFDA/WhatWeDo/History/ProductRegulation/100YearsofBiologicsRegulation/UCM070313.pdf

2. AABB [Internet]. Highlights of transfusion medicine history. Bethesda (MD): AABB; 2010 [cited 4 Oct 2010]. Available from: http://www.aabb.org/resources/bct/Pages/highlights.aspx

3. Centers for Disease Control and Prevention [Internet]. CFR, Title 42, part 403.1–493.25. Atlanta (GA): CDC [cited 1 Dec 2010]. Available from http://wwwn.cdc.gov/clia/regs/subpart_a.aspx

4. U.S. Food and Drug Administration [Internet]. CPG Sec 230.110- Registration of blood banks, other firms collecting, manufacturing, preparing or processing human blood or blood products. Rockville (MD): FDA [cited 3 Dec 2010]. Available from: http://www.fda.gov/ICECI/ComplianceManuals/CompliancePolicyGuidanceManual/ucm073862.htm

5. U.S. Food and Drug Administration [Internet]. Enforcement actions (CBER). Rockville (MD): FDA [cited 3 Dec 2010]. Available from: http://www.fda.gov/BiologicsBloodVaccines/GuidanceComplianceRegulatoryInformation/ComplianceActivities/Enforcement/default.htm

6. U.S. Food and Drug Administration [Internet]. Biological product deviations; Annual summary for fiscal year 2009. Rockville (MD): FDA [cited 3 Dec 2010]. Available from: http://www.fda.gov/BiologicsBloodVaccines/SafetyAvailability/ReportaProblem/BiologicalProductDeviations/ucm214032.htm

7. U.S. Food and Drug Administration [Internet]. Biological product deviation reporting; Blood product codes. Rockville (MD): FDA [cited 27 Nov 2010]. Available from: http://www.fda.gov/BiologicsBloodVaccines/SafetyAvailability/ReportaProblem/BiologicalProductDeviations/ucm129732.htm

8. U.S. Food and Drug Administration [Internet]. Device classification. Rockville (MD): FDA [cited 27 Nov 2010]. Available from: http://www.fda.gov/MedicalDevices/DeviceRegulationandGuidance/Overview/ClassifyYourDevice/default.htm

9. U.S. Food and Drug Administration [Internet]. Overview of device regulation. Rockville (MD): FDA [cited 3 Dec 2010]. Available from: http://www.fda.gov/MedicalDevices/DeviceRegulationandGuidance/Overview/default.htm#510k

10. U.S. Food and Drug Administration [Internet]. How does FDA regulate tissue products? What safeguards are in place for recipients? Rockville (MD): FDA [cited 15 Nov 2010]. Available from: http://www.fda.gov/AboutFDA/Transparency/Basics/ucm194646.htm

11. Centers for Medicare and Medicaid Services [Internet]. Accreditation organizations/ Exempt states. Baltimore (MD); CMS [cited 3 Dec 2010]. Available from: http://www.cms.gov/CLIA/13_Accreditation_Organizations_and_Exempt_States.asp#TopOfPage

12. Castle G, Blaney R. European Union regulation of in vitro diagnostic medical devices. In: Danzis SD, Flannery EJ. In Vitro Diagnostics: The Complete Regulatory Guide. Washington, D.C.: The Food and Drug Law Institute: Washington; 2010. pp. 227–52.

13. Sandid I. European regulation on blood and blood components (Abstract English translation). Transfus Clin Biol Epub 1 Nov 2010.

14. Europa [Internet]. Quality and safety standards for human blood and blood components. Brussels; 1995–2010. [cited 25 Nov 2010)]. Available from: http://europa.eu/legislation_summaries/public_health/threats_to_health/c11565_en.htm

15. Health Canada [Internet]. Medical devices. Ottawa. [cited 25 Nov 2010]. Available from: www.hc-sc.gc.ca/dhp-mps/md-im/index-eng.php.

16. Health Canada [Internet]. Biologics, Radiopharmaceuticals and Genetic Therapies. Ottawa. [cited 25 Nov 2010]. Available from: www.hc-sc.gc.ca/dhp-mps/brgtherap/index-eng.php.

17. Canadian Standards Association. CAN/CSA Z902-10; Blood and blood components. Mississauga: Canadian Standards Association; 2010.

18. Canadian Society for Transfusion Medicine. Standards for hospital transfusion services; version 2. Ottawa: Canadian Society for Transfusion Medicine; 2007.

19. Bureau of Labor Statistics [Internet]. Clinical laboratory technologists and technicians. Washington, D.C. [cited 3 Dec 2010]. Available from: http://www.bls.gov/oco/ocos096.htm#training

20. American Society for Clinical Pathology, Board of Certification. http://www.ascp.org/functionalnavigation/certification.aspx

21. AABB. Accreditation program policy manual. Bethesda (MD): AABB; 2008.

22. AABB. Accreditation information manual. Bethesda (MD): AABB; 2008.

23. International Organization for Standardization [Internet]. Discover ISO. Geneva; 2010. [cited 25 Nov 2010]. Available from: www.iso.org/iso/about/discover-iso_isos-name.htm.

24. Kuert W. Things are going the right way. In: Latimer J. Friendship among equals. Geneva: International Organization for Standardization; 1997. International Organization for Standardization [Internet]. 2010. [cited 25 Nov 2010]. Available from: http://www.iso.org/iso/about/the_iso_story/friendship_equals.htm

25. International Organization for Standardization [Internet]. Stages of the development of international standards. Geneva: ISO; 2010. [cited 25 Nov 2010]. Available from: http://www.iso.org/iso/standards_development/processes_and_procedures/stages_description.htm

26. Canadian Standards Association. The ISO 15189:2003 essentials—A practical handbook for implementing the ISO 15189:2003 standard for medical laboratories. Mississauga: Canadian Standards Association; 2004.

27. International Organization for Standardization. ISO 15189:2007. Geneva: International Organization for Standardization; 2007. p. iii.

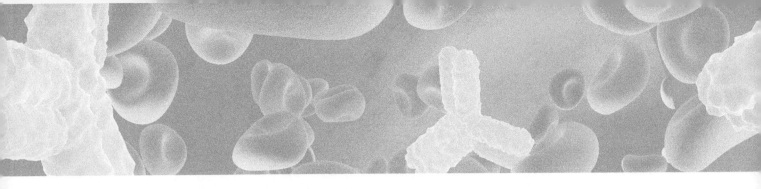

21 Quality Assurance

PATRICIA DAVENPORT

Chapter Objectives

Upon completion of this chapter, the student will be able to:

1. Define the following terms: quality system, quality control, quality assurance, quality management.
2. Describe how the different facets of a quality program interrelate and list examples of components and activities within each facet.
3. Describe at least four methods used in quality assurance activities to assess the performance of the quality system, including how the methods are implemented.
4. Discuss employee training and competency assessment as essential components of a quality assurance program.
5. Describe the functions and responsibilities of a quality assurance unit.
6. Describe equipment requirements, including maintenance, calibration, and validation.
7. Discuss the basic quality assurance requirements for computer systems in blood banks and transfusion services.
8. Define process control and its importance in blood banks and transfusion services.
9. Define document control and describe the elements of a document control system.
10. List the circumstances requiring error reporting and product recall.
11. Identify two major purposes of the lookback process.
12. Describe the internal and external audit process in maintaining a quality system and provide examples for each.
13. Outline a strategy for problem solving, including the tools that can be applied in the process.
14. List elements of a laboratory safety program.

Key Terms

Calibration
Challenge condition(s)
Consignee
Customer(s)
Document control
Event
Lookback
Market withdrawal
Near-miss event
Postdonation information
Process control(s)
Production condition(s)
Proficiency testing (PT)

Quality
Quality assurance (QA)
Quality control (QC)
Quality indicator(s)
Quality management (QM) system
Quality system(s)
Recall
Root cause analysis
Sentinel event(s)
Traceback
Universal precautions
Validation

What's Ahead?

In today's environment of medico-legal, regulatory, and public scrutiny, an effective quality program is of utmost importance to blood banks and transfusion services. A sound quality program is essential for fulfilling the core mission of transfusion medicine: the provision of safe and effective blood products and services.

This chapter explores quality and quality programs by answering the following questions:

- What is quality?
- What are quality systems, quality management, quality assurance, and quality control?
- What is the purpose of a quality program and how is it designed?
- What are the responsibilities of the quality assurance unit and employees within a quality system?

CASE IN POINT

You have just started a new job as the transfusion services manager for a hospital laboratory. This is your first supervisory position and you moved to a new state to take the job. During the interview process the director that you now report to mentioned that the transfusion service was experiencing staffing shortages.

DEFINITION OF QUALITY

There are many definitions of **quality**. Often the definitions talk about characteristics or conformance of a product or service. The characteristics or conformance is usually further defined as satisfaction of needs or meeting requirements, standards or specifications. Quality definitions used in the transfusion medicine community may replace the generic 'product or service' terminology with blood, blood products, blood derivatives and tissue.

No matter what definition is used for quality, the basic idea is the same. To achieve quality, products and services must be consistent, must meet previously established expectations, and must be free from defects.

HISTORICAL BACKGROUND

Quality has been important to both consumers and manufacturers, but in the past has most often been driven by the consumer. When someone buys something that doesn't meet expectations, they probably won't buy it again and they might even tell their neighbors not to buy it. Today, quality is driven by the manufacturer or service provider, including blood establishments and health care industries. In transfusion medicine, there is only one shot at quality: if even one single product is unsuitable, the patient can suffer harm. Moreover, it is often impossible to look at a blood component and determine if there were any defects. Quality must be built into each and every process employed to produce the component.

The notion of organized quality systems has been around for quite some time, but has gained sophistication and complexity only recently. The beginnings of the quality movement date back to medieval times. The concepts of quality evolved slowly over time, but escalated during the 20th century largely due to significant advances of that period.[4] Figure 21-1 ■ illustrates some key developments and leaders in the history of the quality movement.

QUALITY PROGRAM FACETS

The quality program consists of several interrelated facets:

- Quality Control
- Quality Assurance
- Quality System
- Quality Management System

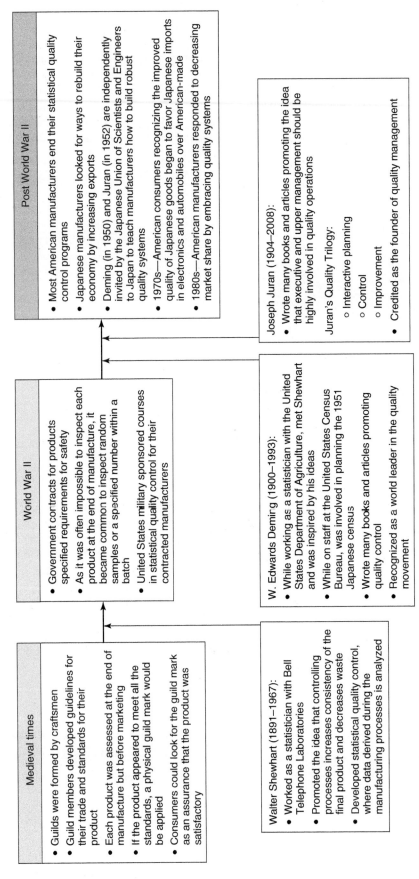

Medieval times

- Guilds were formed by craftsmen
- Guild members developed guidelines for their trade and standards for their product
- Each product was assessed at the end of manufacture but before marketing
- If the product appeared to meet all the standards, a physical guild mark would be applied
- Consumers could look for the guild mark as an assurance that the product was satisfactory

Walter Shewhart (1891–1967):

- Worked as a statistician with Bell Telephone Laboratories
- Promoted the idea that controlling processes increases consistency of the final product and decreases waste
- Developed statistical quality control, where data derived during the manufacturing processes is analyzed

World War II

- Government contracts for products specified requirements for safety
- As it was often impossible to inspect each product at the end of manufacture, it became common to inspect random samples or a specified number within a batch
- United States military sponsored courses in statistical quality control for their contracted manufacturers

W. Edwards Deming (1900–1993):

- While working as a statistician with the United States Department of Agriculture, met Shewhart and was inspired by his ideas
- While on staff at the United States Census Bureau, was involved in planning the 1951 Japanese census
- Wrote many books and articles promoting quality control
- Recognized as a world leader in the quality movement

Post World War II

- Most American manufacturers end their statistical quality control programs
- Japanese manufacturers looked for ways to rebuild their economy by increasing exports
- Deming (in 1950) and Juran (in 1952) are independently invited by the Japanese Union of Scientists and Engineers to Japan to teach manufacturers how to build robust quality systems
- 1970s—American consumers recognizing the improved quality of Japanese goods began to favor Japanese imports in electronics and automobiles over American-made
- 1980s—American manufacturers responded to decreasing market share by embracing quality systems

Joseph Juran (1904–2008):

- Wrote many books and articles promoting the idea that executive and upper management should be highly involved in quality operations

Juran's Quality Trilogy:

- ○ Interactive planning
- ○ Control
- ○ Improvement
- Credited as the founder of quality management

FIGURE 21-1 History of the Quality Movement

Mirroring the history of the quality movement, quality programs in the laboratory began with the smallest facet and then continually expanded and improved. The laboratory began with a strong foundation of quality control, which was later expanded into quality assurance monitoring, then enhanced into a more comprehensive quality system as part of a total quality management program.

CASE IN POINT (continued)

On the first day at your new job, you introduce yourself to the employees you will be supervising and hold a quick, stand-up meeting. You ask the employees to write down their top three concerns by the end of the day. When you review the submissions, you hear multiple times that the employees are unhappy about the amount of overtime they are working. The next day, you meet with a human resources advisor and you also review the previous month's budget report. You discover that there are currently two full-time positions vacant; one has been vacant for 6 months and the other for 3 months. Your department is overbudget on staffing costs.

1. Can you think of any internal factors that you could potentially change that might be contributing to the vacant positions not attracting successful candidates?
2. Can you think of any external factors that might be contributing to the position vacancies remaining open?
3. What part of a robust quality program looks beyond the walls of the organization?

Quality Control

Quality control (QC) is routine testing or activities, often performed daily or during processing of each batch, to ensure that materials, reagents, and equipment are functioning as expected at any given stage of a process. It is the quality control results that indicate to operational staff members whether the process should continue or stop. When QC results identify that a problem exists, the QC is said to be out of control and the problem must be resolved before the process can continue.

Quality Assurance

Quality control and quality assurance terms are sometimes used interchangeably. For the purposes of this chapter, they are distinct processes. **Quality assurance (QA)** is the monitoring performed to ensure that the quality system is being adhered to and is effective. QA includes the following:

• Planning—What will be done?

• Retrospective review processes—What was done or not done?

• Analysis of performance data—Was it done the right way?

Review processes include monitoring, auditing, trend analysis, and *root-cause analysis* of errors. Analysis of performance data is

done to measure how well processes and personnel are functioning through audits, competency assessments, and proficiency testing.

Quality System

AABB defines the **quality system** as, "The organizational structure, responsibilities, policies, processes, procedures and resources established by executive management to achieve quality."[2] It includes everything that is utilized to ensure that products, processes, or services within a department or organization meet or exceed expectations. Box 21-1 lists the components of a quality system.

BOX 21-1 Important Components of a Quality System

Quality System Components

Organization
Personnel and hiring practices
Training
Equipment and supplier qualification
Processes and process control
Procedure manuals
Documentation
Methods to detect errors or deviations
Error correction
Quality controls
Equipment calibration and maintenance
Process and equipment validation
Internal and external audits

Quality system is also sometimes defined as the document that captures the quality program, for example, the quality manual or quality plan of an organization.

Quality Management System

Ideally the quality system, quality assurance, and quality control are all encompassed within a **quality management (QM) system**. The first three facets have an internal focus, whereas QM also looks outward. QM addresses the interrelationship between systems and processes within an organization and between the organization and its suppliers and customers.[5] QM involves strategic and quality planning, validation, training, and implementation with consideration for cost containment and risk management. It ensures that the overall quality program is effective and efficient with a continuous goal of process improvement and customer satisfaction.

Quality has been depicted as a three-legged stool, as illustrated in Figure 21-2.[6] The seat of the stool is quality management. The three legs, all of which are essential to balance the stool, are (1) compliance with government and accreditation requirements, (2) meeting customer requirements and needs, and (3) controlling costs.

The three major components of a quality program are QM, QA, and QC. The activities within each interact with the others, as listed in Table 21-1. For example, QC is a part of QA, which in turn is

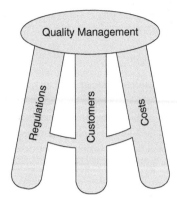

■ FIGURE 21-2 Elements of Quality

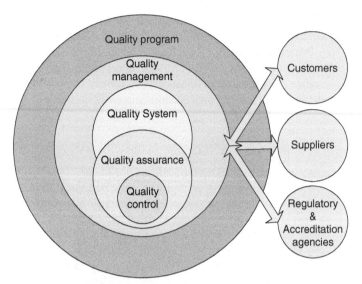

■ FIGURE 21-3 Quality Program Activities

encompassed together with the QS document within QM, as illustrated in Figure 21-3 ■.

QUALITY AND REGULATION

Quality evolution in the health care and transfusion medicine industries included reluctance to change, similar to American manufacturing industries. Often, change within healthcare would be forced through regulation following a public tragedy (Chapter 20). The acquired immunodeficiency syndrome (AIDS) epidemic of the 1980s caused an acute awareness of the need for a more proactive approach to quality and preventive measures. This prompted the health care industry and regulators alike to rethink the way quality activities were viewed. While the need for quality programs was enshrined in the legislation governing blood banks and transfusion services prior to the AIDS epidemic, at that time the programs often existed as paper plans only or if implemented maintained a retrospective approach. Today, both legislative bodies and voluntary accreditation associations expect to see evidence during audits and assessments that quality programs are proactive and are integrated into every aspect of operations (Chapter 20).

Public and political criticism of the actions or inactions of the transfusion industry at the beginning of the AIDS epidemic prompted public inquiries in some countries (Chapter 20) and civil litigation in the United States. Although no test was available for HIV at the time, a patient who was infected with HIV through transfusion in 1984 sued, naming the AABB and others in the lawsuit. The AABB was found partially responsible by the New Jersey Supreme Court, which ruled that the AABB was negligent for failing to recommend surrogate testing for HIV, specifically antibody to hepatitis B core antigen. The AABB was stunned by the decision and there was widespread speculation about the implications for all voluntary standard-setting organizations.[7]

As a result of these events and the pressures of public and governmental criticism, the FDA intensified its surveillance on the blood industry, focusing on enforcement. Blood centers and transfusion services were subject to closer scrutiny, with regularly scheduled inspections and penalties in the form of citations and fines when deficiencies

✶ TABLE 21-1 Example Activities within a Quality Program

Quality Management (QM)	Quality Assurance (QA)	Quality Control (QC)
• Organizational structure planning	• Periodic departmental and process audits	• Record review
• Customer and hospital relations	• Review and approval of procedures and policies	• Positive and negative sample testing
• Vendor selection and relations	• Review and approval of training programs	• Temperature checks
• Quality indicator development	• Review of error reports	• Visual inspection
• Human resources	• Review and approval of corrective action	• Equipment calibration
• Development of job descriptions	• Trend analysis	• Daily reagent reactivity testing
• Development of performance standards	• Review of quality monitoring results	• Adding IgG-coated cells to negative antibody tests, if required by the methodology
• Cost analysis	• Document and record control	• Use of autologous control in antibody identification tests
• Process improvement	• Review and approval of validation plans	• Platelet counts in random or apheresis platelets
		• Expiration date check

in process control and quality assurance were found. As more and more screening tests were licensed and required for blood donors, the FDA began to recognize that overall quality programs in many blood institutions were inadequate to keep up with the advances in technology. In 1992, the FDA made a significant move to further classify blood and blood products as pharmaceuticals. This meant that, in addition to CFR 600, manufacturers of blood products would also have to comply with 21 CFR 210.211, which describes current good manufacturing practices (cGMPs) for pharmaceuticals (Chapter 20).

Regulating, Accrediting, and Certifying Agencies

Transfusion medicine is one of the most closely regulated industries in the world. Table 21-2 ✳ lists the many agencies that influence the operations of blood banks and transfusion services. The activities of the organizations are described in Chapter 20.

Quality Oversight

Although quality is everyone's responsibility, a quality assurance hierarchy is required by both the FDA and AABB.[2, 3] Together, they require one or both of the following:

- An individual appointed for oversight of the quality system who reports to executive management.
- A quality assurance unit or group responsible for oversight of all activities relating to product quality.

In small organizations, the system oversight individual and the QA unit may be represented by one person. QA personnel should not have final oversight of their own work.

In blood manufacturing organizations, the QA unit is responsible for planning and performing appropriate activities to provide confidence that all systems and elements that influence product quality are working as expected. FDA charges the QA unit with ensuring that production personnel follow cGMPs and grants the QA unit the authority to stop production and/or release of product. The QA unit should take

immediate action when data analysis or other events indicate that a process is out of control or may become out of control. Most importantly, proactive measures should be implemented that will prevent processes from going out of control and prevent errors before they happen.

☑ CHECKPOINT 21-2

The individual with oversight of the quality system responsibility reports to _____.

QUALITY PROGRAM GOALS

In today's intricate transfusion medicine environment, an effective and efficient quality program is critical to accomplish compliance with regulation and accreditation standards, to meet customer needs, to ensure safety of the blood products issued, and to contain costs. It ensures workers that they have the knowledge and skills to perform their tasks and that the work environment is as safe as possible. Clearly, these are all specific targets of a quality program, but there are broader missions the program must embrace to be truly successful.

Philosophy

Quality is a word that is hard to define. Some people equate quality with regulatory compliance, but real quality goes far beyond compliance. Box 21-2 lists the potential outcomes from a quality system where the goal stops at regulatory compliance.

BOX 21-2   Outcomes of Ineffective Quality Programs

Focus on meeting minimum regulatory compliance only

Reactive attitude that does not

- Foster constructive outlook among employees
- Encourage creativity in developing preventive measures
- Promote a cooperative relationship with regulatory and accrediting agencies

Same problems and errors can reoccur, which can lead to

- Deteriorating customer relations
- Declining employee morale
- Increasing costs

✳ **TABLE 21-2** Transfusion Medicine Agencies

Agency	Role(s)
U.S. Food and Drug Administration (FDA)	R
Centers for Medicare and Medicaid Services (CMS)	R, C
AABB (formerly the American Association of Blood Banks)	A
The Joint Commission (formerly the Joint Commission on Accreditation of Healthcare Organizations, or JCAHO)	A
College of American Pathologists (CAP)	A, C
Foundation for the Accreditation of Cellular Therapy (FACT)	A
Occupational Safety and Health Administration (OSHA)	R
U.S. Environmental Protection Agency (EPA)	R
U.S. Nuclear Regulatory Commission (NRC)	R
U.S. Department of Transportation (DOT)	R
European Union (EU)	R
State health agencies	R

A, accrediting; C, certifying; R, regulating.

An effective quality program has adoption of a total quality philosophy throughout the organization as a major goal. Everyone views quality activities as an integral part of their normal duties and continually strives for new levels of excellence both as individuals and as team members. Box 21-3 lists the roles of the various groups within an organization during initial implementation and ongoing execution of a total quality program.

BOX 21-3   Total Quality Program

Roles and Responsibilities

Executive and senior leadership:

- Understand the interrelationships between processes, services, customers, suppliers, and employees within their business model.
- Understand that the focus for production processes is conformity, but service processes may require more flexibility.
- Develop a common goal for the organization, which is often stated as a vision or mission statement.
- Develop a quality plan that
  - is focused on the organization's common goal,
  - is as simple as possible,
  - clearly defines accountability and assigns responsibility,
  - incorporates a commitment to quality from every individual in the organization, and
  - allows enough flexibility to adapt to changing circumstances.
- Clearly communicate the quality plan and the common vision to all employees.
- Be seen to utilize the quality plan, for example, applying the vision or mission as the standard that drives strategic decision making.

Senior management:

- Communicate and demonstrate to the employees within their departments a clear commitment to the quality philosophy.
- Implement the quality plan by developing quality systems that
  - are aligned with the common organizational goals,
  - encourage participation of every employee,
  - encourage teamwork among different departments,
  - standardize processes and procedures,
  - incorporate continual surveillance of department operations,
  - monitor all critical operations,
  - identify and correct errors,
  - incorporate continual surveillance of external influences that could affect department operations,
  - promote timely assessment of customer satisfaction,
  - promote process improvement,
  - endorse preventive actions, and
  - incorporate planning and communication as part of process change.

Employees:

- Understand the common goals of the organization.
- Understand how every task and process within their scope of work contributes to the organizational goals.

CASE IN POINT (continued)

You meet with your director and discuss the current human resources crisis. You discover that the local medical laboratory training program closed 3 years ago. All of the employees hired as new graduates in the last 2 years have been from a program in the neighboring state. In the past year the neighboring state has experienced an economic upswing. Unfortunately, this has translated into wage increases for laboratory professionals in the neighboring state that are above what your organization can afford to offer. Your director asks you to come up with alternate solutions to the crisis.

4. What might you consider doing next?

Tools

There are many approaches management can use in developing a quality program. The approaches utilize different tools and change in popularity over time. All the tools strive toward total quality management and continual improvement and historically each new tool generally has built upon the foundation of previous philosophies. It is important that senior management clearly communicate to employees that adoption of a new tool signals a desire to reach the next level of quality and does not negate previous progress. Figure 21-4 ■ illustrates how the various goals, facets, and tools of quality work together.

At the start of the 21st century, Six Sigma and Lean were popular approaches. Six Sigma is a quality approach that strives to eliminate all or nearly all defects from a process and has proven to reduce costs and process time when implemented properly. Lean focuses on eliminating waste. Quality improves because waste includes employee activities not adding value to the process; rework due to errors; and product, reagent, and supply discards.

☑ CHECKPOINT 21-3

What is the name of the quality program approach that focuses on eliminating defects from a process, reducing costs, and increasing efficiency?

The choice of standards upon which to structure the quality program are also numerous. The International Organization for Standards (ISO) is recognized by many as the pinnacle of international quality standards. ISO standards that are popular within the transfusion medicine field include ISO 9000 and ISO 15189 (Chapter 20). AABB Standards remain the most widely used by blood banks and transfusion services. The AABB Standards are consistent with FDA cGMPs, ISO 9000, requirements of the Joint Commission, and the Clinical and Laboratory Standards Institute (CLSI).[8]

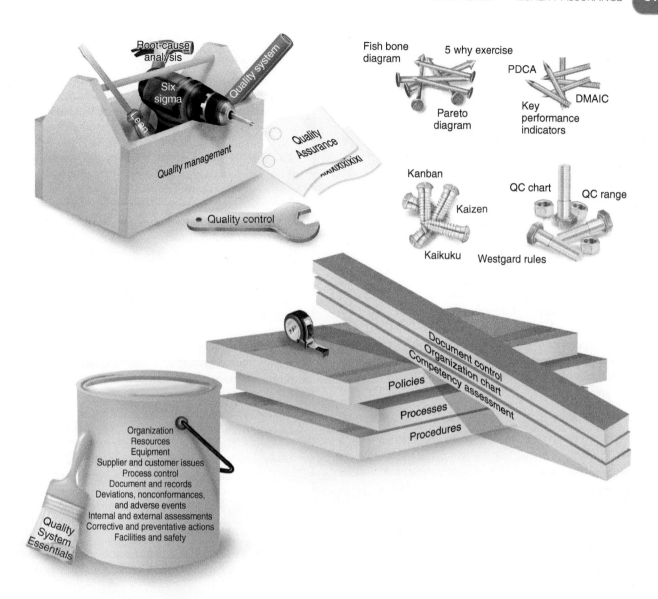

FIGURE 21-4 Quality Program Tools

If we compare building an effective quality program to building a house, the goals are straightforward: affordable shelter in the case of the house and a safe product and regulatory compliance in the case of the quality program. But a well-built house will become a home with outcomes that are much harder to define or quantify, for example, a sense of security and a sense of family for the home. In this metaphor, an engaged, motivated staff with good morale, satisfied customers, and a proactive corporate culture are quality program examples. The well-built house will provide shelter for decades or even centuries, but it does not remain static and the carpenter's tools are never completely retired. The house will need maintenance and occasionally larger renovations. In the quality program this leads to the philosophies of total quality management (TQM) or continuous quality improvement (CQI). Additionally, the expectations of the homeowners or the building inspectors can change over time. Knob-and-tube wiring was okay in 1910 and asbestos insulation was okay in 1950, but neither was acceptable if building or renovating a house in 2010. In transfusion, testing donor blood for hepatitis B surface antigen was state of the art in 1975, but transmissible-disease testing has expanded considerably since that time and will continue to advance. The carpenter as he starts to build a new house or renovate an existing house needs plans and tools and materials. To ensure that he avoids putting a light switch behind a door, or the plumbing on the wrong side of the kitchen, or other, more critical mistakes, he needs a set of blueprints. The quality program's blueprint is the quality system written down in a quality manual or quality plan. As his work progresses, the carpenter must ensure that he has the correct permits and certificates of inspection; quality assurance or monitoring activities is the quality equivalent. In his toolbox or given the large number, more likely his truck with a trailer, the carpenter will have a wide variety of tools and materials. Quality management is equivalent to the carpenter's toolbox, or better yet his truck because it encompasses all of the people, philosophies, data, and analysis involved in achieving quality. The carpenter's tools likely include classics such as hammers, screwdrivers, and paint brushes; and more sophisticated ones such as air compressors, cordless drills, and table saws. In quality, our tools include quality control, Lean, Six Sigma, root-cause analysis, quality system essentials, and other philosophies not developed yet. The carpenter needs building materials, planks of wood, kegs of nails, stacks of brick, pails of mortar, etc. Quality materials can include (quality control) quality control charts, ranges, and rules; (Lean) kanban, kaizen, kaikuku, value added, and continuous flow; (Six Sigma) define/measure/analyze/improve/control (DMAIC) cycle, plan/do/check/act (PDCA) cycle, key performance indicators (KPI), and process maps; (root-cause analysis) Pareto diagrams, fish bone diagrams, and 5 why exercises; (quality system essentials) organization charts, document control systems, policies, processes, and procedures. The variety of tools and materials is almost endless and there is always a new, improved model in the window of the hardware store; or, in the case of quality, on the agenda of conferences or on business management bookshelves.

QUALITY SYSTEM ESSENTIALS

AABB Standards are divided into 10 quality system essentials (QSE)[2]:

1. Organization
2. Resources
3. Equipment
4. Supplier and customer issues
5. Process control
6. Document and records
7. Deviations, nonconformances, and adverse events
8. Internal and external assessments
9. Corrective and preventive action
10. Facilities and safety

Organization

AABB requires that each blood bank or transfusion service define and document its organization, policies, processes, and procedures related both to operational and quality functions.[2] The responsibility for key operational and quality functions should be clearly documented. All personnel must be trained in quality system applications. Examples of items to include in the quality system documentation are:

- Organizational chart
- Statement of intent, or goals and how these goals will be accomplished
- Statement of the responsibilities of management including the executive management, medical director, administrative laboratory director/manager, and the designated quality director
- Statement of parties that will review and approve quality policy
- Statement of parties that will review and approve the facility's quality process descriptions
- Statement of intent that an annual quality assurance summary will be prepared
- Policy documents for each of the 10 QSE
- Process and procedure documents related to quality control, quality assurance, and quality management programs
- Response plans for internal or external emergencies

A requirement specific to blood banks is the quality assurance unit described previously. The QA unit or QA oversight personnel should be involved in developing and approving all the processes implemented to achieve the 10 QSE. Additionally, data generated to document compliance with the 10 QSE often includes the QA unit in the required review and approval process, for example, equipment validation, employee training, and selection of critical suppliers. The QA unit reports directly to upper management, and in licensed firms the unit should report to the responsible head or chief executive officer (CEO). The responsible head is the designated qualified person who exercises control over all matters regarding compliance with FDA requirements and has the authority to implement corrective action and ensure that it is taken. The responsible head also ensures that personnel are appropriately assigned and trained.

CASE IN POINT (continued)

You have networked with some of the laboratory managers in the other departments. Both the microbiology and hematology managers at your laboratory have recently invested in new automation. At a customer focus meeting sponsored by your blood supplier, you meet the managers of the transfusion service laboratories at the other two hospitals in your city. The other two transfusion services are both using the same automation; your laboratory is using manual methods. You have heard about an Internet mailing list for laboratory managers from one of your mentors. You join the list and search the archives for staffing shortage and find discussions about different solutions. You decide to research transfusion medicine automation options and come up with one that you think best meets your laboratory's needs. When you update your director on what you have found, she asks you to write a business case supporting the purchase of the instrumentation. You find a template for the business case in your organization's quality manual. One of the questions on the template is how the proposal will affect human resources.

5. Can you reduce the number of employees your department requires given the following parameters? The department currently performs 30,000 procedures per year and it takes about 25 minutes to complete one procedure. The instrument you have chosen needs about 10 minutes of hands-on tech time per test. Each employee gets 4 weeks of vacation per year.

After your business case is discussed by the executive, your department receives capital funding approval to buy the instrument. Your director asks you to write a change control plan.

6. Part of your change control plan includes a training plan for all employees who will be operating the new instrument. What are some of the methods that may be used to determine initial competency in using the instrument?

Resources

The workforce is the living heart of any organization. Choosing the right people to move the gears of its operations is a key element for success. Successful personnel selection is preceded by the careful analysis of each position to determine qualification requirements, responsibilities, scheduling needs, and compensation. From this analysis, job descriptions are developed for each position. Current job descriptions defining qualifications for each position must be maintained.

The FDA and AABB require that an adequate number of individuals qualified by education, training, and/or experience are employed. Determining the correct number of workers needed can be a daunting task. Hiring too many is not cost-effective and often does not equate to increased production or quality. Hiring too few can be disastrous. A useful tool for predicting the number of employees necessary to carry out the workload in a given operation is the calculation of full-time equivalents (FTEs). Calculated FTEs combined with cost or salary data can also yield information about cost-effectiveness.

To determine FTE requirements, certain data must be gathered:

- Average employee time off per year; include, for example, vacation, sick leave, holidays, continuing education time off—usually 6 weeks
- Average work week, excluding lunch/break time—usually 40 hours
- Productivity—usually 75% or 45 minutes/hour
- Number of procedures performed/year
- Unit value for procedure—for example, time to perform in minutes

The formula and steps for calculating full-time equivalency are as follows.

The formula is: $\dfrac{A \times B}{C}$

Where:

A = Number of procedures performed per year
B = Number of minutes to complete one procedure
C = Number of productive work minutes per year

Step 1: Determine the number of procedures performed per year (A)
Step 2: Determine the number of minutes required to complete one procedure (B)
Step 3: Determine the number of productive work minutes per year

> *Step 3a* Determine the number of productive weeks worked per year, calculated by subtracting the average time off per year in weeks from 52 (the number of weeks in a year)
> *Step 3b* Determine the number of productive hours per year by multiplying the value obtained in step 3a by 40 hours/week
> *Step 3c* Determine the number of productive work minutes per year (C), calculated by multiplying the value obtained in 3b (the number of productive hours worked per year) by the average number of productive minutes in an hour (assume 45 unless otherwise told)

Step 4: Insert the determined values for A, B and C into the formula and solve. The number obtained is the number of full-time equivalency (FTE) requirement. Box 21-4 illustrates an example of an FTE calculation.

Personnel records must be maintained. Each employee should have a unique identifier code. The personnel records for employees performing or reviewing critical procedures should include names, signatures, unique identifiers, and inclusive dates of employment.[2] Training and competency records must be documented and maintained and should be stored separately from other personnel records.

BOX 21-4 Full-Time Equivalency

Example Calculation

Average time off/year:	6 weeks
Average hours/week:	40 hours
Productivity:	45 minutes/hour
Procedures/year:	1,300
Minutes to perform each:	20 minutes

Step 1: Determine the number of procedures performed per year (A)

This value is given and is 1,300 (A)

Step 2: Determine the number of minutes required to complete one procedure (B)

This value is given and is 20 minutes (B)

Step 3: Determine the number of productive work minutes per year

Step 3a Determine the number of productive weeks worked per year, calculated by subtracting the average time off per year in weeks from 52 (the number of weeks in a year)

In this example we are told that the average time off is 6 weeks. To determine the number of productive weeks worked per year, subtract 6 from 52 (weeks in a year)

The calculated value of 52 − 6 = 46 weeks

Step 3b Determine the number of productive hours per year by multiplying the value obtained in step 3a by 40 hours/week

Thus, 46 weeks/year × 40 hours/week = 1,840 hours/year

Step 3c Determine the number of productive work minutes per year (C), calculated by multiplying the value obtained in 3b (the number of productive hours worked per year) by the average number of productive minutes in an hour (assume 45 unless otherwise told)

The value obtained in step 3b is 1,840 hours/year and the average number of productive minutes in an hour is assumed at 45.

Thus, 1,840 hours/year × 45 minutes/hour = 82,800 minutes/year (C)

Step 4: Insert the determined values for A, B and C into the formula and solve. The number obtained is the number of full-time equivalency (FTE) requirement.

The formula is:

$$\frac{A \times B}{C} \quad \frac{1,300 \times 20}{82,800} = \frac{260,000}{82,800} = 3.1$$

In this case, 3.1 FTEs would be required.

Effective training programs must be developed and kept current. The QA unit should assist in developing, reviewing, and ensuring the approval of employee training. Training of employees new to the organization should include:

- New employee orientation
- cGMPs training (blood banks)
- Safety and emergency preparedness
- Operational/technical training
- Quality training
- Supervisory/managerial training, if appropriate

Training specific to the task or tasks performed is also required if:

- An employee transfers to a different department or to a new position
- A new process or procedure is introduced
- A process or procedure is substantially revised

Whereas training relates to a new employee or a new procedure, competency should be measured on an ongoing basis. Initial competency must be established and documented during training for each activity before the employee is allowed to perform the activity independently. After training is complete, employees should be part of a formal competency evaluation program that periodically assesses practical and theoretical knowledge of specific job tasks and procedures. Evaluations should include the following:

- Direct observation of performance
- Review of work sheets, QC records, preventive maintenance records, data entry records
- Written tests
- Internal blind specimens and external proficiency testing, if applicable

A system should be in place that alerts QA oversight personnel to the need for retraining. Sources that indicate problem areas may include:

- Unsatisfactory competency evaluations
- Repeated errors or deviations from procedure noted on error or accident reports
- Incorrect proficiency test results
- Complaints
- Nonconformances identified by internal audits

Thresholds for implementing retraining associated with error or unacceptable competency assessment should be established.[2]

☑ CHECKPOINT 21-4

List three instances when initial training should be undertaken.

CASE IN POINT (continued)

You have developed a validation plan for the instrument and submitted it to the laboratory's quality assurance unit for approval.

7. Into which part of your validation plan will you include each of the following examples? Your validation plan is divided into installation qualification, operational qualification, and performance qualification.

   (a) Compare ABO results from the same specimens when performing the test manually and performing the test on the instrument.
   (b) Do tachometer checks on the centrifuge that is part of the instrument.
   (c) Use the computer interface on the instrument to order antibody screen tests.

8. Your validation plan includes performing crossmatches on the instrument using patient specimens with both crossmatch-compatible and -incompatible units. Why would you intentionally include incompatible crossmatches?

Equipment

Each piece of equipment must have a unique identification. Policies, processes, and procedures must be established to ensure that calibration, maintenance, and monitoring of equipment, including computers, conform to requirements. New equipment should be qualified and validated prior to use.

The FDA defines **validation** as: "Establishing documented evidence which provides a high degree of assurance that a specific process will consistently produce a product meeting its predetermined specifications and quality attributes."[3] Validation may be prospective, concurrent, or retrospective, as defined in Table 21-3 ✶. Both new equipment, including computer hardware and software, and new processes require validation before being implemented. Validation is a series of checks, tests, and challenges that ensure the equipment and/or process function as expected. Revalidation is done whenever a validation fails, a change to a process or procedure is made, equipment is moved or repaired, or if otherwise indicated.

Many facilities develop a template for validation to ensure that necessary steps are taken. The following major steps should at a minimum be carried out to complete a prospective validation protocol:

1. Carefully evaluate, establish, and describe the specifications for the desired product. These are the expected physical and performance end product characteristics. Determine acceptance specifications, which are the limits expressed in measurable terms by which a product or service would be accepted or rejected.

2. List potential risks or factors that could result in failure or nonconformity such as potential for error, undetectable errors, excessive process variation, and insufficient process control.[9]

✷ TABLE 21-3 Validation Definitions

Type of Validation	Definition*	Circumstances
Prospective	Performed prior to equipment or process being implemented	Perform whenever possible. This is the preferred type of validation.
Concurrent	Performed during a live run	Perform when it is not feasible to challenge the equipment or process in a test environment or if the previous equipment or process can no longer be used (e.g., equipment that cannot be repaired, reagents are not available).
Retrospective	Performed after implementation	If process, or less likely, equipment was not adequately validated in the past.

*Definitions apply to both equipment validation and process validation.

3. Establish and document the validation plan. Most validation plans include the following:

- A system or process description
- Purpose, intent, or objectives, sometimes including rationale for change
- Timeline
- Risk assessment
- Responsible parties
- Validation procedures
- Acceptance criteria
- Approval signatures
- Supporting documentation

The validation plan must be reviewed and approved by the QA unit.

4. Train personnel responsible for validation activities.

5. Perform validation. Include sufficient numbers of tests to ensure reliable and statistically valid data. Use **production conditions** (conditions that will be the usual for the equipment) and **challenge conditions** (extreme conditions that could theoretically occur). Validation should be performed by people who are familiar with the process and should be performed in conditions as close to actual operating conditions as possible.

6. Record within the validation plan document or in a separate document:

- Expected and observed results
- Interpretation (acceptable or unacceptable)
- Corrective action and resolution of unexpected results
- Conclusions
- Approval signatures
- Supporting documentation
- Expected implementation date

If the validation is unsuccessful, problem identification and resolution must be carried out and revalidation performed.

7. If a revalidation is required, review and approval steps must be repeated to indicate that the revalidation documentation is complete and results are acceptable.

Three types of validation are specific for new equipment, including computer systems:

1. Installation qualification ensures that manufacturer's specifications have been met for installation within the proper environment. This should include review of calibration methods, maintenance procedures, repair parts list, and inventory. It must be demonstrated that repairs can be made without altering product quality after the repair.

2. Operational qualification establishes the equipment's capability to operate as the manufacturer intended. Installation and operational validation may be performed by supplier personnel, but must be performed on-site.

3. Performance validation provides confidence in the equipment's capability when operated by the facility's own staff under production and challenge conditions. The effectiveness and reproducibility of the process is established by repeated testing.

☑ CHECKPOINT 21-5

What are three types of validation performed on new equipment?

A documented process for monitoring and maintenance of critical equipment must be in place. Procedures should describe the frequency, method, and acceptance criteria for monitoring and maintenance of equipment. Procedures should also specify actions to be taken when unacceptable results are obtained.

Calibration is the standardization of an analytic instrument by comparison against a standard known to be accurate. Correction of error can be performed by determining deviation from the known standard and making adjustments to the instrument being calibrated. For example, a weighing scale is calibrated by weighing an object of known weight in the appropriate range for the intended use of the scale. If the scale measurement deviates from this weight beyond a predetermined specification, then adjustments or possibly repair are necessary. Calibration should be performed before initial equipment use, after activities that may affect calibration, and at prescribed intervals.

In the event of equipment malfunction or calibration failure, investigation steps should include:

- Assess the quality of products or services that may have been affected.
- Remove the equipment from service.
- Investigate the cause of malfunction or failure.
- Requalify or replace the equipment.
- Where indicated, report the problem to the manufacturer.

CASE IN POINT *(continued)*

You are reading the manufacturer's insert for the reagents that will be used on the instrument. You notice that they must be stored at 35.6–46.4° F (2–8° C). You store your reagents on clearly labeled shelves in the same refrigerators that hold your blood products. Your refrigerators are currently set up to store blood products between 33.8 and 42.8° F (1 and 6° C), however they normally run between 37.4 and 39.2° F (3 and 4° C). You decide that it is acceptable to store the reagents in the refrigerators with the current settings.

9. Is your decision correct? Why or why not?

Storage Equipment

Storage temperature is critical for blood, components, tissue, and derivatives. Therefore, there are very specific standards that apply to storage equipment. The temperature of refrigerators, freezers, and platelet incubators must be continuously monitored and recorded at least every 4 hours. The ambient temperature of open areas where blood products are kept or stored must also be recorded every 4 hours at a minimum.

Most facilities use alarms to alert staff when significant variations in refrigerator or freezer temperature occur. Alarms must be set up to activate before unacceptable temperatures are reached. In the event an alarm is activated, there must be a process for immediate investigation and corrective action. There must also be procedures for periodic quality control testing of alarms to ensure they are functioning as expected.

Computer Systems

In transfusion medicine, information technology has allowed growth, precision, speed, and information exchange that would not otherwise be possible. Before laboratory information systems (LIS) were implemented in transfusion medicine, records were kept on paper, index cards, and log books. Record keeping was laborious and lent itself to human error. Even after the advent of practical computer systems, several years passed before the technology could be adapted to the specialized needs of blood establishments.

Laboratory information systems (LIS) and computer systems found in analytic instruments are regulated as medical devices by the Center for Biologics Evaluation and Research (CBER) (Chapter 20).

Important requirements for transfusion medicine computer systems include:

- There must be complete traceability of all products derived from blood or blood components from the collection of the donor through all preparation, distribution, and testing steps to transfusion to the recipient. There must be complete traceability in the reverse from recipient bedside through all testing and manufacturing steps back to the donor. The employee performing each significant step in a process must be identified.

- The software must be thoroughly described, documented, and validated prior to marketing.

- The system, including software, hardware, databases, user-defined tables, and electronic data transfer and receipt, must be described, documented, challenge-tested, and validated in the location where it will be used prior to implementation. Validation records must be maintained.

- There must be documented description of the system maintenance and operation.

- Users must be trained in the operation of the system prior to its use.

- The system must be secure from unauthorized access and must protect the confidentiality of donors and recipients.

- Critical data integrity must be monitored.

- There must be a plan that addresses computer downtime and alternate procedures during such periods.

- Information stored in the system must be backed up in the event data is lost in an unexpected event or during downtime. There must be a documented plan for disaster recovery.

- A process addressing system modification, authorization, and documentation must be in place.

- Personnel responsible for system management are responsible for compliance with applicable regulations.

Supplier and Customer Issues

There should be a defined process for evaluation, selection, and approval of suppliers of critical materials, equipment, and services. Supplier and customer expectations should be defined in a written agreement.

If a blood bank or transfusion service is referring specimens or products to another laboratory for testing, the referral laboratory must meet all required accreditations, certifications, and registrations. In the United States, depending on the service being provided, this can include accreditation by the AABB or an equivalent agency, CLIA certification, or FDA registration.

Blood, tissue products, critical reagents, and materials must be inspected upon receipt and tested as necessary. Collection sets, storage containers, and labels must be inspected to ensure they meet specifications. Receipt of all products and materials must be documented. In the United States, FDA criteria must be met for all containers, solutions, and reagents.

Customers can be defined as anyone who is affected by your processes; generally, customers are divided into internal customers, which include departments and employees within your organization, and external customers, which are the organizations and people who use your product or service. Customer satisfaction data can be gathered by direct communication initiated by the customer, both complaints and compliments, and by conducting anonymous or customer-specific surveys. *Root-cause analysis*, described later in this chapter, of frequent or significant complaints can help prevent recurrences. Frequent review of customer feedback can help an organization recognize the need for change before problems arise. Timely response to feedback lets customers know the organization is attentive to their needs.

☑ CHECKPOINT 21-6

What is the definition of a customer?

Process Control

Processes and products will vary to some degree due to variation of many factors such as reagents, operator technique, and resource materials. The expected outcome of processes must be pre-established in order for personnel to recognize when the process is not functioning as expected. The established, expected outcome may be determined by the manufacturer of a test kit, by regulating agencies, by validation testing, or by data collection.

Process controls are activities or tools used to create a controlled environment for processes and procedures, to standardize processes, or to monitor process outcome. The goal of process controls is to produce a predictable outcome.[2] Many quality activities are process controls. Process controls related to analytic testing, such as quality control and proficiency testing, are similar in transfusion medicine and other medical laboratory disciplines. Process controls in transfusion medicine related to component preparation, such as end labeling and sterility checks, are similar to pharmaceutical requirements.

A primary responsibility of the QA unit is to ensure that written procedures are in place that will adequately instruct employees in operational and quality assurance functions. Additionally, the QA unit monitors that the procedures are effectively carried out. Standard operating procedures (SOP) are discussed later in this chapter. Procedures and processes must be validated before implementation and when substantial changes occur. Process validation is very similar to equipment validation and was discussed previously.

CASE IN POINT (continued)

The instrument you are implementing requires anticoagulated specimens. The manufacturer has validated EDTA as well as the common anticoagulants used in donor units (e.g., ACD). Currently, you test-clotted specimens with your manual method.

10. When you are writing your communication plan, who might you need to notify about the change in patient specimen type?

Your new instrument will be interfaced to your laboratory information system (LIS). During your validation of the LIS interface, you discover that many of your current patient specimen barcodes are having barcode reading errors because the barcodes are not always smooth and not always placed vertically on the specimens.

11. Can you think of some ways that you can address the barcode labeling problems before you complete implementation of the instrument (i.e., before your go-live date)?

Change Control

Change is inevitable and quality systems must not only anticipate change but also control changes in such a way that product quality and safety are not adversely affected. Change may be precipitated by either internal or external factors; examples are listed in Table 21-4 ✳.

The change control process begins even before a change occurs. First, there should be a system that monitors external and internal factors to anticipate change. Then, once a need for change is identified, impacts should be assessed. Assessment can include:

• Timing and resources needed for training
• Laboratory information system maintenance required
• Effect on other departments, for example, when processes interact
• Notification of outside agencies

A communication plan to both external and internal customers is vital. Internally, this allows all affected operations time to assess the impact and make suitable plans. Internal communication may be as simple as a change notification form, which outlines the change and allows for collection of managers' opinions. Externally, some notifications may be required; examples include FDA and/or accreditation agencies. Timely notifications to customers are important for maintaining good customer relations. Additionally, when the change affects component production, the external customer may need lead time to affect their own change control. For example, a transfusion service, as a customer of a blood bank, may need to change their LIS to accommodate an ISBT code for a new product or they may need to educate their clinical staff on appropriate usage of the new or changed product.

Proficiency Testing

Proficiency testing (PT), a program designed to ensure that laboratorians have mastered the skills and tasks related to processing, performing, and interpreting accurate laboratory tests, is required by most accrediting agencies and in the United States is conducted through CMS or by a CMS-approved agency, such as the CAP proficiency program (Chapter 20). As discussed previously, the PT program is part of competency evaluation of personnel and monitoring of equipment performance.

Proficiency testing must be done for each analyte tested by the facility. If no PT program exists for an analyte, CLIA regulations require that there be a method to verify the accuracy of the test performance by other means at least twice annually.[5]

When PT samples are received, the survey kit should be immediately opened and inspected for damage. The supplier should be

✳ **TABLE 21-4** Stimulus for Change

External Factor Examples	Internal Factor Examples
• Regulation or accreditation standard change	• Department or personnel reorganization
• Shift in customer needs or expectations	• Adoption of a new quality philosophy
• Emerging diseases	• New instrumentation
• New product development	

contacted for replacement if necessary. Receipt of the kit should be recorded. The supervisor should assign laboratory staff to perform the testing on a rotating basis or as appropriate. PT should be performed during routine test runs, handling the PT samples as routine specimens. If possible, it should include alternate or back-up methods such as manual and stat testing. Samples for PT should not be tested in duplicate unless it is standard operating procedure to run specimens in duplicate, or unless there is failure in testing or equipment. Results should be recorded in the same manner as routine specimens, if possible; for example, on a routine paper worksheet or in the LIS. If the LIS cannot support recording of PT sample results, the PT program offers an excellent opportunity to assess the downtime procedure, including forms used for documentation during downtime.

In some laboratories, especially if the normal workflow includes a supervisory review of some or all results, the supervisor is responsible for reviewing results and recording them on the provided survey forms or entering them in the electronic survey form. The laboratory manager or director may also review the worksheets and survey form. After appropriate review and signatures, the completed survey form is submitted to the PT program for evaluation. In other laboratories, especially where supervisory review is not part of the path of routine specimen testing, the person performing the tests transfers the results to the appropriate format for submission to the PT program.

In either case, the evaluation summary provided by the PT program supplier must be reviewed by the supervisor and the QA unit. The review must be documented. Some laboratories will also incorporate manager, director, or other levels of review of PT performance into their quality management policies. PT results should be carefully analyzed for trends that could indicate problems. There should be a written plan for remedial action when PT is unsuccessful. Investigation and corrective action taken must be documented. The QA unit should monitor the PT program and ensure that appropriate corrective action, if necessary, has been taken.

Laboratories are prohibited from discussing PT sample results or from sending PT samples to another laboratory for testing, even if that discussion or transfer of samples would be a part of the path of routine specimens. These same prohibitions apply to laboratories that are part of the same organization. This is the one clear exception to the rule that PT samples should be treated in the same manner as routine specimens. Once the PT program has issued the evaluation summary, then discussions or retesting may occur as part of corrective or preventive action, if required.

In addition to external PT, laboratories can make internal PT samples derived from donor or patient blood specimens. These can be tested as unannounced, blind PT or may be announced to staff as internal PT.

Quality Control

Quality controls (QC) are the day-to-day activities and testing done to ensure that equipment, reagents, and materials specific to a procedure are functioning as expected and that the method was performed correctly. For analytic procedures, QC solutions with an expected result range are tested by the same method as the patient or donor specimens. QC is also routinely performed by testing a specified number of each type of manufactured components and products to ensure that they meet the regulatory and accreditation specifications.

Acceptable results or ranges for QC must be predetermined, usually by the kit or reagent manufacturer, by regulation or accrediting agencies and sometimes by internal data. Personnel performing QC must be aware of acceptable results or ranges so they will know when a procedure is out of control and take appropriate steps for correction. Unacceptable QC results may warrant immediate investigation, usually before continuing the process. Results of the investigation and corrective action must be documented. The frequency and method for performance of QC is determined by the manufacturer's requirements and/or regulatory or accreditation requirements. Most laboratory personnel are familiar with QC required to ensure an analytical process or instrument is performing correctly. In transfusion medicine, there is the additional QC of the component preparation; for example, residual white blood cell count in leukoreduced units, hemoglobin levels in apheresis red blood cell units, and bacterial detection of platelet units (Chapter 10).

QC results must be documented immediately after QC is performed or concurrently. Documentation must include:

- QC date
- Identification of individual performing QC
- Identification of reagent, material, or component, including manufacturer and lot number
- Expiration date of above
- Identification of equipment
- Results and interpretation
- Corrective action for unacceptable results

QC results are often plotted on a chart, as illustrated in Figure 21-5 ■. The visual representation of repetitive data can make shifts, spikes, trends, and other patterns more apparent to staff members. Investigation and correction can sometimes occur before a process goes out of control because a shift or trend away from desirable

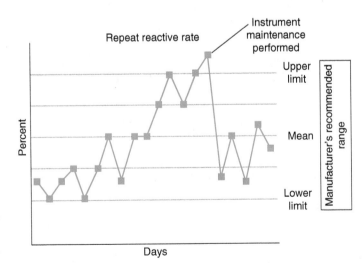

■ **FIGURE 21-5**   Example Control Chart

The repeat reactivity rate for infectious disease testing illustrates an upward shift over several days. When the rate went above recommended levels, unscheduled maintenance was performed, which corrected the problem.

performance was detected early. QC results, error rate, deferral rate, infectious disease test reactivity rate, and product wastage are examples of data that can be collected and mapped by charts.

Supervisory staff should frequently review and monitor QC documentation. The QA unit is responsible for auditing QC records for completeness and performance according to requirements. Regulatory and accreditation requirements determine the length of time that QC records must be retained.

Current Good Manufacturing Practices

Regulations require that current good manufacturing practices (cGMPs) be applied to the manufacture of blood components and plasma protein products (Chapter 20). cGMPs is a form of process control that was developed in the pharmaceutical industry and is now applied to blood banks.

A blood bank example of cGMPs would be the process controls that are instituted to limit the ability of staff members to make an error when affixing the end label to a blood product. Some commonly applied controls in this area include:

- Spatially separating the labeling area from other blood component preparation areas

- Physically segregating blood components that are at different steps along the testing and manufacturing process

- Automating steps that are particularly prone to human error; for example, using scanners to record numbers or check labels

- Requiring multiple independent reviews before the product is released; for example, two reviews happening at different times and/or two reviews conducted by different individuals

CASE IN POINT *(continued)*

You are writing the procedures for the new instrument.

12. What are some examples of the procedures that you might need?
13. How could you validate the procedures?

Documents and Records

Documentation is central to transfusion medicine activities. A document may be any type of recorded and approved information. Table 21-5 ✳ lists some common definitions of document terms and both quality system and operational examples.

Document Control

Document control is a system that standardizes facility documents; ensures that only approved, current documents are in use; and protects documents from unauthorized access or modification. Elements of document control include:

- Current master list of documents, including policies, processes, procedures, labels, and forms

- Standardized format for policies, processes, and procedures

CASE IN POINT *(continued)*

Your new instrument has been up and running for 3 months. A patient experiences a suspected transfusion reaction. Your new procedures specify that employees perform manual methods to check the ABO group and Rh(D) type during a transfusion reaction investigation, in addition to running the specimens on the instrument. Both the pre- and post-transfusion specimens on the patient type as group O by both methods. The ABO confirmation on the donor unit types as group O on the instrument but as a weak positive with anti-A when tested manually. Further investigation reveals that the donor is a weak subgroup of A.

14. If the unit came from an external blood supplier, when should you notify them and why?
15. Should this event be reported to the FDA?
16. What other actions might you consider?

- Documented review and approval of new and revised documents before use

- Periodic documented review of policies, processes, procedures, and associated forms by an authorized individual; some accreditation agencies require annual review

- Distribution of new or revised documents to all areas that require the information

- Removal of obsolete documents from all areas

- Retention of obsolete documents for length of time required by regulation and accreditation

Document control systems may be electronic or hard copy based. Copying of controlled documents in whole or in part should be discouraged to ensure that only current information is being used. If it is necessary to copy a controlled document, the copy should be marked as uncontrolled with an expiration date and should be destroyed after expiration.

Standard Operating Procedures

Standard operating procedures (SOPs) should be written in language that can be easily understood and followed by workers. All critical steps must be included, but excessive detail is unnecessary and can cause confusion. The SOP does not have to be a text document. For example, it can be a flowchart, as long as the formatting of the document is consistent with organizational standards. A flowchart is a pictorial representation of a process or procedure that can help readers visualize the sequence of steps. A well-constructed flowchart can improve clarity and establish boundaries. Flowcharts may be used alone or as a supplement to a text-based procedure or process.

SOPs often include the following:

- Title and, if required by document control system, an identification number

- Date of implementation

✳ **TABLE 21-5** Document Definitions and Examples

Document Type	Definition	FDA Equivalent Term	Quality System Example*	Operational Example*
Policy	What will be done[10]: Principle that guides decision making[2]		All staff will be trained in new procedures prior to the procedure being implemented	Issue group O red blood cells until two ABO group determinations have been made on specimens collected at different times
Process	How it will happen[10]: set of related steps that achieve a goal[2]; often involves multiple departments; often captured in a flowchart	Critical control point**	1. Operational manager implements internal change communication plan 2. Operational unit develops standard operating procedure (SOP), training plan, and procedure validation plan 3. QA unit reviews SOP and plans 4. Operational unit executes procedure validation and training plans 5. QA unit reviews validation and training documents and enter SOP in the document control system 6. Medical director approves SOP 7. QA unit executes communication plan for external stakeholders 8. Operational unit implements new SOP	1. Phlebotomy or nursing staff collect pretransfusion testing specimens 2. Laboratory staff check historical records and record results 3. If no previous ABO group recorded, laboratory staff requests a second collection 4. Laboratory staff performs ABO/Rh on first specimen 5. Laboratory staff issues group O red blood cell units if second specimen is required and not yet tested 6. Laboratory staff perform ABO/Rh on second specimen, if required
Procedure	How to do it[10]: series of tasks performed by one person[2] at one time; often each step in a process with have one or more associated procedures	Key element***	1. Review manufacturers' instructions 2. Open electronic copy of SOP template 3. Insert relevant information and delete unnecessary headings 4. Save as draft SOP 5. Send draft SOP to medical director and QA	1. Inspect ABORH gel card 2. Label ABORH gel card 3. Make cell suspension of patient red blood cells 4. Add plasma and cells to appropriate microtubule well 5. Centrifuge 6. Read results 7. Enter results in laboratory information system
Form	Document used to record data		SOP template; new SOP approval form	Downtime form for manual pretransfusion testing results
Record	Results[10]: Information that provides objective evidence that an activity was completed or a result achieved[2]		Completed SOP approval form with all required signatures	ABO/Rh results in laboratory information system; ABO/Rh results written on downtime form

*Examples are simplified

**Critical control point = steps where failure or loss of control could have an adverse effect on the quality of the finished product and could result in a health risk.[3]

***Key element = individual steps or procedures that if not performed properly could affect the safety and quality of the product or service.[3]

- Current version number or latest revision/review date
- Intent or purpose
- Scope or people responsible for completing the steps
- List of required materials and equipment
- Detailed instructions including calculations
- Documentation requirements and, if applicable, result reporting steps
- References
- Author's or owner's identity
- Identity and signature of approver
- Revision history

☑ **CHECKPOINT 21-7**

What does the acronym SOP mean?

Record Retention

Facilities must comply with all regulatory and accreditation record retention requirements. Some transfusion records must be stored indefinitely; others have a minimum retention period. Many records and documents are stored electronically. If so, there must be a method for backing up all critical data. Back-up data files must be stored offsite. Computerized data integrity must be monitored.

Deviations, Nonconformances, and Adverse Events

Proactive error prevention should be the focus of the quality program. It is inevitable, however, that errors will happen and the quality program should also include processes to detect, evaluate, investigate, and correct errors and accidents. Regulators and accreditation organizations can use similar terms with overlapping definitions when talking about errors. Table 21-6 ✳ lists definitions of error terminology commonly used in blood banks and transfusion services. The term **event** (an unexpected or unintended incident or occurrence related to a process, procedure, or service) is often used as an overarching term that includes errors, accidents, nonconformances, deviations, and complaints.

Product Deviations

Nonconforming products must be quarantined until a determination of the effect of the nonconformance on product quality has been made. If a nonconforming product has been distributed, the blood bank should attempt to **recall** (withdraw a distributed product that has been determined to be unsuitable) the product. Recalls may also be instigated by the FDA (Chapter 20). Even if a unit has already been transfused, the blood bank should still notify the **consignee** (the person who accepted shipment of the blood product) when a nonconforming product is discovered. Transfusion services that distribute to other facilities or that further manipulate blood products must also monitor and report nonconforming products. In the United States, the facility must also complete an FDA biological product deviation report (BPDR) if the safety, purity, or potency of a distributed product may have been affected (Chapter 20).[11] If a facility retrieves a product for a reason unrelated to a violation or for a minor violation that is not subject to legal action by the FDA, this action is called a **market withdrawal**.

> ## ☑ CHECKPOINT 21-8
>
> According to FDA guidelines, under what circumstances must a biological product deviation (BPD) be reported?

Unusual needs of a patient may dictate purposeful deviation from policies or procedures. For example, granulocytes collected by apheresis method for severely neutropenic patients may have to be released prior to completion of infectious disease testing because

✳ TABLE 21-6 Types of Events

Term	Definition	Blood Bank* Example	Transfusion Service** Example
Error	Deviation from cGMPs, applicable regulation, applicable standards, or established specifications	Stock of obsolete labels is discovered in the back of a shelf in the room set aside for final labeling of products	Rh (D)-positive red blood cell unit is issued and transfused to an Rh (D)-negative woman of childbearing age with no prior approval from medical director when this contradicts the facility's written policy
Accident	Unexpected or unforeseeable adverse events	Donor who meets all eligibility criteria suffers a seizure during donation	Transfusion recipient experiences a transfusion-related acute lung injury (TRALI)
Deviation	Departure from policies, processes, procedures, applicable regulations, standards, or specifications	Investigation into a batch of products that failed QC discovers that the processing personnel adjusted centrifuge settings to below optimal relative centrifugal force specified in the standard operating procedure	Investigation into a proficiency test failure discovers that the testing personnel did not incubate antibody screen for the minimum amount of time specified in the standard operating procedure
Biological product deviation	Event that affected the safety, purity, or potency of a distributed product; must be reported to the FDA	Bacterial detection system exhibits bacterial growth after a platelet unit was issued to the transfusion service	Transfusion service irradiates a unit, applies a new label with an incorrect expiration date, and issues the unit after the correct expiration date
Nonconformance	Failure to meet requirements; often specific to an accreditation assessment	During a routine inspection, FDA inspector discovers that monthly QC testing on manufactured platelets was outside limits and was not investigated on two different occasions	AABB accreditor reports that multiple procedures do not have medical director approval documented
Adverse event	Unexpected complication in a donor or patient that occurs in relation to donation, transfusion, diagnostic, or therapeutic procedure	Donor faints upon standing up after whole blood donation	Recipient experiences symptoms of a suspected immediate hemolytic transfusion reaction
Complaint	A statement of discontent made by an external or internal customer	Transfusion service states that an emergency blood shipment ordered after hours did not arrive within the time established in the customer agreement	Operating room states that plasma units were issued when platelet units were ordered

*Blood Bank refers to a blood collection and processing center.

**Transfusion Service refers to the laboratory area responsible for pre-transfusion testing and blood product distribution (typically located in a hospital).

the product expires in 24 hours. Exceptions such as this should be planned and approved in advance by the medical director. The medical director should be consulted to review circumstances and approve each case. Special considerations for patient safety should be a part of the planning, such as choosing a repeat donor as opposed to a first-time donor for this procedure. The patient must be informed of additional risks. In this example, test results would be reported to the transfusion service as soon as completed.

Donor or Recipient Adverse Events

Collection staff must be educated to recognize and respond to adverse events related to donation (Chapter 9). These events must be documented, evaluated, and monitored. Follow-up on the donor should be carried out. Data from donor adverse events should be assessed and evaluated for trends and possible methods to reduce occurrence.

Similarly, nursing and other clinical staff members who are administering blood products must be trained to recognize potential reactions in transfusion recipients (Chapter 12). The transfusion service should be notified if the adverse reaction resulted in discontinuance of the transfusion. Immediate investigation is done to rule out the possibility of immediate hemolytic transfusion reactions. Further investigation may be performed to identify the type of reaction that occurred. If it is suspected the event is related to a donor or manufacturing process, such as suspected bacterial contamination, transfusion-related acute lung injury (TRALI), or transfusion-associated infection, the transfusion service must report the event to the collection facility. Identifying information for administered components should be submitted that will allow the collection facility to investigate possible sources.

Electronic or paper forms should be developed to capture the details of an adverse event when it occurs to ensure that the information needed during the investigation is available. The investigation and corrective action steps may be included on the same form or may be documented elsewhere, but should be formally captured to ensure that all steps were completed. For example, an adverse event form could include:

- Identity of individuals involved in the event and its investigation
- Description of the event
- Location, date, and time of event
- Component number(s) and volume involved
- Donor/patient identification
- Donor/patient signs and symptoms
- Treatment or actions taken
- Donor/patient outcome
- Investigation results
- Follow-up and corrective actions
- Notification to other facilities or agencies

Fatalities of either donors or recipients that are confirmed to be related to the donation or transfusion must be reported to CBER as soon as possible (Chapter 20).

Traceback and Lookback

Transfusion-transmitted infections (Chapter 13) can result in immediate reactions (Chapter 12) or infections that are not detected for months or even years. Transfusion of bacterially contaminated products usually produces an immediate reaction. Investigation includes ruling out other causes of the symptoms, culturing the remaining blood product, and culturing a post-transfusion blood specimen from the recipient. Transfusion services must report suspected bacterial contamination to the collection facility as soon as possible to facilitate immediate quarantine of other products from the same collection. The notification process should not wait for culture results but should occur when the transfusion service identifies that the recipient's symptoms are consistent with exposure to bacteria or bacterial toxins. The culture results are used to confirm or rule out a case of bacterially contaminated product and to decide the final disposition of any quarantined products. Genotyping of any bacteria cultured from the recipient and the blood product can be used in complex cases to confirm or rule out bacterial contamination; for example:

- Patients, such as those in intensive care, who have infections with multiple organisms.
- Patients, such as those who are postoperative, who may have experienced multiple potential exposure points to the implicated organism.
- Organism growth patterns in the remaining blood product that are consistent with testing laboratory contamination.

Conversely, many viral infections do not cause symptoms in the recipient until months or years after the causative transfusion. If a transfusion recipient notifies the transfusion service or blood bank that he has developed a viral infection and suspects it is related to transfusion, an investigation to identify and test all the donors implicated in his treatment will occur. This investigation is often called a **traceback**. If one or more donors are found to currently be carriers of the same virus, this can trigger a lookback. A **lookback** is the process to track the disposition of blood products from previous donations when supplemental or confirmatory tests on a donor are positive for anti-HIV, anti-HCV, or anti–*Trypanosoma cruzi* (Chagas disease–causing parasite). The lookback often does not originate from a recipient complaint, but rather as a result of testing when a donor returns to donate again.

A primary intention of the lookback process is to notify all blood recipients that he or she may be at risk for exposure to infectious disease. The recipient and physician can then determine if the recipient should be tested. The second intent is to retrieve and prevent further distribution of the donor's other in-date products. Figures 21-6 ■ and 21-7 ■ illustrate two relatively simple lookback examples; obviously tracebacks that begin with a multiply transfused recipient or lookbacks that begin with a donor who has made multiple previous donations can be very complex, involve many different facilities, and affect many people.

Regulations specify which screening tests trigger quarantine and notification processes as well as the timelines that need to be met to complete quarantine and notifications. The span of time that prior donations need to be identified and investigated is also determined by regulation; for certain organisms it is all donations for which there are records. Notification of recipients is not required or desired in all cases, but is always required for hepatitis C, HIV, and *T. cruzi* (Chagas disease). Confirmatory testing may be negative when the initial screening test was positive. Test methods with a high sensitivity are explicitly chosen for initial screening to limit the number of false-negative results; test methods that are highly sensitive usually are less

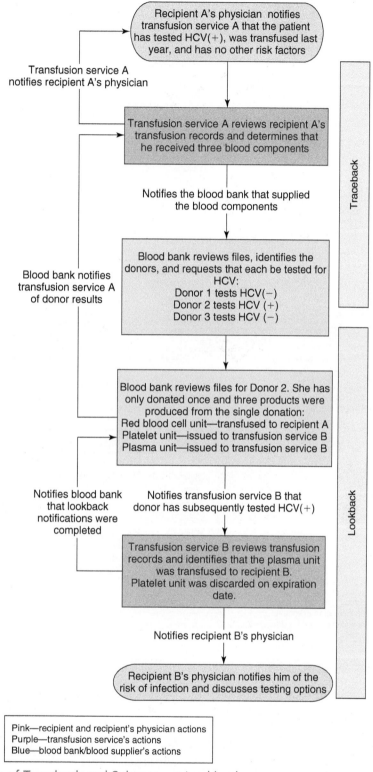

FIGURE 21-6 Example of Traceback and Subsequent Lookback

specific and a certain number of false-positive results are expected. Regulatory and accrediting agencies publish algorithms that define when it may be acceptable to release a previously quarantined product for transfusion or to return a previously deferred donor back to qualified status. The latter is called *donor reentry*. If confirmatory testing is not performed, the quarantined products are always discarded.

If a transfusion service confirms or suspects that a TRALI reaction has occurred (Chapter 12), they should immediately notify their blood supplier. A process similar to a traceback is used to identify potential donors implicated in causing the TRALI. In-date products from any implicated donors should be quarantined during the investigation. Testing for antibodies to human

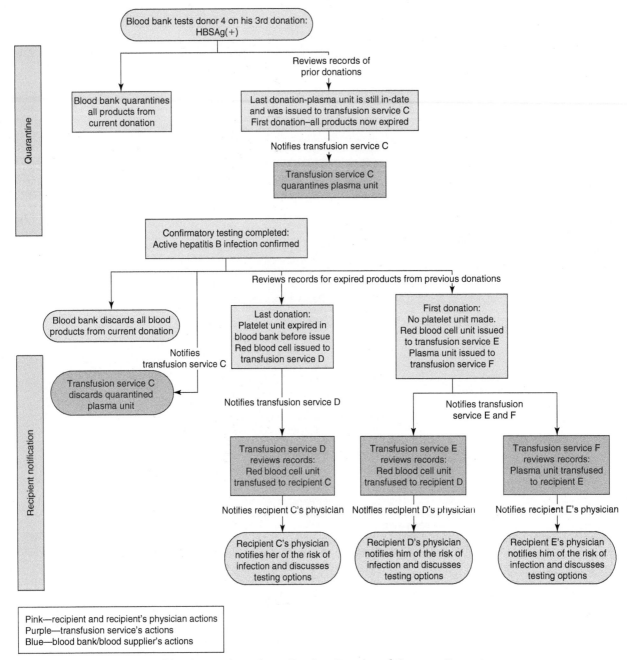

leukocyte antigens (HLA) and/or human neutrophil antigens (HNA) may be performed to help decide if the quarantined products can be released for transfusion and if the implicated donor or donors should be deferred in the future. Many countries, including the United States, have proactively reduced the risk of TRALI by minimizing the preparation of high-plasma-volume components from donors known to be or at increased risk of being leukocyte alloimmunized.[12]

Internal and External Assessments

Assessments try to find objective evidence that policies, processes, and procedures are being followed and are achieving the intended results, including consistently high quality. Conversely, by finding evidence of nonconformance or ineffectiveness, assessments highlight areas where quality initiatives would be most effective.

Internal Audits

Internal audits conducted by the QA unit or others within the same organization are among the most valuable tools in assessing the organization's quality system. Internal audits should be viewed as an opportunity for improvement and should not be punitive in nature. Each facility should have written audit policies and procedures. Audits are planned and performed periodically to assess the effectiveness of the total quality system and to assess the quality system of each operation. Auditing should be planned and scheduled so that the entire system can be assessed at least annually. All audits should begin with an audit plan, which includes:

- The name of the system being audited
- The name of the auditor or audit team
- The purpose and scope of the audit
- The standard used for the audit
- The audit date and schedule

A copy of the audit plan is sent to the management of the system to be audited. Procedures should be established to guide the assessor in the audit and ensure that important aspects of the audit are not left out. A common practice is the development and use of checklists for this purpose. The auditor should have the knowledge, training, and experience to identify problems in the system being audited. The audit should include a review of the following:

- Training and competency records
- Critical control point and key element performance and documentation
- Quality control, calibration, and equipment maintenance records
- Completed records and worksheets
- Facility and storage areas

Process flow and lean audits can also include direct observation of tasks being performed.

The auditor should review an appropriate number of records to effectively evaluate each system. Actual procedure performance should be compared to SOP documents. If nonconformances or areas of concern were observed on a previous audit, careful review of these areas should be made to assess the effectiveness of corrective and preventive actions.

When the assessment is finished, the auditor must prepare a written summary of the audit findings:

- Name of the system being audited
- Date of the audit
- Auditor's name
- Scope of the audit—broad scope of an entire system or narrow scope focusing on a single process
- Auditor's observations, such as nonconformances or deviations from SOP and distinguishing minor and major observations

A copy of the audit is provided to the manager of the system being audited and should be reviewed and discussed with the auditor. The system manager should be provided an opportunity to discuss items of disagreement on the audit report before the final report is prepared. Upon receipt of the final report, the system manager is provided a timeline for preparation of a response. The report is retained consistent with record requirements.

Managers or supervisors in the area being audited are responsible for reviewing and addressing each observation and providing a written response for corrective action, including the date corrective measures will be complete. The QA unit should follow up to make certain these measures are effective and have been completed in a timely manner. To ensure that upper management is aware of problem areas and that measures to rectify them are planned, executive management is required to review and evaluate audit summary reports and written responses to deficiency observations.

Different types of audits can be developed targeting specific processes, products, or systems.

Process audits are particularly effective in spotting errors that may be overlooked by routine record review. A process audit begins by selecting at random a predetermined number of end products produced from the process one wishes to evaluate. The audit traces the entire process from beginning to end for each of the selected products, focusing on records produced by each step of manufacture to determine adherence to policies and procedures. For example, a repeat-reactive process audit traces each step and all records created for a unit found to be repeatedly reactive with an infectious disease test. Records are reviewed from collection, processing, testing, quarantine, and lookback, if applicable, to final disposition, discard, and donor notification, if applicable. In a transfusion service, a process audit may follow a request for a blood product for a neonate from the time of request through to the transfusion of the requested product. Process audits can assess the effectiveness of relationships among different systems or departments when they must interact at different points along the process.

Product audits assess a particular product and can include assessment of customer survey results, *quality indicator* data, and complaint records. A product audit addressing product utilization would yield information useful for the blood utilization or hospital transfusion committee.

Self-audits can be performed for systems, processes, products, or services. A system can be self-audited using checklists developed internally or by using checklists obtained from external assessment agencies. Self-audits are effective in maintaining inspection readiness in a given area.

Blood-utilization monitoring is a type of audit specific to transfusion services. Accreditation agencies require a peer review of transfusion practices within health care facilities. This is usually accomplished by formation of a committee, preferably composed of professionals working in different disciplines involved in the transfusion process, such as nurses, surgeons, transfusion service managers, medical directors, risk management, and quality assurance personnel. Since transfusion is a practice with known risk, a primary purpose of the peer-review committee is improving transfusion safety. Appropriate blood utilization is a key factor in limiting risk by ensuring that patients do not receive unnecessary transfusions and conversely that patients receive blood products when needed. The committee assists in the development of transfusion practice policies for the facility, which must be reviewed and approved by the medical director. The transfusion committee is responsible for developing blood-utilization guidelines. Criteria and methods for monitoring and auditing blood usage should be included in the guidelines.

The blood-utilization review committee should monitor the following areas:

- Ordering practices
- Patient identification
- Sample collection and labeling
- Adverse events

- Sentinel and *near-miss events* (defined later in the "Corrective and Preventive Action" section)
- Administration and discard
- Blood wastage
- Transfusion policies
- Supplier issues

Information learned from data collection and audits should be utilized to determine the effectiveness of the facility's transfusion practices in meeting the needs of patients. The committee should meet regularly to discuss safety issues, quality indicator monitoring results, audit results, and other forms of assessment. Information learned from audits and error reports should be addressed with appropriate personnel for corrective and preventive actions. Feedback from the committee should be provided to medical staff in a continual effort toward process improvement.

☑ CHECKPOINT 21-9

List three specific types of internal audits.

External Assessments

External assessments provide objective insight from individuals outside the organization. These assessments are conducted by regulating and accrediting agencies (Chapter 20). Inspectors can bring new perspectives to the organization regarding quality practice and industry standards. Organizations usually identify individuals, usually QA unit members or supervisors familiar with the system being audited, who will accompany the inspector while on-site. Records should be readily available for the inspector. All employees should be aware that inspectors may ask front-line staff questions and/or directly observe their work performance. Internal audits can help employees become familiar with the types of questions asked by assessors.

CASE IN POINT (continued)

You decide to monitor the number of barcode reading errors on a monthly basis as a quality indicator to assess how well your education and communication efforts during the validation worked. The first month's data showed a high number of errors. Then the number of errors dropped significantly as your employees distributed communication targeted to the collectors involved in labeling the specimens with barcode errors. The error rate remained steady and low for the next 4 months. In the following 4 months you have noticed a slow but steady rise in the number of barcode reading errors.

17. What is the pattern that you noted on your quality indicator data called?
18. What might you do next?

Corrective and Preventive Action

Corrective action occurs in response to a reported event, has a goal of preventing recurrence of the event, and is reactive. Preventive action occurs in response to an identified potential for error, prevents an event from happening, and is proactive. In both cases, action starts with data collection and active surveillance systems. Box 21-5 lists examples of data that should be collected, reviewed, and analyzed.

BOX 21-5 Data Collection

Examples
- Quality control results
- Proficiency testing results
- Validation results
- Postdonation information
- Internal audit reports
- External assessment reports
- Competency assessment reports
- Event/error/occurrence/incident management system reports
- Customer survey results
- Customer complaints
- Quality indicator monitoring reports

Event management systems should detect, identify, and capture information about both errors and near-miss events. **Near-miss events** are unexpected occurrences where an error was identified and corrected before a patient or product was adversely affected. As with other quality systems, while the QA unit may have the primary responsibility for reviewing the data collected by an event management system, all employees should participate in reporting events and near-misses. The reporting system should be nonpunitive to encourage employees to report all incidents. Event management systems usually use standardized forms, either paper or electronic, to capture the essential data around an event:

- Date, time, and location of the event
- People involved
- Description of the event
- Initial corrective actions taken

If the blood bank or transfusion service is part of a larger organization and is using a common event reporting system (e.g., laboratory-wide or hospital-wide), either the reporting form should include places for transfusion-specific data or there should be procedures for where transfusion-specific data will be recorded. For example:

- Product-specific data or actions such as quarantine or recall of the product involved in the incident or of related products; notification of the blood supplier, consignee, and/or FDA.
- Donor-specific data or actions such as future deferral, notification, and/or follow-up testing.

Postdonation information (information learned from the donor or a third party that was unknown or not disclosed at the time of the donation) may either be captured using the same event form or may be captured in a separate, parallel system. Postdonation information is not usually an error unless it resulted from a deviation in policy or procedure, but it may generate similar corrective and preventive actions.

Quality indicators are measureable facets of a process or data collected as a result of a process or service. Each system in an organization should identify quality indicators that can be used to evaluate the effectiveness of the system. Thresholds (acceptable or unacceptable limit) for each quality indicator should be established. Thresholds are determined from regulatory or accreditation requirements, industry standards, or data derived internally. Quality indicator data is collected over a defined period of time and periodically reported. Examples of common quality indicators include:

- Turnaround time between specimen check-in to test completion
- Number of specimens labeled incorrectly and rejected by the laboratory
- Number of incomplete donor records
- Number of donor adverse reactions

New indicators can be added as necessary or if monitoring a different phase of a particular process is desired. Occasionally, a quality indicator can be removed from being monitored if the data has been stable and above the threshold for a long period of time.

Data from different sources and different systems should be analyzed together. By tracking information from the entire organization, the QA unit can see the larger picture, whereas individual system managers may not. For example, the same error could be made in several different departments and might be seen as a random error by individual managers, but when the information is brought together it can be seen as a recurring error, possibly having a common, systemic cause. Data analysis often involves identifying trends, shifts, spikes, or other patterns. Patterns can help identify system weaknesses and opportunities for processes improvements, often before the process goes out of control. Charts and graphs as illustrated in Figure 21-8 ▦ are often used to visualize large amounts of data, making patterns easier to identify.

Root-cause analysis, defined as systematic process designed to determine the flaw at the cores of a problem, is a powerful tool to prevent error recurrence. Sometimes the cause of an error is apparent and easily fixed. For example, quality control results are beyond acceptable limits and when the employee investigates, it is discovered that the test was run using expired reagents. Other times what can be seen on the surface is not really the cause. What if errors caused by expired reagent usage were occurring over and over again or

suddenly spiked? Maybe there are systemic factors that need to be considered, for example, supply chain problems resulting in delays in receiving in-date reagents, storage practices that make it difficult to find in-date reagents, or changes in manufacturer labels causing employees to misread the expiration date. There could be multiple errors that cause an event and some errors may be masked by others. In order to truly correct a problem and bring a process back in line, the *root cause* (flaw at the core of the problem) must be found and corrected.

There are many root-cause analysis methods, but most take time and effort. Not every event needs to be subjected to a full root-cause analysis. An error that is not repeated and that has an obvious solution will not necessarily benefit from root-cause analysis. Conversely, data analysis as described earlier, is often used to identify situations where in-depth investigation will be most beneficial. For example:

- Most common events
- Events with serious consequences
- Sudden increase in a particular type of event
- Alteration in event pattern after implementation of a process change

Organizations or departments within an organization may also periodically target a particular quality indicator as a focus for continuous improvement. **Sentinel events** (events resulting in a donor or patient experiencing a fatal, life-threatening, or serious adverse outcome or where there was potential for such an outcome to occur) should be flagged and acted on immediately. Additionally, sentinel events or near-miss events that could have had similar outcomes often trigger a root-cause analysis.

Two common root-cause analysis methods are *repeating why* and *cause and effect*. In repeating why, sometimes called *5 why*, start at the end point and ask why through each step backward. If the problem is more complex, it may help to put together a team of people who are very familiar with the process for brainstorming. Flowcharts, as illustrated in Figure 21-9 ▦, are useful to visualize the process and identify dead ends, discrepancies, or areas that may need clarification. Another visual tool called the *fish bone chart* or *cause-and-effect diagram* is used in cause-and-effect analysis:

1. First write down the problem or error.
2. Identify all the component parts (category) of the process.
3. Within each part, list the potential causes of the error.
4. Identify which potential causes are most likely and should be investigated first.

A fish bone chart is illustrated in Figure 21-10 ▦.

After the cause of an error is identified, an action plan should be developed. The plan should include:

- Identification of the problem
- Action(s) to eliminate the problem
- Implementation timeline
- Responsible parties

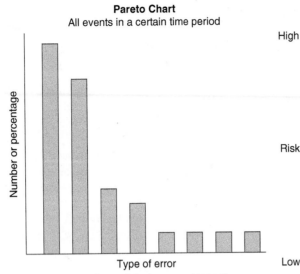

Pareto Chart
All events in a certain time period

The first two types of errors obviously occur most frequently and may therefore be targeted for further investigation.

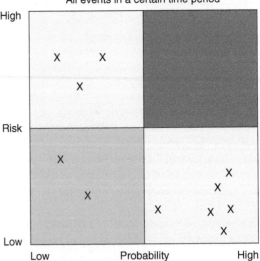

Risk/Probability Chart
All events in a certain time period

Any errors placed in the red high/high quadrant would be addressed immediately.
Errors in the two yellow quadrants are the ones most likely to be targeted for further investigation.
Sentinel events would often fall into the high risk/low probability quadrant.

One type of error over time

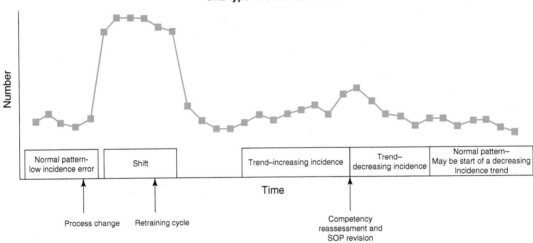

Actions can be added to this type of chart to quickly assess the effect of the action.
For example:
- One type of error was tracked over time because a change in the system where the error occurred was being implemented.
- After the process change was implemented, an upward shift in the number of errors occurring was seen.
- An investigation determined that despite training, staff members were confused about some of the changes.
- A second round of training that targeted the problematic steps was implemented.
- The error rate shows a decrease after the retraining program was complete.
- Several months later, a subtle upward trend is observed.
- Upon investigation, it appears that the majority of errors were made by three staff members.
- During a competency reassessment of these three staff members, an ambiguity in the wording of the standard operating procedure is discovered.
- The procedure is rewritten to clarify the step where the error is occurring.

FIGURE 21-8   Examples of Event Charts

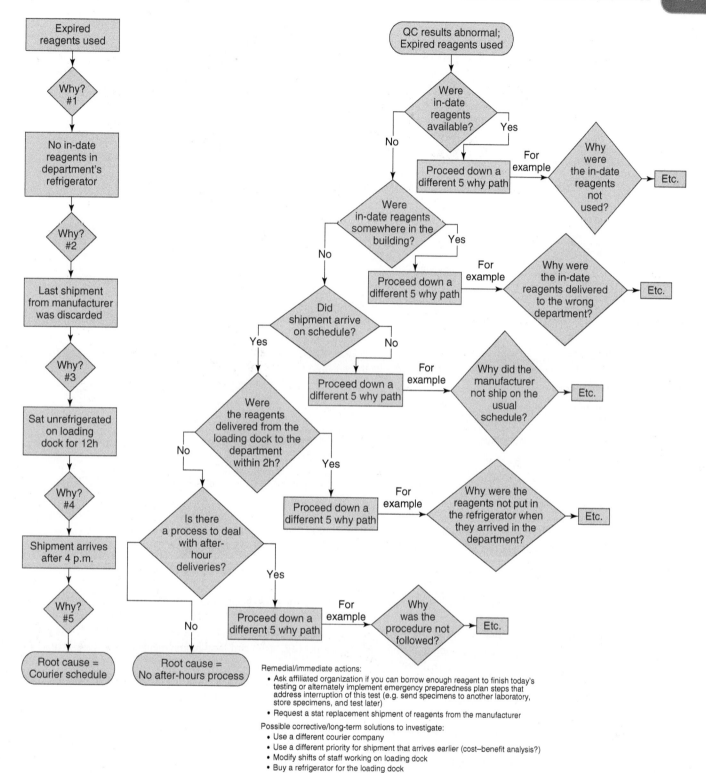

FIGURE 21-9 Examples of Flowcharts in a 5 Why Exercise

The flowchart on the left illustrates how asking why five times can move past the obvious problem into the harder-to-see root causes. The flowchart on the right illustrates how a flowchart can be used to identify dead ends, discrepancies, or areas that may need clarification. For example, in a flowchart for a procedure/process if there is a decision point that only has one arm, this is probably an area of the procedure that needs clarification. Common flowchart symbols include:

- Oval, start or end point
- Diamond, decision point
- Box, process

More complex flowcharts may incorporate symbols for data, records, subprocesses, parallel processes, and predefined processes, and may use swim lanes to identify if different steps are the responsibility of different departments or people.

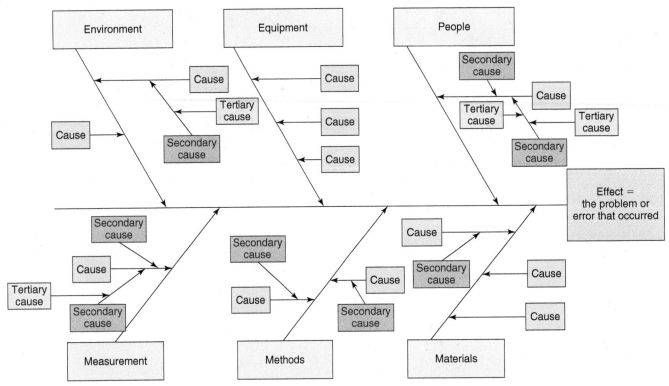

FIGURE 21-10 Example of Fish Bone Diagram

1. Write the effect (error that occurred or problem being investigated) at either the right or left side.
2. Brainstorm possible causes.
3. Organize the causes into categories. Usual categories for a production process are people, materials, equipment, methods, environment, and measurement. Usual categories for a service process are people, policies, procedures, location, and measurement.
4. Add each cause to the appropriate category "bone."
5. For each cause, ask if there is a secondary cause(s), for each secondary cause ask if there is a tertiary cause(s), and so forth. This can be done using the 5 why approach. Stop at a reasonable point or when the group thinks root causes have been identified.
6. Analyze the results. Are there causes that appear more than once? Are there causes that jump out as critical?

Corrective or preventive action plans that will involve large-scale changes may best be implemented in phases rather than all at once. The phases may include implementation in only one department or implementation of a series of changes one at a time. In either case, the effects of the smaller changes can be analyzed before either an organization-wide rollout or before the next steps are implemented.

The final step in both corrective and preventive plans is to monitor and assess the effectiveness of the actions taken. If data analysis supports that the action was effective, then monitoring activities move to a new focus. If data analysis shows that the desired results were not achieved, then new actions need to be undertaken. Sometimes, failure of an action plan can signal that the root cause was not identified. In either case, the return to data monitoring and analysis begins again, which is why corrective and preventive actions are often described as cycles, as illustrated in Figure 21-11 ■.

Facilities and Safety

Facility requirements are part of current good manufacturing processes (cGMPs) and effective quality management programs. Facilities should be clean, orderly, and safe. Box 21-6 lists example elements of a safety

program. In the United States, the Occupational Safety and Health Administration (OSHA) regulates workplace safety (Chapter 20) at the federal level. Employers must be aware of and follow applicable regional (e.g., state) and local requirements as well. Blood banks and transfusion services should have processes and procedures to minimize environmental health risks not only to employees, but also to donors, volunteers, visitors, and patients. The quality system should include proactive monitoring to ensure compliance with biological, chemical, and radiation safety standards. A safety officer is often designated to have the primary responsibility for compliance monitoring, but as with quality, safety is the responsibility of all employees and should be embedded into all procedures.

Employees working in blood banks and transfusion services, like other laboratory professionals, need to be aware of common terminology used in biosafety standards. The Centers for Disease Control and Prevention (CDC) biosafety levels or containment levels are widely accepted both inside and beyond the borders of the United States.[13] Blood banks, transfusion services, and indeed the majority of medical diagnostic laboratories are categorized as Level 2. Table 21-7 ✳ lists definitions and examples of biosafety levels.

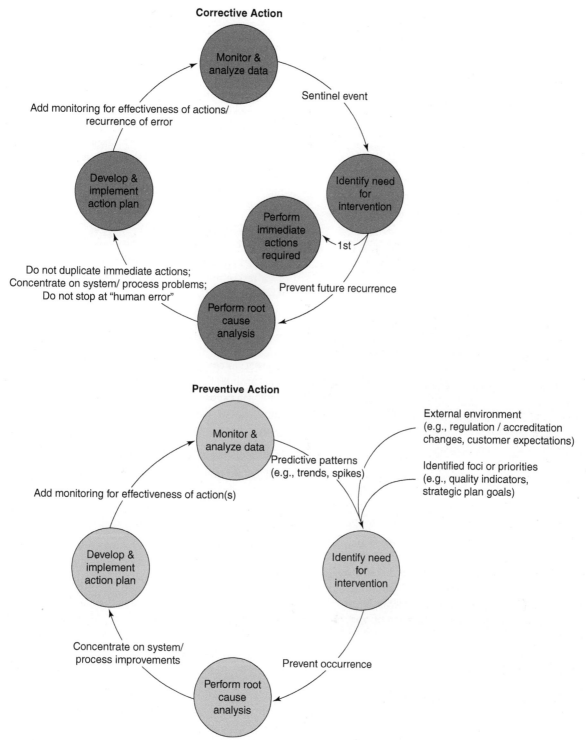

FIGURE 21-11 Corrective and Preventive Action Cycles

BOX 21-6   Safety Policies and Procedures

Examples

- Adequate space, lighting, and ventilation for the tasks being performed
- Facility design details (e.g., dedicated handwashing sinks near exits, eyewash stations close to where splashes are most likely to occur, benchtop materials matched to the exposures likely to occur [water, acid, alkali, solvent, heat])
- Exposure control plans and hazard communication plans developed, documented, implemented, and periodically reviewed (e.g., blood-borne pathogen, chemical, radiation)
- Documented biosafety training before starting work and periodically afterward for all employees whose job potentially exposes them to blood-borne pathogens
- Documented training in chemical safety for all employees whose job potentially exposes them to toxic chemicals, including how to read chemical labels and warning symbols and how to find, understand, and use material safety data sheets
- Fire safety and emergency preparedness processes and training
- Periodic drills in fire safety and emergency preparedness to test processes and procedures
- Clear labeling of rooms or areas where hazards exist as well as labeling of items such as containers for chemicals and biohazard waste receptacles
- Adequate pest control programs
- Procedures for containing and cleaning up spills, especially of biohazards or chemicals
- Periodic safety audits to assess employees (e.g., adherence to safety procedures such as *universal precautions* (a concept defined later in this section); knowledge of personal protective equipment) and the environment (e.g., clear access to emergency exits and safety equipment; minimization of obstructions and trip hazards)
- Policies around working alone and/or communication procedures for employees who may be working alone
- Policies around training required by nonemployee personnel who are in the facility for extended time periods (e.g., volunteers, students, contractors)
- Other job- or task-specific safety training (e.g., drivers may need to take defensive driving courses either periodically or following involvement in an accident; employees who irradiate blood products need to know radiation safety standards, biomedical engineers should have advanced electrical safety knowledge)

Occupational safety professionals use a hierarchy of control systems when discussing ways to make a workplace safer: elimination, substitution, engineering controls, administrative controls, and lastly, personal protective equipment. Personal protective equipment is considered the least effective means of reducing hazards because of the risk that the equipment will fail, for example, a contaminated needle poking through a latex glove. Table 21-8 ✳ lists the definitions and examples of safety control categories.

Universal precautions (treating all blood, body fluids, and tissues as potentially infectious) should be used whenever there is a risk of blood-borne pathogen exposure. Table 21-9 ✳ lists common elements included in universal precautions.

☑ CHECKPOINT 21-11

What work practice control should be used immediately after removing gloves and before leaving a contaminated area?

Health care workers should be offered protective vaccinations at no cost to the employee at the start of their employment. This includes hepatitis B vaccine for workers at risk of blood-borne pathogen exposure. If an exposure occurs, it should be reported to a supervisor as soon as possible. Follow-up to a potential blood-borne pathogen exposure includes:

- Documentation of the circumstances and route of exposure
- Identification of the source individual if possible and if allowed by state or local law
- Testing of the source individual for HBV and HIV, if consent is obtained
- Testing of the employee's blood as soon as possible for baseline HBV and HIV status, if consent is obtained
- Counseling, including discussion of source and employee testing results, and risks and benefits of prophylactic treatment options
- Postexposure prophylaxis, where indicated and if accepted by the employee
- Evaluation of reported illnesses

The identity of the source individual must be protected to the extent required by applicable local, state, and federal privacy laws. Both the employee and the source individual's medical records, including laboratory result testing, must be treated with the usual confidentiality except where privacy and workplace safety legislation allows for exceptions. For example, in the United States, records of exposure incidents, including related medical record information, must be kept by the employer. However, the employer may not disclose the records without the employee's consent. Hepatitis B prophylaxis can include hepatitis B immune globulin if the employee was not previously vaccinated. HIV prophylaxis can include antiviral medications.

✱ **TABLE 21-7** Biosafety Levels

Level	Definition	Example*	Safety Procedures*
1	Little or no risk of exposure to infectious agents, or exposure limited to well-characterized organisms known to not cause disease in healthy humans	Teaching laboratories working with pure cultures of low-risk organisms, such as non-toxin-producing *Escherichia coli*, *Staphylococcus epidermidis*	Minimal: • Good hand hygiene • Cleaning of work surfaces • Waste materials may be autoclaved before disposal depending on the organisms
2	Moderate risk, including potential exposure to organisms that can cause disease in humans	Includes most medical laboratories, as pathogens in this level's definition include hepatitis viruses, human immunodeficiency virus, as well as most bacteria, viruses, and fungi usually encountered in a diagnostic laboratory setting	Level 1 controls plus: • Restricted access • Universal precautions • Decontamination of waste products (often achieved by shipping closed containers to an off-site incinerator) • Use of biological safety cabinets for some higher-risk activities
3	High risk, including potential exposure to organisms that can cause serious disease or death and that can be transmitted through inhalation	Microbiology research and referral laboratories working with organisms such as *Mycobacterium tuberculosis*, *Bacillus anthracis*, *Rickettsia rickettsia*, *Fracisella tularensis*, SARS (sudden acute respiratory syndrome) coronavirus	Levels 1 and 2 plus**: • Positive air flow • Use of biological safety cabinets or equivalent containment devices for all activities • May include use of specialized protective clothing with a separate air supply, depending on the organisms
4	Potential exposure to organisms that are high risk or exotic and that can cause severe or fatal disease, often with no preventative vaccine or disease treatment available	Limited to government and academic facilities conducting research with organisms such as Ebola virus, smallpox virus, Marburg virus	Previous levels plus: • Multiple airlocks on exits • Records of all personnel entering and leaving, often accomplished via electronic security access • Mandatory use of either positive pressure suits with air supply or use of class 3 biosafety cabinets • Series of rooms for clothing changes and showers

*Not inclusive lists; only common examples.

**Level 2 laboratories may occasionally handle level 3 organisms for routine diagnostic procedures (culture, identification, susceptibility testing) when no other safer option exists; in these cases the laboratory director may institute higher levels of safety practice and equipment while the work is being performed.

✱ **TABLE 21-8** Safety Control Categories

Control Category	Definition	Examples
Elimination	Physical removal of the hazard	• Stop performing a test methodology that requires use of a carcinogenic reagent and safely discard any remaining reagent • Remove uneven flooring that is a trip hazard • Use an automated decapper, which eliminates a repetitive motion task and the associated ergonomic risk
Substitution	Replacing a hazard with either something that is not hazardous or that is less hazardous	• Replace a radioimmunoassay method (RIA) with an enzyme-linked immunoassay (EIA) method • Replace mercury thermometers with alcohol-based ones
Engineering controls	Isolating the hazard from the worker, usually via facility design or equipment	• Puncture-resistant waste containers for sharps • Biological safety cabinets
Administrative controls	Changing how workers perform a task to reduce the hazards, also called work practice controls	• Safety policies and safety training • Universal precautions • Warning labels and signs
Personal protective equipment	Garment or equipment designed to protect the worker from the hazard	• Gowns • Gloves • Safety goggles • Face splash guards

★ **TABLE 21-9** Universal Precautions

What	When
Gowns or coats: long-sleeved, often closed at wrists, closed at neck, covering front and fluid resistant	At all times in the laboratory; always removed before leaving the laboratory
Gloves: latex, now more often nitrile or polyvinyl chloride	When performing phlebotomy and, depending on workplace policy, at all times in the laboratory or when handling specimens
Safety goggles, face shields, fume hood sashes, biological safety cabinets	There is a splash risk (e.g., opening specimens, pouring specimens)
Prohibition of eating, drinking, gum-chewing, smoking, mouth-pipetting	At all times in the laboratory
Handwashing	After removing gloves, after handling specimens, before leaving the laboratory

Review of the Main Points

- The AABB defines the quality system as the organizational structure, responsibilities, policies, processes, procedures, and resources established to achieve quality. Others use the term quality program to encompass everything focused on quality and define the quality system as the document that captures the policies, processes, and procedures.
- Quality management is continual system surveillance, monitoring, quality improvement, and cost-containment measures. Quality management looks both within and outside the organization.
- Quality assurance is the activities done to ensure that the quality system policies are being adhered to and that the quality system is effective.
- Quality control is routine testing or activities done to ensure that specific procedures are working as expected.
- Quality is everyone's responsibility, but in organizations that manufacture blood products, there must be a quality assurance unit who has final quality oversight for the procedures and processes that could affect the safety, purity, or potency of the products.
- AABB Standards are divided into 10 quality system essentials.
- The transfusion practice committee monitors errors, adverse events, near-misses, blood utilization/wastage, and transfusion practices. The committee recommends changes to policies as required to improve patient safety.
- Initial competency must be demonstrated before an employee performs a task without supervision. Ongoing competency assessment is also required.
- On-site validation of new equipment includes installation, operational, and performance validations.

- Computer software used in transfusion medicine is considered a medical device and must meet the applicable regulations, including validations.
- Process controls are activities or tools used to create a controlled environment for processes and procedures, to standardize processes, or to monitor process outcome.
- Document control standardizes facility document format, ensures that only approved and current documents are in use, and protects documents from unauthorized access or modification.
- The two major steps in the lookback process are quarantine and recipient notification.
- An event reporting system should identify problems, initiate both corrective and preventive actions, provide data for analysis, and act as both a learning and process improvement tool.
- Audit documentation includes the audit plan, review of records, data and/or products, summary report, response to observations, and verification of corrective-action effectiveness.
- Corrective action is taken to eliminate the causes of an existing nonconformance or other undesirable situation in order to prevent recurrence. Preventive action is changes made or actions taken before a problem occurs to prevent it from occurring.
- Quality indicators are measurable facets of a process that are tracked and used to evaluate the effectiveness of the quality system.

Review Questions

1. A daily check of reagents to ensure that they are functioning as expected is an example of: (Objective #2)

   A. Quality management

   B. Quality system

   C. Quality control

   D. Quality assurance

2. Monitoring performed to ensure that the quality system is effective is the definition of which of the following terms? (Objective #1)

   A. Quality assurance (QA)

   B. Quality control (QC)

   C. Quality management (QM)

   D. Quality program

3. The quality assurance unit in a blood bank is responsible for: (Objective #5)

   A. All human resource activities

   B. Oversight of all activities related to product quality

   C. Oversight of all activities related to donor recruitment

   D. All strategic planning activities

4. The purpose of a document control system includes which of the following? Check all that apply. (Objective #9)

   A. Ensures only current documents are in use

   B. Ensures only executive members change procedures

   C. Protects documents from unauthorized changes

   D. Protects documents from fire or flood

5. When should calibration of equipment be performed? (Objective #6)

   A. At the same time as specimen testing

   B. Prior to initial equipment use

   C. After equipment is taken out of service

   D. Each day of equipment use

6. An effective employee training program includes all of the following elements *except:* (Objective #4)

   A. New employee orientation

   B. Development of threshold limits for retraining

   C. Established competency

   D. Storage of documents with all other personnel records

7. Employee competency can be established through which of the following types of activities? Select all that apply. (Objective #4)

   A. Written exam

   B. Practical exam

   C. Error reporting

   D. Direct observation checklist

8. A transfusion service has just purchased a new computer system. What process must be conducted prior to implementation of the new system at the facility? (Objective #7)

   A. Cost–benefit analysis

   B. Error analysis

   C. Validation

   D. QA audit

9. Which of the following is *not* required for the development of a standard operating procedure (SOP)? (Objective #9)

   A. Written in language that can be understood by all employees

   B. Use of a consistent format

   C. Must be a text document

   D. Must include all critical steps for the procedure

10. Match each validation process with the circumstances for which it should be performed: (Objective #6)

    _____ Concurrent validation

    _____ Prospective validation

    _____ Retrospective validation

    (a) A new process

    (b) Inadequate prior validation

    (c) During a live run

11. The two purposes of the lookback process are: (Objective #11)

    A. Quarantine or recall in-date blood products

    B. Quarantine or recall expired blood products

    C. Notify blood donors of disease risk

    D. Notify blood recipients of disease risk

12. The internal audit process should be: (Objective #12)

    A. Conducted by an accrediting agency such as AABB

    B. Spontaneous and unplanned

    C. Punitive in nature

    D. Performed according to an established plan

13. Which statement regarding the use of quality indicators as part of a quality monitoring process is *false*? (Objective #3)

    A. Each quality indicator is evaluated only once.

    B. There must be an established threshold for each quality indicator.

    C. A quality indicator must be measurable.

    D. A quality indicator may be changed or updated.

14. The governmental agency that sets the standards for safety in the workplace is: (Objective #14)

    A. JCAHO

    B. OSHA

    C. CAP

    D. AABB

15. Which of the following strategies *must* be included in a problem-solving plan in order for it to be successful? (Objective #13)

    A. Use of multiple tools

    B. Start at the beginning point

    C. Put together a team

    D. Determine the root cause

References

1. Daniels, SE, Johnson K, Johnson C. Quality Glossary. *Qual Prog* 2002; 35 (7): 43–61.

2. AABB, 26th edition blood bank/transfusion service standards program unit. *Standards for blood banks and transfusion services*, 28th ed. Bethesda (MD): AABB Press; 2012.

3. Food and Drug Administration. *Guideline for quality assurance in blood establishments. 91N-0450*. Rockville (MD): Food and Drug Administration; 1995.

4. American Society for Quality. The history of quality-the early 20th century [Internet]. Milwaukee (WI): American Society for Quality; 1993–2010 [cited 2010 Feb 10]. Available from: http://www.asq.org/learn-about-quality/history-of-quality/overview/20th-century.html

5. Roback JD, Combs MR, Grossman BJ, Hillyer CD, eds. *Technical manual*, 16th ed. Bethesda (MD): AABB Press; 2008.

6. Berte L. Quality—A 3-Legged Stool. *Lab Medicine* 2005; 36(6): 343.

7. Zacharia M. Supreme Court of New Jersey to AABB (American Association of Blood Banks): "You're guilty and that's final." *MLO Med Lab Obs* 1996; 28(12): 33–4.

8. Smith DM, Otter J. Performance improvement in a hospital transfusion service. *Arch Pathol Lab Med* 1999; 123 (7): 585–91.

9. Taylor WA. *Methods and Tools for Process Validation*. Libertyville (IL): Taylor Enterprises, Inc.; 2005.

10. Berte LM, ed. *A model quality system for the transfusion service*. Bethesda (MD): AABB Press; 1997.

11. Center for Biologics Evaluation and Research. *Guidance for industry. Biological product deviation reporting for blood and plasma establishments*. Rockville (MD): Food and Drug Administration; 2006.

12. AABB. *Association Bulletin #06-07. Transfusion-related acute lung injury*. Bethesda (MD): AABB; November 2006.

13. Chosewood LC, Wilson DE, eds. *Section IV-Laboratory Biosafety Level Criteria in Biosafety in Microbiological and Biomedical Laboratories*, 5th ed. Atlanta (GA): U.S. Department of Health and Human Services; 2009.

Answers to Case In Point Questions

Chapter 1

1. A. Large size; antigens with larger size make better immunogens
   B. Molecular complexity; more complex antigens make better immunogens
   C. Degree of foreignness; the greater the difference between the antigen and the host, the more immunogenic

2. The laboratorian potentially caused a false-negative reaction because she decreased the sensitization of the antigen–antibody reaction. Adequate time is needed for antigen–antibody reactions to reach equilibrium. Addition of an enhancement reagent allows for a shortened incubation time. In this situation, the laboratorian shortened the incubation time but did not add enhancement. This may not have allowed enough time for the antigen–antibody reaction to form.

3. The classical pathway

4. Complement activation and formation of the MAC (membrane attack complex).
   A. Complement activation:
      i. C1s cleaves C4 into C4b and C4a.
      ii. Some of the C4b attaches to cell surfaces.
      iii. C2 binds to the attached C4b in the presence of Mg^{2+}.
      iv. C2 is cleaved into C2a and C2b.
      v. C2a remains bound, which makes C3 convertase.
      vi. C3 convertase cleaves C3 into C3a and C3b.
   B. Formation of the MAC (membrane attack complex):
      i. C3b binds to C3 convertase to form C5 convertase.
      ii. C5 convertase cleaves C5 into C5a and bound C5b.
      iii. C6 and C7 bind to C5b, which creates a rod that is inserted into the lipid bilayer of the red blood cell.
      iv. C8 binds to the structure and creates a small pore.
      v. C9 binds and allows water and solutes to pass freely through the membrane. Sodium and water pass into the red blood cell, which causes swelling and lysis.

Chapter 2

1. Pregnancy or transfusion. Most likely pregnancy because this is her third child.

2. Genotype = CC

3. There is a 100% chance the baby will possess the little-c antigen.

	Mom		
Dad		Big C	Big C
Little c		Cc	Cc
Little c		Cc	Cc

4. There is a 50% chance the baby will possess the little-c antigen.

	Mom		
Dad		Big C	Big C
Big C		CC	CC
Little c		Cc	Cc

5. If the father is homozygous for the little-c antigen, there is a 100% chance that the baby will inherit the antigen that corresponds to the mother's antibody. If the father is heterozygous for the little-c antigen, there is a 50% chance that the baby will not have the little-c antigen. If the baby is negative for the little-c antigen, he or she will be unaffected by the mother's antibody. If the baby is positive for the little-c antigen, the mother's antibody levels will need to be monitored to determine whether the baby is affected by hemolytic disease of the fetus and newborn.

6. Genotype = *Cc* or *CC*

7. Phenotype = C+c+ or C+c−

Chapter 3

1. The DAT will detect *in vivo* sensitization while the IAT detects *in vitro* sensitization.

2. The EDTA-anticoagulated tube should be used. Complement can attach to red cells nonspecifically when serum samples are stored.

3. Positive with 3+ strength. There is one large clump of cells surrounded by a few small clumps and a clear background.

4. IgG and/or complement

5. Test the cells using monospecific reagents (anti-IgG and anti-complement) to determine which is/are coating the cells.

6. The tech made an incorrect choice. Incubating tubes too long can cause bound antibody to dissociate, which may result in false-negative test results. The tech should have discarded the tubes and repeated the testing from scratch.

7. All screen cells are negative and the interpretation is negative. All cells moved freely through the gel and formed a pellet at the bottom of the microtube.

Chapter 4

1. Perform a forward and a reverse ABO grouping to determine the patient's blood type.

2. The ABO results do not correlate and thus cannot be interpreted. The patient's forward type looks like a group A and reverse type looks like a group O.

3. Repeat the ABO testing to rule out technical errors.

4. This could possibly be both (C) unexpected positive reaction in the reverse group or (D) unexpected positive reaction in the forward group. However, answer C is more likely due to the reaction strength of the forward group.

5. Possibilities:
   (a) Patient is an A subgroup with anti-A_1.
   (b) Cold-reactive allo- or autoantibody is present and cross-reacting with A_1 cells.
   (c) Patient has made an antibody to a low-frequency antigen. The corresponding antigen is not located on the antibody screening cells but is present on the A_1 cell.
   (d) The patient is likely a subgroup of A, Rh(D) positive with an anti-A_1. The patient received a transfusion that caused the passive transfer of ABO antibodies (platelet, IVIG, etc.), although this scenario is unlikely due to the patient's history.

6. The patient is likely a subgroup of A, Rh(D) positive with an anti-A_1.

7. The patient should receive A_1-negative or group O red blood cell transfusions because some examples of anti-A_1 react at body temperature and reduce the lifespan of the transfused cells. The patient can receive group A or AB plasma products because they do not contain anti-A.

8. The patient is group A and she received 3 units of group O red blood cells. Mixed-field agglutination is seen because anti-A reacts with the patient's cells but does not react with the donor cells.

9. The patient still requires A_1-negative or O red blood cells.

Chapter 5

1. D, C, c, E, and e.

2. There is no test for the d antigen. The designation "d" refers to the absence of the D antigen. There is no d antigen; it is an amorph.

3. DCce.

4. R_1r or DCe/dce.

5. The donor red blood cells should lack the E antigen.

6. Patients with sickle cell disease may require frequent transfusions, either as treatment during a crisis or as prophylaxis to decrease the risk of stroke. The Rh antigens are very immunogenic. The physician is attempting to minimize the risk of alloantibody formation, which decreases the risk of adverse events associated with the transfusion.

Chapter 6

1. Anti-E, anti-K, anti-Jk^a, and Anti-Fy^a generally all react at 98.6° F (37° C) or AHG.
   Anti-Le^a reacts best at room temperature.
   Anti-M tends to react at room temperature but can react at 98.6° F (37° C) or AHG.

2. Anti-E, anti-K, anti-Jk^a, and anti-Fy^a
   Anti-M rarely causes hemolytic transfusion reaction.
   Anti-Le^a is considered clinically insignificant.

3. Anti-E and Anti-K

4. Anti-Fy^a is destroyed by enzymes. Anti-E and anti-Jk^a are enhanced by enzymes.

5. Anti-M

6. Anti-K

7. Anti-Le^a

8. The patient must receive Jk^a-negative red blood cells. Even though her anti-Jk^a antibody has fallen below detectable levels, the patient has previously been sensitized. This patient should not receive red blood cells that possess the Jk^a antigen. If she is given such red blood cells, she will likely mount an anamnestic response in which her Jk^a antibody levels will rise rapidly and destroy the donor cells.

Chapter 7

1. Two independent patient identifiers such as patient's first and last name, birthdate, hospital number; the date on which the sample was collected; A means to identify the person who collected the sample.

2. The patient may have clinically significant antibodies that have fallen below detectable testing levels. A patient may have a hemolytic transfusion reaction if he or she is transfused red blood cells that possess the corresponding antigens. The patient may also have special transfusion

requirements (e.g., CMV-seronegative blood products, irradiated blood products, IgA-deficient blood products) that were not noted on the current request.

3. ABO type, Rh(D) type, and antibody screen

4. The patient has no current or historical antibodies and has had at least two independent blood types performed. Therefore, the minimum testing requirement is a crossmatch that will identify an ABO mismatch between the donor and recipient. This is generally an electronic or immediate spin crossmatch, but an IAT crossmatch would also be acceptable.

5. The AB units should be issued to the patient. DK is group A. Group O plasma contains anti-A and anti-A,B antibodies that can react with his blood cells. Group AB plasma lacks all ABO antibodies and can be transfused to patients of all blood types.

6. No. Plasma products do not contain Rh(D) antigens.

7. Abnormalities for consideration include:

Visual inspection of blood products.
Turbid, hemolyzed, murky, purple, or brown color to supernatant of red blood cell or plasma products
Black or purple red blood cell mass
Visible clots
Visible blood in ports
Segment color does not match color or red blood cell product

Leaking bag or seams
Uncovered ports
Blood product is past expiration date or time
Debris or particulate matter in blood product

Chapter 8

1. There are several possibilities: anti-K alone, anti-C alone, anti-K, and anti-C. Together, any of the above with or without a previously identified antibody, for example, anti-Le^a.

2. The next step when an antibody screen reacts positively is to test a panel of cells in order to identify the antibody or antibodies that are reacting.

3. Antibodies to D, c, E, e, k, Fy^a, Fy^b, Jk^a, Jk^b, Le^b, P1, S. Antibodies ruled out and the first cell used to rule out each antibody is highlighted in pink in the antigram below.

4. Anti-C and anti-K are reacting as highlighted in green in the antigram below.

5. Antibodies to Le^a, M, N, and s are not ruled out on the initial panel. However, screen cells II and III can be used to rule out anti-M, anti-N, and anti-s. Therefore, only anti-Le^a is not ruled out.

6. No, the positive reaction with cell #9, highlighted in turquoise, is not explained by the anti-C and anti-K (see table below).

Initial panel highlighted:

Donor	D	C	c	E	e	K	k	Fy^a	Fy^b	Jk^a	Jk^b	Le^a	Le^b	P$_1$	M	N	S	s	IS	IAT	CC
1	+	+	0	+	+	+	+	+	+	0	+	0	0	+	+	0	+	0	+	0	3+	
2	+	+	0	0	+	0	+	+	+	0	0	+	+	0	+	+	0	+	+	0	2+	
3	+	0	+	+	0	0	+	0	+	+	0	0	+	0	+	+	+	0	0	0	+
4	+	0	+	0	+	0	+	+	0	+	+	0	+	+	+	+	0	0	0	0	+
5	0	+	+	0	+	0	+	+	0	+	0	+	0	+	+	+	+	+	0	3+	
6	0	0	+	+	+	0	+	+	+	+	0	0	+	+	+	+	+	+	0	0	+
7	0	0	+	0	+	+	+	0	+	0	+	0	+	+	+	+	+	+	0	3+	
8	0	0	+	0	+	0	+	+	0	0	+	0	+	+	+	+	+	+	0	0	+
9	0	0	+	0	+	0	+	+	0	0	+	+	0	0	+	0	0	+	0	1+	

7. Anti-Le^a has been identified in addition to the previously known anti-C and anti-K. Reactions due to anti-C are highlighted in yellow, reactions due to anti-K are highlighted in green, and reactions due to anti-Le^a are highlighted in turquoise in the antigram below.

Additional red blood cell reactions highlighted:

Donor	D	C	c	E	e	K	k	Fy^a	Fy^b	Jk^a	Jk^b	Le^a	Le^b	P$_1$	M	N	S	s	IS	IAT	CC
10	+	+	0	0	+	0	+	0	+	+	+	0	+	+	+	0	0	+	0	1+	
11	+	0	+	+	0	0	+	0	0	+	0	+	0	+	+	0	0	+	0	1+	
12	0	0	+	+	+	0	+	0	+	+	0	+	0	0	+	0	+	+	0	1+	
13	0	0	+	0	+	+	+	0	+	0	+	0	+	+	0	+	0	+	0	3+	
14	0	0	+	0	+	0	+	+	0	+	+	+	0	0	0	+	0	+	0	W+	
15	0	0	+	0	+	+	0	+	+	0	+	0	+	+	+	+	+	0	0	3+	

8. Anti-K has been confirmed with three cells that are K positive and C negative, Le^a negative (cells 7, 13, 15). Anti-Le^a has been confirmed with at least three cells that are Le^a positive and C negative, K negative (cells 9, 11, 12, 14). Full confirmation of the anti-C was not performed by this laboratory on this specimen because the same laboratory had previously identified an anti-C in this patient's plasma (history from 1998). In the testing on this specimen, there is only one cell that reacts solely because of the anti-C (cell 10). There are at least three cells that are negative for C, K, and Le^a and that show a negative reaction (cells 3, 4, 6, 8).

9. Donor units should be C negative and K negative. Anti-Le^a is not clinically significant. Therefore, the crossmatched blood does not need to be antigen-typed for the Le^a antigen.

10. Fifteen donor units should be screened in order to find four compatible donor units determined through completing the following steps:

   Step 1: Determine the percentage of antigen-negative individuals.

   - 70% of the general population is positive for C, therefore **30%** of the general population is negative for C.
   - 10% of the general population is K positive, therefore **90%** of the general population is K negative.

Step 2: Convert each value obtained in step 1 into a decimal.

   - Negative for C: 30% = .30
   - Negative for K: 90% = .90

Step 3: Multiply the decimal values obtained in step 2.

   - .30 × .90 = 0.27

Step 4: Fill in the appropriate values into the formula and calculate the resulting value.

   - The patient needs 4 units of donor blood. Using the formula # of units / value obtained in step 3:
   - 4/0.27 = **15** donor units should be screened to find 4 C-negative, K-negative donor units.

11. The results are most likely caused by a delayed serologic transfusion reaction due to anti-C. All antibodies in the eluate are ruled out on the panel except C and N, as shown by the pink highlights on the following antigram. Anti-N can be ruled out on screen cell II. The pattern obtained fits an anti-C, which is consistent with the patient's history and highlighted in green on the following antigram. The community hospital was not aware of the anti-C previously identified. At the time of their testing, the anti-C had likely dropped to undetectable levels. C-positive donor units were transfused, causing a rise in the level of anti-C.

Donor	D	C	c	E	e	K	k	Fy^a	Fy^b	Jk^a	Jk^b	Le^a	Le^b	P$_1$	M	N	S	s	IS	IAT	CC
1	+	+	0	+	+	+	+	+	0	+	0	0	+	+	0	+	0	+	0	3+	
2	+	+	0	0	+	0	+	+	0	0	+	+	0	+	+	0	+	+	0	3+	
3	+	0	+	+	0	0	+	0	+	+	0	0	+	0	+	+	+	0	0	0	+
4	+	0	+	0	+	0	+	+	0	+	+	0	+	+	+	+	0	0	0	0	+
5	0	+	+	0	+	0	+	+	0	+	0	+	0	+	+	+	+	+	0	3+	
6	0	0	+	+	+	0	+	+	+	+	0	0	+	+	+	+	+	+	0	0	+
7	0	0	+	0	+	+	+	0	+	0	+	0	+	+	+	+	+	+	0	0	+
8	0	0	+	0	+	0	+	+	0	0	+	0	+	+	+	+	+	+	0	0	+
9	0	0	+	0	+	0	+	+	0	0	+	+	0	0	+	0	0	+	0	0	+

Patient Results

Chapter 9

1. A donor may not always reveal the same information at each donation attempt (intentionally or unintentionally). Something that seems unimportant to a donor may have a negative impact on a recipient who receives the donated blood product. Infectious disease testing minimizes but does not completely eliminate the risk of passing on a disease via blood transfusion.

2. It is believed that a donor who is being paid will be more apt to lie or omit information that may disqualify him or her from donating blood. This may put the recipient of the blood product at risk.

3. She should be deferred for 12 months unless the blood center can verify that the tattoo parlor is state-regulated and the tattoos were applied with sterile needles and single-use ink. This is because reused needles and/or ink can transmit infectious diseases. There is a window of time where the donor can be positive for an infectious disease and transmit the disease while infectious disease tests are still negative. The 1-year deferral will minimize any risk posed to the recipient due to this infectious window.

4. The deferral period for visiting a malarial endemic area is 12 months. This donor should not be deferred as long as he has no symptoms of malaria, because his visit was longer than 12 months ago.

5. If the blood floats, the specific gravity of the blood is <1.053, which means the hemoglobin is <12.5% g/dL.

6. No, this donor should be deferred until her hemoglobin is higher. This donor is anemic and the process of donating

blood will make her more anemic, which can cause her harm.

7. The needle must be large enough to prevent hemolysis while allowing blood to flow quickly enough so clotting does not start before the blood mixes with the anticoagulant.

8. 21 days if left in CPD and 35 days if left in CPDA-1

9. Yes, the shelf life would be extended to 42 days.

10. The blood center should investigate whether her blood should be distributed or discarded. Even though she did not have symptoms of illness the previous day, her blood may not be suitable for transfusion.

Chapter 10

1. FFP is processed and frozen within 8 hours of collection. FP24 is processed and frozen within 24 hours of collection. FFP contains normal amounts of all labile and stabile factors. FP24 contains reduced levels of FVIII.

2. No, both are good for 1 year frozen and 24 hours thawed.

3. Thawed plasma has an extended expiration date once thawed (5 days vs. 24 hours), which gives you a longer window to use the plasma prior to expiration.

4. Thawed plasma contains reduced levels of both Factors V and VIII.

5. No, both are converted to thawed plasma.

6. PRP platelets generally have a total volume of 40–70 mL and a minimum platelet count of 5.5×10^{10} whereas apheresis platelet products have a total volume of 100–500 mL and a minimum platelet count of 3.0×10^{11}.

7. 4–8 units

8. 1 unit

9. Information that must be on the blood product label:
   - Donation identification number
   - Blood group and Rh (if applicable) of donor
   - Product code and description
   - Expiration date
   - Results of special testing

10. CPDA-1 red blood cells have an expiration date of 35 days. AS-3 red blood cells have an expiration date of 42 days.

11. Blood products that have been processed to remove white blood cells.

12. 5×10^6

13. Blood product irradiation refers to the process of exposing cellular blood products to gamma or x-ray radiation. This process inactivates T lymphocytes, which can cause graft versus host disease in immunocompromised patients.

14. Cellular blood products such as red blood cells and platelets.

Chapter 11

1. To improve oxygen-carrying capacity (to treat anemia) and to add blood volume in the case of volume depletion.

2. O Rh(D)-negative red blood cells are generally preferred because they lack A, B, and D antigens. However, O Rh(D)-negative red blood cells are not always readily available. O Rh(D)-positive red blood cells may be used for this patient because he is male. When shortages occur, Rh(D)-negative units are saved for women of childbearing age to prevent anti-D formation that could cause hemolytic disease of the fetus and newborn in subsequent pregnancies.

3. The units are issued in a cooler to maintain the appropriate storage temperature. Red blood cells may contain bacteria, which can multiply if the appropriate temperature is not maintained. In addition, the units were ordered before emergency room staff members had the opportunity to evaluate the patient's condition. The units can be kept at the appropriate storage temperature until needed for transfusion or can be returned to inventory if they are not used as long as they were maintained at the proper storage temperature.

4. Any two of the following: infusion rate, filter type, needle size, and infusion solution.

5. Infusion rate: To limit the risk of bacterial contamination, red blood cell units must be transfused within 4 hours. Filter type and needle size: When infusing red blood cells rapidly, a high-volume or high-flow filter and a needle with a larger bore size should be used to help prevent hemolysis. Infusion solution: Only solutions that have been approved for use with blood products should be added. Commonly, either no additional infusion solution or sterile, normal saline is added. Infusion solutions that are not approved may cause hemolysis or clotting in the red blood cell unit.

6. Plasma is transfused to replace coagulation factors and improve hemostasis.

7. This patient is at risk of developing a dilution coagulopathy due to the amount of blood he has lost in addition to the infusion of multiple IV solutions, such as crystalloids and stored red blood cell units.

8. Cryoprecipitate may be indicated when the fibrinogen level is <100 mg/dL (<2.94 μmol/L).

9. Recombinant activated Factor VII (rFVIIa) may be used in trauma to induce platelet aggregation at the site of bleeding, although this is not an FDA-approved use of this product.

10. Platelet and fibrinogen levels are verified and must be adequate prior to administration of rFVIIa. If the patient has a deficiency of platelets or fibrinogen, the rFVIIa will be ineffective.

11. To determine if the medical staff are using the emergency release process in appropriate situations. The

review may also check for opportunities to improve the process, which by definition occurs when the health care providers are under stress. For example, were there any clinically significant delays in delivering the product to the patient's bedside? And if yes, what caused the delay and how can the same issue be prevented in the future? If the identity of the patient was not known, did the emergency identification system work and were all the products linked correctly to the patient once his identity was known?

12. To determine if the medical staff are using the massive transfusion process in appropriate situations and if the medical staff are ordering appropriate type and number of blood products to meet the clinical situation.

13. The physician is not using laboratory values to treat the patient. He is looking at the patient's clinical picture when making the decision to transfuse. Following trauma, laboratory values may not reflect the extent of blood loss the patient is experiencing.

Chapter 12

1. Yes

2. Stop the transfusion.

3. Immediate (or acute); the symptoms occurred during the transfusion.

4. Hemolytic transfusion reaction, febrile nonhemolytic transfusion reaction, transfusion-associated bacterial sepsis, fever due to her underlying condition. Her respiratory symptoms are likely secondary to the discomfort of her fever and distress, but transfusion reactions that involve respiratory symptoms, such as anaphylactic, transfusion-related acute lung injury, and transfusion-associated circulatory overload, should be investigated if her respiratory symptoms persist or worsen.

5. Acute hemolytic transfusion reactions can be life-threatening and are often caused by human error, including misidentification of the patient, specimen, or blood product. A clerical check will help to quickly determine if misidentification of the patient or blood product has occurred and may indicate that another patient is involved (e.g., blood products for two patients were switched).

6. No, a hemolytic reaction is unlikely. No clerical errors were noted and the remaining red blood cell product shows no evidence of hemolysis. There is no visible hemolysis in the postreaction specimen, the postreaction direct antiglobulin test (DAT) is negative, and testing revealed no errors in the ABO grouping or change in the red blood cell antibody screen status.

7. To rule out transfusion-associated bacterial sepsis, which should be treated early and aggressively and which would need to be reported to the blood supplier.

8. Febrile, nonhemolytic transfusion reaction

9. Multiple transfusions can expose the patient to foreign white blood cells, which carry human leukocyte antigens (HLA) different from the patient's phenotype. The patient once exposed to the foreign antigens is more likely to make antibodies to HLA and these antibodies often are the cause of febrile reactions.

Chapter 13

1. *Babesia spp.* is transmitted through the bite of the Ixodes deer tick.

2. The incubation period for the disease is 1–8 weeks. The patient had been hospitalized in a long-term care facility for the previous 3 months. During the period of hospitalization, the patient had not been outdoors and did not have contact with animals, which is the normal means of transmission for this disease.

3. Her age—she is 98 years old.

4. Hepatitis A = rare
Hepatitis B = 1:220,000
Hepatitis C = 1:2 million
HIV I/II = 1:2 million
HTLV I/II = 1: nearly 3 million

5. Bacterial transmission is much more common.

6. The blood supply is currently not being tested for *Babesia spp.* because currently there is no test available that can be adapted to large-scale testing such as with donors. Blood suppliers rely on the donor health history questions to rule out donors with possible infections. However, babesiosis is generally asymptomatic or subclinical in healthy individuals.

Chapter 14

1. G2P1, for two pregnancies and delivery of one live infant

2. During delivery of her first child either through fetal–maternal hemorrhage caused by the ruptured uterus or exposure to donor cells via blood transfusion.

3. Anemia is caused by the destruction of RBCs. Progressive anemia can cause tissue hypoxia, increased cardiac output, hydrops fetalis, and death of the fetus.

4. Increased bilirubin that cannot be metabolized quickly and builds up, causing jaundice, kernicterus, and death.

5. Factors include:
- The woman's genetic makeup
- The dose of antigen presented
- The immunogenicity of the antigen
- How often the antigen is presented
- Whether the fetal RBCs are compatible with maternal plasma

6. If the father is C+c− (where + stands for positive agglutination and − stands for negative agglutination), we know

that there is a 100% chance the baby will possess the C antigen. If the father is C+c+, there is a 50% chance the baby will lack the C antigen.

7. Factors include:

- O-negative red cells
- Negative for the C antigen
- AHG crossmatch compatible with the mother's plasma
- Fresh (<7 days old) or washed
- Leukocyte reduced
- CMV reduced risk
- Irradiated
- Hct of 75–85%

8. Yes, she should receive a prophylactic dose of RhIG at 28 weeks' gestation because she is Rh negative and is not currently sensitized to the D antigen.

9. The anti-D is likely passive anti-D due to the administration of RhIG at 28 weeks' gestation.

10. Benefits include:

- Removes antibody-coated RBCs from neonatal circulation, preventing destruction and increase in bilirubin.
- Removes maternal antibody from neonatal circulation, preventing them from attaching to and causing destruction of neonatal cells.
- Corrects anemia without causing volume overload.

11. Using the formula (% fetal cells in decimal format) × 5,000 mL blood volume / 30 mL (amount of fetal whole blood covered by one vial of RhIG:

Step 1: convert number of fetal cells to % fetal cells: 20 fetal cells/2000 cells counted: 0.01

Step 2: multiple value obtained in step 1 by 5,000 mL blood volume: (0.01) × (5,000) = 50

Step 3: divide value obtained in step 2 by 30 mL: 50/30 = 1.67 = 2

Step 4: add one to the value obtained in step 3: 2 + 1 = 3 vials

Chapter 15

1. IgG because it is only reacting with anti-IgG and not anti-complement

2. Delayed serologic/hemolytic transfusion reaction or autoimmune hemolytic anemia

3. We need to determine whether the patient has been transfused in the previous 3 months to rule out delayed transfusion reaction.

4. Autologous adsorption is always preferred unless the patient had been transfused within the previous 3 months. If autologous adsorption is performed on a transfused patient, the autologous cells are made up of both donor and patient cells. The donor cells can remove alloantibodies in addition to autoantibodies. Autologous adsorption is preferred for this patient because he has not been transfused in >3 months.

5. The patient should receive blood products negative for the E, c, Jk^a, and Fy^a antigens. The patient is positive for the other antigens, so, in theory, he should not make antibodies directed toward any of the antigens.

Chapter 16

1. 3.0×10^{11}

2. $CCI = \dfrac{BSA\ (m^2) \times Platelet\ increment\ (per\ \mu L) \times 10^{11}}{Number\ of\ platelets\ transfused\ \times 10^{11}}$

Note: This formula applies when the measurement units for the BSA is m^2 and the platelet increment is per μL

Step 1: Determine the platelet increment by subtracting the pretransfusion platelet count per μL from the post-transfusion platelet count per μL

Pretransfusion count = 89×10^3 = 89 × 1000 = 89,000 μL

Post-transfusion count = 109×10^3 = 109 × 1000 = 109,000 μL

The 10^3 portions cancel out leaving:
109,000 − 89,000 = 20,000 μL

Step 2: Insert the platelet increment determined in step 1 into the formula as follows:

1.7 (BSA) × 20,000 (platelet increment) × 10^{11}/4.0 × 10^{11} (number of platelets transfused)

The 10^{11} portions cancel out leaving:
1.7 × 20,000/4.0 = 34,000/4.0 = 8,500

3. Since reference to the patient's spleen having been removed, the PPR formula that includes spleen sequestration is used:

$PPR = \dfrac{TBV\ (mL) \times Platelet\ Increment\ (per\ \mu L) \times 10^3}{Number\ of\ Platelets\ Transfused \times F(Sequestration\ factor)} \times 100$

This formula applies when measurement units for the estimated total blood volume (TBV) is mL and the platelet increment is per μL

Step 1: Determine the estimated total blood volume (TBV), calculated by multiplying the assumed amount of blood for an adult female in mL/kg × the weight of the patient in kg
65 mL/kg × 70 kg = 4550 mL

Step 2: Determine the platelet count increment calculated by subtracting the pretransfusion count per μL from the post-transfusion count per μL
Pretransfusion count = 89×10^3 = 89 × 1000 = 89,000 μL

Post-transfusion count = 109×10^3 = 109 × 1000 = 109,000 μL

The 10^3 portions cancel out leaving:
109,000 − 89,000 = 20,000 μL

Step 3: Enter the values obtained into the formula
To determine the numerator:
4550 (estimated TBV) × 20,000 (platelet increment) = 91,000,000 or $0.91 \times 10^8 \times 10^3 = 0.91 \times 10^{11}$

The denominator: given = 3.8×10^{11} (number of platelets transfused) and 0.91 (platelet sequestration factor for an average asplenic individual)

$(3.8 \times 10^{11}) \times 0.91 = (3.8 \times 0.91) \times 10^{11} = 3.458 \times 10^{11}$

Therefore, the calculation is: $0.91 \times 10^{11}/3.478 \times 10^{11}$

The 10^{11} portions cancel out leaving: $0.91/3.478 = 0.262 \times 100 = 26.2\%$

4. The spleen will normally sequester or store some of the circulating platelets. This does not occur in patients who do not have spleens. Therefore, the post-transfusion platelet recovery may be slightly higher in a patient who does not have a spleen.

5. The post-transfusion platelet recovery is not adequate. Her post-transfusion platelet counts are less than the pre-transfusion platelet counts, indicating the platelets are being destroyed for some reason. Both the CCI and PPR result in a negative platelet recovery.

6. Consumption
   - Sepsis
   - DIC
   - Medications
   - Fever
   - Bleeding

   Prothrombotic conditions
   - HIT
   - HUS
   - TTP

   Immune-mediated destruction

7. Suspect immune-mediated destruction because the platelet count is decreased immediately following platelet transfusion.

8. The patient is group O, which means her plasma contains antibodies to both the A and B antigens on platelets. These antibodies can cause increased destruction of platelets that contain the A or B antigen (group A, B, or AB platelet products). ABO-related incompatibility is the second most common cause of refractoriness and accounts for ~20–25% of all refractory cases.

9. Prior exposure to an allogeneic antigen through pregnancy, transfusion, or transplantation; immune status; antigen dose.

Chapter 17

1. Hemoglobin S level of 67.2%; the target hemoglobin S level is 30%.

2. Recipients with sickle cell disease who are frequently transfused will often be given red blood cell units that are phenotypically matched for the antigens in the Rh and Kell systems, most commonly K, C, E, c, e antigens. Go^a is another antigen in the Rh system and anti-Go^a can cause moderate hemolytic transfusion reactions. Transfusing phenotypically matched red blood cell units will decrease the frequency of alloimmunization and the risk of subsequent hemolytic transfusion reactions.

3. AC should receive hemoglobin S negative, leukoreduced red blood cell units. The leukoreduction is indicated because of her history of febrile, nonhemolytic transfusion reactions. And the units should be tested for hemoglobin S because a unit from a donor with sickle cell trait would decrease the efficacy of her transfusion.

4. Cellular blood products, which include both red blood cell and platelet units:
   (a) Leukoreduced due to AC's history of febrile, nonhemolytic transfusion reactions.
   (b) Anti-CMV negative (if available) or CMV reduced risk (leukoreduced, if anti-CMV negative is not available) because AC is seronegative for CMV.
   (c) Irradiated to reduce the risk of transfusion-associated graft versus host disease, which AC is at risk for once her induction chemotherapy or radiation begins.

   Red blood cell units will also have to be negative for hemoglobin S and negative for the Fy^a, Go^a, Jk^a, Js^a, K, C, and E antigens.

5. Group O red blood cell units and either group A or AB plasma products. Red blood cell units must be compatible with antibodies that AC as a group O person could still be producing: anti-A, anti-B, and anti-A,B. Plasma products must not contain anti-A because AC should begin making group A red blood cells once the HPC from the group A donor engrafts.

Chapter 18

1. HLA class I because you need to determine the patient's HLA type for platelet transfusion. Class I antigens are found on almost every nucleated cell in the body and platelets. Class II antigens are only found on some cells lines, but not platelets.

2. The patient is either homozygous for the A2 allele or the patient is positive for an allele for which there was no antiserum on the panel.

3. Blank

4. Platelet 3 first, which is the closest match to the patient. Then platelet 2, which is mismatched at only one of the tested alleles. Finally platelet 1, which only matches at the Cw alleles.

5. Yes, brother 2 is a 10-allele match.

6. GVHD stands for graft versus host disease. It is a disease in which immunocompetent T lymphocytes from the *donor* recognize nonself HLA antigens on the host cells of the *recipient* and attack.

7. This indicates the progenitor cells have engrafted and neither rejection nor GVHD is currently occurring.

Chapter 19

1. TN could check if the testing laboratory has a current, successful accreditation certificate specific for parentage testing from a well-recognized accrediting body (e.g., the AABB).

2. Most recent edition of the AABB Standards for Relationship Testing Laboratories

3. AABB Standards are revised every 2 years.

4. Buccal swabs (or less likely, blood)

5. Short tandem repeat (STR) typing to establish a STR-DNA profile

6. Likelihood ratio (LR) and probability of exclusion (PEx)

7. 50% because then the report is based solely on the laboratory DNA test results

8. Bayes' theorem or Bayesian logic

Chapter 20

1. b

2. a

3. None of the answers are acceptable actions. All of these actions have the potential to announce an unannounced assessment. LD's best course of action is to keep confidential all the information she receives except when absolutely necessary. For example, telling her supervisor the dates of the assessment and that she will be participating on an assessment team in order to ask for educational leave as per her employer's policy. Any communication to the facility being assessed should only come from the lead assessor or the AABB or CAP offices as per the approved processes and policies.

4. c, a, b, d

5. c

6. (a) False. The checklist is likely proprietary and LD cannot share it without the facility's permission. It is irrelevant whether the assessment was voluntary or mandatory.
   (b) False. Both the AABB and CAP ask their assessors to leave all documents at the facility except those that need to be mailed to the AABB or CAP head office. For example, expense reimbursement forms.
   (c) True. A facility can give an assessor permission to share a document or idea. One of the goals of a peer-review process is to share knowledge.
   (d) False. All patient information *must* be kept strictly confidential. Documents that do not contain patient information are also treated as confidential but can be shared *only if* the facility has given their permission.
   (e) True. Asking the facility if they are willing to participate in the AABB's commendable practice program is the best way to share ideas because all AABB members can see the document and the facility that authored the document is recognized for their achievement.

Chapter 21

1. Examples include the style of the supervisor, the work environment, the perception of the department or organization (hospital) to potential employees, the wages and/or benefits being offered. Some potential questions to explore: What do the laboratory professionals in the area think about the department? Is it perceived as being a difficult place to work? If yes, because of the interaction between supervisors/management/executive and front-line staff? Because of interactions among front-line staff? Because competitors for human resources have a newer/nicer facility or more modern equipment? Are the wage and benefits competitive?

2. Examples include the local economy, the number of training programs, and graduates in the area. Some potential questions to explore: Are people moving into or out of the area? What is the vacancy rate at other laboratories in the area? (Many of these questions are part of an "environmental scan" and often aggregate data is available from local, state, and federal agencies.) What training programs are in the area and what changes, if any, have occurred in the recent past?

3. Quality management

4. Examples include the following: You might put together a Six Sigma or a Lean team to identify if there are any non-value-added steps in your department's processes that could be eliminated. You might put together a group to brainstorm possible solutions. You might network with other colleagues who may have dealt with a similar situation.

5. Yes, it may be possible to cut up to 5.2 FTEs from the budget determined by the following calculations:
   To determine the current FTE requirement:

   The formula for calculating full-time equivalency is: $\frac{A \times B}{C}$

   Where:

   A = Number of procedures performed per year
   B = Number of minutes to complete one procedure
   C = Number of productive work minutes per year

   Step 1: Determine the number of procedures performed per year (A)
   The value is given and is 30,000 procedures per year (A)

   Step 2: Determine the number of minutes required to complete one procedure (B)
   This value is given and is 25 minutes (B)

   Step 3: Determine the number of productive work minutes per year
   Step 3a: Determine the number of productive weeks worked per year, calculated by subtracting the average time off per year in weeks from 52 (the number of weeks in a year)
   In this situation we are told that the average time off is 4 weeks. To determine the number of productive weeks worked per year, subtract 4 from 52 (weeks in a year)
   The calculated value is 52 − 4 = 48 weeks
   Step 3b: Determine the number of productive hours per year by multiplying the value obtained in step 3a by 40 hours/week
   Thus, 48 weeks/year × 40 hours/week = 1,920 hours/week

Step 3c: Determine the number of productive work minutes per year (C), calculated by multiplying the value obtained in 3b (the number of productive hours worked per year) by the average number of productive minutes in an hour (assume 45 unless otherwise told)

Thus, 1,920 hours/year × 45 minutes/hour = 86,400 minutes/year (C)

Step 4: Insert the determined values for A, B, and C into the formula and solve. The number obtained is the number of full-time equivalency (FTE) requirement.

The formula is: $\dfrac{A \times B}{C} \quad \dfrac{30,000 \times 25}{86,400}$

$$= \dfrac{750,000}{86,400} = 8.68 = 8.7 \text{ FTEs}$$

To determine the new FTEs required:

Step 1: Determine the number of procedures performed per year (A)

The value is given and is 30,000 procedures per year (A)

Step 2: Determine the number of minutes required to complete one procedure (B)

This value is given and is 10 minutes (B)

Step 3: Determine the number of productive work minutes per year

Step 3a: Determine the number of productive weeks worked per year, calculated by subtracting the average time off per year in weeks from 52 (the number of weeks in a year)

In this situation we are told that the average time off is 4 weeks. To determine the number of productive weeks worked per year, subtract 4 from 52 (weeks in a year)

The calculated value is 52 – 4 = 48 weeks

Step 3b: Determine the number of productive hours per year by multiplying the value obtained in step 3a by 40 hours/week

Thus, 48 weeks/year × 40 hours/week = 1,920 hours/week

Step 3c: Determine the number of productive work minutes per year (C), calculated by multiplying the value obtained in 3b (the number of productive hours worked per year) by the average number of productive minutes in an hour (assume 45 unless otherwise told)

Thus, 1,920 hours/year × 45 minutes/hour = 86,400 minutes/year (C)

Step 4: Insert the determined values for A, B, and C into the formula and solve. The number obtained is the number of full-time equivalency (FTE) requirement.

The formula is: $\dfrac{A \times B}{C} \quad \dfrac{30,000 \times 10 =}{86,400} \quad \dfrac{300,000}{86,400}$

$$= 3.47 = 3.5 \text{ FTEs}$$

The difference between the current and new FTE requirements is 5.2 FTEs (calculated by subtracting the new FTE requirement from the current FTE requirement = 8.7 FTEs (current) − 3.5 FTEs (new) = 5.2). Thus 5.2 FTEs would no longer be necessary.

6. Direct observation of operation, quality control, and maintenance procedures.

   Written tests to ensure understanding of methodology and procedures.

   Testing unknown or blind specimens to ensure results are comparable to results reported by others.

   Records review of quality control results, maintenance forms, validation results.

7. a = performance validation; b = installation qualification; c = operational qualification.

8. The validation should be performed using both "production conditions" and "challenge conditions." Compatible crossmatch tests are the norm on the instrument and represent production conditions; incompatible crossmatches should also be tested to ensure the instrument will determine the results are incompatible. This represents "challenge conditions."

9. No, the refrigerator temperatures and alarms should be adjusted to ensure the acceptable range meets the requirements of all products that will be stored within them. If blood products are stored at 33.8–42.8° F (1–6° C) and reagents at 35.6–46.4° F (2–8° C), the acceptable range should be adjusted to 35.6–42.8° F (2–6° C) to accommodate both.

10. You should notify all the departments who collect specimens for you; for example, your phlebotomy or specimen collection team. Do nurses in some departments such as emergency, obstetrical delivery room, or intensive care units perform phlebotomy in this hospital? If yes, then target communication to those groups. Do nurses everywhere in this hospital perform phlebotomy? If yes, then a wider communication plan is required. Physicians may collect specimens from femoral or jugular veins in emergencies or when other phlebotomies are unsuccessful; you might want to explore what communication processes are in place in this hospital for disseminating information to physician groups. You probably do not have to contact your blood supplier because the segments on their red blood cell units that you will use for crossmatches on the instrument use an anticoagulant that has been validated. If you sometimes refer patient specimens to a referral laboratory for complex antibody investigations, then you will want to communicate with them as well about your patient specimen changes.

11. You might want to analyze the problem to see if you can focus your educational efforts. Are the problematic specimens from everywhere in the hospital or is there a group of collectors you can target? You could distribute a communication, with pictures of correct and incorrect LIS labels, either to your selected target audiences or broadly to all your potential collectors. You could research opportunities to do a live show-and-tell demonstration (e.g., ask for time at the phlebotomy team department meeting;

show the nurse educators and allow them to disseminate the information to all the nurses; ask for 10 minutes at rounds that the physicians who most commonly collect specimens attend). Is there someplace where you could put an educational resource long term? Maybe a video showing proper labeling on your hospital or laboratory's external website, internal intranet, or electronic learning system.

12. Examples of standard operating procedures for an analytic instrument could include start-up, running the instrument, running a stat specimen, reporting results, running quality control, maintenance procedures (weekly, monthly, annual), and troubleshooting common error messages.

13. You could have employees use the procedures to perform the various tasks. If activities will be performed on evening or night shift, you should have employees working on those shifts use the procedures. Who, when, what problems, if any, were encountered should be recorded. There may be a procedure validation form in your laboratory's quality manual for capturing the procedure validation data. You can make any changes to the procedures that were suggested by the employees before submitting the documents for document control. Depending on your organization's policies and processes, you might send the draft procedures to the QA unit for review either before and/or after the validation.

14. You should notify your blood supplier as soon as you discover the discrepant ABO result, even before you confirm the weak A subgroup, because any in-date units from that donor should be quarantined until the donor's true ABO group can be established. If your hospital transfusion service runs a blood bank and the unit was collected there, you should quarantine any in-date products.

15. Yes, the unit was labeled and transfused with the incorrect ABO group. This affects the safety, purity, or potency of the blood product.

16. You probably should review your instrument validation results. Did you include specimens known to be weak subgroups of A? If yes, what were the results? In either case, can you find enough weak A subgroup specimens now to do a targeted revalidation? Can you ask the manufacturer to increase the sensitivity reading on the instrument before the revalidation? If you have no source (e.g., your blood supplier or referral laboratory) for the specialized specimens and you are currently performing electronic crossmatches, will you revert to serological crossmatches for group O patients? Given that it is virtually impossible to detect all variations in blood groups, what policy and/or validation level of error is your medical director willing to accept responsibility for?

17. Trend = steady rise that occurred in the last quarter; spike = large increase that occurred in the first month after implementation

18. You might decide to conduct a root-cause analysis because you are seeing an unfavorable trend in a quality indicator and because this is now a recurring problem where your previous actions may not have been as effective in the long term as you hoped.

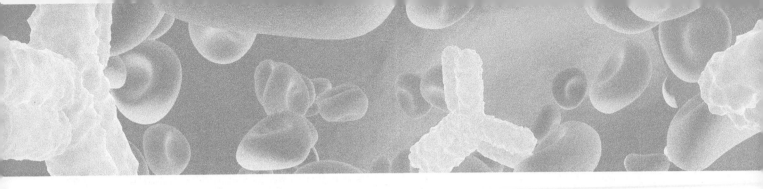

Answers to Checkpoint Questions

Chapter 1

1. C
2. B
3. C, D
4. A
5. D
6. A, D
7. B, C
8. B, D
9. A, B, D
10. B, C
11. C
12. E
13. A, B
14. A
15. 1-C, 2-B, 3-A, 4-B, 5-A
16. A
17. C
18. A, B

Chapter 2

1. Deoxyribonucleic acid
2. Crossover, recombination, nucleotide substitution
3. Messenger RNA
4. Protein
5. Protein-based blood group systems: Kell, Kidd, Duffy, Rh
   Carbohydrate-based blood group systems: ABO, Hh, MNS
6. Linkage occurs when genes are physically so close together on a chromosome that they are inherited as a unit. The human leukocyte antigens (HLA), which are important in transplantation, are an example of linked genes.
7. Antigen is present in <1% of the population.

Chapter 3

1. AHG test
2. IgG is the most abundant immunoglobulin (75%); has two antigen-binding sites; four subclasses; capable of crossing the placenta; predominant in the secondary immune response.
3. A
4. Check cells are IgG-sensitized or complement-coated red blood cells. They are prepared by coating D-positive cells with human anti-D.
5. Polyethylene glycol (PEG)
6. Temperature; ionic strength; plasma-to-cell ratio; incubation time; pH
7. Polyspecific antihuman globulin
8. If AHG is not added immediately after washing, the antibody may elute off the red blood cell. This may result in either too little IgG on cells to be detected or neutralization of the AHG by antibody, which has eluted from the cells. A false-negative reaction may be observed.
9. Gel method

Chapter 4

1. O and h
2. N-acetyl-D-galactosamine
3. Glycoprotein
4. A_3
5. 80%
6. An antibody that occurs without a known antigenic stimulus.

7. Forward and reverse groupings. The forward group tests unknown red blood cells with known commercial anti-A and anti-B reagents. The reverse group tests unknown plasma with known commercial A1 and B cells.

8. When rouleaux is suspected

9. Group O red blood cells; group AB plasma

10. Minor

Chapter 5

1. Anti-Rh(D); anti-LW

2. *RHD* and *RHCE; RHCE, RHcE, RHCe, RHce*

3. Ion channels, although this has not been definitively proven

4. *RHAG*

5. hr′

6. DcE/dce or R_2r

7. D– –

8. Rh(D) positive

9. False-negative reaction

10. Extravascular hemolysis

11. Rh_{null}

Chapter 6

1. Chemical treatment of red blood cells creates either an enhancement or reduction of agglutination reaction. Use of chemical reagents is helpful when identifying multiple antibodies because reactivity can be distinguished.

2. M and N antigen are found on glycoprotein A. S and s are found on glycoprotein B.

3. A biphasic hemolysin attaches to red blood cells at cold temperatures and activates complement at 98.6° F (37° C). The activation of complement initiates hemolysis of red blood cells.

4. Lewis antigens are formed in the plasma and absorbed onto the red blood cell membrane. They are not an integral part of the red blood cell membrane.

5. Fy(a-b-)

6. Suppression of the Lutheran antigens is caused by the presence of a dominant *In(Lu)* suppressor gene, inheritance of a recessive X-linked inhibitor gene, or inheritance of two silent alleles (recessive LuLu genotype).

7. The I antigen is not present at birth.

8. Chloroquin diphosphate; EDTA/glycine acid

9. No, because it is an IgM class antibody.

10. Cromer

Chapter 7

1. A, B

2. B

3. Exposure to foreign red blood cell antigens can occur through blood transfusion or pregnancy.

4. ABO typing, Rh typing, antibody screen

5. The immediate spin crossmatch includes the IS phase of testing. The antiglobulin (IAT) crossmatch includes the IS, 37, and AHG test phases.

6. A hemolytic transfusion reaction can occur when a non–blood group O transfusion recipient is transfused with blood type O single-donor platelets that contain a high titer of anti-A or anti-B.

7. The antiglobulin crossmatch procedure should be selected when a recipient has a clinically significant antibody or has a known history of having an antibody.

8. Electronic crossmatching

9. A platelet product (single-donor platelet) has the highest discard rate because it has the shortest lifespan.

10. C

Chapter 8

1. Antibody screen using an indirect antiglobulin test.

2. D, C, E, c, e, K, k, Fy^a, M, N, S, s

3. Phenotyping should not occur if the patient has been transfused in the last 3 months because the specimen may contain donor red blood cells.

4. The rule-out process excludes antibodies based on a negative reaction occurring with one or more red blood cells that are positive (preferably homozygous positive) for the corresponding antigen.

5. Hardy-Weinberg

6. Fy^a, Fy^b, M, N

7. Anti-Le^a, anti-Le^b, anti-P1, anti-Sd^a, anti-I, anti-Ch, anti-Rg

8. (a) Elution alone: identify antibody attached to the red blood cell, concentrate an antibody, remove antibody from red blood cells so they can be phenotyped. (b) Elution adsorption combination: separate antibody mixtures, detect a weakly reactive antigen.

9. Proteolytic enzyme or ZZAP

10. Anti-B and anti-P1

11. Plasma is serially diluted, usually with saline. The serial dilutions are tested against red blood cell(s) with known phenotype to determine the highest dilution that still has a positive reaction.

12. Panagglutination is when a plasma specimen reacts with all red blood cells tested.

13. Rouleaux is described as a stack of coins.

14. Polyagglutination is when red blood cells react with all adult plasma tested except the person's own.

Chapter 9

1. AABB

2. A document that contains the donor's name and picture identification or a fingerprint scan.

3. Temporary deferral, permanent deferral, and indefinite deferral

4. Hemoglobin must be at least 12.5 g/dL. Hematocrit must be at least 38%.

5. A donor must be given a confidential way to indicate that his or her blood should not be used for transfusion, particularly when more open ways of revealing this information may not be acceptable to the donor.

6. Satellite bags are small bags that are attached to the main blood bag with plastic tubing. The satellite bags are used to make components from a whole blood collection such as platelets, plasma, cryoprecipitate, and red blood cells.

7. 16

8. Vasovagal reaction

9. False

10. A directed donation is a blood donation that is made and identified to be used by a particular patient.

Chapter 10

1. Sodium citrate

2. A tubing sealer maintains a closed system. A closed system ensures that no foreign contaminants, including bacteria, can enter the component.

3. 3 units; each unit contains approximately 80 international units of Factor VIII.

4. A single platelet has a lower risk of transmitting a blood-borne pathogen through blood transfusion because the product is generated from only one blood donor.

5. 5.5×10^{10}

6. A single platelet has a smaller volume that is preferred for the transfusion of a newborn infant.

7. The ISBT 128 labeling system ensures worldwide traceability of blood components back to the original donor, eliminates duplication of identification numbers, and standardizes product codes and blood groups to reduce risk of error.

8. Intracellular potassium returns to normal levels within a few hours of transfusion. Membrane changes due to reduced levels of ATP can be irreversible.

9. Refrigeration prolongs the viability of red blood cells by slowing cell metabolism and inhibiting the growth of contaminating bacteria that can accelerate cellular destruction.

10. Irradiation prevents graft versus host disease (GVHD).

Chapter 11

1. Whole blood, red blood cells, granulocytes

2. 170–260 microns

3. Preoperative autologous donation: units are collected days or weeks before surgery and no volume replacement therapy is done. Acute normovolemic hemodilution: units are collected minutes before surgery begins and crystalloid and/or colloids are infused as volume replacement.

4. Directed donation = specific donor is linked to a specific recipient; often the donor and recipient are related or know each other. Community directed donation = several donors of same or similar phenotype, and therefore often of same ethnicity, are linked to a specific recipient. The donors and recipient usually do not know each other prior to being linked by the donation program.

5. Any two of the following: leukemia, lymphoma, severe aplastic anemia, other hematologic malignancies with poor prognostic indicators, multiple myeloma, severe combined immunodeficiency syndrome, or certain solid organ tumors, hemoglobinopathies, or metabolic disorders.

6. Flow cytometry

7. Any two of the following: febrile nonhemolytic transfusion reaction, transfusion-related acute lung injury, platelet refractoriness, transplant rejection, transfusion-associated immunomodulation, transmission of white blood cell–associated viruses.

8. Leukoreduction and testing donors for antibodies to cytomegalovirus

9. Glycerol

10. To prevent or control bleeding. Platelets may be lost through bleeding, may be decreased due to decreased production or increased destruction, or may be dysfunctional.

11. Immunoglobulin to any two of the following viruses: rabies, rubella, cytomegalovirus, tetanus, varicella zoster, vaccinia, respiratory syncytial, hepatitis B.

12. Replacement of at least one total blood volume with donor components within 24 hours.

Chapter 12

1. Centre for Biologics Evaluation and Research (CBER) of the Food and Drug Administration (FDA)

2. ABO

3. Direct antiglobulin test (DAT) and antibody screen/identification (against red blood cell antigens)

4. Fever and/or chills

5. IgG or IgE

6. 1:700

7. Bilateral infiltrates

8. Transfusion-associated circulatory overload

9. Vasopressors

10. Irradiate cellular products for patients who are at increased risk

11. Anti-HPA-1a

12. Calcium and magnesium

13. Check for visible hemolysis, ABO group, and direct antiglobulin test (DAT). Clerical checks are also performed at the bedside and in the laboratory.

Chapter 13

1. 5%

2. 1990

3. Hepatitis A and Hepatitis E

4. Parenteral, sexual, vertical, and through breast milk

5. Through contact with infected saliva

6. Elderly (> age 50) and immunocompromised patients

7. vCJD

8. Through venipuncture at the time of collection or during the manufacture of blood components

9. Leishmaniasis

10. Heat inactivation and solvent detergent treatment

Chapter 14

1. Rh incompatibility, ABO incompatibility, other IgG antibody

2. Erythroblastosis fetalis

3. Anti-$Rh_0(D)$

4. Antibody titration

5. Amniocentesis; chorionic villus sampling; percutaneous umbilical blood sampling (PUBS)

6. A Liley graph is a predictor of the severity of anemia in HDFN. It is a plot of bilirubin levels measured by optical density (OD) versus gestational age.

7. Plasma exchange; intrauterine transfusion

8. HDFN due to Anti-$Rh_0(D)$. Prevention is achieved through the administration of Rh-immune globulin (RhIg) both during and after pregnancy.

9. Red blood cells are mixed with compatible thawed FFP. RBCs should be compatible with mother and infant, and negative for the offending antigen. RBCs should be less than 7 days old, leukocyte-reduced, CMV-reduced, hemoglobin-S negative, and irradiated.

10. Liver

11. Risk of TA-GVHD is increased for infants with congenital immunodeficiency disorders, hematologic malignancies, or those receiving blood transfusions from blood relatives.

Chapter 15

1. Polyspecific AHG

2. IgM antibodies, IgG auto and alloantibodies, loss of complement-regulating protein

3. No. The two tests serve two different purposes. The DAT detects *in vivo* binding of antibody or complement. The autocontrol determines whether a pattern of antibody reactivity is due to the presence of autoantibodies binding *in vitro*.

4. The alloadsorption uses donor or reagent cells with a phenotype similar to the patient. The autoadsorption technique is performed using the patient's own cells.

5. A biphasic hemolysin is an antibody that has optimal reactivity in two different temperature ranges.

6. A patient history is obtained and lab tests are performed to determine optimal temperature of antibody, complement activation, and idiotype of antibody (IgG or IgM).

7. IgG

8. P

9. Cefotetan, methyldopa, penicillin, quinidine

10. Anti-E

Chapter 16

1. Corrected count increment (CCI) and post-transfusion platelet recovery (PPR)

2. Sepsis, DIC, medications, fever, bleeding, bone marrow transplant

3. Prior exposure, immune status, antigen dose

4. HLA mismatch

5. HLA identical, or "A" match

6. (1) platelet immunofluorescent test by microscopy (PIFT) or flow cytometry (FCIT), (2) modified antibody capture ELISA (MACE), (3) solid-phase red blood cell adherence assay (SPRCA)

7. Heparin-induced thrombocytopenia (HIT)

8. Red blood cell products

9. HPA-1a (anti-Pl^{A1})

Chapter 17

1. 1 IU/kg of Factor VIII will raise the factor activity by approximately 2%. 1 IU/kg of Factor IX will raise the activity rate by approximately 1%.

2. People with sickle cell disease are homozygous (both copies of the gene are the same) for the mutation causing hemoglobin S production. People with sickle cell trait are heterozygous (one mutated gene and one normal gene) for the mutation causing hemoglobin S production.

3. Any two of the following: pneumonia, hepatitis, gastroenteritis

4. Any two of the following: rash, bone marrow failure, liver dysfunction

5. Vitamin K

6. Stimulates red blood cell precursors in the bone marrow to differentiate into mature red blood cells

7. Extravascular

8. Products released during the rapid breakdown of leukemia or tumor cells by chemotherapeutic agents build up and cause electrolyte imbalances and kidney dysfunction.

Chapter 18

1. Multidisciplinary collaboration

2. Adaptive system

3. Class I

4. Chromosome 6 (short arm)

5. To differentiate the HLA-C proteins from complement proteins

6. Sequence of proteins that appears in a large number of HLA antigens, causing the corresponding antibody to react with many HLA antigens (cross-reactivity)

7. Third

8. B lymphocytes

9. To prevent graft (transplant) rejection and graft versus host disease (GVHD)

10. Ten

11. HLA-A, HLA-B, HLA-DR

Chapter 19

1. Red blood cell antigens

2. Accreditation and association with organizations such as the AMA, ABA, and AABB.

3. A short tandem repeat (STR) is a repeated sequence from 2 to 16 base-pairs that is typically in the noncoding intron region.

4. The 13 core loci is a collection of genetic markers for use in identification. They are considered the standard for most crime laboratories and parentage testing laboratories.

5. The likelihood ratio indicates to interested persons how strongly the evidence either supports or contradicts the hypothesis that the alleged parent is the true parent of the child.

6. Hardy-Weinberg formula

Chapter 20

1. Biologics Control Act of 1902

2. Center for Biologics Evaluation and Research (CBER) within the U.S. Food and Drug Administration (FDA)

3. All laboratories performing tests on human specimens with the intent to provide information to assess health or prevent, diagnose, or treat disease

4. 1985

5. Code of Federal Regulations (CFR)

6. Initial inspection within first year of operation and then at least every 2 years thereafter

7. When an error or accident occurs that could potentially affect the safety, potency, or purity of a distributed product.

8. Application process where documentation shows that a new medical device is substantially equivalent to a similar device that is already approved for use.

9. State health departments, CMS-approved accreditation agencies, and licensure programs in exempt states

10. Syphilis, hepatitis B virus, hepatitis C virus, human immunodeficiency virus, West Nile virus

11. AABB, College of American Pathologists (CAP)

12. ISO 15189

Chapter 21

1. Quality system (QS); quality assurance (QA); quality control (QC); quality management (QM).

2. Executive management

3. Six Sigma

4. New employee, employee transferred to a new position, new procedure or process, substantially revised procedure or process

5. Installation qualification, operational qualification, performance validation

6. A customer is anyone who is affected by your processes.

7. Standard operating procedure

8. All licensed and unlicensed blood establishments, including transfusion services, are required to report biological product deviations (BPD) if the event has the potential to affect the safety, purity, or potency of the product involved, and if the product was distributed.

9. Any three of the following: process audit, product audit, self-audit, blood utilization.

10. All levels of employees should participate.

11. Handwashing

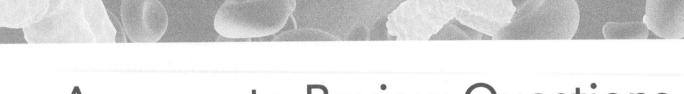

Answers to Review Questions

Chapter 1

1. Matching
   A – 4
   B – 5
   C – 1
   D – 3
   E – 2

2. A, B, D

3. A

4. B

5. A

6. B

7. B, D

8. B, C, D

9. A, B, C

10. A, B, C, D

11. A, C

12. A, B, C, D

13. C

14. A, B, C, D

15. A, B, D

16. A, C, D

17. A, D

Chapter 2

1. a, b, b, a

2. B

3. D

4. A, C

5. B

6. C

7. C

8. B

9. A

10. A, B, C

Chapter 3

1. A, B, C

2. B

3. A, D

4. B

5. D

6. D

7. A, B, D

8. A

9. B, C

10. A

11. 1. b, 2. a, 3. b, 4. b, 5. a

12. D

13. B

14. B, C

15. B

Chapter 4

1. C

2. A

3. C

4. D

5. B

6. A
7. D
8. A
9. B
10. C
11. D
12. B
13. A
14. C
15. D

Chapter 5

1. A
2. B
3. A, B, C
4. D
5. A, B
6. A, B, C
7. A, B, C, D
8. B
9. A
10. B, C, A, D
11. B, D
12. B
13. D
14. A, B, C
15. B
16. A, B, B, A
17. A
18. B, C
19. A
20. C

Chapter 6

1. A, B, C
2. B
3. A

4. D
5. C
6. B, A, B, A, C
7. A
8. C
9. A, B, C
10. B
11. C
12. C
13. A, C
14. C, D
15. A, B, C, D

Chapter 7

1. A, B
2. A, B, C, D
3. A, B, C
4. A, C
5. A, B, C, D
6. B
7. A, B, C, D
8. A
9. A, B, C
10. C
11. A
12. D
13. B
14. B
15. A
16. A, B, C, D
17. B

Chapter 8

1. C
2. C
3. D

4. D

Step 1: Determine antigen *negative* frequencies

Jk^b: 100 − 73 = 27% | K: 100 − 10 = 90%

Step 2: Convert % values obtained in step 1 to decimals

Jk^b: 27% = .27 | K: 10% = .90

Step 3: Multiply the values obtained in step 2

.27 × .90 = 0.243

Step 4: Fill-in appropriate values into the formula

3 units desired/0.243 = 12.3 or 12

5. A

6. C

7. B

8. D

9. 1. D; 2. A; 3. B; 4. C

10. C

11. B

12. C

13. A

14. C

15. D

Chapter 9

1. A, B, C, D

2. C

3. A, D

4. 1. A, 2. B, 3. B, 4. A, 5. A

5. A, C

6. 1. A, 2. C, 3. A, 4. B

7. B

8. A

9. B

10. A

11. B, D

12. A, B, C

13. C

14. D

15. B

Chapter 10

1. D

2. B

3. D

4. B

5. B

6. A

7. C

8. A

9. D

10. B

11. C

12. B

13. A

14. D

15. C

16. C

17. B

18. A

19. D

20. C

Chapter 11

1. B, C, E, D, A

2. C

3. A, B, C

4. B, C, F

5. A, C, D

6. C

7. B, C

8. B

9. A, C, D

10. D

11. A, B, C, D

12. A, A, C, B

13. C

14. A

15. A, B, C

Chapter 12

1. A, B, C, D

2. A, B, D, F

3. B

4. D

5. c, d, f, b, a, e

6. A, C

7. B

8. B

9. B, C, D, F

10. A

11. C

12. D

13. A, B

14. A

15. D

Chapter 13

1. B

2. D

3. C

4. C

5. A

6. B

7. D

8. B

9. D

10. C

11. D

12. C

13. A, B, C

14. A, D, C, B

15. D

Chapter 14

1. A, D

2. C

3. B

4. D

5. B, C

6. A

7. C

8. A

9. B, D

10. D

11. B, A, A, B

12. D

13. C; using the formula (% fetal cells in decimal format) $\times$ 5,000 mL blood volume/30 mL (amount of fetal whole blood covered by one vial of RhIG):

   Step 1: convert % fetal cells to decimal : 3.2% = 0.032
   Step 2: multiple value obtained in step 1 by 5,000 mL blood volume: (0.032) $\times$ (5,000) = 160
   Step 3: divide value obtained in step 2 by 30 mL: 160/30 = 5.33 = 5
   Step 4: add one to the value obtained in step 3: 5 + 1 = 6 doses

14. A, D

15. C

Chapter 15

1. D

2. B

3. D

4. C

5. A

6. False

7. B

8. A, C, E, F

9. C

10. B

11. C

12. C, A, A, C, B

13. D

14. C

15. B

Chapter 16

1. B

2. D

3. C

$$CCI = \frac{BSA\ (m^2) \times \text{Platelet increment (per } \mu L) \times 10^{11}}{\text{Number of platelets transfused} \times 10^{11}}$$

Note: This formula applies when measurement units for the BSA is m^2 and the platelet increment is per μL

Step 1: Determine the platelet increment by subtracting the pretransfusion platelet count per μL from the post-transfusion platelet count per μL

Pretransfusion count $= 5 \times 10^3$
$= 5 \times 1000 = 5{,}000\ \mu L$

Post-transfusion count $= 45 \times 10^3 = 45 \times 1000$
$= 45{,}000\ \mu L$

$45{,}000 - 5{,}000 = 40{,}000\ \mu L$

Step 2: Insert the platelet increment determined in step 1 into the formula as follows:

1.7 (BSA) $\times$ 40,000 (platelet increment) $\times 10^{11}/4.0 \times 10^{11}$ (number of platelets transfused)

The 10^{11} portions cancel out leaving:

$1.7 \times 40{,}000/4.0 = 68{,}000/4.0 = 17{,}000$

4. A, B, C

5. A, B

6. D

7. B

8. C

9. D

10. A

11. A, C

12. B

13. A

14. C

15. B

Chapter 17

1. A, C

2. C

3. B

4. A, B, C, D

5. B

6. A, B

7. C

8. C

9. A, B

10. B

11. C

12. A, B, C, D

13. C

14. B

15. B, D

Chapter 18

1. B

2. A, B, C

3. A, B

4. A

5. B

6. D

7. C

8. 3rd, 1st, 4th, 2nd

9. C

10. B

11. A

12. A

13. C

14. A

15. D

Chapter 19

1. B

2. A, B, C

3. D

4. A

5. C

6. B

7. A

8. C

9. D

10. False

Chapter 20

1. A, B, C, D

2. C

3. B

4. A

5. C

6. C, A, B

7. A, B, C

8. C, A, D, B

9. C

10. A

11. C

12. A

13. A, C, D

14. A, B, C, D

15. B

Chapter 21

1. C

2. A

3. B

4. A, C

5. B

6. D

7. A, B, D

8. C

9. C

10. c, a, b

11. A, D

12. D

13. A

14. B

15. D

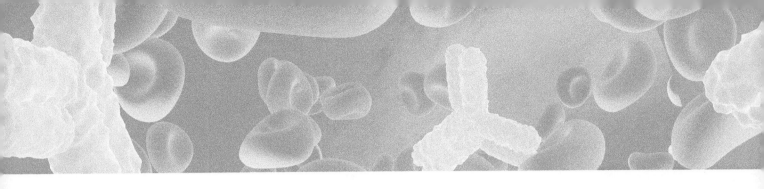

Glossary

α helix (helices) *(Ch 18)*—Protein chains arranged into right-handed coils.

ABO discrepancy (discrepancies) *(Ch 4)*—When the results of the forward and reverse groupings do not correlate.

ABO incompatibility (incompatibilities) *(Ch 7)*—An antigen–antibody reaction that takes place as a result of two different blood types being mixed together that cannot coexist. The antigens of one blood type typically react with their corresponding antibodies associated with the other blood type, resulting in red blood cell hemolysis, may be deadly.

Acquired immunodeficiency syndrome (AIDS) *(Ch 13)*—A potentially fatal disease caused by the presence of the HIV virus, resulting in a weakened immune system of infected patients that makes them susceptible to numerous infectious agents.

Absorption *(Ch 4)*—A process by which unwanted antibodies are removed from red blood cells.

Activation of complement *(Ch 1)*—A function of antibody molecules that enhances the bactericidal actions of phagocytes.

Acute normovolemic hemodilution (ANH) *(Ch 11)*—A process in which just before surgery begins, whole blood is removed from a patient while simultaneously replacing the volume with crystalloid and/or colloid solutions. The main goal of ANH is to reduce the volume of red blood cells that are lost during a surgical procedure by decreasing the patient's hematocrit. The collected blood is returned when the patient needs it most.

Acute reaction *(Ch 12)*—An adverse transfusion reaction that occurs within 24 hours within the time of transfusion.

Adaptive immunity (acquired immunity) *(Ch 1)*—A specific response to an antigen accomplished by cells of the immune system known as B and T lymphocytes; adaptive immunity has the property of immunological memory so that when an antigen is reintroduced to the host, the response to the antigen the second and subsequent times is significantly faster.

Adsorption *(Ch 8, 15)*—A process used to selectively remove an antibody from plasma or serum by adding red blood cells with the corresponding antigen under conditions that will enhance the antibody–antigen binding. Adsorption may aid in detecting any coexisting antibodies.

Adult T-cell leukemia/lymphoma (ATL) *(Ch 13)*—A rare leukemia that occurs in a small percentage of patients infected with HTLV.

Affinity *(Ch 1)*—The initial force of attraction between one binding site on an antibody molecule and the portion of an antigen molecule where an antibody binds and a complex is formed (known as an *epitope*).

Agglutination *(Ch 1)*—The visualization of antigen–antibody reactions typically seen in the form of one or more clumps or aggregates.

Allele(s) *(Ch 2)*—One of two or more different forms of a gene at a specific locus on a chromosome

Alloadsorption *(Ch 15)*—A technique that removes antibodies by using donor or reagent red blood cells with known phenotypes; also known as *allogeneic adsorption*.

Alloantibody (alloantibodies) *(Ch 1)*—An antibody that is produced as a result of red blood cell exposure through pregnancy or transfusion.

Allocating *(Ch 7)*—A process of applying a label or tag that contains the recipient information and usually also the donor unit information to the selected donor unit; also known as *tagging*.

Allogeneic adsorption *(Ch 15)*—A technique that removes antibodies by using donor or reagent red blood cells with known phenotypes; also known as *alloadsorption*.

Allogeneic donation(s) *(Ch 9)*—Donations made for use by someone other than the donor.

Allotype(s) *(Ch 3)*—A variant within immunoglobulin classes that is typically of heavy chain regions.

Alternative pathway *(Ch 1)*—Activation of complement as part of the body's natural defense system that does not require the presence of the specific antibody to be activated; this pathway is linked to the innate immune system.

Amorphic/amorph *(Ch 2)*—Refers to being silent or hidden.

Amplification loop *(Ch 1)*—Another name for the alternative pathway that primarily responds to charged and neutral sugar targets such as fungal cell walls, endotoxins, or membranes of microorganisms.

Anamnestic *(Ch 1)*—Another name for a secondary immune response that occurs upon re-exposure to an antigen.

Anaphylactoid *(Ch 12)*—A term that refers to a scenario in which reactions to plasma proteins result in the production of non-IgE-class antibodies with non-IgE-mediated release of mast cell mediators.

Anisopoikilocytosis *(Ch 15)*—Red blood cells that show variation in both size and shape.

Antibody (antibodies) *(Ch 1)*—Proteins that are designed to attack a specific foreign particle when present; some antibodies are produced by the body (via plasma cell secretion) whereas others are transferred to the body from another source; also known as *immunoglobulins*.

Antigen profile(s) *(Ch 6)*—A grid that indicates the antigen makeup of commercial red blood cells used for antibody detection and identification.

Antigen typing *(Ch 8, 15)*—A test that is designed to determine the antigens present on patient or donor red blood cells, also known as the *phenotype*. This test can also be used to help prove an antibody is present and to rule out antibodies that are not present. The test consists of mixing either patient or donor red blood cells with commercial (known) antisera. The red blood cells lack the corresponding antigen if they do not react with the antiserum.

Antigen(s) *(Ch 1)*—Any substance that the body recognizes as foreign and is subsequently capable of triggering an immune response; antigens are chemically complex, are foreign because they are nonself, and are usually of a high molecular weight. As related to blood banking, antigens primarily consist of proteins that reside on the surface of red blood cell membranes.

Antiglobulin crossmatch *(Ch 7)*—The testing of donor red blood cells with patient plasma or serum following an IAT procedure using the antihuman globulin (AHG) test phase. Also known as an *IAT crossmatch*.

Antigram *(Ch 6, 8)*—A chart provided by the manufacturer that shows the antigenic makeup of each cell (*antigen profile*) in the panel. The results that are obtained when the panel cells are tested against the patient's plasma are compared to the antigram to determine the identity of antibody(ies) in the specimen.

Antihuman globulin (AHG) technique *(Ch 3)*—A procedure that involves adding a reagent containing antibodies with specificity for human proteins (globulins), called antihuman globulin, to agglutinate sensitized red blood cells.

Antithetical *(Ch 2, 6)*—Antigens that represent different forms of a gene product from the same locus.

Apheresis *(Ch 9, 10, 11)*—A procedure in which whole blood is removed from the body and a specific component is retained, while the remainder of the blood is returned to the donor.

Aplastic crisis *(Ch 13)*—An occurrence in which the bone marrow ceases production of red blood cells due to a number of conditions, including the presence of parvovirus B19.

Apoptosis *(Ch 10)*—Preprogrammed cell death.

Autoabsorption *(Ch 4)*—The process of removing autoantibodies against using patients own red blood cells.

Autoadsorption *(Ch 15)*—A technique that consists of adding patient red blood cells to remove patient autoantibodies; also known as *autologous adsorption*.

Autoantibody (autoantibodies) *(Ch 15)*—Antibodies that individuals make against their own red blood cells.

Autocontrol (AC) *(Ch 8)*—The testing of patient plasma against patient cells by the same method used to perform other transfusion service testing on the patient. The purpose of the autocontrol is to screen for the presence of autoantibodies.

Autoimmune hemolytic anemia (AIHA) *(Ch 15)*—A condition that results when individuals make autoantibodies with resultant hemolysis.

Autologous adsorption *(Ch 15)*—A technique that removes autoantibodies by using the patient's own red blood cells; also known as *autoadsorption*.

Autologous control (autocontrol; AC) *(Ch 7)*—A test that involves mixing patient cells with patient serum/plasma that is designed to detect the presence of autoantibodies.

Autologous donation(s) *(Ch 9)*—Donations made by donors for their own use.

Avidity *(Ch 1, 8)*—The sum of all attractive forces between antigens and antibodies, which keeps antigens and antibody molecules together once binding has occurred. To determine avidity, also known as the titration score, a value is assigned to each positive reaction in a titration. These scores reflect the total binding strength of antigen and antibody molecules. The resulting titration score can be useful for comparing how an antibody reacts to different red blood cells or comparing how different antibodies react to the same red blood cell.

β-pleated sheet *(Ch 18)*—An almost fully extended and folded protein chain whose folds are fixed with lateral hydrogen bonds.

Babesiosis *(Ch 13)*—A parasitic infection caused by the protozoan *Babesia microti*. The parasite is transmitted to humans through tick bites where the organisms invade red blood cells.

Biologic(s) *(Ch 20)*—A substance that is used to treat illness and that is isolated from a naturally occurring source.

Biphasic hemolysin *(Ch 15)*—An antibody (usually an anti-P) whose IgG component will bind optimally to red blood cells at cooler temperatures, such as 39.2° F (4° C), but will activate complement and cause hemolysis nearer body temperature of 98.6° F (37° C).

Blood group system(s) *(Ch 6)*—A collection of antigens shown to be related by biological testing and genetic studies and distinct from all other previous antigens.

Bromelin *(Ch 6)*—An enzyme that when added to red blood cells destroys some structures from the cell membrane and enhances others.

C:T ratio *(Ch 7)*—Crossmatched-to-transfused ratio; considered a common metric used to assess inventory management.

C3 convertase *(Ch 1)*—An enzyme in the complement cascade that catalyzes the proteolytic cleavage of C3 into C3a and C3b; considered a pivotal step in the process of complement activation.

C5 convertase *(Ch 1)*—An enzyme in the complement cascade that catalyzes the proteolytic cleavage of C5 into C5a and C5b.

Calibration *(Ch 21)*—The standardization of an analytic instrument by comparison against a standard known to be accurate.

Catabolize *(Ch 1)*—A process of breaking down molecules.

Cation(s) *(Ch 1)*—Positively charged particles from saline.

Cell culture(s) *(Ch 5)*—A cell line that is capable of growing outside a body in a liquid medium.

Certification *(Ch 20)*—A designation issued by a professional society to indicate that a person has met a set of qualifications and is therefore qualified to perform a particular job.

Chagas disease *(Ch 13)*—A parasitic infection caused by the parasite *Trypanosoma cruzi*. The parasite is transmitted to humans when the reduviid bug defecates during a blood meal on an unsuspected human. The motile parasites migrate from the insect feces into the bloodstream by entering the body at the site of the insect blood meal.

Challenge condition(s) *(Ch 21)*—An extreme condition that could theoretically occur.

Check cells *(Ch 3)*—IgG or complement-coated red blood cells used to confirm that an AHG technique is performed correctly.

Chemokine(s) *(Ch 1)*—Small proteins that attract and cause the migration of cells with specific chemokine receptors such as neutrophils and monocytes from the bloodstream to the site of infection; along with cytokines, they initiate the process of inflammation.

Chromosome(s) *(Ch 2)*—A linear thread of deoxyribonucleic acid (DNA).

Chronic granulomatous disease (CGD) *(Ch 6)*—An X-linked hereditary condition that results in malfunctioning phagocytes that make them unable to produce NADH-oxidase, an enzyme necessary in the formation of H_2O_2. Without the production of H_2O_2, affected individuals are unable to fight off bacteria and are thus susceptible to severe and ongoing infections.

Circular of Information *(Ch 10)*—A document provided to anyone involved in blood transfusions that provides critical information about each blood component and how it is to be used.

Cis *(Ch 2)*—A term used to describe two or more alleles present on the same chromosome. This term is considered the opposite of the term *trans*.

Classical pathway *(Ch 1)*—The activation of complement by the presence of an antigen–antibody complex. This pathway is linked to the adaptive immune system.

Clonal deletion *(Ch 1)*—A process involved in developing lymphocytes that are potentially self-reactive being eliminated prior to release into the bloodstream.

Clonal selection theory *(Ch 1)*—A theory that when naive lymphocytes enter the bloodstream, only those that encounter an antigen to which their receptor binds will be stimulated to proliferate and differentiate into effector cells. Upon binding of antigen to their receptors, the lymphocyte is activated, divides, and produces many identical offspring, or clones.

Closed system(s) *(Ch 10)*—An entire blood collection set, which is sterile on the inside and may contain satellite containers that allow whole blood to be separated into individual blood components. A closed system ensures that no foreign contaminants in the outside environment, such as bacteria, can enter the system.

Co-dominant *(Ch 2)*—The expression of the traits on both alleles independent of each other.

Codon *(Ch 2)*—A genetic code consisting of three base-pairs of material that typically result in the translation of an amino acid or stop codon (a signal for stopping the translation).

Cold agglutinin(s) *(Ch 4, 8, 15)*—An antibody, primarily of the IgM variety, that reacts at temperatures between 39.2° F (4° C) and 77° F (25° C), with optimal reactivity at cooler temperatures. Cold agglutinins may be autoantibodies or alloantibodies. These antibodies are usually not clinically significant unless there is reactivity at body temperature.

Cold agglutinin disease (CAD) *(Ch 15)*—A condition in which a patient has clinically significant hemolysis in association with a cold agglutinin that is weaker but still reactive at or near 98.6° F (37° C); also known as *cold agglutinin syndrome (CAS)*.

Cold agglutinin syndrome (CAS) *(Ch 15)*—A condition in which a patient has clinically significant hemolysis in association with a cold agglutinin that is weaker but still reactive at or near 98.6° F (37° C); also known as *cold agglutinin disease (CAD)*.

Cold autoagglutinin *(Ch 6)*—An antibody against self that reacts best at room temperature or lower.

Cold autoimmune hemolytic anemia (CAIHA) *(Ch 15)*—A form of anemia mediated by autoantibodies that react optimally at room temperature or below.

Colloid solution(s) *(Ch 11)*—Solutions containing larger insoluble molecules such as gelatin or starch used to treat volume depletion.

Community directed donation(s) *(Ch 11)*—The process of collecting blood from targeted community donors for a specific blood need such as to treat those with sickle cell anemia or thalassemias.

Community donation(s) *(Ch 9)*—A donation made for any recipient.

Compatibility test (testing) *(Ch 7)*—A test that is performed prior to release of red blood cells for transfusion. The compatibility test uses *in vitro* testing results to try to predict if patient/recipient plasma will react *in vivo* with donor RBCs if transfused. Also known as a *crossmatch*.

Compatible *(Ch 7)*—The interpretation of a crossmatch test in which there is no reaction between donor red blood cells and patient serum/plasma. Compatible results indicate that there will likely be no adverse reactions if the donor cells are given to the patient, assuming that all other pretransfusion testing meets the required guidelines.

Complement *(Ch 1)*—A group of proteins that when activated trigger a series of reactions that ultimately cause damage to cell membranes; in blood bank reactions, the presence of select red blood cell antibodies triggers this cascading event, which results in red blood cell destruction (hemolysis).

Conditional probability *(Ch 19)*—Refers to the post genetic testing phase of parentage investigation. It is at this phase that the level of certainty of relatedness will be modified downward or upward.

Confidential unit exclusion (CUE) *(Ch 9)*—A confidential way for donors to indicate that their blood should not be used for transfusion.

Consignee *(Ch 21)*—The person who accepts merchandise, in the case of a blood bank, for example, the person who receives a blood product shipment.

Continuous exchange *(Ch 14)*—A term associated with an exchange transfusion, defined as a process by which there are two points of venous access allowing for the removal of the newborn's blood and transfusion of the replacement blood to occur simultaneously.

Cordocentesis *(Ch 14)*—The extraction of fetal blood in the umbilical cord with the assistance of advanced imaging ultrasound technology. Subsequent genetic testing designed to detect fetal abnormalities is then performed; also known as *percutaneous umbilical blood sampling (PUBS)*.

Corrected count increment (CCI) *(Ch 16)*—A calculated value designed to assess platelet transfusion effectiveness. The CCI takes into account the transfused platelet dose and the patient's blood volume, which are assumed to be proportional to the body surface area (BSA). The latter is calculated from a conventional nomogram based on body weight and height. The calculated CCI in patients who have a spleen cannot be higher than 26,600, since that would correspond to more than 100% recovery and indicates an error in data or calculations. The CCI is one of two such methods, the other being post-transfusion platelet recovery (PPR). The formula for calculating the CCI is:

$$CCI = \frac{BSA\ (m^2) \times Platelet\ increment\ (per\ \mu L) \times 10^{11}}{Number\ of\ platelets\ transfused \times 10^{11}}$$

Creutzfeldt-Jakob disease (CJD) *(Ch 13)*—A disease transmitted through human growth hormone products and contains a known hereditary component. The onset of symptoms in CJD is sudden and often includes rapidly progressing dementia, poor coordination, visual problems, and involuntary movements. All cases of CJD are eventually fatal, with death usually occurring within 1 year of the onset of symptoms.

Crossmatch (crossmatches) *(Ch 7)*—An *in vitro* test performed prior to transfusion designed to predict whether donor red blood cells will react with potential patient plasma *in vivo*. A reaction obtained in any test phase indicates an incompatibility and thus the donor blood should not be transfused to the patient. In instances when no reaction is obtained and all other pretransfusion testing performed meets the appropriate requirements, the donated blood is generally considered safe for transfusion. Also known as *compatibility testing*.

Crossmatch compatible *(Ch 6)*—The interpretation of the scenario when donor red blood cells that when tested with patient/recipient plasma or serum suggest that no reaction will take place *in vivo* if the cells are transfused to this patient. Synonymous with the term *compatible*.

Crossmatch incompatible *(Ch 6)*—The interpretation of the scenario when donor red blood cells that when tested with patient/recipient plasma or serum suggest that a reaction will take place *in vivo* if the cells are transfused to this patient. Synonymous with the term *incompatible*.

Crossmatching *(Ch 7)*—The act of performing a crossmatch test. Also known as a *compatibility test*.

Cryptantigen(s) *(Ch 4)*—An antigen located on the RBC membrane that is typically hidden.

Cryptic autoantigen(s) *(Ch 8)*—A red blood cell (RBC) membrane protein that emerges in the presence of viral or bacterial enzymes. Antibodies to these cryptic autoantigens are naturally formed in adult plasma in response to environmental exposures similar to the formation of ABO antibodies.

Crystalloid solution(s) *(Ch 11)*—Aqueous solutions of water-soluble molecules such as normal saline, dextrose, or Ringer's lactate solutions used to treat volume depletion.

Customer(s) *(Ch 21)*—A person who is affected by your processes; generally customers are divided into internal customers, that include departments and employees within your organization, and external customers, which are the organizations and people who use your product or service.

Cyanosis *(Ch 15)*—A bluish discoloration of the skin due to buildup of deoxygenated blood that affects the extremities such as fingertips, toes, ears, and nose; it is associated with diminished flow in cutaneous capillaries in the cold.

Cytokine(s) *(Ch 1)*—Proteins released by cells that affect the behavior of other cells. Cytokines, along with chemokines, initiate the process of inflammation.

Cytomegalovirus (CMV) *(Ch 13)*—A DNA virus that is a member of the *Betaherpesvirinae* subfamily. The mode of transmission of CMV may be through direct contact of blood and body fluids with infected leukocytes, transfusion transmission, or from mother to fetus. CMV infection, in most cases, causes a mild or asymptomatic illness in healthy individuals.

Deferred donor directory (DDD) *(Ch 9)*—A list of donors who have been deferred from donating blood on a previous donation or donation attempt; also referred to as the *donor deferral registry (DDR)*.

Deglycerolization *(Ch 11)*—A washing process performed on select previously frozen units of red blood cells that removes glycerol.

Delayed reaction *(Ch 12)*—An adverse transfusion reaction that occurs between 1 day and 2 weeks following transfusion.

Designated donation(s) *(Ch 9)*—A donation made for a specific recipient; also known as a *directed donation*.

Direct antiglobulin test (DAT) *(Ch 3)*—A test designed to demonstrate a visual reaction of red blood cells, which have already been sensitized *in vitro*, that is, antibodies are already on the RBC surface.

Direct transfusion(s) *(Ch 11)*—A process that takes the patient's blood used in cardiopulmonary bypass machines and transfuses it back to the patient as whole blood.

Directed donation(s) *(Ch 9, 11)*—The process that occurs when blood from a specific donor is drawn and set aside for a specific recipient; also known as *designated donation*.

Discontinuous exchange *(Ch 14)*—A term associated with exchange transfusion in which there is only one point of venous access resulting in a small amount of blood being slowly removed and then replaced.

Discriminatory power *(Ch 19)*—An ability to discriminate two samples coming from different sources. This capability is proportional to both the number of alleles exhibited by that marker in the population as well as the degree to which those alleles are evenly distributed in terms of their frequency.

Disseminated intravascular coagulation (DIC) *(Ch 12)*—A process in which microvascular thrombi form causing organ and tissue damage due to blockage of capillaries and uncontrolled bleeding due to consumption of coagulation factors and platelets.

Dithiothreitol (DTT) *(Ch 6)*—A reducing agent that breaks disulfide bonds, destroying antigens that rely on a bond to maintain their structure.

DNA replication *(Ch 2)*—A process in which chromosomes within a cell nucleus duplicate prior to cell division.

Document control *(Ch 21)*—A system that standardizes facility documents; ensures that only approved, current documents are in use; and protects documents from unauthorized access or modification.

Dominant *(Ch 2)*—The expression of a trait coded by allele on one chromosome that does not allow for the expression of a trait encoded by an alternative allele at the same locus on the other chromosome.

Donath-Landsteiner test *(Ch 6)*—A test that mimics the temperature changes that occur as blood flows into and out of the extremities of the body. This test is used to confirm the diagnosis of paroxysmal cold hemoglobinuria (PCH).

Donor cell antigen typing(s) *(Ch 7)*—A test performed to determine if a specific antigen is on donor red blood cells. This test is performed by mixing donor red blood cells and commercial antisera. A reaction indicates the presence of the antigen being tested for whereas no reaction indicates that the cells lack the specific antigen.

Donor deferral registry (DDR) *(Ch 9)*—A list of donors who have been deferred from donating blood on a previous donation or donation attempt; also known as *deferred donor directory (DDD)*.

Donor History Questionnaire (DHQ) *(Ch 9)*—A full-length set of questions that individuals must answer prior to donating blood to ensure that the donor gets a consistent message and that the questions asked are thorough and meet the AABB Standards as well as the FDA regulations.

Donor lookback *(Ch 9)*—A process in which a blood center checks which patient(s) received the blood products from a donor's previous donation and whether the patient(s) contracted the disease for which the donor now tests positive.

Dosage *(Ch 8)*—The designation for when an antibody reacts differently with cells that have homozygous (visualized as stronger reactions) versus heterozygous antigen expression (visualized as weaker reactions).

Dosage effect *(Ch 2)*—The serologic difference encountered with heterozygous (producing weaker antigen–antibody reactions) versus a homozygous antigen expression (producing stronger antigen–antibody reactions).

Drug(s) *(Ch 20)*—A chemical used to treat, cure, prevent, or diagnose disease.

Drug-induced immune hemolytic anemia (DIIHA) *(Ch 15)*—A condition that results when an individual experiences anemia as a result of certain medications.

Electronic crossmatch *(Ch 7)*—A test that uses logic tables located in a laboratory information system (LIS) to detect ABO incompatibilities between a patient and donor. The recipient's plasma is not physically tested against the donor cells but requires the entry of select information and other transfusion medicine test results. The electronic crossmatch is also called a computer crossmatch or computer-assisted crossmatch.

Eluate *(Ch 15)*—The supernatant liquid recovered from an elution procedure that can be tested for the presence of antibodies. The antibody specificity found in the eluate can help distinguish a delayed hemolytic transfusion reaction from an autoimmune hemolytic anemia.

Elution *(Ch 8, 15)*—A process that removes/frees antibodies bound to red blood cells. The resulting eluate (substance containing the free antibody) may then be further tested.

Endothermic *(Ch 1)*—A reaction between antigen and antibody that requires free environmental energy to occur; this type of reaction typically occurs at 98.6° F (37° C), the temperature that IgG antibodies prefer.

Enzyme(s) *(Ch 8)*—A protein that increases the rate of a chemical reaction. In transfusion medicine, enzymes are used to alter red blood cell antigens.

Epitope *(Ch 1)*—Another name for the antigenic determinant, that is, the portion of an antigen molecule where an antibody binds and a complex is formed.

Eplet(s) *(Ch 16)*—Another name for short (ranging from two to five amino acid residues long), adjacent, antibody-accessible amino acid sequences.

Epstein-Barr virus (EBV) *(Ch 13)*—A member of the *Herpesviridae* family, first identified in 1964. EBV is mainly acquired through contact with infected saliva thus it is often referred to as the kissing disease. EBV is the causative agent of *infectious mononucleosis*.

Erythroblastosis fetalis *(Ch 14)*—The release of immature nucleated red blood cells (RBCs) into fetal circulation from the bone marrow.

Erythropoietin (EPO) *(Ch 14, 17)*—A growth factor that stimulates the proliferation and differentiation of stem cells into red blood cell precursors.

Event *(Ch 21)*—An unexpected or unintended incident or occurrence related to a process, procedure, or service; includes errors, accidents, nonconformances, deviations, and complaints.

Exchange transfusion *(Ch 14)*—A process consisting of replacing one or more volumes of an infant's blood with compatible red blood cells and plasma.

Exclusion *(Ch 8)*—A process used to rule out antibodies that consists of crossing off the antigens that did not react with the patient specimen; generally only antigens that are homozygous are used to exclude an antibody.

Exon *(Ch 5)*—A sequence of DNA that codes for a protein.

Exothermic *(Ch 1)*—A reaction that results in released energy that appears as heat when antibodies bind to their targeted antigens.

Extracorporeal membrane oxygenation (ECMO) *(Ch 14)*—A form of cardiopulmonary bypass providing artificial oxygenation into an infant with severe respiratory failure or congenital heart disease.

Extravascular *(Ch 1)*—Pertains to areas outside the circulation.

Extravascular hemolysis *(Ch 6)*—Destruction of red blood cells outside of the blood vessel via antibodies, such as those in the Duffy blood group, that do not bind complement.

Fetomaternal hemorrhage (FMH) *(Ch 14)*—Fetal red blood cells entering maternal circulation; the number of fetal cells entering maternal circulation is typically small under normal circumstances. There are times when the number of cells increases dramatically, such as after amniocentesis or spontaneous or induced abortion.

Ficin *(Ch 6)*—An enzyme that when added to red blood cells, destroys some structures from the cell membrane and enhances others.

Forward group (grouping) *(Ch 4)*—The results of the testing performed on "unknown" patient red blood cells with "known" commercial antibody (anti-A and anti-B). This test is designed to determine the presence of A and/or B antigens on patient RBCs and combined with a reverse group (grouping) constitutes a blood type test.

Fractionated product(s) *(Ch 7)*—A product that is made up of select plasma proteins that does not require pretransfusion testing prior to administration to a patient.

Gene(s) *(Ch 2)*—A basic unit of heredity composed of deoxyribonucleic acid.

Genotype(s) *(Ch 2)*—An actual genetic makeup.

Glycoprotein(s) *(Ch 6)*—A carbohydrate substance, made up specifically of glycol, that is attached to proteins; many red blood cell antigens consist of glycoproteins.

Gravid *(Ch 14)*—A pregnant woman.

Gravida *(Ch 14)*—A term that expresses the number of pregnancies experienced by a woman regardless of whether they resulted in birth or not.

Haplotype(s) *(Ch 2, 18)*—A group of gene units (alleles) on the same chromosome that are transmitted together.

Hapten *(Ch 15)*—A small molecule that only when attached to a larger molecule, such as a protein, is capable of eliciting an immune response.

Hapten(s) *(Ch 1)*—A substance that is too small to be recognized on its own, but can potentially combine with a carrier molecule to create a new antigenic determinant able to elicit the formation of an antibody.

Hemagglutination *(Ch 4)*—An instance when antigen on red blood cells is the same antibody specificity in the plasma/serum that is visualized by clumping of the cells.

Hematoma(s) *(Ch 9)*—The leaking of blood out of the vessels and subsequent pooling in surrounding tissues.

Hemoglobinemia *(Ch 12)*—The presence of free hemoglobin circulating in plasma.

Hemoglobinuria *(Ch 12)*—The presence of hemoglobin in the urine.

Hemolysis *(Ch 1, 15)*—Destruction/lysis of red blood cells.

Hemolytic disease of the fetus and newborn (HDFN) *(Ch 6, 14)*—A condition in which antibodies in maternal circulation target and attach to corresponding antigens on fetal red blood cells. HDFN can occur only if the maternal antibody is IgG that can cross the placenta and the fetal or neonatal red blood cells express the corresponding antigen.

Hemolytic transfusion reaction(s) *(Ch 6)*—An adverse reaction in which recipient antibody typically destroys transfused RBCs, causing them to hemolyze.

Hemophagocytosis *(Ch 15)*—A process resulting in red blood cells being found within phagocytic cells (in this case, neutrophils).

Hemophilia A *(Ch 17)*—An inherited bleeding disorder due to a deficiency in coagulation Factor VIII.

Hemophilia B *(Ch 17)*—An inherited bleeding disorder due to a deficiency in coagulation Factor IX.

Hemostasis *(Ch 11)*—The ability to stop bleeding.

Hemovigilance *(Ch 20)*—The reporting of adverse events in blood donors and recipients.

Hepatitis A virus (HAV) *(Ch 13)*—A small, nonenveloped RNA virus in the *Picornaviridae* family. HAV is transmitted when unsanitary conditions result in contaminated food or water, which is then ingested. HAV is the most common of all the hepatitis viruses and is transmitted mainly through the fecal–oral route.

Hepatitis B virus (HBV) *(Ch 13)*—An enveloped DNA virus in the *Hepadnaviridae* family. The prevalence of HBV in the United States has also decreased during the last couple of decades as a result of available vaccination.

Hepatitis C virus (HCV) *(Ch 13)*—A small enveloped RNA virus in the *Flaviviridae* family. HCV is transmitted parenterally, particularly through contaminated sharp objects such as infected needles.

Hepatitis D virus (HDV) *(Ch 13)*—A small RNA virus that is sometimes referred to as the "delta hepatitis" virus. HDV infection can only occur as a co-infection with HBV or with a preexisting HBV infection.

Hepatitis E virus (HEV) *(Ch 13)*—A nonenveloped RNA virus in the *Hepeviridae* family. The mode of transmission for HEV is similar to HAV because it is transmitted mainly through the fecal–oral route.

Hepatitis G virus (HGV) *(Ch 13)*—An enveloped RNA virus in the *Flaviviridae* family. Although HGV is transmitted through blood transfusion, the virus does not appear to cause disease in humans.

Hepatosplenomegaly *(Ch 14)*—Enlargement of the liver and spleen.

Heterozygous *(Ch 2)*—When alleles at a given locus on both chromosomes are not identical.

Histocompatibility *(Ch 18)*—The ability of tissues to exist together.

Homozygous *(Ch 2)*—When alleles at a given locus on both chromosomes are identical.

Human herpes virus 8 (HHV-8) *(Ch 13)*—A gamma herpes virus that is transmitted parenterally and is present in blood, saliva, and semen. It is associated with Kaposi's sarcoma and is not a common virus in the general population.

Human immunodeficiency virus (HIV) *(Ch 13)*—An enveloped virus in the *Retroviridae* family. HIV is composed of an outer envelope of proteins around an inner core of RNA and reverse transcriptase enzyme.

Human leukocyte antigen(s) (HLA) *(Ch 6, 16, 18)*—An antigen present on the surface of white blood cells, platelets, and many tissue cells that is genetically determined by the *major histocompatibility complex*.

Human platelet antigen(s) (HPA) *(Ch 16)*—An antigen that is platelet-specific.

Human T-cell lymphotrophic virus (HTLV) *(Ch 13)*—A group (HTLV-I and HTLV-II) of delta retroviruses whose modes of transmission are parenteral and sexual. HTLV is also transmitted through breast milk. Active infection is usually asymptomatic and infection is lifelong.

Humoral immunity *(Ch 1)*—A type of response against foreign particles present that the body initiates through the production and secretion of targeted antibodies.

Hybridoma *(Ch 5)*—Two or more cell types merged into a new cell.

Hydrops fetalis *(Ch 14)*—A serious complication of *hemolytic disease of the fetus and newborn (HDFN)* involving significant fluid build-up characterized by respiratory and circulatory distress, hepatosplenomegaly, and cardiac decompensation.

Hyperhemolysis *(Ch 12, 15, 17)*—A delayed transfusion reaction where both donor and recipient red blood cells are destroyed, resulting in a profound anemia that occurs most often in multiply transfused patients such as those with sickle cell disease.

Hypoxemia *(Ch 12)*—The inadequate oxygenation of the blood.

IAT crossmatch *(Ch 7)*—The testing of donor red blood cells with patient plasma or serum following an IAT procedure using the anti-human globulin (AHG) test phase. Also referred to as an *antiglobulin crossmatch*.

IgA *(Ch 1)*—A class of immunoglobulins whose principal residence is in mucosal secretions; IgA does not activate complement.

IgD *(Ch 1)*—A class of immunoglobulins found predominantly bound to the surface of naive B lymphocytes (B cells that have not yet been exposed to antigen) along with surface IgM whose function remains unclear.

IgE *(Ch 1)*—A class of immunoglobulins that is officially recognized as the factor in serum that causes allergies.

IgG *(Ch 1)*—A class of immunoglobulins found in blood and extracellular fluid that can readily cross the placenta; three of the four known subclasses are able to activate complement. IgG reacts best at 98.6° F (37° C).

IgM *(Ch 1)*—A class of immunoglobulins, bound to the surface of naive B lymphocytes along with IgD that is the first antibody produced in a primary immune response and is mainly found in blood and lymph; the pentameric structure of IgM makes it especially effective in activating complement. IgM reacts best at room temperature 71.6° F (22° C) or at refrigerated temperatures 39.2° F (4° C).

Immediate spin crossmatch *(Ch 7)*—The testing of donor red blood cells and patient serum/plasma at room temperature that is designed to detect ABO incompatibilities.

Immune hemolysis *(Ch 15)*—Hemolysis due to an immune process.

Immune-mediated hemolytic anemia *(Ch 15)*—A general term that refers to anemia that results in the destruction of RBCs and are immune based; includes both autoimmune hemolytic anemia (AIHA) and drug-induced immune hemolytic anemia (DIIHA).

Immunodominant sugar(s) *(Ch 4)*—A sugar molecule that makes one antigen different from another antigen.

Immunogen(s) *(Ch 1)*—A substance capable of eliciting the formation of an antibody. An antigen is a substance that reacts with an antibody, but may or may not be able to evoke an immune response. Therefore, all immunogens are antigens, but not all antigens are immunogens. The best immunogens are proteins.

Immunogenicity *(Ch 1)*—The ability of an antigen to elicit the formation of an antibody.

Immunoglobulin(s) (Ig) *(Ch 1)*—An antigen recognition molecule of B lymphocytes; also known as *antibody*.

Incompatibility (incompatibilities) *(Ch 7)*—The term given to compatibility test results in which a reaction occurs between donor red blood cells and patient serum/plasma and thus the RBCs are not safe for transfusion to the patient.

Incompatible *(Ch 7)*—An interpretation of a crossmatch test in which there is reaction between donor red blood cells and patient serum/plasma at any test phase. The donor cells used in this testing should not be used for transfusion.

Incubation period *(Ch 13)*—The time between primary infection and onset of symptoms.

Indefinite deferral *(Ch 9)*—A term that describes a scenario that occurs when a prospective donor is unable to give blood to someone else for an unspecified period of time due to current regulatory requirements that could change in the future, allowing the donor to give blood. An example of an indefinite deferral in the United States is having spent 3 months or more in England during the years 1980–1996.

Indirect antiglobulin test (IAT) *(Ch 3)*—A test designed to demonstrate a visual *in vitro* reaction where IgG antibodies sensitize but do not agglutinate cells that express the corresponding antigen.

Infant *(Ch 14)*—A baby during the first year of life.

Infectious mononucleosis *(Ch 13)*—The condition caused by EBV, also known as the kissing disease, that can be asymptomatic but can demonstrate symptoms of sore throat, enlarged lymph nodes, fever, lethargy, and malaise.

Infiltration(s) *(Ch 9)*—The result of fluid going into the interstitial tissue instead of the vein, resulting in fluid entering the surrounding tissues.

Informed consent(s) *(Ch 7)*—A cornerstone of transfusion safety that involves the education of patients regarding the risks and benefits of transfusion as well as any available alternatives. This information is presented at an easy-to-understand level with the opportunity for patients to ask questions prior to the patient being asked to give his or her consent.

Inhibitor(s) *(Ch 17)*—An antibody to human Factor VIII or IX.

Innate immunity *(Ch 1)*—Immunity that occurs within the body naturally utilizing the body's physiologic capabilities as opposed to that which is triggered by a previous infection or vaccination.

Intraoperative blood salvage *(Ch 11)*—A process in which blood is collected from the surgical site during or after surgery and reinfused. Blood salvage may involve whole blood or packed cells. Blood salvage may reduce allogeneic blood use during surgical procedures where large blood loss is experienced or expected, for example, vascular aneurism repair or liver transplantation.

Intrauterine transfusion (IUT) *(Ch 14)*—The infusion of red blood cells into the fetus *in utero*.

Intravascular *(Ch 1)*—Pertaining to the vasculature.

Intravascular hemolysis *(Ch 4)*—The destruction of red blood cells that occurs inside the veins and arteries.

Ion channel(s) *(Ch 5)*—A structure that forms pores that establish and control the small-voltage gradient that exists across the lipid bilayer of the red blood cell, thus allowing the flow of ions down their electrochemical gradient.

ISBT 128 *(Ch 10)*—A global standard, developed in 1994, for blood component labeling. This document provides standards for the information that must be present on the blood component label. It also defines the structure of the barcodes used to code the information for computer systems.

Isotype switching *(Ch 1)*—A process, involving a biochemical mechanism, in which B cells are able to switch the class of antibody molecules they produce.

Isotype(s) *(Ch 1)*—Pertaining to the different classes of antibody molecules: IgA, IgD, IgE, IgG, and IgM.

Issue *(Ch 7)*—The release of a blood product for clinical use; considered as the last step for a laboratory to catch a mistake before the unit moves outside their realm of influence.

Karyotype(s) *(Ch 2)*—A normal set of human chromosomes.

Kernicterus *(Ch 14)*—The presence of indirect bilirubin in the brain that becomes deposited in the cells of the basal ganglia and hippocampus that ultimately leads to cell death.

Labile plasma protein(s) *(Ch 10)*—A protein that breaks down easily during refrigerated storage or standing at room temperature.

Lattice formation *(Ch 1)*—The second step of the agglutination process that involves the formation of a lattice structure that allows for the visualization (agglutination) of the formed complex.

Law of mass action *(Ch 1)*—A law based on the premise that the rate of a chemical reaction is directly proportional to the molecular concentrations of the reacting substances.

Lectin(s) *(Ch 4)*—A plan extract reagent that binds to a specific red blood cell membrane carbohydrates.

Lectin-binding pathway (mannose-binding pathway) *(Ch 1)*—A pathway that is similar to that of the classic, but is not antibody-dependent. Mannose-binding lectins bind with mannose residues on glycoprotein or carbohydrate located on a variety of microorganisms (including select bacteria, viruses, and yeast) in this pathway.

Leishmaniasis *(Ch 13)*—An infection that is caused by the parasite *Leishmania*, which is transmitted to humans by the bite of an infected sandfly. The parasite is known to be transmitted in blood and body fluids as well as through blood transfusion. Rare cases of transfusion transmitted *Leishmania* have been reported. Presently there is no recommended blood donor screening test for *Leishmania*.

Licensure *(Ch 20)*—A designation issued typically by a government department or regulatory body to indicate that a person has met a set of qualifications and is therefore qualified to perform a particular job that is mandated by law.

Likelihood ratio (LR) *(Ch 19)*—As it relates to genetic parentage testing, the likelihood ratio is the expression of the comparison between a child's alleles with the alleged parent's. The LR indicates to the court or other interested persons how strongly the evidence either supports or contradicts the hypothesis that the alleged parent is the true parent of the child. Also known as the *parentage index*.

Liley graph *(Ch 14)*—A means by which amniotic fluid can be analyzed for the concentration of bilirubin present via spectrophotometry; the information provided by the three-zoned graph is helpful in predicting the severity of anemia of the fetus and whether or not intrauterine transfusion or early delivery is warranted.

Linkage *(Ch 2)*—The tendency for genes that are close together on the same chromosome to be inherited as a unit.

Locus (loci) *(Ch 2)*—The site of a gene on a chromosome.

Lookback *(Ch 21)*—A process designed to track the disposition of blood products from previous donations when supplemental or confirmatory tests are positive for an infectious agent such as anti-HIV, anti-HCV, or anti-*Trypanosoma cruzi*; in this case, the process typically originates as the result of testing when a donor returns to donate blood again.

Lyme disease *(Ch 13)*—A bacterial illness that is spread by a tick bite. The causative agent is the spirochete *Borrelia burgdorferi*. In the United States, no cases of transfusion-transmitted Lyme disease have been reported, but the disease is present in the general population and in the donor population.

Lymphocyte(s) -T, B, and NK *(Ch 1)*—A category of white blood cells whose primary function is to assist the body in fending off unwanted foreign particles (a process completed by an immune response). T lymphocytes, which mature either after thymic hormone interaction or as the cells pass through the thymus, function in both humoral and cellular immunity. Lymphocytes that are different in terms of function and morphology and do not develop or migrate like the T-lymphocytes but rather develop into antibody-secreting plasma cells are known as B lymphocytes. NK lymphocytes (NK stands for natural killer) differ from T and B lymphocytes in that they are found in bone marrow and the spleen and are capable of destroying virus-infected and select tumor cells.

Major ABO incompatible/incompatibility *(Ch 7)*—A term used in platelet transfusion testing when recipient anti-A and/or anti-B bind to platelet ABH antigens present that cause the platelets to be cleared from the patient's circulation. This term is used because the causative ABO antibody is in the recipient's plasma and will continue to be produced.

Major histocompatibility complex (MHC) *(Ch 1, 18)*—A complex containing multiple genes located on chromosome 6 that are found in all mammals. The MHC genes code for targets of rejection (antigens) involved in blood and tissue compatibility.

Malaria *(Ch 13)*—A disease caused by the parasite *Plasmodium*. Mosquitoes serve as the vectors in the *Plasmodium* life cycle and thus inject the parasites into the bloodstream of unsuspecting humans during a blood meal. The parasites ultimately invade red blood cells. The symptoms of malaria include intermittent fevers, lethargy, and hemolysis of red blood cells with resulting anemia. Only a few cases of transfusion-transmitted malaria are reported in the United States each year.

Market withdrawal *(Ch 21)*—The removal of a blood product by a facility for a reason unrelated to a violation or for a minor violation that is not subject to legal action by the FDA.

Massive transfusion *(Ch 11)*—The replacement of a patient's total blood volume with donor components within 24 hours.

McLeod phenotype *(Ch 6)*—A very rare phenotype associated with a hereditary form of chronic granulomatous disease (CGD). This phenotype occurs in individuals in which there is a deletion of the XK gene or inheritance of a nonfunctional XK gene, resulting in no expression of the Km antigen and weak expression of the other Kell antigens.

Medical device(s) *(Ch 20)*—A health or medical instrument used in the treatment, mitigation, diagnosis, or prevention of a disease.

Meiosis *(Ch 2)*—Sexual cell division, yielding four daughter cells each containing half of the number of chromosomes found in the parent cell.

Membrane attack complex (MAC) *(Ch 1)*—A complex that forms as a result of complement cascade activation that is formed on the surface of bacterial cells; the complex consists of the complement factors C5b and C6–C9.

Minor ABO incompatible/incompatibility *(Ch 7)*—A term used in platelet transfusion testing when an anti-A or anti-B is present in the platelet component and can potentially react with A and B antigens on a patient's red blood cells. This term is used because the causative ABO antibody is in the blood component and is therefore in a limited quantity.

Mitosis *(Ch 2)*—Somatic or nonsexual division yielding two diploid daughter cells that contain the same number of chromosomes as the parent cell.

Mixed autoimmune hemolytic anemia (MAIHA) *(Ch 15)*—Patients with an autoimmune hemolytic anemia who simultaneously have two types of autoantibodies causing both warm autoimmune hemolytic anemia (WAIHA) and cold agglutinin syndrome (CAS); also referred to as combined warm and cold autoimmune hemolytic anemia.

Monoclonal *(Ch 5)*—Originating from a single group of identical cells called clones.

Monospecific AHG *(Ch 3)*—A reagent that contains either anti-IgG *or* anti-C3d.

Myeloablative *(Ch 11)*—Complete destruction of the bone marrow.

Native *(Ch 16)*—A term that describes a patient's own platelets.

Naturally occurring antibody (antibodies) *(Ch 4)*—An antibody that occurs without any apparent stimulus.

Near-miss event *(Ch 21)*—An unexpected occurrence in which an error was identified and corrected before a patient or product was adversely affected.

Neonate *(Ch 14)*—A newborn from birth to 4 months of age.

Neutralization *(Ch 1, 8)*—A function of antibody molecules in which antibodies bind to pathogens or toxins and prevent their entry into cells. Also referred to as the inactivation of an antibody by combining it with a soluble form of the corresponding antigen.

Nonconformance *(Ch 20)*—A term that describes the situation when a facility is not meeting an applicable standard.

Noncovalent bond(s) *(Ch 1)*—A type of bonding through decentralized electromagnetic interactions as opposed to bonding that involves electron pair sharing.

Nonglycosylated *(Ch 5)*—A term associated with proteins that means absence of an attached carbohydrate molecule, also known as a sugar molecule.

Nonsecretor(s) *(Ch 4)*—A person who does not produce any A, B, or H antigen in his/her secretions.

Nucleotide(s) *(Ch 5)*—A molecule that when present in aggregate makes up DNA.

Null phenotype *(Ch 6)*—A red blood cell that has no detectable antigens in a given blood group system.

Open system(s) *(Ch 10)*—A blood system that has been exposed to the outside environment, which creates an increased risk of bacterial contamination. Products in an open system must be used within a very short time after modification to decrease this risk.

Opsonization *(Ch 1)*—A function of antibody molecules consisting of a process in which the antibodies bind to bacteria, coating them and allowing phagocytes to recognize the Fc portion of the antibody molecule and eliminate the bacteria.

Panagglutination *(Ch 8)*—A name that describes the scenario in which an antibody causes all cells tested to agglutinate.

Panagglutinin *(Ch 8)*—An antibody that causes all cells to agglutinate.

Panel reactive antibody (PRA) *(Ch 16)*—An assay that gives a good estimate of the degree of alloimmunization, which is reported as a percentage; it does not allow for accurate antibody specificity indentification in HLA alloimmunized patients with PRA approaching 100%.

Panel reactive antibody (PRA) level *(Ch 18)*—Antibody screen results in HLA that are often expressed as a percentage of the cells that reacted.

Panreactive pattern *(Ch 15)*—A pattern of reactions that typically includes positive autocontrol, positive DAT, and positive antibody screen with all reagent screen and panel cells reacting upon indirect antiglobulin test phase testing. The eluate is usually panreactive as well.

Papain *(Ch 6)*—An enzyme that when added to red blood cells destroys some structures from the cell membrane and enhances others.

Para *(Ch 14)*—Delivery of a live infant.

Parentage index *(Ch 19)*—Another name for the *likelihood ratio* and refers to the expression of the comparison between a child's alleles with the alleged parent's. The parentage index indicates to the court or other interested persons how strongly the evidence either supports or contradicts the hypothesis that the alleged parent is the true parent of the child.

Parentage testing (Ch 19)—The testing performed on a mother, child, and alleged father to determine the probability that the alleged father is the biological parent of the tested child.

Parenterally *(Ch 13)*—Transmission via injection through a route other than the gastrointestinal tract.

Paroxysmal cold hemoglobinuria (PCH) *(Ch 6, 15)*—A rare autoimmune hemolytic anemia historically associated with syphilis infections, but now more commonly encountered as an acute, temporary hemolytic episode in children following a viral infection. PCH is attributable to an IgG autoantibody usually directed against the P carbohydrate antigen. This antibody is also known as a biphasic hemolysin.

Paroxysmal nocturnal hemoglobinuria (PNH) *(Ch 6)*—A rare red blood cell membrane protein defect that results in an acquired hemolytic anemia. Affected patients experience pain in the back and extremities, fever, chills, abdominal pain, and when enough RBCs have been destroyed, hemoglobinuria.

Parvovirus B19 *(Ch 13)*—A nonenveloped single-stranded DNA virus. It infects red blood cells and therefore is classified as an erythrovirus. It is the only known pathogenic human parvovirus.

Passenger lymphocyte syndrome *(Ch 17)*—A self-limiting process associated with transplantation involving hemagglutinin-producing lymphocytes in a transplanted organ that subsides with donor lymphocyte death.

Passive immunity *(Ch 1)*—The type of response against foreign particles present that the body acquires by the transfer of targeted antibodies from another source other than itself.

Paternity testing *(Ch 19)*—Testing performed to determine the biological father of a child.

Pathogen inactivation *(Ch 13)*—The process by which blood and blood products are treated to remove or inactivate infectious agents.

Patient cell antigen typing(s) *(Ch 7)*—A test performed to determine if a specific antigen is on a patient's red blood cells. This test is performed by mixing patient red blood cells and commercial antisera. A reaction indicates the presence of the antigen being tested for, whereas no reaction indicates that the cells lack the specific antigen.

Pedigree chart *(Ch 2)*—A mechanism for recording a family tree in which a trait is mapped through several generations.

Percutaneous umbilical blood sampling (PUBS) *(Ch 14)*—The extraction of fetal blood in the umbilical cord with the assistance of advanced imaging ultrasound technology. Subsequent genetic testing designed to detect fetal abnormalities is then performed; also known as *cordocentesis*.

Perinatal *(Ch 14)*—The period beginning as early as the 20th week of gestation or as late as the 28th week of pregnancy and ending 28 days after birth.

Permanent deferral *(Ch 9)*—A term that describes a scenario that occurs when a donor has a condition or exposure that causes them to never be eligible to donate blood for someone else again. An example would be having a positive laboratory test result for certain viruses, such as HIV or hepatitis C.

Phagocytosis *(Ch 1)*—Literally means "cell-eating" and refers to the process by which a cell called a phagocyte ingests foreign particles.

Phase-change material(s) *(Ch 10)*—A compound that shifts between a solid and a liquid state at a very specific temperature. It stores and releases large amounts of energy in the form of heat, acts as an interceptor of heat energy in a container, and provides protection to blood components during shipping.

Phenotype *(Ch 2)*—The observable expression of inherited traits.

Phototherapy *(Ch 14)*—Light-based treatment used to treat infants suffering from high serum bilirubin levels resulting in jaundice; phototherapy works by converting toxic unconjugated bilirubin in the skin to a nontoxic isomer, called lumirubin, that is water-soluble and excreted in the urine.

Plasma cell(s) *(Ch 1)*—A cell that is derived from B lymphocytes whose primary function is to secrete antibodies.

Plasma fractionation *(Ch 11)*—A term referring to the general processes required to separate plasma components for subsequent transfusion.

Plasma press(es) *(Ch 10)*—A device, also called an expresser, that is designed to apply firm, even pressure to a blood bag, forcing plasma out through the connection tubing into an empty satellite container.

Plasmapheresis *(Ch 9)*—Plasma collected by automation.

Platelet crossmatch *(Ch 16)*—An alternative to HLA-based selection that involves 12–18 randomly selected, preferable ABO-identical platelet units that may be performed using a variety of techniques. Testing involves combining recipient (patient) plasma with donor platelets.

Platelet refractoriness *(Ch 16)*—An inadequate response to platelet transfusion.

Platelet sequestration *(Ch 16)*—An instance in which platelets that are removed from circulation and stored by the spleen and/or increased platelet consumption are the predominant factors in non-immune refractoriness.

Plateletpheresis *(Ch 9)*—The removal of platelets from the whole blood with the plasma and RBCs being returned to the donor.

Polyagglutinable *(Ch 8)*—A term that describes the scenario in which an individual's red blood cells agglutinate with all sera.

Polyagglutination *(Ch 4, 8)*—Changes to the red blood cell membrane surface that causes the cells to agglutinate with all plasma. In this state a person's red blood cells are altered in a way that exposes carbohydrates that are not normally seen. In this state, affected patient red blood cells react with all adult plasma except that of self.

Polygenic *(Ch 18)*—Multiple genes expressed in an individual that produce similar products.

Polymorphic *(Ch 18)*—The presence of multiple alleles of a given gene in a species.

Polymorphism *(Ch 2)*—Refers to a genetic system that expresses two or more phenotypes.

Polyspecific AHG *(Ch 3)*—A reagent that contains *both* anti-IgG *and* anti-C3d.

Post-donation information *(Ch 21)*—Information learned from the donor or a third party that was unknown or not disclosed at the time of the donation

Post-transfusion platelet recovery (PPR) *(Ch 16)*—A calculated value designed to assess platelet transfusion effectiveness. The PPR formula normalizes the increment by the platelet dose, the blood volume, and optionally the spleen status. The total blood volume (TBV) is derived from body weight assuming 75 mL/kg for adult men and 65 mL/kg for women. The spleen sequestration factor (F) is optional and assumed to be 0.62 in an average person, 0.91 in an asplenic individual, and 0.23 in a patient with hypersplenism. The PPR is one of two such methods, the other being the corrected count increment (CCI). The formula for PPR when taking the spleen into account is:

$$PPR = \frac{TBV~(mL) \times Platelet~Increment~(per~\mu L) \times 10^3}{Number~of~Platelets~Transfused \times F(Sequestration~factor)} \times 100$$

Posterior probability *(Ch 19)*—A value determined by creating a ratio comparing the evidence favoring parentage with the probability or both and against parentage. Using a combination of the *prior* and *conditional* probabilities, the posterior probability results in the determination of a revised level of biological parent certainty.

Potentiator (s) *(Ch 8)*—A substance added to a mixture of antigen and antibody in tube testing designed to enhance antigen–antibody complex formation when present; also known as an *enhancer*.

Preoperative autologous donation (PAD) *(Ch 9, 11)*—Donating blood (typically one or more units 1–3 weeks before potential use) for one's own use, such as for surgery.

Prion(s) *(Ch 13)*—An infectious self-regulating protein that converts normal proteins into abnormal structures.

Prior probability *(Ch 19)*—The level of certainty of a relationship before the genetic testing is performed.

Probability of exclusion (PE$_X$) *(Ch 19)*—A concept indicative of the proportion of the population who would have been excluded from parentage because they lacked the obligate allele(s). Stated another way, the PEx is the probability the alleged parent would be excluded if they were falsely accused.

Process control(s) *(Ch 21)*—An activity or tool used to create a controlled environment for processes and procedures, to standardize processes, or to monitor process outcome; the goal is to produce a predictable goal.

Production condition(s) *(Ch 21)*—A condition that will be the usual for the equipment.

Proficiency testing (PT) *(Ch 21)*—A program designed to ensure that laboratorians have mastered the skills and tasks related to processing, performing, and interpreting accurate laboratory tests.

Prothrombotic *(Ch 16)*—Refers to conditions that lead to clot formation.

Pruritus *(Ch 12)*—Another term for itching.

Punnett square *(Ch 2)*—A method of predicting genotype frequencies of offspring that show the different ways that genes can separate and combine.

Pyrogen *(Ch 12)*—A substance that causes fever.

Quality *(Ch 21)*—The characteristics of a product or service that bear on its ability to satisfy stated or implied needs; a product or service free of deficiencies.

Quality assurance (QA) *(Ch 21)*—The monitoring performed to ensure that the quality system is being adhered to and is effective.

Quality control (QC) *(Ch 21)*—The routine testing or activities often performed daily or during processing of each batch to ensure that materials, reagents, and equipment are functioning as expected at any given stage of a process.

Quality indicator(s) *(Ch 21)*—A measurable facet of a process, or data collected as a result of a process or service.

Quality management (QM) system *(Ch 21)*—An entity that addresses the interrelationship between systems and processes within an organization and between the organization and its customers and suppliers; the quality system, quality assurance, and quality control are all components of this system.

Quality system(s) *(Ch 21)*—A general umbrella term that refers to all aspects of ensuring quality (includes policies, procedures, resources, processes, and responsibilities).

Quantity not sufficient (QNS) *(Ch 9)*—Occurs when there is not enough blood collected to utilize and may be due to a number of reasons such as when the flow of blood is very slow and a clot forms in the needle with subsequent blocking of blood flow.

Recall *(Ch 21)*—The withdrawal of a distributed product that has been determined to be unsuitable.

Recessive *(Ch 2)*—A trait that does not express itself in the presence of a dominant allele.

Recombination *(Ch 2)*—Genetic material formed during meiosis following the intertwining, breaking, and exchanging of material and repairing of chromosomes.

Red cell storage lesion(s) *(Ch 10)*—A red blood cell change that results from it being out of the body.

Reflex test(s)|testing *(Ch 7)*—Automatically performed laboratory tests as a result of inconclusive or unexpected results during mandatory testing.

Refractory *(Ch 7, 11)*—The failure of a patient to demonstrate an incremental increase in platelet count post transfusion.

Regulation(s) *(Ch 7)*—A mandatory rule made by governments that support implementation of laws.

Relative centrifugal force (RCF) *(Ch 10)*—A measure of how much gravitational force (*g*-force) is applied to a blood bag during centrifugation and is a function of the speed of rotation, the amount of time that the centrifugal force is applied, and the radius of centrifugation.

Retrovirus *(Ch 13)*—A category of viruses that use reverse transcriptase to convert their viral single-stranded RNA into double-stranded DNA that is then inserted into the host genome and replicated.

Reverse group (grouping) *(Ch 4)*—The results of the testing performed on "unknown" patient serum or plasma with "known" commercial A and B red blood cells. This test is designed to determine the presence of A and/or B antibodies in patient plasma and combined with forward group (grouping) constitutes a blood type test.

Rh-immune globulin (RhIg) *(Ch 7, 14)*—A commercially available product consisting of purified anti-Rh(D) antibody that when given to an Rh(D) negative mom carrying an Rh(D)-positive baby prevents the mother from making her own anti-Rh(D). Rh-immune globulin appears to attach to the baby's Rh(D) positive cells, thus masking the Rh antigen sites. The mother does not recognize the baby's cells as foreign and thus does not mount an immune response. The benefits of RhIg are temporary and thus more than one dose is often required for maximum protection.

Root cause analysis *(Ch 21)*—A systematic process designed to determine the flaw at the core of a problem.

Rouleaux *(Ch 4, 8)*—Unusual properties in a patient's plasma (such as an intravenous injection or abnormal concentration of serum proteins due to the patient's clinical condition) that can aggregate red blood cells and mimic agglutination; often resembles a stack of coins.

Satellite bag(s) *(Ch 9, 10)*—A section of a blood collection system, typically a smaller bag, that is typically connected to the main collection bag with hollow tubing. Satellite bags become the storage containers for the blood components prepared from the donation; also known as *satellite container(s)*.

Satellite container(s) *(Ch 10)*—A section of a blood collection system, typically a smaller bag, that is typically connected to the main collection bag with hollow tubing. Satellite containers become the storage containers for the blood components prepared from the donation; also known as *satellite bag(s)*.

Secretor(s) *(Ch 4)*—A person who has ABO antigens in his/her fluids.

Sensitization *(Ch 1)*—The first step that occurs when antigen and antibody come together to form a complex; also known as an *immune complex*.

Sentinel event(s) *(Ch 21)*—An event resulting in a donor or patient experiencing a fatal, life-threatening, or serious adverse outcome or when there is a potential for such an outcome to occur.

Sepsis *(Ch 13)*—Infection of the blood; also known as blood poisoning.

Serologic crossmatch *(Ch 7)*—Testing that occurs when donor red blood cells are physically tested against the recipient/patient plasma.

Sickle cell disease (SCD) *(Ch 17)*—A disease caused by a single amino acid substitution from valine to glutamic acid (Val $\rightarrow$ Glu) in the sixth position on the β-hemoglobin chain, resulting in the production of hemoglobin S (HbS).

Somatic hypermutation *(Ch 1)*—A process that occurs via cellular mechanism that allows the immune system to adapt to the antigens that confront it.

Standard(s) *(Ch 7)*—A mandatory or voluntary guideline issued by an accreditation organization that outlines an expected level of quality.

Sterile docking *(Ch 10)*—A process used in buffy coat production through which pooling is accomplished. This process is accomplished by using a small benchtop device that welds connection tubing together while maintaining a closed system. The four to six buffy coats and the plasma or additive solution are all pooled together into one satellite container.

Surveillance network *(Ch 12)*—A large-scale system designed to track and monitor adverse transfusion events. National surveillance systems allow for aggregate data, which can identify systemic problems much earlier than may be seen within individual facilities.

Syncytiotrophoblast *(Ch 14)*—The outer layer of cells in contact with maternal blood that cover the chorionic villi in the placenta.

Syntenic *(Ch 5)*—Refers to location of genes; located on the same chromosome but not linked.

Syphilis *(Ch 13)*—An infection caused by the spirochete *Treponema pallidum*. Syphilis is most commonly spread through sexual contact. Transfusion-transmitted syphilis is now rare as a result of strategies that have improved the blood donor screening process, transmissible disease testing, and available antibiotic therapies.

Tachyphylaxis *(Ch 11)*—A rapidly decreasing response to a drug after administration of a few doses.

Tagging *(Ch 7)*—A process of applying a label or tag that contains the recipient information, and usually also the donor unit information, to the selected donor unit. Also known as *allocating*.

Temporary deferral *(Ch 9)*—A term that describes a scenario that occurs when a donor has had an exposure that results in a risk to the potential recipient for a limited period of time. An example would be a donor who is vaccinated for yellow fever, which results in a 2-week deferral for the prospective donor.

Therapeutic apheresis *(Ch 17)*—A process that involves the removal of whole blood from a patient, machine-facilitated extraction of a select whole blood component such as plasma, red blood cells, platelets, or white blood cells and the return of the remaining blood components back to the patient.

Therapeutic phlebotomy *(Ch 9)*—A procedure to remove blood from a patient, generally with a myeloproliferative disorder or neoplasm causing a high hematocrit.

Titration *(Ch 8)*—A technique used to measure the strength (concentration) of an antibody. Serial dilutions are made of the antibody containing plasma and tested against selected red blood cells to determine the highest dilution causing a positive reaction.

Titration score *(Ch 8)*—The sum of scores assigned to each positive reaction in a titration reflects the total binding strength of antigen and antibody molecules. Also known as *avidity*, this score can be useful for comparing how an antibody reacts to different red blood cells or comparing how different antibodies react to the same red blood cell.

Toxoplasmosis *(Ch 13)*—A parasitic infection that is caused by the protozoan *Toxoplasma gondii*. The parasite can be transmitted to humans through undercooked meats and feces from farm animals and household pets, particularly cats after eating infected rodents. Fetal demise can result in pregnant women infected early in the gestational period. The parasite invades white blood cells and remains viable for several weeks in stored blood. Rare transmissions of toxoplasmosis via blood transfusion have been reported. Blood donor screening is not currently recommended.

Traceback *(Ch 21)*—The investigation performed to identify and test all donors implicated when a patient develops symptoms, such as a viral infection, months or years after the causative transfusion.

Trans *(Ch 2)*—A term used to describe one or more alleles present on opposite chromosomes of a homologous pair. This term is considered the opposite of the term *cis*.

Transfusion-associated graft versus host disease (TA-GVHD) *(Ch 17)*—A complication of transfusion therapy that occurs when transfused T lymphocytes engraft in the bone marrow of immunosuppressed patients, such as HPC transplant recipients. The resulting clinical symptoms include bone marrow failure, rash, and liver dysfunction.

Transfusion trigger(s) *(Ch 11, 15)*—Diagnostic parameters (a condition or change) that when considered with the entire patient picture guide transfusion decisions.

Transmissible spongiform encephalopathy (TSE) *(Ch 13)*—The group of diseases caused by *prions*.

Trypanosomiasis *(Ch 13)*—Another name for the diseases caused by infections with *T. brucei gambiense* and *T. brucei rhodesiense* that are both transmitted by the tsetse fly. Following invasion in the bloodstream, irreversible neurologic damage called sleeping sickness and death may result if untreated.

Trypsin *(Ch 6)*—An enzyme that when added to red blood cells destroys some structures from the cell membrane and enhances others.

Tubing sealer(s) *(Ch 10)*—A contraption designed to close off blood collection system connection tubing that allows each bag (each typically consisting of a separated blood component) of a multiple bag system to be detached for later transfusion. Tubing sealers ensure that the system remains closed and that sterility is maintained.

Tumor lysis syndrome *(Ch 17)*—A complication of chemotherapy in which a large number of cells are broken down in a short period of time. The influx of breakdown products results in electrolyte changes and dysfunction of the kidneys.

Type and screen (T & S) *(Ch 7)*—An orderable laboratory test that consists of three components: (1) ABO typing, (2) Rh(D) testing, and (3) antibody screen (a test that screens for the presence of unexpected antibodies).

Unexpected antibody (antibodies) *(Ch 8)*—Any antibody, other than those connected with the ABO blood system, found in human serum or plasma that are directed against red blood cells. These antibodies have the ability to cause harm to the patient when the patient is exposed to their corresponding antigens and thus must be identified before blood transfusion.

Universal precautions *(Ch 21)*—The practice of treating all blood, body fluids, and tissues as potentially infectious.

Urticaria *(Ch 12)*—Refers to hives or rash that appear on the surface of the skin.

Valency *(Ch 3)*—Refers to the number of potential binding sites present on a given structure.

Validation *(Ch 21)*—A process that is designed to ensure that specific processes consistently meet established criteria related to quality; the process may be prospective, concurrent, or retrospective.

Variance *(Ch 20)*—An alternate way to meet the intent of a particular standard without actually meeting the letter of the standard.

variant Creutzfeldt-Jakob disease (vCJD) *(Ch 13)*—A fatal neurological disease with symptoms believed to be caused by prions. Unlike CJD, vCJD is transmissible through blood transfusion.

Vertically *(Ch 13)*—Transmission from a mother to her fetus through the placenta.

Warm autoantibody (antibodies) *(Ch 8)*—An antibody that reacts with the patient's own red blood cells at body temperature.

Warm autoimmune hemolytic anemia (WAIHA) *(Ch 15)*—A form of anemia mediated by autoantibodies (usually directed against an Rh antigen) that react optimally at 98.6° F (37° C). Causes of WAIHA include lymphoproliferative disorders, autoimmune conditions, and viral infections.

West Nile virus (WNV) *(Ch 13)*—A single-stranded enveloped RNA virus of the *Flaviviridae* family. WNV is transmitted to humans through infected mosquitoes. Peak times of transmission of the virus are in late summer and early fall when mosquitoes are abundant. People with symptomatic infection, called WNV fever, develop flu-like symptoms that includes fever, rash, headache, and vomiting. Symptoms usually last from 3 to 6 days and only supportive care is needed. Rare complications include encephalitis and meningitis.

Window period *(Ch 13)*—The time between infection and detection of serological markers.

Xenotransfusion(s) *(Ch 11)*—Transfusion across species lines.

X-linked *(Ch 2)*—Pertaining to the sex of an individual (male vs. female).

Yersinia enterocolitica *(Ch 13)*—A bacteria considered as one of the most identified in contaminated donor red blood cell components and can actually grow in refrigerated RBC products; most other bacteria die or fail to thrive in refrigeration.

Zeta potential *(Ch 1)*—The force of repulsion between red blood cells in physiologic saline.

Zymogen(s) *(Ch 1)*—A protein in the complement system that remains inactive until it is acted upon by another protein.

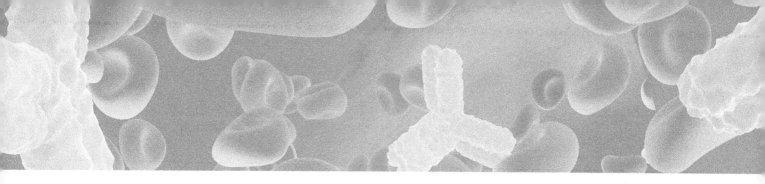

Index

Note: page numbers with *f* indicate figures, those with *t* indicate tables, and those with *b* indicate boxes.